Complications in
Vascular Surgery

Complications in
Vascular Surgery

Edited by

Victor M. Bernhard, M.D.

Professor and Chairman, Vascular Surgery Section,
Department of Surgery, University of
Arizona College of Medicine,
Tucson, Arizona

Jonathan B. Towne, M.D.

Professor of Surgery and Chairman, Department of
Vascular Surgery, Medical College of Wisconsin,
Milwaukee, Wisconsin

QUALITY MEDICAL PUBLISHING, INC

ST. LOUIS, MISSOURI   1991

Printed in the United States of America.

EDITOR   Beth Campbell

PROJECT MANAGER   Linda Kocher

PRODUCTION   Judy Bamert

BOOK DESIGN   Susan Trail

COVER DESIGN   Diane M. Beasley

Quality Medical Publishing, Inc.
2086 Craigshire Drive
St. Louis, Missouri 63146

LIBRARY OF CONGRESS CATALOGING-IN-PUBLICATION DATA

Complications in vascular surgery / Victor M. Bernhard, Jonathan B.
    Towne, editors.
        p.   cm.
        Based on a symposium held in Tucson, Ariz. in 1991.
        Includes bibliographical references and index.
        ISBN 0-942219-20-1 (hardcover)—ISBN 0-683-14511-8
(International)
        1. Blood-vessels—Surgery—Complications and sequelae—Congresses,
I. Bernhard, Victor Montwid, 1927-   . II. Towne, Jonathan B.
        [DNLM: 1. Intraoperative Complications—congresses.
2. Postoperative Complications—congresses.   3. Vascular Surgery—
congresses.   WG 170 C7371 1991]
RD598.5.C64   1991
617.4'1301—dc20
DNLM/DLC
for Library of Congress   91-21826
                                                                    CIP

CT/PC/PC
5   4   3   2   1

Contributors

Chapter 30

Mark B. Adams, M.D., M.S.

Professor and Chairman, Department of Transplant Surgery, Medical College of Wisconsin, Milwaukee, Wis.

Chapter 37

William H. Baker, M.D.

Professor of Surgery, Stritch School of Medicine; Head, Section of Peripheral Vascular Surgery; and Director, Peripheral Vascular Laboratory, Loyola University, Chicago, Ill.

Chapter 24

Jeffrey L. Ballard, M.D.

Resident in General Surgery, Maricopa Medical Center, Phoenix, Ariz.

Chapters 2 and 17

Dennis F. Bandyk, M.D.

Professor of Surgery, Department of Vascular Surgery, Medical College of Wisconsin, Milwaukee, Wis.

Chapter 34

Michael Belkin, M.D.

Assistant Professor of Surgery, New England Medical Center, Tufts University School of Medicine, Boston, Mass.

Chapter 19

Thomas M. Bergamini, M.D.

Instructor in Surgery, University of Louisville School of Medicine, Louisville, Ky.

Chapter 27

John J. Bergan, M.D., Hon. F.R.C.S. (Engl.)

Clinical Professor of Surgery, University of California, San Diego, San Diego, Calif.; Clinical Professor of Surgery, Uniformed Services University of the Health Sciences, Bethesda, Md.; Attending Surgeon, Scripps Memorial Hospital, La Jolla, Calif.

Chapter 29

R. Thomas Bergman, M.D.

Fellow, Section of Vascular Surgery, Mayo Medical School, Mayo Clinic, Rochester, Minn.

Chapters 15 and 18

Victor M. Bernhard, M.D.

Professor and Chairman, Vascular Surgery Section, Department of Surgery, University of Arizona College of Medicine, Tucson, Ariz.

Chapter 3

David C. Brewster, M.D.

Associate Clinical Professor of Surgery, Massachusetts General Hospital and Harvard Medical School, Boston, Mass.

Chapter 6

David A. Bull, M.D.

Vascular Fellow, Section of Vascular Surgery, University of Arizona College of Medicine, Tucson, Ariz.

Chapter 5

Alexander W. Clowes, M.D.

Professor, Department of Surgery, University of Washington, Seattle, Wash.

Chapter 15

Earl D. Cottrell, M.D.
Instructor in Surgery, University of Arizona College of Medicine, Tucson, Ariz.

Chapter 13

Chris Cunningham, M.D.
Clinical Fellow, Vascular Surgery, University of California, San Francisco, San Francisco, Calif.

Chapter 4

Richard H. Dean, M.D.
Director, Division of Surgical Sciences; Professor and Chairman, Department of General Surgery, Bowman Gray School of Medicine, Wake Forest University, Winston-Salem, N.C.

Chapter 35

Robert DeFrang, M.D.
Chief Resident, Department of Surgery, Oregon Health Sciences University, Portland Ore.

Chapter 20

Magruder C. Donaldson, M.D.
Assistant Professor of Surgery, Harvard Medical School; Attending Vascular Surgeon, Brigham and Women's Hospital, Boston, Mass.

Chapter 3

John D. Edwards, M.D.
Assistant Professor of Surgery and Chief, Division of Vascular Surgery, Creighton University School of Medicine, Omaha, Neb.

Chapter 10

Calvin B. Ernst, M.D.
Clinical Professor of Surgery, University of Michigan Medical School, Ann Arbor, Mich.; Head, Division of Vascular Surgery, Henry Ford Hospital, Detroit, Mich.

Chapter 29

Peter Gloviczki, M.D.
Assistant Professor of Surgery, Section of Vascular Surgery, Mayo Medical School, Mayo Clinic, Rochester, Minn.

Chapter 27

Mitchel P. Goldman, M.D.
Assistant Clinical Professor of Medicine/Dermatology, University of California, San Diego, San Diego, Calif.; Consulting Medical Staff, Scripps Memorial Hospital, La Jolla and Encinitas, Calif.

Chapter 7

Jerry Goldstone, M.D.
Professor and Vice Chairman, Department of Surgery; Chief, Division of Vascular Surgery, University of California, San Francisco; Staff Surgeon, Department of Veterans Affairs Medical Center, San Francisco, Calif.

Chapter 28

Lazar J. Greenfield, M.D.
Frederick A. Coller Professor and Chairman, Department of Surgery, University of Michigan; Surgeon-in-Chief, University of Michigan Hospitals, Ann Arbor, Mich.

Chapter 21

Sushil K. Gupta, M.D.
Professor and Associate Chief of Vascular Surgery, Montefiore Medical Center, Albert Einstein College of Medicine, New York, N.Y.

Chapter 26

Robert W. Hobson II, M.D.
Professor of Surgery and Chief, Section of Vascular Surgery, Department of Surgery, UMDNJ-New Jersey Medical School; Director, Department of Surgery, St. Michael's Medical Center, Newark, N.J.

Chapter 9

John R. Hoch, M.D.
Resident in Vascular Surgery, Department of Surgery, University of Missouri-Columbia School of Medicine, Columbia, Mo.

Chapter 11

Larry H. Hollier, M.D.
Chairman, Department of Surgery, Ochsner Clinic and Alton Ochsner Medical Foundation; Clinical Professor of Surgery, Tulane University Medical Center and Louisiana State University Medical Center, New Orleans, La.

Chapter 6

Glenn C. Hunter, M.D.
Associate Professor of Surgery, Section of Vascular Surgery, University of Arizona College of Medicine; Chief, Vascular Surgery Section, Veterans Administration Medical Center, Tucson, Ariz.

Chapter 5

Arkadiusz Jawien, M.D.
Senior Fellow, Department of Surgery, University of Washington School of Medicine, Seattle, Wash.

Chapter 30

Christopher P. Johnson, M.D.
Assistant Professor of Surgery, Department of Transplant Surgery, Medical College of Wisconsin, Milwaukee, Wis.

Chapter 32

K. Wayne Johnston, M.D., F.R.C.S.(C)
Professor of Surgery and Chairman, Vascular Surgery, University of Toronto, Toronto, Ontario, Canada

Chapter 12

Richard F. Kempczinski, M.D.
Professor of Surgery and Chief, Vascular Surgery, Department of Surgery, University of Cincinnati Medical Center, Cincinnati, Ohio

Chapter 21

Ross T. Lyon, M.D.
Assistant Professor and Attending Vascular Surgeon, Montefiore Medical Center (Weiler Division), Albert Einstein College of Medicine, New York, N.Y.

Chapter 24

James M. Malone, M.D.
Chairman, Department of Surgery, Maricopa Medical Center, Phoenix, Ariz.; Clinical Professor of Surgery, University of Arizona College of Medicine, Tucson, Ariz.

Chapter 20

John A. Mannick, M.D.
Moseley Professor of Surgery, Harvard Medical School; Surgeon-in-Chief, Brigham and Women's Hospital, Boston, Mass.

Chapter 16

Walter J. McCarthy III, M.D.
Assistant Professor of Surgery, Division of Vascular Surgery, Northwestern University Medical School, Chicago, Ill.

Chapter 22

Kenneth E. McIntyre, Jr., M.D.
Associate Professor of Surgery, Section of Vascular Surgery, University of Arizona College of Medicine, Tucson, Ariz.

Chapter 35

Gregory L. Moneta, M.D.
Assistant Professor of Surgery, Department of Surgery, Oregon Health Sciences University and Portland Veterans Affairs Hospital, Portland, Ore.

Chapter 36

Wesley S. Moore, M.D.
Professor of Surgery and Chief, Section of Vascular Surgery, UCLA Center for Health Sciences, Los Angeles, Calif.

Chapter 11

Thomas C. Naslund, M.D.
Fellow in Vascular Surgery, Ochsner Clinic and Alton Ochsner Medical Foundation, New Orleans, La.

Chapter 34

Thomas F. O'Donnell, Jr., M.D.
Chief, Vascular Surgery, New England Medical Center; Professor of Surgery, Tufts University School of Medicine, Boston, Mass.

Chapter 21

Thomas F. Panetta, M.D.
Associate Professor and Director of Vascular Surgery Research, Montefiore Medical Center, Albert Einstein College of Medicine, New York, N.Y.

Chapter 16

William H. Pearce, M.D.
Associate Professor of Surgery, Division of Vascular Surgery, Northwestern University Medical School, Chicago, Ill.

Chapter 25

Malcolm O. Perry, M.D.
The H. William Scott, Jr. Professor of Surgery and Chief, Division of Vascular Surgery, Vanderbilt University School of Medicine, Nashville, Tenn.

Chapter 18

Joseph J. Piotrowski, M.D.
Assistant Professor of Surgery, Department of Surgery, Case Western Reserve University, Metro-Health Medical Center, Cleveland, Ohio

Chapter 35

John M. Porter, M.D.
Professor of Surgery, Chief of Vascular Surgery, Oregon Health Sciences University, Portland, Ore.

Chapter 11

Charles D. Procter, Sr., M.D.
Staff, Vascular Surgeon, Department of Surgery, Ochsner Clinic and Alton Ochsner Medical Foundation, New Orleans, La.

Chapter 21

Steven P. Rivers, M.D.
Assistant Professor and Attending Vascular Surgeon, Montefiore Medical Center (Weiler Division), Albert Einstein College of Medicine; Vascular Surgeon in Charge, Bronx Municipal Hospital Center, New York, N.Y.

Chapter 30

Allan M. Roza, M.D.
Assistant Professor of Surgery, Department of Transplant Surgery, Medical College of Wisconsin, Milwaukee, Wis.

Chapter 1

Robert B. Rutherford, M.D.
Professor of Surgery, Department of Surgery, Vascular Surgery Division, University of Colorado Health Sciences Center, Denver, Colo.

Chapter 13

Peter A. Schneider, M.D.
Clinical Fellow, Vascular Surgery, University of California, San Francisco, San Francisco, Calif.

Chapter 31

Gary R. Seabrook, M.D.
Assistant Professor of Surgery, Department of Vascular Surgery, Medical College of Wisconsin, Milwaukee, Wis.

Chapter 9

Donald Silver, M.D.
Professor and Chairman, Department of Surgery, University of Missouri-Columbia School of Medicine, Columbia, Mo.

Chapter 32

Kenneth W. Sniderman, M.D., F.R.C.P.(C)
Associate Professor, Department of Radiology, University of Toronto; Chief, Cardiovascular Radiology, The Toronto Hospital; Attending Radiologist, The Toronto General Hospital, Toronto, Ontario, Canada

Chapter 14

James C. Stanley, M.D.
Professor of Surgery and Head, Section of Vascular Surgery, Department of Surgery, University of Michigan, Ann Arbor, Mich.

Chapter 13

Ronald J. Stoney, M.D.
Professor of Surgery, Department of Surgery, University of California, San Francisco, San Francisco, Calif.

Chapter 39

D. Eugene Strandness, Jr., M.D.
Professor and Head, Section of Vascular Surgery, Department of Surgery, University of Washington School of Medicine, Seattle, Wash.

Chapter 38

David S. Sumner, M.D.
Professor of Surgery and Chief, Section of Peripheral Vascular Surgery, Southern Illinois University School of Medicine, Springfield, Ill.

Chapter 10

David F.J. Tollefson, M.D.
Senior Fellow, Vascular Surgery, Henry Ford Hospital, Detroit, Mich.

Chapters 8, 19, and 23

Jonathan B. Towne, M.D.
Professor of Surgery and Chairman, Department of Vascular Surgery, Medical College of Wisconsin, Milwaukee, Wis.

Chapter 4

Reid W. Tribble, M.D.
Clinical Assistant, Department of General Surgery, Bowman Gray School of Medicine, Wake Forest University, Winston-Salem, N.C.

Chapter 21

Frank J. Veith, M.D.
Professor and Chief of Vascular Surgical Services and Acting Chairman, Department of Surgery, Montefiore Medical Center, Albert Einstein College of Medicine, New York, N.Y.

Chapter 21

Kurt R. Wengerter, M.D.
Assistant Professor, Attending Vascular Surgeon, and Director of Vascular Registry, Montefiore Medical Center, Albert Einstein College of Medicine; Vascular Surgeon in Charge, North Central Bronx Hospital, New York, N.Y.

Chapter 33

Rodney A. White, M.D.
Chief, Vascular Surgery, Harbor-UCLA Medical Center, Torrance, Calif.; Associate Professor of Surgery, UCLA School of Medicine, Los Angeles, Calif.

Chapter 20

Anthony D. Whittemore, M.D.
Associate Professor of Surgery, Harvard Medical School; Chief, Division of Vascular Surgery, Brigham and Women's Hospital, Boston, Mass.

Chapter 16

James S.T. Yao, M.D., Ph.D.
Magerstadt Professor of Surgery, Division of Vascular Surgery, Northwestern University Medical School, Chicago, Ill.

To our wives

Suzan and **Sandy**

who have provided
important insight, helpful suggestions,
and infinite patience

Preface

Under the best of circumstances, competent vascular surgeons will encounter a myriad of complications in the management of their patients. These problems reflect the complexity of surgical care that must be provided to individuals who are usually beyond their sixth decade and who are afflicted with a variety of associated diseases involving major organ systems, which places them at high risk. In 1980, and again in 1985, we asked a group of colleagues to participate in symposia specifically directed toward the management of vascular surgery complications. It was our perception that frank, objective, and timely appraisals of these problems would lead to more opportune and accurate diagnosis and effective therapy and would point the way to methods of prevention. Since the last symposium, many new procedures have been added to the armamentarium of the vascular surgeon. These procedures have in some instances replaced certain forms of therapy or have altered our perspective in the design of the most appropriate management course. It is well established that these interventions, as well as the more classic methods of management, may result in a variety of adverse outcomes due to the nature of the procedure itself or to the manner in which it is performed. Continued scrutiny of old and new techniques provides the basis for scientific management of these problems and offers a wider opportunity to develop and explore alternate forms of therapy.

Six years have passed since the last symposium, and we believed that the time was ripe for reassessment of the current status of vascular surgery complications in light of our broader understanding of the disease processes encountered and recent advances in technology. As in the past, we have invited experienced senior vascular surgeons whose published experiences identify them as experts in the field. It is our hope that this volume, which embodies the discussions at our third symposium, will serve as a useful reference for the clinical practitioner.

We wish to thank Ann Hopkins, who supervised the details of organization and took major responsibility for overseeing manuscript preparation and editorial review. We would also like to thank Lynne Mascarella of the Office of Continuing Medical Education at the University of Arizona College of Medicine for her help in organizing this symposium.

Victor M. Bernhard
Jonathan B. Towne

Acknowledgment

The symposium

Complications in Vascular Surgery III
Tucson, Arizona
February 28–March 2, 1991

was generously supported by the following corporations:

C.R. Bard, Inc., Vascular Systems Division
Billerica, Mass.

W.L. Gore & Associates, Inc.
Elkton, Md.

Impra, Inc.
Tempe, Ariz.

Meadox Medicals, Inc.
Oakland, N.J.

Contents

XII

Interventional Radiologic Techniques

XIII

Cerebrovascular Surgery

Complications in
Vascular Surgery

I General Considerations

1

Suggested Standards for Reporting Complications in Vascular Surgery

Robert B. Rutherford

It would seem axiomatic that vascular surgeons should report the complications of vascular operations just as conscientiously as the successful outcomes; however, whereas patency and limb salvage rates are the central focus of reports on lower extremity arterial reconstructions, often only the operative mortality is offered on the risk side of the ledger. Similarly, for other procedures, the reader is more likely to be informed of the percentage and/or the mean time interval free of stroke, venous ulceration, aneurysm, hypertension, or whatever was the primary goal of operative intervention than of the percentage of complications of the procedure performed. It must be conceded that this is a natural perspective, with no intent to deceive. Furthermore, we do not have accepted standards, or even a commonly used approach, for reporting the complications of vascular surgery. However, ad hoc committees of the Joint Council of the Society for Vascular Surgery and the North American Chapter of the International Society for Cardiovascular

Surgery (SVS/ISCVS) have recommended standardized reporting practices for studies dealing with lower extremity ischemia and venous, cerebrovascular, and aneurysmal disease[1-4] and have made some worthwhile suggestions regarding complications. This chapter will attempt to bring together some of these recommendations along with other suggestions to provide an overall framework for reporting complications of vascular surgery. In doing so, I will discuss in order the categorization of complications, suggest an approach to grading complications according to their severity, consider a temporal frame of reference for reporting purposes, and discuss the appropriate application of these methods to different types of studies in which complications are reported.

CATEGORIZATION

In broadest terms, complications of vascular surgery can be characterized as being either fatal (mortality) or nonfatal (morbidity), early (perioperative) or late, major or minor, tempo-

---

**POSSIBLE CATEGORIES FOR
COMPLICATIONS OF VASCULAR
SURGERY**

Fatal/nonfatal (mortality/morbidity)
Early/late
Major/minor
Permanent/temporary
Disabling/nondisabling
Specific/nonspecific
Systemic/local
Vascular/nonvascular

---

rary or permanent, disabling (to a variable degree) or not, nonspecific (generic) or specific (to a particular procedure), systemic or local, and vascular or nonvascular (see box). Beyond this, complications may be attributable to errors in diagnosis, technique, judgment, management, or, in the absence of such, to the patient's disease. However, these latter distinctions usually are more applicable in morbidity and mortality conferences than in journal articles.

It is not suggested that a categorization system be based on separation by *each* of the paired characteristics mentioned above, if for no other reason than the combinations and permutations of these outcome characteristics would produce too many categories to adequately evaluate. However, each of these particular characteristics can provide a useful perspective in certain settings and can significantly aid in characterizing complications *if* these descriptive terms are used in standardized fashion. With that in mind, a number of recommendations for categorizing complications are made.

Early vs. Late Complications

To define early and late deaths or complications the division point should be the traditional 30 days (inclusive) rather than the time from hospital discharge because the latter is variable and allows a significant number of relatively early complications directly related to an operation to go unrecorded. This uniform, albeit arbitrary, cutoff point in time allows inclusion

of the vast majority of complications directly relatable to operation and is preferable. Specifically, the time of *onset* of nonfatal complications or the time of death itself should be used to determine whether complications are designated as early or late. Theoretically, a patient might have an *early* onset of a complication resulting in a *late* death, but this situation is a minor consequence. However, this brings up the potential problem of double listing of deaths and complications. For example, an investigator might report a 2% mortality and a 3% permanent stroke rate in a patient group following carotid endarterectomy yet claim only a 4% combined risk of mortality or permanent neurologic deficit *if* 1% had suffered fatal strokes. It is important in most instances for the reader to know (and therefore for the author to report) the operative mortality as well as the overall incidence of permanent complications, but fatal complications should *not* be counted twice (as both complication and death) because this yields a false high mortality and permanent morbidity rate.

Fatal Complications

On the other hand, the designation of *fatal* complication should *not* have an arbitrary temporal cutoff point. That is, if a complication directly or indirectly leads to a fatal outcome, even if it is a *late* death, that complication should be listed as fatal. Examples include a major wound hematoma, requiring return to the operating room for drainage and resulting in an unexpected anesthetic-associated death; a graft infection, resulting in death from complications of graft removal several months later; and an unsuccessful graft thrombectomy, resulting in death from pulmonary embolus following subsequent below-knee amputation. Thus, if the patient ultimately dies following a series of events reasonably connected to the original complication, the original complication should be classified as fatal. No benefit of doubt is given and there are no temporal restrictions. Again, however, statistical duplication should be avoided; that is, no more than one fatal complication should be attributed to each death. If a series of complications leads to death, the most significant event is identified as the fatal complication, or if a particular complication does not stand out as such, then that designation goes to the first of the series.

Major vs. Minor Complications

A *major* complication is one that results in death or permanent disability, requires reoperation or other invasive intervention, delays hospital stay, or results in significant pain or disability beyond the hospital stay, even if the disability can ultimately be listed as temporary. All other complications may be considered minor with the important proviso that *failure to achieve the main goal of the operation must always be considered a major complication*, even though the procedure itself may not have been "complicated" in the usual sense or did not cause the patient any new or more severe symptoms. Some examples of operative failure as major complication follow: a femoral venous valvuloplasty was performed but does not result in valve competency; in an attempted percutaneous balloon angioplasty the guidewire or a laser probe cannot be passed; on exploration a pedal artery is found to be unsuitable for bypass; or lumbar sympathectomy does not relieve the patient's ischemic pain or heal an ischemic ulcer. In each case the patient could have been discharged after a brief convalescence without new symptoms occurring and without requiring reoperation, but *as long as the surgical intervention was undertaken with intent to treat*, failure to successfully complete the intended procedure or achieve its stated goals constitutes a major complication. Nor should these cases be excluded from calculations of the cumulative success rates as has recently been practiced in reports on endovascular procedures. In some sports there is a "no harm, no foul" rule in assessing penalties. Surgery is not a sport, but the patients are penalized to some extent (time, expense, disappointment) for any procedure, however justified and well carried out (i.e., without "complications"), in which its primary goal is not achieved.

Nonspecific Complications

Authors are not expected to report all *nonspecific* complications, that is, those that might be considered "generic" to any operation in that region (e.g., atelectasis, ileus, wound infection, dehiscence, hematoma, urinary tract infection, phlebitis). However, such complications should be reported *if their rate is excessive and could conceivably be related to the conduct or design of the procedure*. For example, hematomas are a "generic" risk of all surgical wounds and are not uncommon after vascular surgical procedures carried out through a groin incision; however, if major hematomas develop in 15% of patients who underwent femoral thrombectomies in which either heparin administration was prolonged or dextran 40 was used to avoid rethrombosis, this complication should be reported. A 10% major hematoma rate for a percutaneous technique in which multiple or large-caliber introducing sheaths and/or catheters were employed, or an 8% wound infection rate following infrainguinal bypass performed for limb salvage in the face of necrotic or septic foot lesions are other examples of nonspecific complications that should be reported. The guiding principle here is clear, even if it is not feasible to assign "acceptable limits" in percentage figures for such generic complications for each procedure.

In a similar vein, *if it is claimed* that a particular (new) operation is *safer* or *better tolerated* than another (older) approach, it is recommended that nonspecific complications be reported along with the specific complications to allow proper comparison and to justify this conclusion.

Permanent vs. Temporary Complications

For reporting purposes a "permanent" complication ordinarily can be defined as one that persists *at the time the patient was last examined* rather than beyond an arbitrary time limit. The fact that the problem seems to be improving and is expected to resolve does not mean it can be categorized as temporary. However, in regard to one particular complication, an arbitrary time limit has been recommended. If, after carotid endarterectomy, postoperative neurologic dysfunction persists for over 1 month (e.g., an expressive aphasia caused by postoperative stroke), the patient is considered to have had a *permanent stroke* and this complication is included under permanent neurologic morbidity[3] even though this dysfunction might have completely disappeared several months later. This policy has a specific purpose (to gauge relative degrees of disability), and the use of such arbitrary temporal cutoff points (e.g., 1 month, 1 year) may have valid application in other settings, particularly with neurologic complications. Otherwise, the time of last follow-up seems to be the most appropriate end-point and should be applied to those complications in which the likelihood of complete resolution *is not obvious* (e.g., peroneal palsy or reflex sympathetic dystrophy, but not wound hematoma or secondary lymphedema following infrainguinal bypass). When this approach is used, the mean follow-up time interval should also be supplied for it provides valuable perspective.

Disabling Complications

Whether a complication is *disabling* or not is admittedly a subjective opinion, and, in a given instance, the patient and the surgeon may legitimately disagree on this designation. Similarly, the same limitation (e.g., a claudication distance of one block) may disable one patient and not another. Therefore for general purposes a patient should be considered disabled by a complication if he cannot return to his former level of activities (e.g., vocation, recreation, ambulation, communication) or does so only with significant limitations *because of the complication*. Examples include blindness in one eye, the need to use a cane, speech impairment resulting in loss of job, reassignment of work responsibilities, or being forced to give up a major retirement activity such as golf.

Ideally, a graded disability scale such as the neurologic deficit (stroke) severity scale[3] should be used (Table 1-1), but such scales have not been developed for the complications of most vascular operations. Most surgeons are familiar with the often complex disability rating systems required by various health care agencies, which usually are too specific for reporting purposes and often separately grade several functional

Table 1-1. Neurologic Event Severity Scale*

Severity grade	Impairment[†]	Neurologic symptoms	Neurologic signs
1	None	Present	Absent
2	None	Absent	Present
3	None	Present	Present
4	Minor, in one or more domains	Present	Present
5	Major, in only one domain	NA[‡]	NA
6	Major, in any two domains	NA	NA
7	Major, in any three domains	NA	NA
8	Major, in any four domains	NA	NA
9	Major, in all five domains	NA	NA
10	Reduced level of consciousness	NA	NA
11	Death	NA	NA

NA, not applicable.

*Modified from The EC/IC Bypass Study Group. The international cooperative study of extracranial/intracranial arterial anastomosis (EC/IC Bypass Study): Methodology and entry characteristics. Stroke 16:397-406, 1985. Reproduced by permission of the American Heart Association.

†Impairment in the domains of swallowing, self-care, ambulation, communication, and comprehension. If independence is maintained despite the impairment, it is classified as minor; if independence is lost, it is classified as major.

‡Neurologic signs and symptoms are integrated into the higher grades of impairment.

capabilities (e.g., ability to lift weights, duration of uninterrupted activity in certain positions). Disability severity grading is not often needed in reporting vascular surgical complications, but, if required, the common three-level grading system could be used as follows:

1 = *Mild disability*—patient has detectable function loss that does not prevent his return to preoperative activity level

2 = *Moderate disability*—patient is able to perform only part of previous activities and may require assistance or supporting devices but is still capable of independent existence

3 = *Severe disability*—patient can perform only very limited activities, requires assistance or special devices, and is *not* capable of significant independent activity or solo existence

Severity Grading

All specific complications of a vascular operation ordinarily do not need to be reported separately, but only when the complications are a major focus of the report and its conclusions. Otherwise, an overall major and minor complication rate might suffice, with a breakdown of the former if particular complications stand out. However, when there is a focus on particular complications, they should be graded according to severity as suggested below. When reports on the same procedure or reports on different procedures directed at the same condition or with the same treatment goals are compared, it is valuable to know more than an overall complication rate and/or frequency of specific complications. Unlike death, which is an absolute event, complications may vary significantly in severity and the reader may not be able to gauge the relative merits (i.e., safety) of a particular procedure or treatment if provided only with an overall complication rate. For example, in the case of amputation rates, not only are major and minor amputations vastly different, but so are the disabilities associated with different major amputations (e.g., above-knee vs. below-knee amputation). Similarly, two operative approaches to thoracoabdominal aneurysm may carry approximately the same

incidence of permanent paraplegia/paresis, but in one series the majority of permanent paraplegia/paresis complications may have been mild to moderate and allowed most of the patients to return home and function with assistance, whereas in the other series the majority of paraplegia/paresis complications may have been severe and required institutionalization or ultimately resulted in the patient's demise. By the same token, stroke after carotid endarterectomy may leave patients with complications ranging from clumsiness of the nondominant hand or a mild expressive aphasia to almost complete aphasia and a dense hemiplegia on the dominant side. It is for this reason that the neurologic deficit severity scale was devised,[3] but such elaborate severity scales are not available for most other types of complications or surgery. The main advantage of a simple severity grading system is that it can be applied to all complications and then be combined with the overall complication rate to give a *complication severity score* much like the relative severity scores used in reports on trauma.[5] Again, for general purposes a simple three-level severity scale (1 = mild, 2 = moderate, and 3 = severe) is recommended. *Mild* would include a transient complication, requiring no interventional treatment and resulting in such minor dysfunction or loss of function that it does not significantly affect the patient's basic lifestyle. At the other extreme, a *severe* complication would be one resulting in a major or complete loss of tissue, organ mass, or limb; loss of significant function to interfere with the patient's independence and/or cause the patient to require major assistance or artificial support; or any complication ultimately resulting in death. With these outer limits defined, *moderate* severity would be applied to any complications in between.

Such a gradation need not necessarily apply to the patient as a whole; it can apply to the extremity or organ whose circulation was the focus of the surgical intervention. This can be illustrated by applying this grading system to three examples: the lower extremity, the kidney, and the gut. For a revascularized lower extremity, a typical *mild* complication would include a hematoma or lymphedema that ultimately resolved without treatment or a measurable hemodynamic deterioration without change in clinical status.[1] *Moderate* complications would include symptomatic deterioration with worsening of clinical classification, the unexpected "minor" loss of tissue (e.g., amputation at or below the transmetatarsal level), or ischemia resulting in a mild foot drop manageable by a cock-up splint and ambulation with the aid of a cane. *Severe* complications would include any major amputation (i.e., in which a functional foot was not salvaged) or loss of useful (independent) limb function because of pain or paralysis.

When this severity scale is applied to the kidney, a *mild* complication would include transient loss of function or dysfunction stabilizing at a level that does *not* require special treatment (e.g., creatinine level around 2 to 3 mg%). A *moderate* complication would involve partial loss of parenchymal mass or function, a degree of dysfunction requiring special diet and/or control of salt and fluid intake or transient dialysis, or a complication resulting in the new onset of renovascular hypertension. Partial nephrectomy would therefore be listed as a moderate complication. *Severe* complication would include either nephrectomy or loss of overall renal mass or function to such a degree as to require permanent dialysis or transplantation.

For the gut, a *mild* complication would include a *transient* period of dysfunction requiring hyperalimentation or resulting in intermittent mild bowel dysfunction but without loss of bowel. A *moderate* complication would include partial loss of bowel, segmental resection of bowel, or permanent change in bowel function and need for modification of diet but without significant restrictions on lifestyle. A *severe* complication would include such extensive resection of bowel as to require indefinite or prolonged hyperalimentation just to sustain nutritional balance.

These same basic principles can be applied to almost all complications following the revascularization of any organ, extremity, or tissue. Table 1-2 presents a modified list of graded complications similar to those originally recommended by the SVS/ISCVS subcommittee report.[1] Here again, each complication is graded in severity from 1 to 3. A *complication severity score* can then be calculated by adding these scores and multiplying by the complication rate. For example 20% of 50 cases of a new procedure suffer a complication. If the highest rated complication for each of the ten cases is used, the scores (1, 3, 1, 1, 2, 1, 3, 3, 2, 3) add up to 20. The complication severity score (CSS) would be arrived at using the following equation:

$$CSS = \frac{20}{10} \times \frac{10}{50} \times 100 = 40$$

The highest possible CSS is three times the complication rate; the lowest CSS is one time the complication rate. This approach will allow valid intergroup comparisons.

Categories of Deaths

It may be appropriate to subdivide perioperative deaths into (1) those directly attributable to the operation or *surgical management* itself (including errors in diagnosis, judgment, and technique), (2) those caused primarily by the patient's *underlying disease* (e.g., a second, fatal *cerebral* embolus in a patient who has undergone *femoral* embolectomy), or (3) those considered "*unrelated*" (e.g., an anesthetic complication like malignant hyperthermia). This practice may seem, and be, arbitrary and often would serve little useful purpose. However, it may be justified because of the added perspective it offers. This is particularly true for late deaths, which, with the same approach, would include a breakdown into those caused by (1) delayed complications of operation, (2) the patient's underlying vascular disease, and (3) unrelated causes. An example of the perspective this analysis of late deaths could give is, if 5 years after a particular operation for peripheral atherosclerotic occlusive disease, there was a 40% incidence of late deaths, with only 2% caused by delayed complications of operation and 8% unrelated, one would have to consider more aggressive preoperative screening and treatment of associated coronary disease. If, on the other hand, there was a 30% late mortality rate but 15% of the deaths were related to the

Table 1-2. Types of Complications With Suggested Grading for Outcome and Severity

Complication	Severity/outcome grading*
Systemic/Remote	
Cardiac	1 = little/no hemodynamic consequence
Ectopic/arrhythmia	2 = symptomatic: treatment required
Congestive failure	3 = cardiac arrest, fatal outcome
Myocardial infarction	
Stroke/TIA	1 = TIA: temporary deficit
	2 = permanent: minor deficit
	3 = permanent: major deficit or fatal outcome
Deep vein thrombosis	1 = hospitalization, not prolonged
Suspected	2 = treatment, prolonged hospitalization
Confirmed	3 = operation/interventional therapy required
Pulmonary embolism	1 = mild: antithrombotic drugs required
Suspected	2 = serious: resuscitation required
Confirmed	3 = severe: embolectomy required or resulted in fatal outcome
Coagulation complications (including drug induced)	1 = resolved without treatment
Spontaneous hemorrhage	2 = drug therapy required
Thrombocytopenia	3 = operation required or resulted in loss of limb/organ/life
White clot syndrome	
Thrombosis from antithrombin III, protein C or S deficiency	
Renal insufficiency	1 = transient: dialysis not required or resulted in mild, permanent dysfunction not requiring treatment
Contrast media–induced	
Thromboembolic	2 = transient dialysis required or resulted in moderate, permanent dysfunction requiring special care
Ischemic (acute tubular necrosis)	
Obstructive	3 = permanent dialysis or transplant required or resulted in death
Local/Vascular	
Graft infection	1 = successful local treatment
Early (<30 days)/late (>30 days)	2 = graft removal/bypass required
Culture positive/negative	3 = loss of limb/life
Noninvasive (exposed, contaminated)	
Invasive, involves graft or anastomoses	
Complications of graft/vessel interaction	1 = observed; no treatment required
Intimal hyperplasia (arteriographic, intraoperative, or pathologic diagnosis)	2 = local treatment sufficed (dilation/revision, local resection)
Proximal anastomosis	3 = "redo" operation required
Distal anastomosis	
Anastomotic pseudoaneurysm	1 = observed; no treatment required
Mechanical	2 = local treatment sufficed (dilation/revision, local resection)
Infectious	3 = "redo" operation required
Graft complications (exclusive of anastomotic changes)	1 = observed; no treatment
Dilation/aneurysm	2 = local treatment sufficed (dilation/revision, local resection)
Stenosis, focal/diffuse	
Elongation/kinking	3 = "redo" operation required
Intrinsic, structural defect†	
Arteriosclerotic change†	
Technical†	
Anastomotic hemorrhage	1 = observed
External bleeding	2 = aspiration, drainage required
Internal (hematoma)	3 = anastomotic repair, revision required

TIA, transient ischemic attack.
*0, none; 1, mild; 2, moderate; 3, severe.
†These features apply to all subgroups of graft complications exclusive of anastomotic changes.

Continued.

Table 1-2. Types of Complications With Suggested Grading for Outcome and Severity—cont'd

Complication	Severity/outcome grading*

Graft thrombosis
  Early/late
  Cause found
  Cause not found
	1 = not corrected or corrected with restorative procedure
	2 = revision or ''redo'' operation required
	3 = limb loss (unexpected tissue loss)

Unsatisfactory hemodynamic result (despite patency)
  Insufficient inflow
  Insufficient outflow
  Steal
	1 = >+1 (but less than expected)
	2 = +1
	3 = <+1

Graft-enteric reaction
  Anastomotic (fistula) vs. nonanastomotic
    (erosion)
  Primary infectious cause vs. no secondary
    infection
	1 = successfully treated without permanent sequelae
	2 = permanent sequelae (e.g., limb loss, ostomy)
	3 = fatal outcome

Unexpected tissue loss/amputation	1 = minor tissue loss without amputation 2 = minor amputation 3 = major amputation
Atherothromboembolism	1 = without tissue loss 2 = minor tissue loss with amputation 3 = major tissue loss with amputation
Colon ischemia	1 = no operation required 2 = colon resection or temporary colostomy 3 = permanent colostomy required or resulted in fatal outcome
Spinal cord ischemia	1 = transient or mild paresis 2 = minor permanent deficit: returned home with assistance 3 = major permanent deficit: institutionalized, died
Local/Nonvascular	

Noninfectious wound fluid accumulation
  Hematoma
  Seroma
  Lymphocele
	1 = observed, resolved
	2 = aspiration required
	3 = surgical drainage/closure required

Wound infections
  Superficial
  Deep
  Exposed/contaminated graft
	1 = treated with antibiotic
	2 = drainage required
	3 = graft removal or bypass required

Lymphatic disruption
  Lymphedema
  Lymphocele
  Lymph fistula
	1 = no treatment required
	2 = aspiration, drainage required
	3 = exploration with closure of lymphatics

Ureteral injury
  Partial obstruction
  Complete obstruction
  Urinoma (closed leak)
	1 = resolved spontaneously
	2 = temporary drainage, diversion required
	3 = surgical correction or nephrectomy required

Sexual dysfunction
  Affecting ejaculation (e.g., retrograde)
  Affecting fertility
  Affecting erection (potency)
	1 = mild or no permanent effect on sexual activity
	2 = reduces sexual activity
	3 = prevents or eliminates sexual activity

Complications of sympathectomy
  Disturbance in ejaculation/potency
  Neuralgia after sympathectomy
  No demonstrable therapeutic benefit
	1 = transient: no operative treatment required
	2 = permanent, not disabling: operative treatment required
	3 = no demonstrable therapeutic effect or worsening: permanent injury to adjacent structure

original operation, the major focus should be on operative management.

TEMPORAL CONSIDERATIONS

Many if not most complications are not discrete events that appear at one point in time after operation and continue unchanged thereafter. Generally the longer and more carefully one follows up patients after operation, the higher the frequency of late complications (e.g., recurrence, restenosis, anastomotic aneurysm, graft structural changes) and the lower the incidence or severity of early complications, at least those that tend to improve with time either by spontaneous improvement or compensatory change (e.g., collateral flow). Therefore it is important when reporting complications *to report a mean follow-up time for each group or series of patients undergoing a particular operation.* Any temporal perspective that can be supplied to the reader regarding such complications is valuable. If the complication in question is an important focus of a report and there is a significant trend towards either increase in frequency or decrease in persistence with time, life-table projections can be employed if the numbers permit. In such projections the endpoint can be either an absolute (percentage) frequency or a percentage of the total patients observed to have this complication. For instance, the former approach might allow the observation that "no anastomotic aneurysms appeared before 18 months postoperatively and a 10% incidence had occurred by 10 years." The latter approach would allow such observations as "following lumbar sympathectomy 40% of patients experienced postsympathectomy neuralgia, but 90% of these had no significant residual pain beyond 3 months and 75% experienced improvement by 6 weeks postoperatively." Such perspective is valuable enough in certain settings that this method of reporting is encouraged.

APPLICATION OF THESE REPORTING STANDARDS TO DIFFERENT TYPES OF STUDIES

Reports in which one or more complications is the major focus of a study require special comment. One might wish in such a study to call attention to an unusual complication by detailed reporting of one or more cases in which it has occurred. Here a review of the literature, speculation as to cause, and recommendations regarding diagnosis and treatment with a critique of previous experiences are, of course, appropriate. Nevertheless, *a denominator should be supplied*, if possible, for the sake of perspective. For example: "We have seen this complication only three times in the last 12 years, during which time a total of 314 of these operations have been performed."

For reports in which an extended experience with more common and well-recognized complications is the major focus, it is appropriate to document the overall incidence of the complication and discuss diagnostic methods and therapeutic options based on an analysis of this experience. However, more information is necessary if the report is to significantly add to our perspective of this complication. Detailed characterization by gradation according to severity and temporal relationships (onset, duration, changing incidence with time) is desirable, if not essential. If claims are made regarding a change in incidence, better diagnostic accuracy of this complication, or improved outcome by treatment, these must be documented by detailed comparison with other experiences or subgroup analysis within the series being reported. If possible, the natural history of untreated cases should also be supplied.

Finally, if the focus of the report is on the overall results of a particular operation and includes a description of complications for the sake of completeness, these complications can be detailed in the manner recommended, but it is usually not necessary or desirable to detail *each* complication in this manner. Instead, one can simply list the total major complication rate, broken down as to complication type, in addition to providing a combined mortality and permanent/disabling complication rate. Grading the severity of all complications to produce a complication severity score is indicated if any comparative statements are made about the superiority or safety of a new or modified technique relative to previous approaches.

REFERENCES

1. Rutherford RB, Flanigan DP, Gupta SK, et al. Suggested standards for reports dealing with lower extremity ischemia. J Vasc Surg 4:80-94, 1986.
2. Porter JM, Rutherford RB, Clagett GP, et al. Reporting standards in venous disease. J Vasc Surg 8:172-181, 1988.
3. Baker JD, Rutherford RB, Bernstein EF, et al. Suggested standards for reports dealing with cerebrovascular disease. J Vasc Surg 8:721-729, 1988.
4. Johnston KW, Rutherford RB, Tilson MC, et al. Suggested standards for reporting on arterial aneurysms and their treatment. J Vasc Surg (accepted for publication).
5. Champion HR, Sacco WJ, Copes WS, et al. A revision of the Trauma Score. J Trauma 29:623-629, 1989.

2

Pitfalls of Noninvasive Vascular Testing

Dennis F. Bandyk

Accurate evaluation of patients with diseases of the circulatory system requires a thorough understanding of the anatomy and flow dynamics of the arterial and venous circulations. Although physical examination and arteriography are indispensable in the management of patients with suspected vascular disease, noninvasive testing methods have assumed a prominent role in the diagnostic process. The accuracy of this technology to monitor arterial and venous system function is superior to clinical evaluation, and the hemodynamic information gleaned by noninvasive testing complements anatomic morphology demonstrated by invasive diagnostic techniques such as arteriography or contrast-enhanced computed tomography. Methods that use Doppler ultrasound and plethysmography form the cornerstone of noninvasive diagnosis of cerebrovascular and peripheral arterial occlusive disease, deep vein thrombosis (DVT), and chronic venous insufficiency. The development of duplex ultrasonography, and more recently color flow imaging, has resulted in a greater emphasis on direct anatomic studies that not only can identify disease, but also can assess its extent, determine the severity, and characterize the underlying pathologic state.

Noninvasive testing methods measure biophysical properties of the circulation (e.g., pressure, pulse contour, blood flow velocity, turbulence); these measurements then can be used for disease localization and classification of severity. The diagnostic accuracy of each technique depends on the precision and reproducibility of the measurements. A measurement should not be assumed to be accurate just because it has been recorded. The results of noninvasive testing are affected by factors including biologic variability, instrumentation used, skill and bias of the examiner, pathologic process studied, and conditions under which the measurement is made. It is critical that the user of noninvasive diagnostic techniques appreciate the associated limitations and pitfalls for appropriate use in patient evaluation and clinical decision-making. To this end, this chapter reviews common pitfalls of noninvasive vascular testing related to instrumentation, testing procedures, and diagnostic criteria.

CLASSIFICATION OF NONINVASIVE TESTING PITFALLS

When noninvasive testing is applied for the detection of vascular disease, diagnostic errors can result from procedural, interpretative, or statistical pitfalls. *Procedural pitfalls* can be the consequence of the instrumentation used, deviations from the testing protocol, or the result of biologic variability of the measurement. *Interpretative pitfalls* also decrease diagnostic accuracy and occur when the measurement or outcome acquired by testing does not agree with a recognized "gold standard" test (e.g., arteriography). Interpretative errors can occur despite the recording of a measurement that is both precise and reproducible. The accuracy of noninvasive testing methods is commonly expressed in terms of statistical parameters such as sensitivity, specificity, and positive (PPV) and negative (NPV) predictive values. Although these parameters are useful to compare the diagnostic accuracy of different testing methods, they are subject to *statistical pitfalls* introduced by the reliability of the gold standard, disease prevalence in the population studied, bias in selection of the study population, and the symptomatic or asymptomatic state of the population. For example, the sensitivity (ability to detect the presence of disease) and specificity (ability to recognize absence of disease) of a test are not affected by the prevalence of disease in a study population, but predictive values, which are better measures of clinical utility in studying individual patients, are highly dependent on disease prevalence to reflect the data accurately. It is recommended that testing with a high sensitivity (high NPV) should be used to rule out disease, and testing with a high specificity (high

PPV) should be used to confirm the presence of disease.[1] It is impossible to eliminate all sources of measurement error when noninvasive testing methods are used to diagnose vascular disease because of inherent variability in anatomy, pathologic process, and examination technique. Despite this caveat, noninvasive diagnostic techniques, in particular duplex ultrasonography, demonstrate sufficient accuracy to permit medical or surgical management of a vascular problem with a near 100% certainty as to its presence and extent.

An assortment of instruments is typically available in the noninvasive vascular laboratory with which to measure vascular system function (see box). The most widely used devices rely on ultrasound to assess vessel patency, demonstrate blood flow patterns, or image vascular structures, but plethysmographic instruments remain an integral part of vascular laboratories, providing comprehensive testing capability. The recent development of a voluntary accreditation process for noninvasive vascular laboratories has emphasized the use of specific instrumentation in the areas of peripheral arterial, cerebrovascular, venous, and abdominal visceral disease (Table 2-1). For each testing area, primary and secondary diagnostic devices have been defined. To comply with accreditation standards, primary instrumentation must be provided and used appropriately. Secondary instrumentation can also be utilized to supplant the primary devices and enhance the diagnostic

---

INSTRUMENTS FOR NONINVASIVE MEASUREMENT OF VASCULAR DISEASE

Ultrasound imagers
Continuous-wave Doppler
Duplex ultrasonography (color-coded flow mapping)

Plethysmography
Air (pulse volume recorder)
Impedance
Photosensitive

Pressure transducers
Aneroid manometer
Segmental limb blood pressure cuffs

Table 2-1. Primary and Secondary Instrumentation Relative to Vascular Testing Area

Testing area	Primary instrumentation	Secondary instrumentation
Cerebrovascular	Duplex ultrasonography	Color flow imaging Transcranial Doppler Oculopneumoplethysmography
Peripheral arterial	Segmental cuffs/manometer Continuous-wave Doppler Air plethysmography (PVR) Duplex ultrasonography	Photoplethysmography Laser Doppler Transcutaneous oximetry
Peripheral venous	Duplex ultrasonography Impedance plethysmography Phleborheography	Continuous-wave Doppler B-mode ultrasonic imaging
Abdominal visceral	Duplex ultrasonography	

PVR, pulse volume recording.

process, but these devices should not be used alone because of limited diagnostic capability. Since duplex ultrasonography is a primary diagnostic device in all testing areas and the only acceptable instrumentation for cerebrovascular and visceral vascular testing, it is appropriate that the pitfalls of this diagnostic technique be discussed in detail. Continuous-wave Doppler and plethysmography are primary diagnostic instrumentation in testing for peripheral arterial and venous disease. Compared with duplex scanning, these indirect noninvasive techniques are prone to unique diagnostic pitfalls.

Procedural Pitfalls
Instrumentation

Quality noninvasive testing requires the use of appropriate instrumentation that is maintained in good operating condition and undergoes periodic calibration. Repeated measurements of ankle/brachial systolic pressure index (ABI), treadmill walking time, and pulsatility index, when carefully performed with proper instrumentation, demonstrate reproducibility that compares favorably with other clinical (pulse rate), hematologic (hemoglobin level, white blood count), and biochemical (blood urea nitrogen, creatinine) measurements.[2] At a 95% confidence level, a significant change between two measurements has been found to be greater than 14% for ABI, greater than 120 seconds for treadmill walking time, and greater than 3.4 for pulsatility index. Use of pressure cuffs of improper width relative to limb size, measurement with defective manometers, and variation in testing conditions decrease measurement precision and reproducibility, leading to the erroneous conclusion that serial measurements are "significantly" different. The interpretation of high-thigh pressures is highly dependent on the size of the limb relative to the width of cuff used. When narrow (10 cm) thigh cuffs are used, normal high-thigh pressure is at least 20 to 30 mm Hg higher than brachial pressure because of the artifact associated with the relatively narrow cuff. Theoretically, cuff width should be 20% greater than the diameter of the limb to which it is applied.[3]

Careful attention to instrument calibration is particularly important when plethysmographic techniques are used to record pulse volume waveforms (air plethysmography) or to perform venous occlusion plethysmography (air, strain gauge, or impedance plethysmography). Standardization of cuff inflation pressure is mandatory to obtain reliable, reproducible air plethysmographic data for the assessment of arterial occlusive disease or the identification of acute venous thrombosis. Similarly, the internal resistance of impedance plethysmographic instruments must be balanced to equal the resistance in the patient's leg before recording maximal venous filling and venous outflow. Improper cuff, electrode, or photocell application can also produce artifacts and result in erroneous measurements.

When ultrasound is used to image blood vessels or to study blood flow within them, a variety of pitfalls can arise and result in erroneous data or an inadequate study. These problems can be minimized greatly by the examiner having a thorough understanding of the physics of ultrasound and the design features of the instrumentation. Many factors relating to the ultrasound scanhead, Doppler system, frequency analyzer, and display devices affect image resolution and the Doppler data of duplex instruments (see box). Inappropriate selection

---

FACTORS AFFECTING ULTRASONIC IMAGING AND DOPPLER DATA OF DUPLEX SCANNING

Scanhead design
Ultrasound frequency
Scan format
Method of beam steering (mechanical, electronic)

Doppler system
Sample volume size
Pulse repetition frequency
Sample gate number

Frequency analyzer
Method of spectrum analysis
Characteristic frequency and width

Display devices
Gray-scale spectral waveforms
Compensation for aliasing
Doppler sample volume superimposed on B-mode
Real-time color Doppler in vessels

of the ultrasound frequency for vessel imaging or Doppler measurements is a common pitfall. High ultrasound frequencies allow superior lateral and depth resolution but are strongly attenuated by tissue, limiting the ability to adequately image or record Doppler signals from deeply positioned vessels. To date, ultrasound systems have been developed for transcutaneous application in vascular testing, with emitting Doppler frequencies from 2 to 10 MHz. Selection of the optimal Doppler frequency should be based on the depth of the vessel examined and the composition of overlying tissue. Table 2-2 lists the transducer ultrasound frequency for the strongest Doppler signal from vessels viewed through different tissues based on equations that account for scattering of ultrasound by blood cells, tissue attenuation, and vessel depth.[4] For example, examination in an obese individual of the carotid artery or a peripheral vessel that lies under fat and muscle at a depth of 5 to 7 cm may require an ultrasound frequency of 3 MHz to achieve the strongest Doppler signal.

Variation in focusing and pointing the ultrasound beam using mechanical or electronic methods can also be a source of measurement error. A recent study demonstrated significant overestimation of recorded velocity when linear array multielement scanheads were used to measure a known peak velocity generated by a velocity-calibrated string phantom.[5] Errors exceeding 50% were observed when end-element-

ments of the scanhead were used to record the Doppler signal. Errors of this magnitude are worrisome since measurements of peak systolic and end-diastolic frequency and velocity are used extensively in predicting the degree of stenosis in arterial occlusive disease. The reasons for velocity overestimation are complex and are related to characteristics of the Doppler measuring system including beam width, aperture size, transmitting frequency, and angle of Doppler beam insonation. These concerns should motivate manufacturers of duplex systems with linear array Dopplers to modify their instrumentation, as well as provide test phantoms for periodic instrument calibration. At present, careful selection of ultrasound scanheads, image views, and Doppler spectral measurements relative to the vessel being interrogated should be exercised to optimize the diagnostic results of duplex scanning. In clinical situations in which peak velocity measurements approach threshold levels for significant disease categories (e.g., peak systolic velocity of 125 cm/sec for 50% to 75% diameter-reducing arterial stenosis), linear Doppler scanheads should be used in the steered configuration, with the Doppler cursor positioned at the end of the transducer face so that the Doppler signal recording will be made at the lowest angle of incidence to the axis of flow.

Real-time two-dimensional color Doppler instruments allow display of color-coded Doppler flow data within a high-resolution B-mode tissue image. This newer duplex technology greatly facilitates vessel imaging and the recognition of sites of disordered flow compared with that possible with conventional duplex scanning, but caution is advised when interpreting the color-coded flow data in the display. The images generated by color Doppler are not analogous to contrast angiography. When contrast media is injected into the vascular system, opacification of the vessel will occur if blood is moving or stopped. In color Doppler, changes in direction and velocity of blood cause the color to appear and disappear in the image. Regions of slow blood flow or vessel segments insonated at high Doppler beam angles (greater than 80 degrees) may be coded as black, indicating no flow in a color flow image despite the presence of flowing blood. When areas of

Table 2-2. Ultrasound Frequency for the Strongest Doppler Signal Relative to Depth of Vessel and Type of Overlying Tissue*

	Ultrasound frequency (MHz)			
Depth (cm)	**Blood (0.18)†**	**Fat (0.63)**	**Muscle (1.2)**	**Bone (20)**
0.5	97	28	5	0.9
2	24	7	7	0.2
5	10	3	0.5	0.1
8	6	2	0.3	
15	3	1	0.5	

*Modified from Beach KW. Physics and instrumentation for ultrasonic duplex scanning. In Strandness DE Jr, ed. Duplex Scanning in Vascular Disorders. New York: Raven, 1990, pp 196-227.
†All values for attenuation equal dB/cm/MHz.

apparent no flow are examined, it is essential to scan from at least two lines of sight to improve the angle at which the scanlines intersect the vessel and thereby increase the likelihood of color coding low-flow regions if present. Similarly, distortions in the direction and streamlines of flow can occur with color flow imaging as a result of varying angles of insonation when blood flow is viewed from an off-axis direction with a linear array transducer[6] (Fig. 2-1). There also exists a space-time distortion in color Doppler imaging. The time required to compose a single "real-time" color image varies but is in the range of 30 to 50 msec; this results in the instrument generating a color flow image on a video display like a windshield wiper, with a sweep speed of 100 cm/sec. Since arterial systole last only 0.12 sec and the pulse wave velocity is over 16 m/sec, the spatial-temporal relationships of blood flow cannot be correctly depicted in a single color flow image.

Examination Technique

Obtaining satisfactory ultrasound images, Doppler signals, or plethysmographic waveforms requires skill, concentration, and experience. Lack of expertise on the part of the examiner is the most important cause of measurement error and variability. Transcutaneous Doppler arterial and venous surveys require the examiner to prepare the patient properly, manipulate the probe with care, and develop a standard sequence of examination with testing of both limbs for comparison. Because of the multiple potential pitfalls of Doppler surveys (see box), interpretation of the Doppler signals must be performed by an experienced observer and used in conjunction with careful clinical examination. By comparison, plethysmographic techniques are less subject to examiner error and are the preferred indirect methods when experienced technologists are not available. When hemodynamic data from the arterial and venous circulations are recorded, it is important the patient be rested before examination and be positioned appropriately for the testing method and for the indication for testing. A pitfall of venous outflow plethysmography when used to detect acute DVT is extrinsic vein compression produced by leg positioning, wound dressings

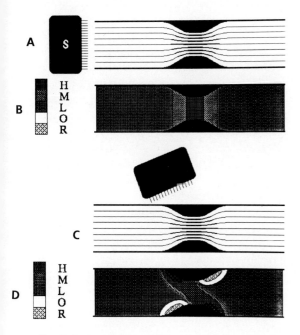

Fig. 2-1. Anomalous coding of streamlines in color flow imaging. **A,** Streamlines in a stenosis viewed in an axial direction with a linear array. Streamline spacing and thickness indicate increased velocity. **B,** Schematic of color display from top arrangement. **C,** Streamlines in a stenosis viewed from an off-axis direction with a linear array. **D,** Color display resulting from the lower scanplane. The high Doppler angles cause the impression of flow separation and of a high-angle jet at the inlet and outlet of the stenosis. *H,* Highest color Doppler frequencies; *M,* medium frequencies; *L,* lower frequencies; *O,* minimal frequencies; *R,* Doppler frequencies in the reverse direction. (From Beach KW. Physics and instrumentation for ultrasonic duplex scanning. In Strandness DE Jr, ed. Duplex Scanning in Vascular Disorders. New York: Raven, 1990, pp 196-227.)

POTENTIAL PITFALLS OF DOPPLER ARTERIAL AND VENOUS SURVEYS

Improper probe position or emitting frequency
Inadvertent probe motion
Incorrect incident probe angle
Inadequate amount of conduction gel
Excessive probe pressure on skin
Insufficient patient preparation or positioning

or hematoma, or a gravid uterus. To avoid false-positive findings when recording Doppler signals and plethysmographic waveforms for quantitative analysis or when measuring systolic blood pressure, it is recommended that when abnormal measurements are obtained, the examination should be repeated several times, with particular attention directed at measurement technique.[5,7]

Duplex scanning requires considerable learned expertise in ultrasound physics, vascular anatomy, and the recording of velocity spectra. This is particularly apparent when color duplex scanning is performed. These instruments allow simultaneous viewing of both flow and soft tissue information in real-time. Color coding of Doppler frequency shifted information from samples taken in a portion or all of the B-mode image is based on single characteristic frequency (e.g., mean frequency) rather than on all the frequencies that are present at that specific time, as in a spectral waveform. This accounts for the lower frequency scales that appear in the color display and the inability to classify accurately occlusive lesions based on inspection of the color image alone. To achieve the high level of agreement that has been reported between duplex scanning and contrast angiography in classifying carotid and peripheral artery stenosis, a variety of pitfalls must be avoided[4,8-12] (see box). The two most prominent problems, particularly when using color duplex instruments, are (1) assignment of the Doppler angle and true direction of blood flow and (2) aliasing. An understanding of these two

---

POTENTIAL PITFALLS OF COLOR DUPLEX ULTRASONOGRAPHY

Vessel misidentification
Improper Doppler angle assignment
Aliasing
Calcified atherosclerotic plaque
Vessel tortuosity
Tandem occlusive lesions
Incorrect sample volume placement
Improper scanning technique
Overinterpretation of flow image

---

concepts is essential to perform accurate duplex examination, particularly when tortuous or kinked arterial segments are examined. The vascular group at the University of Washington has recommended that an examination angle of 60 degrees is ideal for signal processing, should be used in all examinations, and should remain consistent for repeated studies of the same artery.[11,13,14] Because modern duplex instruments utilize linear array transducer and electronic steering of the Doppler beam, Doppler data commonly must be recorded at various transducer scanlines ranging from 30 to 60 degrees. In this range, an angle assignment error of ±5 degrees will cause a 10% to 20% error in the calculated velocities. By contrast, at an angle of insonation of 70 degrees, this level of uncertainty results in a 25% error in the calculated velocities. There is concern regarding the calculation of velocity since classification of arterial stenoses is based primarily on measurements of peak systolic and end-diastolic velocities. Reports that analyzed the variability of velocity measurements obtained by duplex scanning have concluded that the variability is within clinical acceptable levels and is caused mainly by problems with the examination technique (failure to record the Doppler signal downstream of a stenosis, difficulty distinguishing between a kink and a stenosis, failure to recognize an improper Doppler angle) rather than inaccurate measurement of waveform parameters or changes in patient hemodynamics.[14,15]

In color Doppler systems, color coding of flow is based on the direction of the frequency shift (velocity) either toward or away from the transducer. Since the anatomy of blood vessels is complex with curves, branches, and dilatations, attention to the insonation angle of transducer scanlines is critical for defining patency, directionality, and flow characteristics. For optimal imaging, scanlines should be perpendicular to vessel walls, but this results in minimal Doppler shifts that produce erroneous areas of "no flow," necessitating insonation of blood vessels at an angle or electronic steering of scanlines for Doppler data recording. The percentage change in velocity relative to a velocity measured at 60 degrees increases dramatically at an angle of insonation of 70 degrees or more (Fig. 2-2). The small Doppler frequency shifts recorded at high angles of insonation decrease the sensitivity of color flow imaging in detecting flow and make velocity readings and measurements of volume flow unreliable.[16] As the angle of insonation decreases toward zero, the Doppler frequency shift will increase. When the detected frequency shift exceeds one half the pulse repetition frequency (known as the Nyquist limit) of the instrument, aliasing occurs. Aliasing in color flow imaging results in an improper assignment of both direction and velocity data, with the resulting flow pattern erroneously interpreted as abnormal or turbulent flow. Aliasing is easily recognized on pulsed Doppler spectral analysis, and the phenomenon can be decreased or eliminated by increasing the angle of insonation or the pulse repetition frequency of the instrument, or by changing the scanplane of the transducer to decrease the depth at which the vessel is being examined. Accurate color flow imaging compels the examiner to be vigilant constantly to keep an appropriate angle (60 degrees or less) between the axis of blood flow and the transducer scanlines. To avoid the pitfalls of color duplex scanning, vessels must be imaged in multiple planes and the technologist must learn to think three-dimensionally, a skill acquired only through experience.

Interpretative and Statistical Pitfalls

All noninvasive vascular diagnostic techniques are subject to interpretation errors independent of problems related to the instrumentation or the testing procedure. Measurements from both indirect and direct methods can produce false-positive results because of variation in vascular anatomy, presence of bilateral disease or tandem lesions, or concomitant medical problems (congestive heart failure, hypertension, hypotension), which alter arterial and venous circulation. Heavily calcified vessels can artificially elevate segmental pressure measurements, as well as impair the ability of duplex scanning to image and record Doppler data from arterial segments with circumferential disease. Calcification, which severely attenuates ultrasound transmission, leads to blind areas (acoustic shadowing) in the B-mode image, sometimes rendering the study uninterpretable. Direct measurements of arterial stenosis from conventional and color duplex images have been shown to be inaccurate in the presence of calcified plaque when compared with those obtained with angiography.[17,18] Ultrasonic imaging can accurately characterize minimal disease (<50% diameter reduction), but red thrombus, with an acoustic density similar to blood, may escape detection. The incorporation of sensitive Doppler flow sensing capability in current-day color flow imagers has mark-

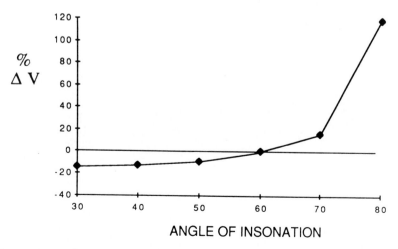

Fig. 2-2. Percentage change in calculated velocity relative to velocity calculated at an angle of insonation of 60 degrees.

edly decreased the likelihood of missing a total vessel occlusion.

An abnormal hemodynamic state that produces an increase in basal flow is another interpretative pitfall of duplex scanning that can result in overestimation of stenosis severity. In patients with an intact circle of Willis, contralateral carotid stenosis or occlusion can lead to an overreading of ipsilateral disease since diagnostic criteria depend on the levels of peak systolic and end-diastolic velocity, which are increased because of compensatory collateral flow.[19,20] This effect appears most evident in the misclassification of lesions in the 50% to 75% diameter reduction category.[18] Similarly, the severity of peripheral arterial or infrainguinal vein graft stenoses will be overclassified in the presence of a downstream arteriovenous fistula or in the presence of a postrevascularization hyperemic state.

The interpretation of the results of various noninvasive test methods is also complicated by the absence of uniform diagnostic criteria. In order to grade peripheral arterial occlusive disease, a multitude of criteria have been published using segmental pressure measurements alone or in combination with pulse volume recordings or, in the case of duplex scanning, the use of imaging criteria alone and in combination with pulsed Doppler spectral analysis. The national vascular societies have addressed the problem of nomenclature by the development of suggested standards of reporting for peripheral arterial, cerebrovascular, and venous disease.[21-23] With the vascular laboratory accreditation process, it is anticipated that minimum standards with respect to the elements of diagnostic criteria will be adopted by testing facilities. Users of sophisticated Doppler instrumentation must realize that the results obtained by one group of investigators with a particular instrument may not be duplicated when a different instrument is utilized. A recent review of current practice in the assessment of diagnostic tests noted that a gold standard was used in only 68% of the studies reported and its use was a major factor contributing to the difficulty in interpreting the value of such tests.[24] Directors of noninvasive vascular laboratories are responsible for quality assurance, which includes implementation of an independent, blinded review of the results of noninvasive tests against gold standard tests performed for clinical reasons. Such a review process should expose pitfalls of testing related not only to inadequate diagnostic criteria but also to instrumentation and technologist performance.

Contrast studies such as angiography and venography have been considered the reference standard of vascular diagnosis, although these techniques are know to have considerable interobserver variability and can miss significant lesions as a result of imaging in only one plane, patient motion, and timing of contrast injection. Investigators have shown that the agreement between duplex scanning and angiographic classification of occlusion in both the cerebrovascular and peripheral arterial systems has a variability similar to the agreement of two radiologists' readings of the same angiograms (sensitivity 87%, specificity 94%).[8,11] Reliability of the gold standard remains an unresolved problem of confirming the accuracy of noninvasive testing. In selected clinical situations, such as nonoccluding venous thrombosis and severe peripheral arterial ischemia, the accuracy of duplex scanning has been judged by the investigators to be superior to contrast studies.[12,25] Interobserver and intraobserver variability of ultrasonic duplex examinations can be minimized by the recording of velocity waveforms using a standardized testing procedure and the use of diagnostic criteria based on quantitative data. As in angiographic studies, classification of disease into minimal to moderate categories accounts for most of the variability.[14]

PERIPHERAL ARTERIAL TESTING

Tests used to investigate peripheral arterial disease should identify, locate, and grade the severity of the obstructive process. Measurement of systolic blood pressure at one or more levels, in combination with pulse (Doppler, plethysmographic) waveform analysis, is an essential component of peripheral arterial testing. Segmental pressure measurements are used primarily to establish the severity of limb ischemia, either at rest or following stress testing. Localization of disease to the aortoiliac, superficial femoral, and popliteal-tibial arterial segments by segmental pressure measurements alone is not accurate, with only one half to three fourths of limbs correctly classified using angiography as a gold standard.[26] Multilevel and isolated tibial disease, as well as vessel wall calcification producing vessel incompressibility, lessens the accuracy of the test. To achieve a diagnostic accuracy greater than 90%, segmental limb pressure must be evaluated together with pulse volume recordings or quantitative Doppler signal analysis.[27,28] An important limitation of indirect hemodynamic noninvasive tests is that they provide no information as to the nature (stenosis vs. occlusion) of the pressure-reducing lesions. This factor limits their clinical usefulness in the postoperative period for the detection of vein graft stenosis or the evaluation of peripheral angioplasty unless limb pressures and pulse waveforms were normalized following the procedure.

Duplex scanning can be used to provide detailed morphologic and hemodynamic information regarding disease processes in specific arterial segments. Important applications of duplex scanning in peripheral arterial testing include study of patients who, based on clinical indications, appear to be candidates for either percutaneous transluminal angioplasty or direct arterial surgery; screening of high-risk patients for aneurysmal disease; and surveillance of arterial reconstructions for restenosis or anastomotic pseudoaneurysm formation. Since individual lesions are graded based on proximal and distal changes in velocity spectra, duplex scanning can be used to assess patients with multilevel disease. Prospective studies have demonstrated an overall sensitivity of 80% to 87%, specificity of 92% to 99%, PPV of 80% to 91%, and NPV of 91% to 93% in the determination of >50% diameter reduction stenosis using angiography as the gold standard.[11,12] The addition of color flow imaging permitted accurate identification of both the presence and length of occlusion in 94% of extremities.[12] The reported accuracy of color flow imaging is sufficient to permit planning for endovascular vs. direct surgical treatment of symptomatic lower extremity occlusive disease manifest as claudication. In patients presenting with critical limb ischemia, angiography remains an essential component of patient evaluation before surgical intervention. In cases of severe, multilevel disease, duplex scanning is plagued by a variety of pitfalls that impair obtaining the necessary detailed anatomic and hemodynamic definition of the arterial tree, including artifacts produced by vessel calcification, difficulty in imaging of the tibioperoneal trunk, and the requirement for extensive examiner experience to achieve an interpretable study.

CEREBROVASCULAR TESTING

Evaluation of cerebrovascular problems differs from peripheral arterial testing in that lesions with embolic potential, in addition to pressure- and flow-reducing lesions, must be identified. To adequately identify, locate, and grade obstructive or aneurysmal lesions in the extracranial carotid and vertebral arteries, cerebrovascular testing requires the use of duplex instrumentation. The diagnostic accuracy of carotid duplex scanning has improved with modifications in instrumentation, examination technique, and spectral criteria.[9] For distinguishing between normal and diseased carotid bifurcations, conventional duplex scanning has a specificity of 84% and sensitivity of 99%. The accuracy for detecting 50% to 99% diameter stenosis or occlusion exceeds 93%.[9,28-30] The addition of color flow imaging reportedly decreases the frequency of errors encountered in classifying lower grades (<50% diameter reduction) of stenosis.[10] Although NPVs exceed 95% for all categories of stenosis or occlusion, PPVs for the detection of >80% diameter stenosis or occlusion of the internal carotid artery (ICA) was 90% and 88%, respectively.[10] Acoustic shadowing produced by plaque calcification, slow flow in the distal ICA, and compensatory collateral flow via the external carotid artery are diagnostic pitfalls limiting the certainty with which duplex scanning can exclude patency of the ICA in a patient with hemispheric symptoms. A high-grade (>90% diameter) ICA stenosis can escape detection when either conventional or color duplex scanning is used despite both scanning methods fulfilling the imaging and hemodynamic criteria to demonstrate an ICA occlusion (Fig. 2-3). When less severe stenoses are being graded,

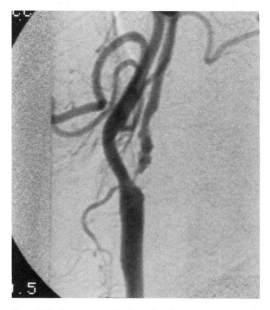

Fig. 2-3. Intra-arterial digital subtraction angiography of the left carotid bifurcation with a >90% stenosis of the proximal ICA. Duplex scanning detected no flow in the ICA with low peak systolic flow in common carotid artery (35 cm/sec) and flow to zero during diastole. At the time of carotid endarterectomy, peak systolic velocity in the distal portion of the artery was measured at 8 cm/sec by high (20 MHz) pulsed Doppler spectral analysis.

proper assignment of the angle-correction cursor avoids most mismatches between duplex interpretations and arteriographic readings.

PERIPHERAL VENOUS TESTING

Diagnosis of acute lower limb DVT can be made accurately by using duplex ultrasonography or by measuring outflow resistance with plethysmography. Sensitivities are reported in the 90% to 100% range (mean, 97%), with specificities in the range of 78% to 100% (mean, 93%).[7,17,25,31-33] Color flow imaging shows promise in increasing the accuracy of duplex studies by facilitating the examination of veins below the knee and intra-abdominal veins (iliac, vena cava). Venous duplex imaging has the potential to become the diagnostic standard for acute DVT, given the difficulties with contrast venography (interpretation error, failure to visualize the deep venous system, and the risk

of precipitating DVT). As in other areas of vascular testing, duplex imaging results depend on examiner experience and technical quality of the examination. Erroneous or equivocal studies can be minimized by meticulous infrapopliteal vein examination, better estimation of the age of the thrombotic process, and recognition of segmental incompressibility of the superficial vein within the adductor canal as a normal finding, especially in the absence of abnormal Doppler flow or imaged thrombus. The ability of venous duplex imaging to diagnose nonocclusive and infrapopliteal thrombus makes it the preferred method for surveillance of patients at high risk for DVT. By comparison, plethysmography has been shown to have a decreased diagnostic capability in this patient group.[25] Impedance plethysmography has demonstrated greatest efficacy in the evaluation of patients with clinically suspected DVT. In this patient group the accuracy of impedance plethysmography in the detection of above-knee occluding thrombus is 100%.[34] Importantly, management decisions can be made safely even though this test fails to detect calf vein thrombosis. Positive results with impedance plethysmography are sufficient to justify initiation of anticoagulant therapy. Normal or equivocal findings with impedance plethysmography in a symptomatic patient mandate the performance of serial studies (several times over the next 10 to 14 days) to exclude the development of calf vein propagation into the popliteal vein. This approach has been demonstrated to be safe. The development of a fatal pulmonary embolus was not observed, but proximal DVT developed in 2% of patients based on serial testing.[34] Pitfalls of venous testing are largely caused by anatomic (duplicated popliteal or superficial venous segments) or Doppler signal variants, nonoccluding thrombus, chronic DVT, or thrombus outside the scanfield. Because of these limitations, if duplex or impedance plethysmographic findings are negative but there is convincing evidence of DVT, it is recommended that venography be performed.

GOALS FOR DIAGNOSIS

A primary requirement of noninvasive testing is the ability to detect the clinical spectrum of vascular disease involved in the causation of symptoms. Although the instrumentation utilized in the various testing areas may be similar, testing procedures and diagnostic criteria must be focused to provide measurements that characterize the pathologic features of disease such as location, extent, severity, and morphology. An important pitfall of the application of noninvasive vascular testing is the failure to consider the clinical background of the patient with the type of testing performed and the interpretation of the examination. For example, an abnormal carotid duplex study in an asymptomatic patient should focus primarily on the degree of stenosis, with the issues of plaque surface characteristics and plaque composition being of more clinical importance in evaluating the embolic potential of lesions in symptomatic patients. The decision as to what to measure in the arterial or venous circulations is complex and can vary depending on the need to establish a diagnosis, determine a treatment plan, assess the results of intervention, or determine the natural history of a disease process. Regardless of the goal, precision and reproducibility of measurements are important. Avoiding the known and suspected pitfalls of noninvasive testing results in improved diagnostic accuracy and patient care.

REFERENCES

1. Sumner DS. Evaluation of noninvasive testing procedures: Data analysis and interpretation. In Bernstein EF, ed. Noninvasive Diagnostic Techniques in Vascular Disease, 3rd ed. St. Louis: CV Mosby, 1985, pp 861-889.
2. Johnston KW, Hosang MY, Andrews DF. Reproducibility of noninvasive vascular laboratory measurements of the peripheral circulation. J Vasc Surg 6:147-151, 1987.
3. Kirkendall WM, Burton AC, Epstein FH, et al. Recommendations for human blood pressure determination by sphygmomanometers: Report of a subcommittee of the post-graduate education committee, American Heart Association. Circulation 36:980-988, 1978.
4. Beach KW. Physics and instrumentation for ultrasonic duplex scanning. In Strandness DE Jr, ed. Duplex Scanning in Vascular Disorders. New York: Raven, 1990, pp 196-227.
5. Bridges RA, Barnes RW. Segmental limb pressures. In Kempczinski RF, Yao JST, eds. Practical Noninvasive Vascular Diagnosis, 2nd ed. Chicago: Year Book, 1987, pp 112-126.
6. Daigle RJ, Stavros AT, Lee RM. Overestimation of velocity and frequency values by multi-element linear array Doppler. J Vasc Technol 14:206-213, 1990.
7. Wheeler HB, Anderson FA Jr. Impedance plethysmography. In Kempczinski RF, Yao JST, eds. Practical Noninvasive Vascular Diagnosis, 2nd ed. Chicago: Year Book, 1987, pp 407-437.
8. Fell G, Phillips DJ, Chikos PM, et al. Ultrasonic duplex scanning for disease of the carotid artery. Circulation 64:1191-1195, 1981.
9. Roederer GO, Langlois YE, Chan AW, et al. Ultrasonic duplex scanning of extracranial carotid arteries—Improved accuracy using new features from the common carotid artery. J Cardiovasc Ultrasonog 1:373-379, 1982.
10. Sumner DS. Use of color-flow imaging technique in carotid artery disease. Surg Clin North Am 70:201-211, 1990.
11. Jager KA, Phillips DJ, Martin RL, et al. Noninvasive mapping of lower limb arterial lesions. Ultrasound Med Biol 11:515-521, 1985.
12. Cossman DV, Ellison JE, Wagner WH, et al. Comparison of contrast arteriography to arterial mapping with color-flow duplex imaging in the lower extremities. J Vasc Surg 10:522-529, 1989.
13. Beach KW, Lawrence R, Phillips DJ, et al. The systolic velocity criterion for diagnosing significant internal carotid stenosis. J Vasc Technol 13:65-68, 1989.
14. Kohler T, Langlois Y, Roederer GO, et al. Sources of variability in carotid duplex examination—A prospective study. Ultrasound Med Biol 11:571-576, 1985.
15. Kohler TR, Langlois Y, Roederer GO, et al. Variability in measurement of specific parameters for carotid duplex examination. Ultrasound Med Biol 13:637-642, 1987.
16. Rizzo RJ, Sandager G, Astleford P, et al. Mesenteric flow velocity variations as a function of angle of insonation. J Vasc Surg 11:688-694, 1990.
17. Comerota AJ, Cranley JJ, Katz ML, et al. Real-time B-mode carotid imaging: A three-year multicenter experience. J Vasc Surg 1:84-95, 1984.
18. Erickson SJ, Mewissen MW, Foley WD, et al. Stenosis of the internal carotid artery: Assessment using color Doppler imaging compared with angiography. Am J Radiol 152:1299-1305, 1989.
19. Cato RF, Bandyk DF, Livigni D, et al. Carotid collateral circulation decreases the diagnostic accuracy of duplex scanning. Bruit 10:68-73, 1986.
20. Spadone DP, Barkmeier LD, Hodgson KJ, et al. Contralateral internal carotid artery stenosis or occlusion: Pitfall of correct ipsilateral classification—A study performed with color flow imaging. J Vasc Surg 11:642-649, 1990.
21. Rutherford RB, Flanigan DP, Gupta SK, et al. Suggested standards for reports dealing with lower extremity ischemia. J Vasc Surg 4:80-94, 1986.
22. Porter JM, Clagett PG, Cranley JJ, et al. Reporting standards in venous disease. J Vasc Surg 8:172-181, 1988.

23. Thiele BL. Standards in noninvasive cerebrovascular testing. In Bernstein EF, ed. Recent Advances in Noninvasive Diagnostic Techniques in Vascular Disease. St. Louis: CV Mosby, 1990, pp 15-24.

24. Sheps S, Schecter MT. The assessment of diagnostic tests—A survey of current medical research. JAMA 252:2418-2422, 1984.

25. Comerota AJ, Katz ML, Greenwald LL, et al. Venous duplex imaging: Should it replace hemodynamic tests for deep venous thrombosis. J Vasc Surg 11:53-61, 1990.

26. Rutherford RB, Lowenstein DH, Klein MF. Combining segmental systolic pressures and plethysmography to diagnose arterial occlusive disease of the legs. Am J Surg 138:211-218, 1979.

27. Kempczinski RF. Segmental volume plethysmography in the diagnosis of lower extremity arterial occlusive disease. J Cardiovasc Surg 23:125-129, 1982.

28. Johnston KW. Peripheral arterial Doppler blood flow—Velocity waveform analysis. In Kempczinski RF, Yao JST, eds. Chicago: Year Book 1987, pp 154-177.

29. Cardullo PA, Cutler BS, Wheeler HB, et al. Accuracy of duplex scanning in the detection of carotid artery disease. Bruit 8:181-186, 1984.

30. Daigle RJ, Gardner M, Smazal SF, et al. Accuracy of duplex ultrasound in the evaluation of carotid artery disease. Bruit 7:17-21, 1983.

31. Langsfeld M, Hersey FB, Thorpe L, et al. Duplex B-mode imaging for the diagnosis of deep venous thrombosis. Arch Surg 122:587-591, 1987.

32. Persson AF, Jones C, Zide R, et al. Use of the triplex scanner in diagnosis of deep venous thrombosis. Arch Surg 124:593-596, 1989.

33. Wright DJ, Shepard AD, McPharlin M, et al. Pitfalls in lower extremity venous duplex scanning. J Vasc Surg 11:675-679, 1990.

34. Hull RD, Hirsh J, Carter CJ, et al. Diagnostic efficacy of impedance plethysmography for clinically suspected deep-vein thrombosis—A randomized study. Ann Intern Med 102:21-28, 1985.

II Associated Diseases

3

Cardiopulmonary Complications Related to Vascular Surgery

David C. Brewster **John D. Edwards**

As a result of the well-known high incidence of coexistent cardiac and pulmonary pathologic conditions in patients with vascular disease, cardiopulmonary complications are among the most frequent and significant perioperative problems affecting the patient undergoing vascular surgery. As is true of all complications, potential problems are best avoided in the first place rather than waiting to treat them after they occur. Hence, careful preoperative assessment of cardiopulmonary function and identification of patients at high risk of perioperative difficulties in these areas is an important aspect of management of the vascular surgery patient.

ISCHEMIC HEART DISEASE

Because atherosclerosis is a systemic disease process, it is well recognized that coronary artery disease (CAD) is highly prevalent in patients with peripheral vascular disease. Coronary atherosclerosis is responsible for the majority of both early and late deaths following peripheral vascular surgery.[1-3] Acute myocar-

dial infarction (MI) is the cause of approximately 50% or more of perioperative deaths in patients undergoing vascular operations.[4] In two large series reported from the Cleveland Clinic,[5,6] fatal MI accounted for a 3.3% perioperative mortality rate (52% of the deaths) following lower extremity revascularization and a 6% mortality rate (37% of the early postoperative deaths) for aortic aneurysm resection. In the United States 50,000 perioperative MIs occur annually, resulting in more than 20,000 deaths per year.[7]

The value of accurate and reliable methods of screening vascular surgery patients for CAD is further emphasized when one reviews data concerning the incidence of CAD in this patient group. Studies using routine coronary angiography before aortic surgery report that 85% of patients have some degree of CAD, whereas severe (2- or 3-vessel or left main) disease is found in 31%.[8,9] In the epic report by Hertzer et al.[8] of 1000 patients subjected to mandatory coronary arteriography before undergoing indicated vascular operations, severe CAD was present in 36% of patients with abdominal aortic aneurysms, in 32% of patients with cerebrovascular disease, and in 28% of patients with lower extremity ischemia. It is important to note that these studies revealed that 14% to 22% of patients without any previous clinical evidence of CAD (negative cardiac history and normal ECG) had severe disease revealed by coronary angiogram.[8] In light of the prevalence of associated CAD, the incidence of clinically apparent perioperative MI of 2% to 8% reported in most vascular surgical series is not surprising.[10,11] In fact, when careful prospective studies are performed using serial ECG and creatine phosphokinase (CPK)-isoenzyme analyses in the postoperative period, the incidence of perioperative MI increases to 10% to 17%.[12-14]

Although the pathophysiology of perioperative MI has not been fully elucidated, numerous factors are probably involved. Both surgery and anesthesia trigger a number of processes that place added stress on the myocardium. Catechol release, increased myocardial sensitivity to catechols, fluid shifts, swings in blood pressure, decreased oxygen transport, transient hypercoagulable states, and tachycardia may compromise the ability of the diseased coronary circulation to supply adequate oxygen to the myocardium.[15] Tachycardia may be particularly deleterious since it decreases the duration of diastole, which is the period during which the majority of coronary arterial flow occurs. Many of these factors tend to be most problematic in the first 2 to 3 postoperative days, which corresponds with the timing of 60% to 90% of perioperative MIs.[12,15]

PREOPERATIVE CARDIAC RISK ASSESSMENT

The high prevalence of CAD in peripheral vascular surgery patients and the 50% mortality rate associated with postoperative MI in this population justify and in fact necessitate aggressive and dedicated preoperative evaluation in order to identify high–cardiac risk patients. Once identified, it is hoped that proper precautions and specific interventions may be used to reduce the risk of perioperative MI.

A wide variety of methods are currently

METHODS OF CARDIAC RISK ASSESSMENT

Clinical risk factor indices
Coronary angiography
Exercise-stress ECG testing
Radionuclide ventriculography (MUGA scan)
Echocardiography
Dipyridamole-thallium scan
Ambulatory ECG monitoring

---

available for cardiac risk assessment including clinical risk factor indices, coronary angiography, exercise-stress ECG testing, radionuclide ventriculography (MUGA scan), echocardiography, dipyridamole-thallium scanning, continuous portable ECG monitoring, duplex aortic velocimetry, and positron emission tomography (PET scanning) (see box). Such tests are particularly valuable in those situations in which the clinical assessment may underestimate the severity of a patient's CAD.[16] Unfortunately, despite the availability of numerous testing modalities and extensive data concerning evaluation of cardiac risk in vascular surgery patients, no consensus currently exists regarding the best methods of accomplishing this goal. Determination of a clear-cut algorithm is impossible because of the differences in clinical circumstances in each individual patient and the considerable variability of study populations, methodologies, and end-point definitions in prior published reports.[12] Nonetheless, it is important for the vascular surgeon to be familiar with available approaches, know their potential strengths and weaknesses, and gain insight into the logical and practical application of such tests in the preoperative evaluation and management of the patients before vascular operation. Thus this discussion focuses on the current status of available methods of cardiac risk assessment.

Clinical Risk Assessment

Clinical assessment of cardiac risk may be sufficient in an active individual with no history of angina or MI, a normal physical examination, and a normal ECG. In this scenario a patient can probably safely undergo vascular surgery without further cardiac evaluation.[17,18] However, the presence of specific clinical risk factors including history of previous MI, congestive heart failure, unstable angina, abnormalities on the preoperative ECG, diabetes mellitus, and advanced age (over 70 years) place the patient at increased risk for postoperative cardiac events.[3,10,17,19]

The difficulty with traditional clinical cardiac risk assessment arises in the typical peripheral vascular surgery patient who often leads a sedentary lifestyle. In this setting the absence of a history of cardiac problems cannot safely be assumed to imply the absence of severe CAD. In fact, numerous studies have shown that clinical assessment using traditional clinical criteria to develop a weighted scoring system, such as the widely known Goldman risk index,[20,21] underestimates cardiac risk in many vascular surgery patients.[22,23] This lack of sensitivity of clinical assessment alone has made surgeons turn to other methods to improve cardiac risk stratification.

Coronary Angiography

Routine coronary angiography has been used in the preoperative assessment of vascular surgery patients.[8,9,11] The Cleveland Clinic experience with this protocol revealed that 34% of patients with a clinical history suggesting CAD were found to have severe CAD on preoperative coronary angiogram, whereas 14% of patients with no clinical history demonstrated severe disease on angiogram.[24] Thus, although the incidence of disease is significant, some 66% to 86% of patients would undergo unnecessary coronary angiography if this protocol were used, severely limiting the cost effectiveness of such an approach. In addition, the cumulative risks of coronary angiography, a coronary revascularization procedure, and then the indicated vascular operation may well exceed the risk of the vascular operation alone.[25] Finally, since coronary angiography provides anatomic definition but no functional information, it may not necessarily be predictive of perioperative cardiac ischemic events or clearly improve perioperative survival.[11,24,26,27]

For these reasons, routine preoperative screening of vascular surgery patients for CAD by means of preoperative coronary angiography is not recommended. Rather, angiography should be used in the relatively small subset of patients identified by other, less invasive and less costly screening tests. A variety of noninvasive techniques have been developed that provide functional and/or metabolic definition regarding the status of the myocardium. These tests should be used to stratify patients with regard to coronary risk and thus selectively direct the preoperative use of coronary angiography and possibly prophylactic coronary bypass or percutaneous transluminal coronary angioplasty (PTCA) only in the truly high-risk cohort.

Exercise-Stress ECG Testing

Exercise-stress ECG testing was one of the earliest methods employed for screening for CAD and may be valuable in assessing cardiac risk if ischemic ECG changes develop in the patient during the exercise protocol.[13,28-31] However, because of severe claudication, ischemic ulcerations, prior amputation, stroke, severe lung disease, arthritis, or other infirmities, many peripheral vascular surgery patients are incapable of adequate exercise to achieve 75% to 85% of maximal predicted heart rate required by the test protocol; only 30% of patients from one series were able to do so.[31] With exercise-stress ECG testing, submaximal effort may yield false-negative results. It is this very population, with its sedentary lifestyle or associated debilitating conditions that limit the ability to achieve adequate exercise levels, who may harbor severe silent CAD and therefore have the greatest need for accurate preoperative cardiac evaluation.

Dipyridamole-Thallium Myocardial Scintigraphy

Although exercise is the best known and most widely employed stimulus for producing coronary vasodilatation and thereby maximization of regional blood flow abnormalities, many patients with peripheral vascular disease cannot exercise sufficiently for a meaningful test. Dipyridamole, administered intravenously, provides a pharmacologic stimulus to increase coronary blood flow and thereby "stress" coronary perfusion. The agent produces coronary vasodilatation even greater than that produced by exercise but without a concomitant increase in myocardial oxygen consumption. The effectiveness of oral dipyridamole has also been evaluated but oral administration was found to be much less satisfactory than the intravenous preparation because the time to onset of effect and time to peak effect are less predictable, and therefore appropriate timing of initial and delayed scintigrams is much less precise.

The mechanism of action of dipyridamole involves increasing cellular concentrations of adenosine.[32] This results in coronary vasodilatation and increased flow through normal coronary arteries, while atherosclerotic coronary arteries fail to vasodilate. This produces a preferential flow through the normal, low-resistance coronary bed and away from the myocardium supplied by the stenotic coronary arteries. The preferential flow results in areas of hypoperfusion (ischemic regions of myocardium) in the distribution of the severely diseased coronary arteries. Thallium-201 is used as a marker for viable myocardium. The presence of any ischemic regions can be documented by using thallium-201 myocardial perfusion scintigraphy. The uptake of thallium-201 by the heart is linearly related to blood flow. The myocardium normally has homogeneous thallium uptake unless there are regions of hypoperfusion.

The dipyridamole-thallium scanning technique involves the intravenous administration of dipyridamole followed within a few minutes by the intravenous injection of thallium-201. Scans are obtained at 15 minutes (initial) and 3 hours (delayed) in three projections (Fig. 3-1). Normally perfused myocardium absorbs thallium-201 promptly and is visualized on the initial scan. Ischemic myocardium, beyond a fixed degree of coronary artery stenosis that cannot dilate normally, takes up the thallium-201 more slowly than areas supplied by normal vessels and is therefore only visualized on delayed images (Fig. 3-2). Hence, any areas of hypoperfusion appear on the initial scan as areas of decreased thallium uptake ("cold spots"). If these initially underperfused areas show more homogeneous uptake of the marker ("fill-in") on the delayed images, this is referred to as thallium redistribution.[33] A scan is considered positive if areas of redistribution are confirmed. These areas indicate regions of ischemic but viable myocardium at risk for infarction. Regions of persistent decreased thallium uptake on both initial and delayed images represent previously infarcted (i.e., scarred) myocardium not likely to be at jeopardy of further ischemic insult, and hence the scan is not considered positive (Fig. 3-3).

The sensitivity of the test may be enhanced by low-level exercise following dipyridamole

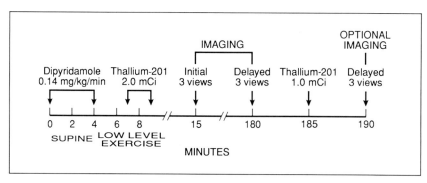

Fig. 3-1. Protocol of dipyridamole-thallium scanning. Dipyridamole is infused over a 4-minute period followed by injection of the marker, thallium-201. Initial scans are obtained at 15 minutes and delayed images at approximately 3 hours. Sensitivity may be enhanced by low-level exercise during dipyridamole administration or by a second injection of thallium followed by a third scan. (From Cutler BS. Cardiac evaluation prior to aortic surgery. In Bergan JJ, Yao JST, eds. Arterial Surgery: New Diagnostic and Operative Techniques. Orlando, Fla.: Grune & Stratton, 1988, pp 243-256.)

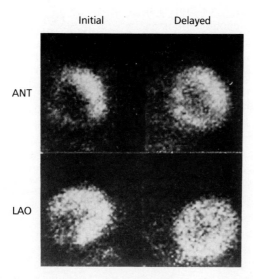

Fig. 3-2. Thallium fill-in (redistribution) on delayed scans of perfusion defect seen in both anterior *(ANT)* and left anterior oblique *(LAO)* views of initial images. This indicates a sizable area of ischemic but viable myocardium at risk of ischemic event.

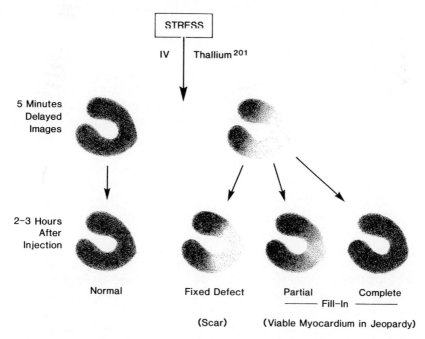

Fig. 3-3. Schematic representation of possible scan results. Homogeneous perfusion on initial scan without change on delayed images indicates normal coronary artery perfusion. A cold spot on initial scans, which does not change on later scan, indicates area of scar, whereas fill-in (redistribution) on delayed scans suggests areas of viable ischemic myocardium.

administration. Side effects of intravenous dipyridamole administration are common but rarely life threatening. Adverse reactions may be attenuated with the intravenous administration of aminophylline, which competes for adenosine receptors. Obviously patients taking aminophylline medication must discontinue its use before testing.

Numerous clinical studies have identified thallium redistribution as an especially sensitive marker for those patients likely to suffer postoperative cardiac morbidity or mortality.[13,17,33-36] The finding of thallium redistribution identifies patients with a 30% to 50% risk of suffering a postoperative cardiac event. However, the dipyridamole-thallium test specificity is low, resulting in a positive predictive value (for suffering a postoperative cardiac event) of 22%.[12] This low specificity results in part from thallium redistribution occurring in the face of coronary stenoses in the 40% to 60% range, which is a degree of stenosis that may not result in any significant postoperative MI.[35,37] Thus, although a negative dipyridamole-thallium study identifies a patient with very low cardiac risk, the implication of a positive study is more difficult to define for a particular individual.

Clinical studies from the Massachusetts General Hospital by Eagle et al.[17] report that the specificity of thallium redistribution for predicting postoperative cardiac ischemic events can be significantly increased by combining the thallium scan results with five clinical markers. The clinical markers are advanced age (over 70 years), history of angina, presence of Q wave on the ECG, insulin-dependent diabetes, and history of ventricular ectopic activity requiring treatment (see box). The study categorized patients into three risk groups based on the presence of the clinical markers. The low-risk group consisted of patients with no clinical markers. The presence of one or two markers placed the patient in the intermediate-risk group, and the presence of three or more markers defined the high-risk category. As illustrated in Fig. 3-4, the study found that the risk of a cardiac ischemic event (acute ischemic pulmonary edema, unstable angina, MI, cardiac death) in the low-risk group is so small (3% events, no deaths) that thallium scanning is

---

CLINICAL PREDICTORS OF POSTOPERATIVE CARDIAC ISCHEMIC EVENTS*†

Q waves on electrocardiogram
History of angina
History of ventricular ectopic activity
    requiring treatment
Diabetes requiring other than dietary therapy
Advanced age (>70 years)

---

*From Eagle KA, Coley CM, Newell JB, et al. Combining clinical and thallium data optimizes preoperative assessment of cardiac risk before major vascular surgery. Ann Intern Med 110:859-866, 1989.
†Cardiac ischemic events include cardiac death, acute MI, ischemic pulmonary edema, or unstable angina.

---

probably not warranted in such patients. Similarly, thallium scanning may not be helpful or indicated in the high-risk group since the cardiac ischemic event rate (50%) is so high that scan results would not improve the risk prediction nor alter the preoperative workup or management. Such patients may often be better managed by having cardiac catheterization and coronary angiography, or considering alternative surgical approaches or even deferral of surgery if it is not mandatory. However, in the moderate-risk group the scan is most useful since a negative dipyridamole-thallium scan predicts a perioperative ischemic risk similar to that in the low-risk group (3%), whereas a positive scan indicates a 30% risk and suggests the advisability of more detailed preoperative assessment. Eagle et al.[17] concluded that by combining the five clinical markers with dipyridamole-thallium scanning, the specificity of the scan result for predicting a perioperative cardiac ischemic event was increased from 66% to 81%. The Massachusetts General Hospital group further concluded that if this protocol were used, less than half of the peripheral vascular surgery patients would require dipyridamole-thallium testing and less than one third of those patients would require further evaluation with coronary angiography.[17] This method of assessment seems to have widespread applicability to the vascular surgery pa-

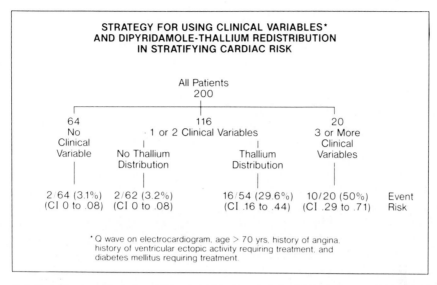

Fig. 3-4. Stratification of cardiac risk by combination of clinical risk markers and dipyridamole-thallium scanning. Event refers to postoperative cardiac ischemic events, including unstable angina. *CI*, cardiac index. (From Eagle KA, Coley CM, Newell JB, et al. Combining clinical and thallium data optimizes preoperative assessment of cardiac risk before major vascular surgery. Ann Intern Med 110:859-866, 1989.)

tient population. It does not require exercise and is not influenced by medications that limit the heart rate or ST-segment response to exercise. It is minimally invasive, is relatively risk-free, can be performed on an outpatient basis, and has sufficient sensitivity to reliably detect the presence of disease. If applied only in those patients with positive clinical markers, it is likely to be quite cost effective since only the relatively small subset of patients with positive clinical risk factors *and* a positive scan needs further evaluation.

Overall accuracy and reduction of interpretation difficulties encountered by many clinicians who have used the technique may hopefully be improved by further quantification of the degree of thallium redistribution, which is under current investigation. Preliminary evidence suggests that the presence of increasing numbers of ischemic segments on the thallium scan or ischemia in a number of views or in several coronary territories correlates with an increased likelihood of cardiac events.[38] As shown in Table 3-1, patients with redistribution in only one view were much less likely than patients with redistribution in two or three such

Table 3-1. Maximizing Thallium Interpretation*

Variables	Probability of cardiac events
Ischemic segments	
<3	12% ($p = .03$)
>4	38%
No. of views with ischemia	
<1	0% ($p = .005$)
>2	36%
No. of coronary territories with ischemia	
<1	13%[†] ($p = .007$)
>2	43%

*From Levinson JR, Boucher CA, Coley CM, et al. Usefulness of semiquantitative analysis of dipyridamole-thallium-201 redistribution for improving risk stratification before vascular surgery. Am J Cardiol 66:406-410, 1990.

†No patients with MI or death.

views to have an event (0% vs. 36%). In fact, no patient with redistribution in only a single view had any cardiac complications of vascular surgery in the study by Levinson et al.[38] Patients with redistribution in 3 or fewer segments were much less likely than patients with 4 or more such segments to suffer a perioperative cardiac event (12% vs. 38%). Finally, patients with thallium redistribution in only one cardiac territory were less likely than patients with redistribution in two or three territories to have an ischemic event (13% vs. 43%). Intravenous dipyridamole has just been approved by the Food and Drug Administration (FDA), which should markedly improve the availability of this test. This was previously a significant limitation to the value of this method of evaluation of CAD.

Radionuclide Ventriculography

Radionuclide ventriculography (gated blood pool scan, MUGA scan) is a noninvasive technique that provides quantitative assessment of left ventricular ejection fraction (LVEF) and qualitative evaluation of ventricular wall motion. The technique involves intravenous injection of technetium-99m pertechnetate, which labels red blood cells with radioactive technetium. Scintigraphic computer analysis of the cardiac images then allows calculation of the LVEF, and real-time study of the images permits evaluation of ventricular wall motion. A normal LVEF is 55% or greater. Abnormalities in wall motion include areas of hypokinesia, akinesia, or dyskinesia, which may represent areas of ischemia or prior infarction.

Several studies have shown that radionuclide ventriculography may be useful in preoperative cardiac risk stratification in the vascular surgery patient population.[14,39-41] A study from New York University Medical Center stratified patients undergoing aortic aneurysm surgery into three risk categories. The low-risk group had an LVEF greater than 56% and in this group no patient suffered a perioperative MI. The moderate-risk group had an LVEF ranging from 36% to 55%, and the perioperative infarction rate in this group was 20%. The high-risk group had an LVEF less than 35% and an 80% incidence of MI.[39] A University of Washington study reported that an LVEF less than 35% was

predictive of an increased risk of perioperative MI associated with carotid surgery.[42] Radionuclide ventriculography, with an LVEF value of 35%, has a specificity of 94%, with a positive predictive value of 52% for perioperative MI. However, the test lacks sensitivity (44%), that is, a normal test does not eliminate the risk of perioperative MI.[43] This is hardly surprising, as the finding of a normal ejection fraction is no assurance that the patient does not have severe CAD and is not at risk for a perioperative cardiac ischemic event. The prognostic value of the test may be increased by combining exercise testing with such functional measurements of left ventricular performance. A decrease in the LVEF or an increase in wall motion abnormalities following exercise is indicative of regional hypoperfusion caused by CAD and has been shown to correlate with the risk of infarction.[44,45] In addition to CAD, this response is also observed in patients with significant valvular and hypertensive heart disease.

Continuous Portable ECG Monitoring

The literature has shown that 75% to 85% of all cardiac ischemic episodes occur without any accompanying angina or anginal equivalents.[46-48] Angina pectoris occurs only after development of ventricular wall motion and ECG abnormalities. This progression may account for the sizable subset of patients in whom ECG abnormalities develop when the patient is either at rest or on the treadmill and not experiencing symptoms. Patients with diabetes or elevated pain thresholds may have considerably more ischemia before symptomatic myocardial dysfunction develops. The recognition of the frequency and significance of silent ischemia underscores the need for reliable and noninvasive methods of preoperative assessment.

Several recent reports have examined the ability of continuous portable ECG monitoring to detect silent ischemia.[49-51] When ambulatory ECG monitoring is performed, the findings of ischemia based on 2 mm or more of ST-segment depression and the presence of six or more episodes of ischemia per day are considered high-risk criteria associated with adverse outcomes. A Duke Medical Center study used continuous portable ECG monitoring to identify patients suffering "silent myocardial ischemia" to determine if the occurrence of these silent events correlated with the incidence of perioperative MI.[49] The study reported a significantly greater incidence of perioperative cardiac morbidity and mortality in patients with evidence of silent ischemia. Interestingly, the monitoring revealed that most ischemic events occurred in the postoperative rather than the preoperative or intraoperative periods. Thus the advantage of this testing modality may lie in its use for postoperative monitoring to identify silent events that might benefit from various types of pharmacologic intervention (e.g., nitrate, calcium channel blockers, β-blockers). Pasternack et al.[50] found a significant correlation between the presence of asymptomatic ischemia during preoperative monitoring and the likelihood of an untoward cardiac postoperative event in patients undergoing vascular surgery procedures. In the recent study of Raby et al.,[51] 176 consecutive patients scheduled for elective peripheral vascular surgery procedures wore a portable Holter monitor for 24 to 48 hours within 9 days of their surgery. Preoperative ischemia was detected in 32 patients (18%) for a total of 75 episodes (mean, 2.3 per patient; range, 1 to 9). Of 75 episodes, 73 (97%) were asymptomatic. The episodes lasted from 1 minute to 12 hours; the overall average duration was 36 minutes and the average duration per patient was 85 minutes. Postoperative cardiac events occurred in 13 patients, all within 48 hours of surgery. Of the 32 patients who had preoperative ischemia, 12 (38%) had postoperative events. Of 144 patients without preoperative ischemia, only one suffered an event. Thus 12 of 13 postoperative events occurred in patients who had preoperative ischemia detected by ambulatory monitoring.[51]

It is noteworthy, however, that 10% of patients originally selected for inclusion in the study were taking digoxin or had baseline ECG abnormalities that precluded monitoring because of interpretational difficulties. This problem was also encountered by McCann and Clements[49] and Pasternack et al.[50] In addition, false-positive ST-segment shifts have been noted by some investigators, clouding cost-benefit analysis.

Although the sensitivity of this approach is good, the results of Raby et al.[51] had a relatively poor positive predictive value: only 38% of patients demonstrating ischemia suffered a postoperative ischemic event. Nonetheless, this method of assessment is a relatively simple, available, and fairly inexpensive method of evaluation. Further experience with this and dipyridamole-thallium scanning will be of major importance.[52]

Transcutaneous Aortic Velocimetry

Transcutaneous aortic velocimetry (TAV) is a noninvasive technique that can be used to assess exercise-related cardiac stroke volume changes, abnormalities of which correlate with CAD. The technique of TAV uses a 2 MHz continuous-wave Doppler to transcutaneously measure flow velocities in the aorta. The flow velocities are calculated from the Doppler frequency shift data using fast Fourier transform and are displayed as a spectral waveform on a monitor. The area under the spectral waveform is directly proportional to the stroke volume. The normal response to exercise is an increase in stroke volume of 5%. Abnormal results correlate with an LVEF less than 60% and are indicative of CAD.[53] Further studies are required to assess the application of TAV as a predictor of perioperative cardiac events in vascular surgery patients.

VALVULAR HEART DISEASE

Valvular heart disease significantly increases the risk of vascular surgery procedures. Studies by Goldman and associates[20,21] reported a 20% incidence of postoperative congestive heart failure in patients with valvular heart disease. In the presence of aortic valvular stenosis, there is a 10% mortality rate for extracavitary operations and a 20% mortality rate for thoracic or abdominal procedures.[54] The presence of significant aortic valvular stenosis may be suspected on the basis of the patient's clinical history, physical examination, and abnormalities on the ECG and/or chest x-ray film. Symptoms of congestive heart failure, angina, or syncope in a patient with a murmur of aortic valvular stenosis are indications for cardiac catheterization as part of the preoperative evaluation for vascular surgery. Cardiac catheterization allows measurement of any pressure gradient across the aortic valve. An aortic gradient of 35 to 40 mm Hg confirms hemodynamically significant aortic valvular stenosis. In this setting patients should undergo aortic valve replacement before undergoing any elective vascular surgery procedure.[55]

Mitral valve stenosis represents a significant risk because any fall in left atrial filling pressure can produce deleterious effects on cardiac output. Very close monitoring of the fluid status in the perioperative period using Swan-Ganz monitoring is required to prevent hypovolemia. The importance of any existing mitral valve insufficiency depends on the status of the left ventricular function. Patients with coexisting mitral valve insufficiency and poor left ventricular function should be considered for mitral valve replacement before any vascular surgery is performed.

CARDIAC RISK MANAGEMENT— AN OVERVIEW

Either of two extreme positions might be taken in response to the clinical dilemma of identifying significant CAD in the perioperative vascular surgery patient. On the one hand, it could be argued that significant CAD is so prevalent in patients with overt vascular disease in other arterial beds (approximately 30%) that all such patients should be evaluated regardless of whether they have clinical symptoms of cardiac disease or ECG abnormalities. Conversely, some authorities maintain that current perioperative anesthesia and monitoring are so good and corresponding cardiac morbidity and mortality so low that screening studies have little value. As usual, the truth probably lies somewhere in between, and a simplistic all-or-none approach is not reasonable.

Currently, there is fairly uniform agreement that it is too hazardous and expensive to perform coronary angiography on all preoperative patients. Similarly, it is not cost effective to employ various noninvasive tests to assess cardiac risk in all patients. Some systematic approach that relies on selective application of one or more simple and reliable screening tests is optimal. The best approach needs to take into consideration the type of surgery, the clinical likelihood of a perioperative cardiac event, knowledge about the relative usefulness of various tests, and the therapeutic options available in management.[52]

The most important harbinger of perioperative cardiac ischemic complications is the number and location of diseased coronary arteries and the status of left ventricular function. The various methods of cardiac risk assessment should be used, along with thoughtful evaluation of clinical risk factors, to stratify patients according to their risk of having severe two- or three-vessel and/or left main disease, with or without significant left ventricular dysfunction. Those patients identified as high risk should be considered for further evaluation with coronary angiography if they are potential candidates for revascularization. In addition, it may be advisable in patients with severe CAD to consider modification of the planned vascular surgery procedure and/or utilization of specific perioperative hemodynamic monitoring and pharmacologic interventions during the following operation designed to minimize cardiovascular physiologic disturbances.

At present, available data appear to support the appropriateness of proceeding with the indicated vascular operation without further cardiac assessment in patients without a positive clinical history or ECG abnormality (absence of clinical markers). Experience suggests this is both safe and cost effective.[17,18,56] Conversely, patients with three or more clinical markers and obviously at high risk should probably undergo coronary angiography at the outset, provided they would be reasonable candidates for coronary revascularization if severe CAD were confirmed. The various screening studies described appear most useful in patients between these two extremes, in whom risk is much more difficult to determine at the bedside.

To stratify risk in this cohort of patients and identify those who may be best served by further, more intensive preoperative evaluation and/or coronary revascularization, use of exercise-stress testing is probably the most available and well-studied approach. For the sizable number of patients with vascular disease who cannot exercise adequately, however, use of dipyridamole-thallium scanning would appear the best strategy. Further experience with portable ECG monitoring may also confirm that this is a reasonable alternative. If such tests indicate a low probability of a perioperative ischemic event, the surgeon can confidently proceed with the indicated vascular surgery procedure.

If the presence of significant CAD is confirmed, several management options exist. Modification of the planned operation may be considered, or operation may be avoided entirely. For instance, operation might be deferred in a claudicant in whom the relief of claudication symptoms might only unmask underlying CAD or in whom the risk of operation is significantly increased or the patient's life expectancy significantly decreased. Similar logic could be applied to the management of the patient with a small aortic aneurysm or severe but asymptomatic carotid stenosis. Or the surgeon might elect a "lower risk" procedure if circumstances allowed and a more pressing need for arterial reconstruction were present. Such options are most often available in the management of patients with aortoiliac disease. For example, one might recommend axillobifemoral grafting instead of aortobifemoral operation for limb salvage, consider iliac percutaneous transluminal angioplasty (PTA) more seriously, or combine iliac PTA on one side to allow a femorofemoral extra-anatomic procedure for the other leg.[15,57] Similarly, for infrainguinal disease, one could consider performing a required femoropopliteal bypass graft using PTFE rather than vein to reduce operative time and complexity and save the vein for potential coronary bypass.

Preliminary coronary artery bypass grafting (CABG) clearly reduces the risk of perioperative MI events in patients undergoing subsequent vascular surgery procedures and improves their survival.[1,24,58-60] On the basis of these observations, a number of researchers have recommended preliminary (prophylactic) coronary artery surgery before a major vascular operation for patients with severe associated CAD.[11,61,62] Although long-term survival seems improved by this approach, preliminary CABG remains controversial since the early mortality

of the combined cardiac and vascular surgery procedures often exceeds that of the vascular operation alone.[25,27,63] Unfortunately, patients with peripheral vascular disease are often also at high risk for CABG because of factors such as advanced age, severe multivessel disease, reduced left ventricular function, or diabetes.[64] The operative mortality for CABG in these patients probably exceeds 5%.[8] Therefore in some patients the short-term risk of cardiac catheterization and coronary revascularization may actually exceed the risk reduction hoped to be achieved by successful coronary surgery.[56] The Cleveland Clinic experience suggests that among vascular surgery patients nondiabetic men derived the greatest benefit from CABG.[65] Analysis of data therefore suggests that CABG immediately before an elective vascular operation should be considered only in those patients who are excellent candidates for such cardiac surgery. The role of PTCA in this setting has yet to be determined. Although appealing in concept, most patients in the high-risk category have diffuse three-vessel disease, which is poorly suited to treatment by PTCA. In addition, the restenosis rate is acknowledged to be significant (approximately 30% to 40% at 6-month follow-up). At present, insufficient data and experience exist to firmly establish the application of PTCA in the preoperative vascular surgery patient.

In the patient with severe CAD who absolutely needs a specific vascular operation that cannot be modified by a lesser procedure (e.g., carotid endarterectomy for symptomatic lesion, lower extremity revascularization for rest pain or tissue necrosis, aortic aneurysm repair for large or symptomatic aneurysm) but who is not a good candidate for preliminary CABG or whose coronary anatomy is not considered amenable to bypass, the surgeon may have little choice but to proceed with operation with intensive hemodynamic monitoring. Appropriate anesthetic management requires invasive monitoring of those physiologic parameters that are related to the balance of myocardial oxygen supply and demand. A variety of modalities are available for monitoring the patient's cardiovascular status during and after surgery. These monitoring techniques include intra-arterial blood pressure monitoring; ECG monitoring of limb and a precordial lead; pulmonary artery pressure (Swan-Ganz) catheter monitoring of the pulmonary capillary wedge pressure (PCWP), cardiac output, systemic vascular resistance, and mixed venous oxygen saturation; and periodic measurement of core temperature.

Several studies have shown the efficacy of using pulmonary artery catheter pressure monitoring to preoperatively assess and optimize ventricular function. These studies examined the effects of sequential intravenous fluid challenges on cardiac output and related these data to the simultaneous PCWP measurements, thus determining what PCWP correlated with the best cardiac output. The results can then be used to direct intraoperative fluid management.[66,67]

One of the primary functions of the various monitoring techniques is to detect myocardial ischemia and thus direct therapeutic interventions to correct the ischemia before infarction occurs. However, studies have shown that standard ECG and PCWP measurements may be inadequate to detect early ischemic events. Several investigators have shown that the technique of *transesophageal echocardiography* can detect myocardial dysfunction subtle enough not to be detected by standard monitoring techniques.[68,69]

The technique of transesophageal echocardiographic monitoring involves the placement of a cardiac ultrasonic transducer in the esophagus positioned at the level of the left ventricle. The cardiac ultrasound then provides a real-time two-dimensional image of the ventricle. Segmental cardiac wall motion abnormalities can be detected and have been shown to be early signs of ischemia. The wall motion abnormalities can be detected even while the ECG and PCWP are still normal.[70] In addition to revealing regional wall motion abnormalities, transesophageal echocardiography can be used to assess volume status by visualizing the ventricle cavity size. Continuous monitoring of the real-time image can be used to direct intraoperative fluid management and specific pharmacologic therapy to modify MI episodes, such as administration of intravenous nitroglycerin, use

of nitroprusside at the time of aortic cross-clamping, use of vasopressors at the time of aortic unclamping, or use of intravenous β-blockers if segmental wall motion abnormalities seem to be caused by tachycardia. The increased sensitivity of this form of monitoring will allow earlier recognition of MI and more precise regulation of the therapeutic interventions, which should result in a decreased complication rate.[71]

The perioperative monitoring techniques discussed above should be used to direct specific pharmacologic interventions to prevent or treat myocardial ischemia. The goal of pharmacologic therapy is to increase myocardial blood flow and decrease myocardial oxygen demand. Increased myocardial perfusion can be obtained by inducing coronary artery dilatation, reducing left ventricular end-diastolic pressure, and prolonging diastole by reducing the heart rate. Decreased myocardial oxygen demand results from decreasing the heart rate, systolic blood pressure, cardiac contractility, and left ventricular dimension. Intravenous nitroglycerin augments coronary vasodilatation and decreases preload by causing venodilatation and thus lower venous return. This reduces ventricular wall tension and thus reduces oxygen demand. The reduction in left ventricular end-diastolic pressure also enhances subendocardial perfusion. Nitrates also result in coronary artery vasodilatation, thus increasing myocardial perfusion. Several studies have reported reduced incidence of perioperative myocardial ischemia and/or infarction with the use of routine intravenous nitroglycerin.[72]

β-blockers reduce the heart rate and decrease the cardiac contractility, thereby increasing myocardial perfusion and decreasing oxygen demand. Several studies have shown that β-blockers reduce infarct size and mortality when administered early during acute MI.[73] Studies have also shown a decrease in perioperative ischemic events and MIs that correlated with perioperative β-blocker therapy.[74,75]

At many centers epidural anesthesia is being employed more frequently, often in conjunction with a general anesthetic, for patients undergoing aortic surgery. Although it is the impression of many that epidural anesthesia offers significant overall advantages in the high-risk cardiac patient, this practice remains somewhat controversial and not firmly established. Many of the studies relevant to the benefit of epidural anesthesia have focused on its role in terms of reduced pulmonary function impairment and postoperative pain relief. A randomized study by Yeager et al.[76] of epidural anesthesia/analgesia in 53 high-risk surgical patients noted a significant reduction in postoperative complications, a reduced stress response, and a significantly lower incidence of postoperative cardiac failure. Another recent prospective study comparing use of combined epidural and light general anesthesia (n = 30) and general anesthesia alone (n = 19) in patients undergoing infrarenal abdominal aortic surgery was reported by Her et al.[77] Their results indicated that combined epidural/general anesthesia is associated with more stable intraoperative hemodynamics and significantly lower postoperative morbidity than general anesthesia alone. After cross-clamping of the aorta, cardiac index and PCWP did not change in the combined technique group, whereas cardiac index decreased and PCWP increased in the general anesthesia group. After unclamping, cardiac index increased in both groups. Postoperatively, the need for ventilatory support, incidence of respiratory failure, and duration of ICU stay were reduced in the combined technique group. All differences were statistically significant. Although these data and other similar reports are encouraging, it should be pointed out that no prospective randomized study comparing epidural anesthesia to general anesthesia has demonstrated any difference in their effect on the incidence of MI or cardiac death.[12]

In rare circumstances when severe unstable CAD exists but revascularization by CABG or PTCA is not feasible for whatever reason, cardiac risk may be reduced with counterpulsation using an intra-aortic balloon pump inserted just before the vascular operation and maintained during the perioperative period.[78,79] Similarly, in some patients with both unstable vascular problems and advanced CAD, the two procedures may need to be done simultaneously. This is by far most often considered in the patient with symptomatic carotid disease and unstable CAD.[80,81] Myocardial revascularization combined with aneurysm repair has also been reported in a few instances.[62,82,83]

PULMONARY COMPLICATIONS

Risk factors for pulmonary complications include advanced age, obesity, chronic obstructive pulmonary disease (COPD), cigarette smoking, type of surgical procedure and technique, and duration of anesthesia.[84] Pulmonary complications are not unique to vascular surgery procedures. However, because of the high incidence of cigarette smoking and COPD in the atherosclerotic population and the frequent extensive nature of major vascular surgery procedures, vascular surgery patients are often at increased risk for pulmonary complications.

Preoperative Pulmonary Risk Assessment

A detailed history and physical examination are invaluable in identifying patients with significant pulmonary disease. Although the degree of dyspnea on exertion may be an indicator of significant pulmonary insufficiency, many of these patients have sedentary lifestyles, thus potentially limiting the usefulness of this historical information. It is most important to ascertain any history of cigarette abuse. Cigarette smoking, especially in patients with a history of >20 pack years, is associated with increased postoperative atelectasis and pneumonia, even in the absence of any detectable lung disease.[85,86] Physical examination should detect hypoventilation in weak or debilitated patients, and wheezing, rhonchi, and hyperinflation in patients with COPD. The quantity and nature of sputum production may provide a sense of the chronicity and severity of lung disease and allow distinction between chronic bronchitis and emphysema. Routine anteroposterior and lateral chest x-ray films may contribute to impressions gained from patient history and physical examination.

If the clinical findings suggest that a patient is at increased pulmonary risk, pulmonary function tests (PFTs) are often useful in directing further management. Spirometry (Fig. 3-5) provides important information regarding lung volumes and flow rates, whereas arterial blood gas determination of room-air Pa_{O_2} and Pa_{CO_2}

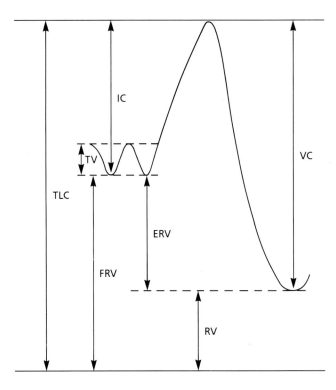

Fig. 3-5. Lung volumes as measured by spirometry. *ERV*, expiratory volume; *IC*, inspiratory capacity; *FRV*, functional residual volume; *RV*, residual volume; *TLC*, total lung capacity; *TV*, tidal volume; *VC*, vital capacity.

Table 3-2. Preoperative Pulmonary Assessment*

	Normal	**High Risk**
Vital capacity	30-50 cc/kg; >80% predicted	<30%-50%
Forced expiratory volume, 1 second (FEV$_1$)	>80% predicted	<40%-50%
Maximal midexpiratory flow (FEF$_{25\%-75\%}$)	150-200 L/min; >80% predicted	<35%-50%
Maximal voluntary ventilation	150-500 L/min; >80% predicted	<35%-50%
Pao$_2$, room air	85 ± 5 mm Hg	<50-55 mm Hg
Paco$_2$, room air	40 ± 4 mm Hg	>45-55 mm Hg

*From Stanley JC, Wakefield TW. Cardiopulmonary assessment for major vascular reconstructive procedures. In Haimovici H, ed. Vascular Surgery: Principles and Techniques, 3rd ed. Norwalk, Conn.: Appleton & Lange, 1989, pp 195-203.

indicates the current status of compensation. In COPD (emphysema, bronchitis) the forced expiratory volume in 1 second (FEV$_1$) and the ratio of the FEV$_1$ to the forced vital capacity are the most important components of PFTs. An FEV$_1$ greater than 2 L is not associated with an increased risk. An FEV$_1$ less than 2 L but greater than 1 L is associated with a moderate risk, whereas an FEV$_1$ less than 800 cc is associated with very high risk of postoperative pulmonary failure[87-89] (Table 3-2). In addition to these abnormal flow rates, arterial blood gas analysis revealing evidence of CO$_2$ retention (hypercarbia) in the COPD patient places that patient at markedly increased risk.[90]

Perioperative Risk Management

Vascular surgery procedures on the thoracic or abdominal aorta require the use of thoracotomy or laparotomy incisions. These incisions alter chest wall and diaphragmatic mechanical function, and postoperative incisional pain causes splinting, which produces hypoventilation. This splinting results in decreased tidal volume and functional residual capacity. The splinting also prevents the patient from coughing effectively and from taking deep breaths. The cumulative effects of these mechanical problems is small airway closure (microatelectasis) resulting from the decreased functional residual capacity and bronchial occlusion and regional atelectasis (macroatelectasis) from poor pulmonary toilet.[91]

In addition to the effects of the surgery, anesthesia itself has adverse effects on ventilatory mechanics. General anesthesia alters the mechanical properties of the chest wall and the lungs. The anesthetics used decrease bronchial ciliary mucus transport. Mechanical ventilation uses positive pressure, which fails to adequately ventilate the dependent portions of the lungs where the airways are the smallest and are the least compliant, leading to further atelectasis.

When preoperative clinical and laboratory evaluation identifies a patient with significant risk of postoperative pulmonary complications, modifications in management are often necessary, and usually additional preoperative pulmonary preparation and careful attention to postoperative pulmonary mechanics are required. Cessation of smoking well in advance of an elective surgical procedure is helpful, if possible. For patients with COPD, asthma, or chronic bronchitis, respiratory flow measurements should be obtained before and after the use of bronchodilators. Intensive preoperative preparation of the patient with nebulized bronchodilators until pulmonary status is improved as determined by spirometric measurements is frequently helpful. Both theophyllines and steroids may be administered to patients with significant reversible obstructive defects. Such measures, together with vigorous chest physiotherapy, respiratory exercises, humidified air, and often a course of broad-spectrum antibiotics, can reduce the postoperative complication rate in patients with COPD by more than half.[92]

In addition, avoidance of conventional abdominal incisions may be helpful in minimizing pulmonary function disturbance in the high-risk patient. As already described for the high-risk cardiac patient, this may be possible by modifying the revascularization technique employed by the surgeon if anatomy and the nature of the problem allow (e.g., substitution of extra-anatomic grafts vs. direct aortic reconstruction, increased consideration of PTA). If direct aortic surgery is unavoidable, a retroperitoneal approach may be used. This is believed by many to have fewer adverse effects on pulmonary mechanics and a lower incidence of pulmonary complications than a conventional midline transabdominal approach,[93,94] although our own prospective randomized study did not reveal statistically significant differences in this regard.[95] Without question, use of epidural anesthetic technique, either as the sole means of anesthesia for infrainguinal surgery or as a combined epidural/light general anesthesia technique for abdominal vascular surgery, is helpful in minimizing pulmonary problems postoperatively, principally by continued use for postoperative analgesia following operation.[76,77,96,97] Epidural narcotics and local anesthetics postoperatively provide both analgesia and muscle relaxation, thereby avoiding large doses of systemic narcotics and paralyzing agents and reducing the incidence of postoperative hypoventilation and muscle splinting. This currently allows extubation in the operating room in approximately 90% of our patients undergoing aortic operation and appears to be a major factor in reducing postoperative complications and lessening the need for prolonged mechanical ventilatory support.[95] Therefore pulmonary insufficiency is rarely a major contraindication to indicated vascular surgery procedures in current practice.

In those patients who do require postoperative mechanical ventilation, aggressive pulmonary toilet can reduce the incidence of atelectasis and pneumonia. The techniques involved include frequent position changes of the patient to prevent atelectasis in the dependent portions of the lungs, endotracheal suctioning as needed for clearance of secretions, and the use of positive end-expiratory pressure (PEEP) on the ventilator. PEEP is used to reduce the small-airway collapse that occurs with positive pressure ventilation. Rapid ventilator weaning using intermittent mechanical ventilation mode will prevent ventilator dependence in COPD patients.

CONCLUSION

The typical vascular surgery patient presents at surgery following a lifetime of cigarette smoking, which has usually resulted in the systemic disease process of atherosclerosis, including CAD, and pulmonary disease of varying severity. The prevalence of cardiopulmonary disease in this population places these patients at increased risk for postoperative complications related to these disorders. A dedicated approach to the preoperative evaluation of the patient will stratify patients according to their risk, thus identifying those patients who will benefit from an alternative surgical approach, changes in management strategies, and/or special perioperative monitoring techniques that may reduce the incidence of cardiopulmonary complications in this patient population.

REFERENCES

1. Jamieson WR, Janusz MT, Miyagishima RT, Gerein AN. Influence of ischemic heart disease on early and late mortality after surgery for peripheral occlusive vascular disease. Circulation 66(Suppl I):I92-I97, 1982.
2. Crawford ES, Bomberger RA, Glaeser DH, Saleh SA, Russell WL. Aortoiliac occlusive disease: Factors influencing survival and function following reconstructive operation over a twenty-five year period. Surgery 90:1055-1067, 1981.
3. Cooperman M, Pflug B, Martin EW Jr, Evans WE. Cardiovascular risk factors in patients with peripheral vascular disease. Surgery 84:505-509, 1978.
4. Hertzer NR, Avellone JC, Farrell CJ, et al. The risk of vascular surgery in a metropolitan community, with observations on surgeon experience and hospital size. J Vasc Surg 1:13-21, 1984.
5. Hertzer NR. Fatal myocardial infarction following lower extremity revascularization. Ann Surg 193: 492-498, 1981.
6. Hertzer NR. Fatal myocardial infarction following abdominal aortic aneurysm resection. Ann Surg 192:667-673, 1980.
7. Mangano DT. Preoperative assessment. In Kaplan JA, ed. Cardiac Anesthesia, vol. 1, 2nd ed. Orlando, Fla.: Grune & Stratton, 1987, pp 341-392.
8. Hertzer NR, Beven EG, Young JR, et al. Coronary artery disease in peripheral vascular patients. A classification of 1000 coronary angiograms and results of surgical management. Ann Surg 199:223-233, 1984.
9. Hertzer NR. Clinical experience with preoperative coronary angiography. J Vasc Surg 2:510-514, 1985.
10. Yeager RA, Weigel RM, Murphy ES, McConnell DB, Sasaki TM, Vetto RM. Application of clinically valid risk factors to aortic aneurysm surgery. Arch Surg 121:278-281, 1986.
11. Blombery PA, Ferguson IA, Rosengarten DS, Stuchbery KE, Miles CR, Black AJ, Pitt A, Anderson ST, Harper RW, Federman J. The role of coronary artery disease in complications of abdominal aortic aneurysm surgery. Surgery 101:150-155, 1987.
12. Yeager RA, Moneta GL. Assessing cardiac risk in vascular surgical patients: Current status. Perspect Vasc Surg 2:18-39, 1989.
13. Leppo J, Plaja J, Gionet M, Tumolo J, Paraskos JA, Cutler BS. Noninvasive evaluation of cardiac risk before elective vascular surgery. J Am Coll Cardiol 9:269-276, 1987.
14. Pasternack PF, Imparato AM, Riles TS, Baumann FG, Bear G, Lamparello PJ, Benjamin D, Sanger J, Kramer E. The value of the radionuclide angiogram in the prediction of perioperative myocardial infarction in patients undergoing lower extremity revascularization procedures. Circulation 72(Suppl II):II13-II17, 1985.
15. Cutler BS. Cardiac evaluation prior to aortic surgery. In Bergan JJ, Yao JST, eds. Arterial Surgery: New Diagnostic and Operative Techniques. Orlando, Fla.: Grune & Stratton, 1988, pp 243-256.
16. Calvin JE, Kieser TM, Walley VM, McPhail NV, Barber GG, Scobie TK. Cardiac mortality and morbidity after vascular surgery. Can J Surg 29:93-97, 1986.
17. Eagle KA, Coley CM, Newell JB, Brewster DC, Darling RC, Strauss HW, Guiney TE, Boucher CA. Combining clinical and thallium data optimizes preoperative assessment of cardiac risk before major vascular surgery. Ann Intern Med 110:859-866, 1989.
18. Golden MA, Whittemore AD, Donaldson MC, Mannick JA. Selective evaluation and management of coronary artery disease in patients undergoing repair of abdominal aortic aneurysms: A 16-year experience. Ann Surg 212:415-423, 1990.
19. McPhail N, Menkis A, Shariatmadar A, Calvin J, Barber G, Scobie K, White P. Statistical prediction of cardiac risk in patients who undergo vascular surgery. Can J Surg 28:404-406, 1985.
20. Goldman L, Caldera DL, Nussbaum SR, Southwick FS, Krogstad D, Murray B, Burke DS, O'Malley TA, Goroll AH, Caplan CH, Nolan J, Carabello B, Slater EE. Multifactorial index of cardiac risk in noncardiac surgical procedures. N. Engl J Med 297:845-850, 1977.
21. Goldman L. Cardiac risks and complications of noncardiac surgery. Ann Intern Med 98:504-513, 1983.
22. Detsky AS, Abrams HB, McLaughlin JR, Drucker DJ, Sasson Z, Johnston N, Scott JG, Forbath N, Hilliard JR. Predicting cardiac complications in patients undergoing noncardiac surgery. J Gen Intern Med 1:211-219, 1986.

23. Jeffrey CC, Junsman J, Cullen DJ, Brewster DC. A prospective evaluation of cardiac risk index. Anesthesiology 58:462-464, 1983.

24. Hertzer NR, Young JR, Beven EG, O'Hara PJ, Graor RA, Ruschhaupt WG, Maljovec LC. Late results of coronary bypass in patients with peripheral vascular disease. I. Five-year survival according to age and clinical cardiac status. Cleve Clin Q 53:133-143, 1986.

25. Brown OW, Hollier LH, Pairolero PC, Kazmier FJ, McCready RA. Abdominal aortic aneurysms and coronary artery disease: A reassessment. Arch Surg 116:1484-1487, 1981.

26. Brewster DC, Okada RD, Strauss HW, Abbott WM, Darling RC, Boucher CA. Selection of patients for preoperative coronary angiography: Use of dipyridamole-stress thallium myocardial imaging. J Vasc Surg 2:504-510, 1985.

27. Reigel MM, Hollier LH, Kazmier FJ, O'Brien PC, Pairolero PC, Cherry KJ Jr, Hallett JW Jr. Late survival in abdominal aortic aneurysm patients: The role of selective myocardial revascularization on the basis of clinical symptoms. J Vasc Surg 5:222-227, 1987.

28. Cutler BS, Wheeler HB, Paraskos JA, Cardullo PA. Applicability and interpretation of electrocardiographic stress testing in patients with peripheral vascular disease. Am J Surg 141:501-506, 1981.

29. Arous EJ, Baum PL, Cutler BS. The ischemic exercise test in patients with peripheral vascular disease. Arch Surg 119:280-283, 1984.

30. Gage AA, Bhayana JN, Balu V. Assessment of cardiac risk in surgical patients. Arch Surg 112:1488-1492, 1977.

31. McPhail N, Calvin JE, Shariatmadar A, Barber GG, Scobie TK. The use of preoperative exercise testing to predict cardiac complications after arterial reconstruction. J Vasc Surg 7:60-68, 1988.

32. Shub C. Stable angina pectoris: 2. Cardiac evaluation and diagnostic testing. Mayo Clin Proc 65:243-255, 1990.

33. Boucher CA, Brewster DC, Darling RC, Okada RD, Strauss HW, Pohost GM. Determination of cardiac risk by dipyridamole-thallium imaging before peripheral vascular surgery. N Engl J Med 312:389-394, 1985.

34. Cutler BS, Leppo JA. Dipyridamole thallium 201 scintigraphy to detect coronary artery disease before abdominal aortic surgery. J Vasc Surg 5:91-100, 1987.

35. Eagle KA, Singer DE, Brewster DC, Darling RC, Mulley AG, Boucher CA. Dipyridamole-thallium scanning in patients undergoing vascular surgery. Optimizing preoperative evaluation of cardiac risk. JAMA 257:2185-2189, 1987.

36. McPhail NV, Ruddy TD, Calvin JE, Davies RA, Barber GG. A comparison of dipyridamole-thallium imaging and exercise testing in the prediction of postoperative cardiac complications in patients requiring arterial reconstruction. J Vasc Surg 10:51-56, 1989.

37. Josephson MA, Brown BG, Hecht HS, et al. Noninvasive detection and localization of coronary stenoses in patients: Comparison of resting dipyridamole and exercise thallium-201 myocardial perfusion imaging. Am Heart J 103:1008-1018, 1982.

38. Levinson JR, Boucher CA, Coley CM, Guiney TE, Strauss HW, Eagle KA. Usefulness of semiquantitative analysis of dipyridamole-thallium-201 redistribution for improving risk stratification before vascular surgery. Am J Cardiol 66:406-410, 1990.

39. Pasternack PF, Imparato AM, Bear G, Riles TS, Baumann FG, Benjamin D, Sanger J, Kramer E, Wood RP. The value of radionuclide angiography as a predictor of perioperative myocardial infarction in patients undergoing abdominal aortic aneurysm resection. J Vasc Surg 1:320-325, 1984.

40. Jones RH, Douglas JM Jr, Reryeh SK, Newman GE, Sabiston DC Jr. Noninvasive radionuclide assessment of cardiac function in patients with peripheral vascular disease. Surgery 185:59-70, 1979.

41. Foster ED, Davis KB, Carpenter JR, et al. Risk of noncardiac operation in patients with defined coronary disease: The coronary artery surgery study (CASS) registry experience. Ann Thorac Surg 41:42-50, 1986.

42. Kazmers A, Cerqueira MD, Zierler RE. The role of preoperative radionuclide left ventricular ejection fraction for risk assessment in carotid surgery. Arch Surg 123:416-419, 1988.

43. Yeager RA. Basic data related to cardiac testing and cardiac risk associated with vascular surgery. Ann Vasc Surg 4:193-197, 1990.

44. Beller GA, Gibson RS. Sensitivity, specificity, and prognostic significance of noninvasive testing for occult or known coronary artery disease. Prog Cardiovasc Dis 29:241-270, 1987.

45. Cheitlin MD. Finding the high-risk patient with coronary artery disease. JAMA 259:2271-2277, 1988.

46. Epstein SE, Quyyumi AA, Bonow RO. Myocardial ischemia—Silent or symptomatic. N Engl J Med 318:1038-1043, 1988.

47. Gottlieb SO, Weisfeldt ML, Ouyang P, et al. Silent ischemia as a marker for unfavorable outcomes in patients with unstable angina. N Engl J Med 314:1214-1219, 1986.

48. Rocco MB, Nabel EG, Campbell S, et al. Prognostic importance of myocardial ischemia detected by ambulatory monitoring in patients with stable coronary artery disease. Circulation 78:877-884, 1988.

49. McCann RL, Clements FM. Silent myocardial ischemia in patients undergoing peripheral vascular surgery: Incidence and association with perioperative cardiac morbidity and mortality. J Vasc Surg 9:583-587, 1989.

50. Pasternack PR, Grossi EA, Baumann FG, et al. The value of silent myocardial ischemia monitoring in the prediction of postoperative myocardial infarction in patients undergoing peripheral vascular surgery. J Vasc Surg 10:617-625, 1989.

51. Raby KE, Goldman L, Creager MA, Cook EF, Weisberg MC, Whittemore AD, Selwyn AP. Correlation between preoperative ischemia and major cardiac events after peripheral vascular surgery. N Engl J Med 321:1296-1300, 1989.

52. Eagle KA, Boucher CA. Cardiac risk of non-cardiac surgery [editorial]. N Engl J Med 321:1330-1332, 1989.

53. Nicolaides AN. The diagnosis and assessment of coronary artery disease in vascular patients. J Vasc Surg 2:501-504, 1985.

54. Skinner JR, Pearce ML. Surgical risk in the cardiac patient. J Chronic Dis 17:57, 1964.

55. Hirshfeld JW Jr. Surgery in the patient with valvular heart disease. In Goldman DR, Brown FH, Levy WK, et al., eds. Medical Care of the Surgical Patient —A Problem-Oriented Approach to Management. Philadelphia: JB Lippincott, 1982, pp 99-112.

56. Coley CA, Eagle KA, Singer DE, Mulley AG, Boucher CA. Decision analysis for preoperative cardiac risk evaluation before vascular surgery. Clin Res 35:342A, 1987.

57. Brewster DC, Cambria RP, Darling RC, Geller SC, Waltman AC, Moncure AC, Athanasoulis CA, Abbott WM. Long-term results of combined iliac balloon angioplasty and distal surgical revascularization. Ann Surg 210:324-331, 1989.

58. Crawford ES, Morris GC Jr, Howell JF, Flynn WF, Moorhead DT. Operative risk in patients with previous coronary artery bypass. Ann Thorac Surg 26:215-221, 1978.

59. Edwards WH, Mulherin JL Jr, Walker WE. Vascular reconstructive surgery following myocardial revascularization. Ann Surg 187:653-657, 1978.

60. McCollum CH, Garcia-Rinaldi R, Graham JM, DeBakey ME. Myocardial revascularization prior to subsequent major surgery in patients with coronary artery disease. Surgery 81:302-304, 1977.

61. DeBakey ME, Lawrie GM. Combined coronary artery and peripheral vascular disease: Recognition and treatment. J Vasc Surg 1:605-607, 1984.

62. Reul GJ Jr, Cooley DA, Duncan JM, et al. The effect of coronary bypass on the outcome of peripheral vascular operations in 1093 patients. J Vasc Surg 3:788-798, 1986.

63. Hollier LH. Advocates in vascular controversies: The case against prophylactic coronary bypass. Surgery 96:78-87, 1984.

64. Cosgrove DM, Loop FD, Lytle BW, Baillot R, Gill CC, Golding LAR, Taylor PC, Goormastic M. Primary myocardial revascularization: Trends in surgical mortality. J Thorac Cardiovasc Surg 88:673-684, 1984.

65. Hertzer NR, Young JR, Beven EG, O'Hara PJ, Graor RA, Ruschhaupt WR, Maljovec LC. Late results of coronary bypass in patients with peripheral vascular disease. II. Five-year survival according to sex, hypertension, diabetes. Clev Clin J Med 54:15-23, 1987.

66. Bush HL Jr, LoGerfo FW, Weisel RD, Mannick JA, Hechtman HB. Assessment of myocardial performance and optimal volume loading during elective abdominal aortic aneurysm resection. Arch Surg 112:1301-1306, 1977.

67. Whittemore AD, Clowes AW, Hechtman HB, Mannick JA. Aortic aneurysm repair. Reduced operative mortality associated with maintenance of optimal cardiac performance. Ann Surg 192:414-421, 1980.

68. Roizen MF, Beaupre PN, Albert RA, et al. Monitoring with two-dimensional transesophageal echocardiography. J Vasc Surg 1:300-305, 1984.

69. Smith JS, Benefiel DJ, Lurz FW, et al. Detection of intraoperative myocardial ischemia ECG vs 2-D transesophageal echocardiography. Anesthesiology 61:A158, 1984.

70. Beaupre PN, Kremer PF, Cahalan MK, et al. Intraoperative detection of changes in left ventricular segmental wall motion by transesophageal two-dimensional echocardiography. Am Heart J 107: 1021, 1984.

71. Gewertz BL, Kremser PC, Zarins CK, et al. Transesophageal echocardiographic monitoring of myocardial ischemia during vascular surgery. J Vasc Surg 5:607-613, 1987.

72. Coriat P, Daloz M, Bousseau D, Fusciardi J, Echter E, Viars P. Prevention of intraoperative myocardial ischemia during noncardiac surgery with intravenous nitroglycerin. Anesthesiology 61:193-196, 1984.

73. Frishman WH, Skolnick AE, Lazar EJ, Fein S. Beta-adrenergic blockade and calcium channel blockade in myocardial infarction. Med Clin North Am 73:409-436, 1989.

74. Pasternack PF, Grossi EA, Baumann FG, Riles TS, Lamparello PJ, Giangola G, Primis LK, Mintzer R, Imparato AM. Beta blockade to decrease silent myocardial ischemia during peripheral vascular surgery. Am J Surg 158:113-116, 1989.

75. Pasternack PF, Imparato AM, Baumann FG, Laub G, Riles TS, Lamparello PJ, Grossi EA, Berguson P, Becker G, Bear G. The hemodynamics of beta-blockade in patients undergoing abdominal aortic aneurysm repair. Circulation 76(Suppl III):III1-III7, 1987.

76. Yeager MP, Glass DD, Neff RK, Brinck-Johnsen T. Epidural anesthesia and analgesia in high-risk surgical patients. Anesthesiology 66:729-736, 1987.

77. Her C, Kizelshteyn G, Walker V, Hayes D, Lees DE. Combined epidural and general anesthesia for abdominal aortic surgery. J Cardiothorac Anesth 4:552-557, 1990.

78. Grotz RL, Yeston NS. Intra-aortic balloon counterpulsation in high-risk cardiac patients undergoing noncardiac surgery. Surgery 106:1-5, 1989.

79. Hollier LH, Spittell JA, Puiga RJ. Intraaortic balloon counterpulsation as an adjunct to aneurysmectomy in high-risk patients. Mayo Clin Proc 56:565-567, 1981.

80. Cambria RP, Ivarsson BL, Akins CA, Moncure AC, Brewster DC, Abbott WM. Simultaneous carotid and coronary disease: Safety of the combined approach. J Vasc Surg 9:56-64, 1989.

81. Brewster DC, Cambria RP. Evaluation and management of patients with combined carotid and coronary artery disease. In Veith FJ, ed. Current Critical Problems in Vascular Surgery, vol. 2. St. Louis: Quality Medical Publishing, 1990.

82. Ruby ST, Whittemore AD, Couch NP, Mannick JA. Coronary artery disease in patients requiring abdominal aortic aneurysm repair. Ann Surg 201:758-764, 1985.

83. David TE. Peripheral vascular disease. Combined cardiac and abdominal aortic surgery. Circulation 72:18-21, 1985.

84. Harman E, Lillinton GA. Pulmonary risk factors in surgery. Med Clin North Am 63:1289, 1979.

85. Buist AS, Sexton GJ, Nagy JM, Ross BB. The effect of smoking cessation and modification on lung function. Am Rev Respir Dis 114:115, 1976.

86. Buczko GB, Day A, Vanderdoelen JL, Boucher R, Zamel N. Effects of cigarette smoking and short-term smoking cessation on airway responsiveness to inhaled methacholine. Am Rev Respir Dis 129:12, 1984.

87. Burrows B, Knudson RJ, Kettel LJ. Respiratory Insufficiency. Chicago: Year Book, 1975.

88. Peters RM. Identification, assessment and management of surgical patients with chronic respiratory disease. Probl Gen Surg 1:432-444, 1984.

89. Stanley JC, Wakefield TW. Cardiopulmonary assessment for major vascular reconstructive procedures. In Haimovici H, ed. Vascular Surgery: Principles and Techniques, 3rd ed. Norwalk, Conn.: Appleton & Lange, 1989, pp 195-203.

90. Wolfe WG, Hopkins RA. Clinical and physiologic evaluation of respiratory function. In Sabiston DC, ed. Textbook of Surgery, 13th ed. Philadelphia: WB Saunders, 1986, pp 1973-1989.

91. Meyers JR, Lembeck L, O'Kane H, Baue AE. Changes in functional residual capacity of the lung after operation. Arch Surg 110:576, 1975.

92. Gracey DR, Divertie MB, Didier EP. Preoperative pulmonary preparation of patients with chronic obstructive pulmonary disease. A prospective study. Chest 76:123-129, 1979.

93. Sicard GA, Freeman MB, Van Der Woude JC, Anderson CB. Comparison between transabdominal and retroperitoneal approach for reconstruction of the infrarenal abdominal aorta. J Vasc Surg 5:19-27, 1987.

94. Leather RP, Shah DM, Kaufman JL, Fitzgerald KM, Chang BB, Feustel PJ. Comparative analysis of retroperitoneal and transperitoneal aortic replacement for aneurysm. Surg Gynecol Obstet 168:387-393, 1989.

95. Cambria RP, Brewster DC, Abbott WM, Freehan M, Megerman J, LaMuraglia G, Wilson R, Wilson D, Teplick R, Davison JK. Transperitoneal versus retroperitoneal approach for aortic reconstruction: A randomized prospective study. J Vasc Surg 11:314-325, 1990.

96. Cullen ML, Staren ED, El-Ganzouri A, Logas WG, Ivankovich AD, Economou SG. Continuous epidural infusion for analgesia after major abdominal operations: A randomized, prospective, double-blind study. Surgery 98:718-728, 1985.

97. Jayr C, Mollie A, Bourgain JL, Alarcon J, Masselot J, Lasser P, Denjean A, Truffa-Bachi J, Henry-Amar M. Postoperative pulmonary complications: General anesthesia with postoperative parenteral morphine compared with epidural analgesia. Surgery 104:57-63, 1988.

4

Renal Failure and Fluid Shifts Following Vascular Surgery

Richard H. Dean   **Reid W. Tribble**

The factors affecting fluid shifts and renal functions have interested scientists and physicians for 300 years.[1] As in other fields in the life sciences, however, much of our knowledge about renal function has been accumulated and applied to the management of the surgical patient only in the past 50 years. Our understanding remains fragmentary and therapeutic regimens for prevention or correction of renal dysfunction remain imperfect. Examination of the nomenclature used for description of renal dysfunction underscores the relative simplicity with which the medical community views renal injury and its management. For instance, the term "acute tubular necrosis (ATN)" is commonly used by the clinician as the single term to describe the kidney's response to injury. The implication that an insult to renal function must produce tubular cell death in order to be considered clinically important connotes a level of understanding that is both naive and erroneous.

To address fluid shifts after operation and the potential renal insults associated with vascular surgery, first one must understand normal renal physiology. From this reference point a better appreciation of the spectrum of aberrations in renal function that can be induced by the stress of major vascular surgery can be achieved.

NORMAL RENAL FUNCTION

A complete discussion of normal renal physiology is beyond the scope of this text; excellent reviews of normal anatomy and physiology are available for the reader in standard surgical texts.[2,3] However, an understanding of certain components of intrarenal and extrarenal regulatory mechanisms governing excretory renal function is germane to comprehending the effects of insults on the functions.

The kidney serves as the dominant site for maintenance of normal intravascular volume and solute constituency. Under normovolemic baseline states the kidneys receive approximately 25% of the cardiac output. Based on a 5 L/min cardiac output, this means that the kidneys receive 900 L/day of plasma flow. Given the fact that the glomeruli filter 20% of the renal plasma flow into the tubular space within Bowman's capsule and that the normal 24-hour urinary output for a 70 kg man is less than 1.8 L, then the kidneys must reabsorb greater than 99% of the 180 L/day of filtered water to maintain homeostasis. Similarly, the initial composition of the tubular fluid is essentially an ultrafiltrate of plasma with a concentration of electrolytes and other solutes similar to that in plasma. Therefore these electrolytes and other solutes such as glucose must also be almost totally reabsorbed. For the purposes of this discussion the mechanisms of sodium, potassium, and water reabsorption will primarily be reviewed.

Reabsorption of electrolytes from the tubular fluid occurs both by active transport and passive back-diffusion. The sodium ion is reabsorbed in the early proximal tubule by its cotransportation with organic solutes, bicarbonate, and divalent cations through an active transport mechanism. Similarly, sodium is actively transported in the late proximal tubule in linkage with chloride transport. Since water freely follows this movement of solutes and ions, the tubular fluid is isosmotic to plasma as it enters the loop of Henle (Fig. 4-1).

The tubular cells of the loop of Henle vary in permeability depending on their location in the loop. This establishes a hypotonic tubular fluid and medullary osmotic gradient. Whereas the descending loop of Henle is permeable to water but relatively impermeable to sodium and chloride, the ascending loop of Henle is impermeable to water but actively transports the chloride ion, with sodium passively following. The resulting *countercurrent mechanism* produces a medullary osmotic gradient that regulates urine osmolarity from 50 to 1200 mOsm.[4] Distal tubular reabsorption of sodium is also active. In the distal tubule and in the proximal collecting ducts sodium is actively reabsorbed under the control of aldosterone. Sodium is almost completely reabsorbed through these mechanisms. Of the approximately 25,000 mEq of sodium filtered daily, only 50 to 200 mEq is ultimately excreted through urination (less than 1%).

Filtered potassium is almost totally reabsorbed in the proximal tubule and the loop of Henle. However, influenced by the electronegativity of the tubular fluid and the intracellular concentration of potassium, potassium is also passively secreted by the distal tubules and early collecting ducts into the tubular lumen. Essentially all of the potassium in the urine is transported there through this process.

Neuroendocrine Modulators of Renal Function

Intravascular volume is regulated primarily by a series of stretch receptors or baroreceptors located in systemic and renal arteries and the atria. Since these receptors not only sense pressure or volume changes (atrial receptors), but also monitor their rate of change during the cardiac cycle, they predominantly sense what might be called the effective circulating volume. Factors that decrease cardiac performance will alter the intravascular volume perceived by these receptors and thereby will also alter the

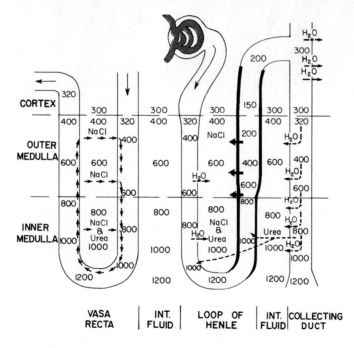

Fig. 4-1. Depiction of the loop of Henle demonstrating the development of the countercurrent mechanism.

renal response to retain water and increase the effective circulating volume. Similarly, when the concentration of circulating plasma proteins is reduced, there is a net diffusion of intravascular water into the extracellular space secondary to the decreased intravascular oncotic pressure. This net decrease in circulating volume is sensed by these same receptors, and the neuroendocrine regulators of urinary output inhibit excretion of water in order to correct the perceived deficiency.

When the baroreceptors perceive a reduction in circulating volume, a reduction in their afferent signals occurs, which decreases their tonic inhibition over the neuroendocrine system. This leads to increased secretion of vasopressin, β-endorphins, growth hormone, and adrenocorticotropic hormone through the CNS and to the increased release of epinephrine. Likewise, when baroreceptors within the juxtaglomcrular apparatus of the kidney perceive a decreased intravascular pressure, they are stimulated to increase renin release.

Other monitors and regulators of intravascular volume include the macula densa of the juxtaglomerular apparatus, osmoreceptors located near the hypothalamic ventricles of the CNS and in the liver, and sensors of plasma potassium concentration in the adrenal cortex. The primary hormonal regulators of fluid and electrolyte balance are aldosterone, cortisol, vasopressin, and angiotensin. However, the interactions between insulin, epinephrine, plasma glucose concentration, acid-base balance of the plasma, and other factors also play a vital role in modulating the release of these hormones as well as directly affecting the renal tubular management of water and the respective filtered solutes. Further discussion of their interactions and their impact on renal function and fluid shifts will be limited here to the effects of major vascular surgery. A more detailed description of their respective roles and integrated functions is provided elsewhere.[3,4]

FLUID SHIFTS ASSOCIATED WITH SURGERY

We will address fluid shifts associated with vascular surgery within the context of aortic and/or other major intra-abdominal vascular surgery exclusive of procedures requiring temporary interruption to visceral or renal perfusion. The impact of ischemia on the viscera or kidneys provides additional and peculiar factors influencing the body's management of fluid and electrolyte balance. Therefore the influence of suprarenal aortic cross-clamping and renovascular surgery is reviewed later in the context of causes and prevention of renal failure.

Intra-abdominal vascular surgery appropriately can be considered a major insult, trauma, or injury. To appreciate the response to such an insult and the impact on the fluid balance within the respective fluid compartments of the body, one must examine the factors influencing transcapillary and transcellular migration of fluid.

Normally water and its respective solutes move from the plasma into the interstitial space at the precapillary level because of the net hydrostatic pressure at that level. Reentry into the intravascular space at the distal capillary level is predominantly governed by the net intravascular oncotic pressure produced by plasma proteins. Among these proteins, albumin is the most plentiful and important. Normally, approximately 7% of intravascular albumin arriving at the capillary level crosses the capillary membrane into the interstitial space. This is a unidirectional flow of albumin; it ultimately returns to the intravascular pool by transport through the lymphatic system.

Following trauma to a specific tissue and as a net result of multiple complex hemodynamic mechanisms triggered by any major insult, capillary membrane permeability to albumin is dramatically increased. This net egress of albumin into the interstitial space is further enhanced by interruption or alteration of poorly understood complex mechanisms governing the lymphatic transport of albumin following systemic or local trauma.[5-7] Therefore the excess albumin transported across the capillary membranes stays in the interstitial space longer. In response to the increased migration of albumin into the interstitial space, distal capillary oncotic pressure falls and a resultant decrease in the reabsorption of water into the intravascular compartment occurs. This in turn decreases intravascular volume and causes the neuroendocrine mechanisms to reduce the renal excretion of sodium and free water.

The normal homeostatic response to contend with a decreased circulating intravascular volume is to mobilize the extracellular fluid in the interstitium (third space). Indeed, the extracellular fluid space is expanded as a consequence of the aforementioned response to the stress of major intra-abdominal surgery. One might conceptually describe this excess extracellular third-space fluid as "entrapped" by its greater oncotic pressure, and the functional reserve of fluid available for return to the plasma for expansion of the contracted intravascular volume is severely reduced. When one considers the added impact of temporary ischemia to tissue beds during major vascular surgery, the ensuing shift in the acid-base balance within the involved tissue beds, the adverse impact of unreplaced blood loss, the potential reductions in cardiac performance during aortic cross-clamping, and the stimulation of stress-response neuroendocrine mechanisms, one can easily understand the vicious cycle of events leading to a shift of total body water out of the functional circulating blood volume into the *third space*.[8,9]

This obligatory loss of circulating free water and associated solutes following major surgery has only recently been appreciated. This knowledge has been dramatically beneficial in the intraoperative and early postoperative fluid management of patients undergoing major vascular surgery. Recognition of increased obligatory losses of intravascular volume associated with major surgery has led to the current use of balanced salt solutions for replenishment.[10] Although formulas for calculating required intraoperative and postoperative fluid administration are available,[11] of greatest importance is the appreciation that hourly parenteral fluid replacement requirements during surgery are several-fold that which is required during a resting state and may vary from 100 to 500 ml/hr. Even this range of additional replacement fluids is inadequate during and after acute blood loss. These increased fluid replacement requirements continue to be necessary in the immediate postoperative period as a result of continued sequestration of fluid into the operative site.

Mobilization of the sequestered third-space fluid is delayed for a variable number of days depending on the magnitude of ongoing postoperative stress, cardiac performance, and intravascular oncotic pressure. Usually the reabsorption of this third-space fluid begins on the second or third postoperative day. If not managed with appropriate reduction in maintenance parenteral fluid administration and/or addition of diuretic therapy, this mobilization phase of third-space fluid can lead to intravascular volume overload and acute congestive heart failure.

RENAL DYSFUNCTION AFTER VASCULAR SURGERY

The severity of renal dysfunction following vascular surgery may range from minor inappropriate loss of sodium in the urine to anuric acute renal failure. Similarly, its causes span a wide range of prerenal, postrenal, and parenchymal causes (Table 4-1). Thankfully, the incidence of clinically severe acute renal failure after major surgery has dramatically decreased over the last 50 years as knowledge of the factors affecting fluid and electrolyte balance has increased and as early intervention to abort

Table 4-1. Sites and Causes of Acute Renal Failure

Prerenal	Parenchymal	Postrenal
Low cardiac output/cardiogenic shock	Nephrotoxic drugs	Catheter kinking
Increased vascular space	Radiologic contrast	Catheter clot
Septic shock	Myoglobinuria	Bladder clot
Hypovolemia	Acute tubular necrosis	Ureteral obstruction
Blood loss	Any cause	Renal pelvic obstruction
Dehydration		
Third-space sequestration		

underlying causes has been implemented. Nevertheless, the mortality of postoperative acute renal failure remains high and varies from 10% to 80% depending on the associated presence of multiorgan system failure.

Prerenal Causes

Prerenal causes are the most frequent source of acute renal dysfunction in the early postoperative period. Usually renal failure from a prerenal cause is a direct result of a contracted intravascular volume secondary to inadequate fluid replacement following intraoperative and immediate postoperative fluid losses or fluid sequestration into the third space. Less commonly it is secondary to reduced cardiac performance, which likewise triggers the neurohormonal reflexes to increase intravascular volume by increasing tubular reabsorption of sodium and water. In their pure forms, these two causes of reduced renal function are easily discernible. Whereas hypovolemia is associated with flat neck veins, dry mucous membranes, reduced central venous pressure, and reduced pulmonary artery wedge pressure, renal dysfunction secondary to poor cardiac performance is associated with distended neck veins, apparent fluid overload (evident when the lungs are auscultated), elevated central venous pressure, and elevated pulmonary artery wedge pressure. Obviously, therapy for hypovolemic prerenal azotemia is to increase intravascular volume by administration of a balanced salt solution and red blood cells as needed. Conversely, therapy for renal dysfunction of a cardiogenic origin is directed at improving myocardial performance by administering afterload reducing agents and inotropic agents, and instituting diuretic therapy as needed to diminish preloading of the failing myocardium.

Unfortunately the diffusely atherosclerotic patient who is submitted to major vascular surgery frequently has associated coronary artery disease and impaired myocardial function. Segregation of the two causes of renal dysfunction (hypovolemic vs. cardiogenic) can be problematic. In this circumstance preexisting heart disease may alter the euvolemic level for an individual at higher central filling pressures and apparently normal or low normal cardiac filling

pressures may in fact reflect hypovolemia. In this clinical setting we maintain a constant infusion of afterload reducing agents (e.g., nitroprusside or nitroglycerine) and inotropic agents (e.g., dobutamine) and cautiously administer sequential boluses of balanced salt solutions while monitoring cardiac output and left atrial filling pressure (pulmonary artery wedge pressure). If no urinary response is noted once filling pressures begin to rise, we then begin diuretic therapy as an added measure to treat the cardiac origin of the reduced urinary output.

The final variety of prerenal causes is occlusive disease of the renal arteries. Because occlusive disease is initially a diagnosis made by exclusion of other causes, one should first evaluate the patient for other sources of renal failure. When other causes have been excluded, our initial study to determine if there is occlusive disease of the renal arteries is a technetium-99m pertechnetate perfusion scan of the kidneys. Since intense interstitial swelling from parenchymal causes of ATN may dramatically increase renal parenchymal resistance, a slow renal perfusion as determined by isotope renography may be misleading. In all instances in which correction of a renovascular occlusion may be contemplated we perform contrast arteriography to clarify the presence of the occlusion and to plan its correction.

Postrenal Causes

Although an uncommon cause of postoperative oliguria and apparent renal failure, postrenal obstruction to urine flow may be the easiest to correct or exclude. Kinking or obstruction of the indwelling urinary catheter may produce sudden cessation of urinary flow. For this reason the catheter should be irrigated as the first maneuver for diagnostic evaluation and potential therapy. Obstruction by clotted blood in the bladder can follow a traumatic catheter insertion. Therefore one should be especially aware of this possibility following a difficult bladder catheterization.

Finally, ureteral or renal pelvic obstructions also can cause postrenal oliguria. If other causes of oliguria have been excluded, preliminary screening of their cause can be obtained with isotope renography. Definitive diagnosis is obtained by retrograde urography. When the cause is identified, placement of an ureteral stent frequently can relieve such an obstruction.

Renal Parenchymal Causes

Parenchymal causes of acute renal dysfunction represent a wide range of etiologies and pose the greatest potential for permanent compromise of renal function. The pathophysiology of the dysfunction depends on the specific etiology.

Ischemic Injury

Caused by either temporary periods of interruption of perfusion to the kidney or periods of shock during or after major vascular procedures, ischemic injury is twofold. First, as a consequence of the magnitude and duration of ischemia, tubular cell swelling occurs following reperfusion. This in turn can cause tubular obstruction and lead to further reduction or cessation of glomerular filtration in the nephron. Second, tubular cells can either lose their basement membrane attachment secondary to interstitial edema, which develops after reperfusion, or undergo cell death during ischemia and subsequently be sloughed into the tubule. The finding of tubular cells in the urinary sediment is the genesis of the term "acute tubular necrosis (ATN)." Although this term is a poor pathologic description of this form of injury, ATN is commonly used to describe all renal parenchymal causes of acute renal failure. The medullary thick ascending loop of Henle and the pars recta of the proximal tubule appear to be the segments of the tubular epithelium most sensitive to ischemia.[12,13] Following loss of the tubular cell, a back-leak of glomerular filtrate into the renal parenchyma develops.[14]

Toxic Injury

Chemical injury to the kidney can result from many sources. The most common compounds responsible for such an injury in the postoperative period are aminoglycosides, yet myoglobin and radiologic contrast media have also been implicated. Aminoglycosides appear primarily to exert their toxicity on the tubular cell in relationship to their trough level of plasma concentration.[15] Because of this relationship and the frequent history of reduced renal function in postoperative vascular surgery patients requiring the administration of aminoglycosides, it is important to monitor the peak and trough levels of the antibiotic to establish appropriate dosing levels.

Myoglobinuria is an important cause of renal failure in patients submitted to revascularization of limbs with prolonged extreme ischemia. Circulating as a breakdown product of muscle death, myoglobin is freely filtered by the glomerulus. Myoglobin exerts its toxicity through direct tubular cell injury and through precipitation and obstruction of the tubule.[16,17] Therefore prevention of injury to the kidney is directed toward maximizing urine flow rate with intravenous crystalloid infusion and diuretics and by alkalinization of the urine.

Although there are a multitude of other parenchymal causes of acute renal failure, most are infrequent in surgical patients. Causes that are peculiar to vascular surgery and vascular contrast imaging have special pertinence and are discussed separately.

RENAL FAILURE ASSOCIATED WITH AORTIC SURGERY

Acute renal failure following aortic surgery continues to be a complication associated with an extremely high mortality. Although acute renal failure is reported to have an incidence ranging from 1% to 13% in elective aortic surgery,[18-25] its occurrence depends on the clinical circumstances of the operation, intraoperative and postoperative events, and the overall prior health status of the patient.

The incidence of acute renal failure following elective abdominal aortic aneurysm surgery and operations performed for ruptured abdominal aortic aneurysms in several series is summarized in Tables 4-2 and 4-3. As shown by the dates of these reports, no measurable impact on the incidence of acute renal failure has occurred in the past 20 years despite major efforts to identify and diminish the frequency and magnitude of precipitating causes. Similarly, the mortality rate associated with postoperative renal failure has remained formidable. Nevertheless, recognition of the clinical syndrome of

Table 4-2. Acute Renal Failure After Elective Aortic Surgery

Series	No. of patients	Type of procedure	Incidence (%)
Gardner et al.[18] (1970)	56	AAA	1
David et al.[25] (1974)	69	AAA	13
Thompson et al.[20] (1975)	108	AAA	8
Volpetti et al.[21] (1976)	585	AAA	4
McCombs and Roberts[23] (1979)	361	AAA	2
Diehl et al.[24] (1983)	350	AAA	6
	173	AIO	5
Bergqvist et al.[22] (1983)	221	AIO	8

AAA, abdominal aortic aneurysm; AIO, aortoiliac occlusion.

Table 4-3. Acute Renal Failure in Ruptured Aneurysm Surgery

Series	No. of patients	Incidence (%)	Mortality (%)
Tilney et al.[29] (1973)	18	100	95
Hicks et al.[26] (1975)	56	18	70
Sink et al.[27] (1976)	28	46	69
McCombs and Roberts[23] (1979)	38	21	50
Gornick and Kjellstrand[28] (1983)	30	—	64

multiorgan system failure has shed some light on factors that increase the mortality rate associated with postoperative renal failure. In patients with postoperative renal failure as an isolated system failure, the associated mortality rate is low. In contrast, when renal failure is only one of several system failures, the mortality is extremely high.[29] It might be surmised that one simply needs to prevent or provide improved treatment of multiorgan system failure in order to improve the probability of survival in that group with renal failure. To date, however, the prevention of multiorgan system failure has been an unachieved goal of allied research and clinical care.

Pathophysiology of Postaortic Surgery Renal Failure

The development of acute renal failure following procedures involving the juxtarenal aorta seldom parallels pure pathophysiologic models, but rather stems from a mixture of underlying causes. However, for the sake of understanding, the respective causes are ad-dressed here as independent sources of acute renal failure, with the knowledge that all of these mechanisms may be active in the production of postoperative renal failure in an individual patient.

A temporary, isolated period of renal ischemia caused by suprarenal aortic cross-clamping, temporary renal artery occlusion, a single episode of hypovolemic shock, declamping hypotension, or cardiogenic shock in the perioperative period is the most common cause of acute renal dysfunction and renal failure associated with aortic surgery. Through observations of patients and use of investigative models, Myers and associates[30-33] have postulated that the pathophysiologic cascade of events following temporary renal ischemia leads to acute renal failure. The observation that renal biopsies and autopsy studies in patients with postischemic acute renal failure showed minimal if any disturbance in glomerular architecture yet demonstrated profound disruption of tubular morphology led Oliver, MacDowell, and Tracy[34] to conclude that this form of acute renal failure was initiated through tubular luminal obstruction caused by sloughed tubular cells. The resultant tubular obstruction is postulated to first cause a transtubular back-leak of glomerular filtrate. Since obstruction of tubular flow also leads to an increase in the tubular luminal hydrostatic pressure above the obstruction, less hydrostatic pressure differential exists between the glomerular capillary lumen and the tubular space within Bowman's capsule. This reduced hydrostatic pressure differential leads to reduction in glomerular filtration. Then, because of the increased permeability of the tubular lining and the resultant increased interstitial oncotic pressure, further back-diffusion of filtered water occurs. This increased back-diffusion of glomerular filtrate further spurs the progression of oliguria. The final mechanism that leads to filtration failure and oliguria is the impact of an increased solute load presented to the macula densa as a consequence of the dramatic back-diffusion of fluid. This solute load is believed to stimulate the macula densa to activate the renin-angiotensin-aldosterone system. Through this mechanism, afferent or preglomerular arteriolar vasoconstriction is triggered, which decreases the glomerular capillary hydrostatic pressure and further encourages filtration failure. The magnitude and duration of the ischemic result are the predominant factors that determine the clinical severity and duration of this type of acute renal failure.

An alternate cause of acute renal failure in aortic surgery that might be considered a permanent form of ischemic insult is microscopic embolization of cholesterol-rich atheromatous debris into the renal vasculature during the act of cross-clamping and/or declamping the juxtarenal aorta. Although this cause receives much less attention in the literature than the pathophysiologic consequences of temporary ischemia, we suspect that it is the dominant cause of acute renal failure in patients without prolonged renal ischemia, excessive blood loss and hypotension, or other recognized nephrotoxic insults to renal function. Obviously, the quantity of microemboli produced by clamping or declamping the aorta and by manipulation of the juxtarenal aorta during

dissection depends on the embologenic potential of the atheromatous debris and the operative techniques employed to prevent such an event. Furthermore, the clinical impact of such renal microembolization depends on the quantity of functioning renal parenchyma embolized and the presence of other causes of acute renal failure. In the absence of other causes of acute renal failure and with a normal mass of functioning nephron units, relatively large amounts of atheromatous microemboli can occur without having an immediate impact on the adequacy of renal function. In contrast, if there is a minimal renal reserve as in the azotemic patient, then the added insult of even minor losses of nephron units by microembolization can lead to decompensation and acute renal failure.

Protection of Renal Function

Several fundamental concepts for protection of renal function during aortic surgery are widely understood and practiced. These include provision of adequate circulating blood volume before operation by preoperative intravenous fluid hydration, adequate blood volume replacement during and immediately after surgery, avoidance of repetitive or prolonged renal ischemia, and maintenance of maximal parameters of cardiac performance. Additional modalities include the use of mannitol and other diuretics, renal hypothermia, renal vasodilatory drugs, and other more investigational techniques.[35-40] Conceptually, all of these modalities are directed toward reduction of the severity or duration of renal tubular ischemia, reduction of renal tubular metabolic needs during periods of ischemia, or prevention of tubular obstruction by sloughed tubular cells. No single modality or combination prevents the insult of aortic surgery on renal function; yet by maximizing the impact of each of these preventive measures, one can often significantly lessen the severity and duration of renal dysfunction.

The intravenous administration of mannitol, 12.5 to 25 gm, before aortic cross-clamping is widely practiced as a routine measure to prevent acute renal failure. Extensive investigation of its actions suggests that mannitol not only acts as an osmotic diuretic to increase urine flow rate, but also may attenuate the reduction in cortical blood flow that occurs during and immediately after aortic cross-clamping and beneficially function as a free radical scavenger.[35]

Regional renal hypothermia has been used sporadically for many years to protect renal function during periods of ischemia. Its use is based on the valid premise that even modest decreases in core temperature will create major reductions in metabolic needs and that it is these unmet metabolic needs during ischemia that lead to the cascade of events producing acute renal failure. The technique usually employs the infusion of 500 ml to 1 L of cold (4° to 5° C) crystalloid solution with or without other additives into the isolated segment of the aorta containing the renal arteries or directly into the renal artery ostia using a handheld cannula. Although one cannot argue against the logic of this preventive measure, studies proving the benefit of renal hypothermia in humans primarily have been testimonial only and we currently do not routinely use it for aortic or standard renal artery procedures.

Finally, one cannot overstate the importance of operative technique in prevention of microembolization of atheromatous debris during juxtarenal aortic manipulation or clamping. Since the embologenic potential of the debris cannot be judged definitively until after the aorta is opened, one should assume the worst until it is proved otherwise. For this reason we temporarily occlude renal artery flow immediately before the application of the aortic clamp whenever the aortogram suggests the presence of succulent atheromatous debris. This applies to both cross-clamping immediately below the renal arteries and suprarenal aortic cross-clamping. For infrarenal cross-clamping we "flash unclamp" the proximal aortic clamp after opening the aorta to flush out any loose debris. Then we reapply the aortic clamp, remove the renal artery occluding device, and reestablish renal perfusion. Although we can provide only anecdotal support for this maneuver, we believe it has been an important adjunct in minimizing the incidence of postoperative acute renal failure among our patients.

RENAL FAILURE ASSOCIATED WITH ARTERIOGRAPHY

Contrast arteriography is the gold standard of diagnostic studies used in the evaluation of vascular disease. Conventional contrast agents have iodine incorporated into their structure to absorb x-ray photons and in this way achieve visualization of the vasculature. Nephrotoxicity of such iodinated contrast agents has been recognized for many years.[41] The ionization and high osmolarity of these agents may contribute to their nephrotoxicity. New agents, nonionic contrast agents (e.g., iopamidol), are now available that provide comparable absorption of x-ray photons yet are significantly less charged than the traditional agents. This reduction in ionization was hoped to decrease nephrotoxicity,[42] but significant alterations in the incidence of nephrotoxicity have not been achieved.[43]

The incidence of acute renal dysfunction following contrast arteriography depends on several factors: the quantity of contrast material injected, the patient population, and the prearteriographic preparation of the patient; the reported incidence varies from 0% to 92%.[44-46] The incidence of acute renal failure requiring dialysis for management in patients with no risk factors is very low, probably less than 1%. A number of factors, however, have been identified that increase the risk of contrast-induced acute renal failure (Table 4-4). Among these, diabetes and preexisting renal issue insufficiency are of the greatest concern for they are both common and unavoidable. Risk factors such as dehydration, volume depletion, volume of contrast used, and simultaneous exposure to other nephrotoxins are common yet should be avoidable through proper patient preparation. Other risk factors such as multiple myeloma or severe proteinuria are uncommon and may be lesser risk factors in the absence of secondary renal insufficiency.

The impact of diabetes on the risk of acute renal failure following arteriography appears to depend on the type of diabetes and the magnitude of secondary diabetic nephropathy. Type I diabetic patients appear to be more susceptible to contrast-induced acute renal failure than

Table 4-4. Factors Implicated in Arteriography-Induced Renal Failure

Advanced age	Hyperuricemia
Renal insufficiency	Exposure to other nephrotoxins
Diabetes mellitus	Repeated exposure to radiocontrast material
Multiple myeloma	Excessive volume of contrast material
Anemia	Intra-arterial vs. intravenous administration of contrast material
Proteinuria	Cardiovascular disease
Abnormal liver function	Hypertension
Dehydration	Renal transplantation

type II diabetic patients.[47,48] Harkonen and Kjellstrand[47] found that in 22 of 26 diabetic patients (76%) with a prestudy serum-creatinine level greater than 2 mg/dl who underwent excretory urography, acute renal failure developed. Weinrauch et al.[46] reported that in 12 of 13 patients (92%) with juvenile onset diabetes and severe diabetic nephropathy, acute renal failure developed following coronary arteriography. The cause of chronic renal insufficiency also appears to affect the permanency of contrast-induced acute renal failure. Whereas both diabetic and nondiabetic patients with renal insufficiency are at increased risk for contrast-induced acute renal failure, diabetic patients appear to recover less often and are at a much greater risk of permanent dialysis dependence as a consequence of contrast-induced acute renal failure.

The cause of acute renal failure following angiography is probably multifactorial. In contrast to the widely known potential for the nephrotoxicity of contrast agents, there are relatively little experimental data confirming the pathogenesis. This is partially explained by the difficulty in creating animal models that mimic the human conditions known to predispose to the injury. Factors considered important in the pathogenesis include the osmolality of the contrast material,[49] presence of proteinuria,[50] tubular obstruction,[51] allergic reactions,[52] enzymuria,[53] direct toxicity of the agent,[54] and altered glomerular permeability.[55] Although the newer nonionic contrast materials have been developed to address some of these potential causes (e.g., osmolality and

magnitude of ionic change), they are significantly more expensive. They appear to diminish the pain experienced by the patient immediately following injection, yet prospective and controlled comparative trials have not demonstrated a significant reduction in the risk of acute renal failure with their use.[43,56]

Prevention of Contrast-Induced Renal Failure

Specific measures used to minimize the risk of contrast-induced acute renal failure remain controversial and without controlled studies available to confirm their efficacy. Nevertheless, experimental parallels and the understanding of factors that increase the risk of this complication have led to generally accepted tenets of prevention. The basic relationship between the use of contrast material and the risk of induced acute renal failure for any of the currently used agents in the higher risk patient population appears to be related to the duration of time the kidney is exposed to a given concentration of contrast material. For this reason maximizing urine flow rate during and immediately after arteriography and limiting the quantity of agent used during an arteriographic session are important considerations. Insurance of a maximal urine flow rate should be achieved by preliminary intravenous hydration of the patient and the use of diuretic therapy. We routinely admit any patient with recognized risk factors 12 hours before arteriography to administer intravenous hydration and infuse D_5 ¼N saline solution at 1.5 ml/kg/hr during this period. Immediately before arteriography the patient usually receives a bolus of intravenous fluid (3 to 5 ml/kg). In addition, 12.5 gm of mannitol and/or 20 to 40 mg of furosemide is given intravenously at the time of arteriography. Finally, intravenous hydration is continued for 4 to 6 hours after completion of the study.

No definitive formula exists for establishment of the upper safe limit of administered contrast material in patients with respective levels of risk for induced acute renal failure. Even small doses (30 to 60 ml) may induce decompensated renal failure in patients with extreme renal insufficiency (glomerular filtration rate less than or equal to 15 ml/min). In contrast, more than 300 ml of contrast material may be safely administered to other patients with no risk factors for acute renal failure. Our practice is to limit the quantity of a contrast agent, a nonionized material, to less than 50 to 75 ml in patients with significant reductions in glomerular filtration rate (less than 20 to 30 ml/min). If additional contrast material is required to evaluate other areas of the vasculature, we postpone such studies and approach the total evaluation in a sequential manner after having confirmed that no adverse effect from the prior study has occurred. The introduction of digital subtraction techniques has been useful in limiting the quantity of contrast material used in patients with renal insufficiency. Digital subtraction techniques are especially useful when the areas to be viewed would require multiple injections if conventional radiologic techniques were employed. Nevertheless, we have found a single midstream aortic injection using 30 ml of nonionic contrast material and standard radiologic techniques to be equally safe when compared with digital subtraction techniques. We believe that this technique provides superior visualization of the renal vasculature and related aortic anatomy in renal insufficiency patients in whom the presence of ischemic nephropathy is being evaluated.

Finally, we believe that future advancements in the safe visualization of the vasculature will not come from further modification of the chemical composition of the contrast agents. Rather, we believe the greatest innovation and progress will be made in the application of noncontrast agent studies. The reported use of carbon dioxide is generally overlooked but can be a viable alternative to the use of standard contrast agents for limited studies.[57] Most important, however, is the development of nuclear magnetic imaging of the vasculature.[58] Through further technologic modification, this field holds the greatest promise for providing excellent visualization of the vascular anatomy without the risks induced by injection of any noxious chemical.

REFERENCES

1. Harvey W. Exercitatio Anatomica de Motu Cordis et Sanguinis, 1628. Quoted in The Works of William Harvey. London: The Syndenham Society, 1847.
2. Shires TG, Canizaro PC, Shires TC III, Lowry SF. Fluid, electrolyte, and nutritional management of the surgical patient. In Schwartz SI, ed. Principles of Surgery, 5th ed. New York: McGraw-Hill, 1989, pp 68-104.
3. Gann DS, Amaral JF. Preoperative electrolyte management. In Sabiston DC Jr, ed. Sabiston's Essentials of Surgery. Philadelphia: WB Saunders, 1987, pp 29-61.
4. Valtin H. Renal function: Mechanisms preserving fluid and solute balance in health. In Valtin H, ed. Renal Dysfunction: Mechanisms Involved in Fluid and Solute Imbalance. Boston: Little, Brown, 1983.
5. Carey LC, Lowery BD, Cloutier CT. Hemorrhagic shock. Curr Probl Surg 8:1-48, 1971.
6. Granger H, Dhar J, Chen HI. Structure and function of the interstitium. In Squoris JT, Rene A, eds. Proceedings of the Workshop on Albumin. Bethesda, Md.: National Institutes of Health, 1976, pp 114-123.
7. Taylor AE, Granger DN. A model of protein and fluid exchange between plasma and interstitium. In Squoris JT, Rene A, eds. Proceedings of the Workshop of Albumin. Bethesda, Md.: National Institutes of Health, 1976, pp 93-113.
8. Lucas CE, Ledgerwood AM. The fluid problem in the critically ill. Surg Clin North Am 63:439, 1983.
9. Dawson CW, Lucas CE, Ledgerwood AM. Altered interstitial fluid space dynamics and post-resuscitation hypertension. Arch Surg 116:657, 1981.
10. Baxter CA. Balanced salt solutions as renal prophylaxis. In Brown BR Jr, ed. Fluid and Blood Therapy in Anesthesia. Philadelphia: FA Davis, 1983, pp 137-150.
11. Thorén L, Wiklund L. Intraoperative fluid therapy. World J Surg 7:581, 1983.
12. Glaumann B, Glaumann H, Trump BF. Studies of cellular recovery from ischemia: III. Ultrastructural studies on the recovery of the pars recta of the proximal tubule (P_1 segment) of the rat kidney from temporary ischemia. Virchows Arch [B] 25:281, 1977.
13. Brezis M, Rosen S, Silva P, Epstein FH. Renal ischemia: A new perspective. Kidney Int 26:275, 1984.

14. Jones DB. Ultrastructure of human acute renal failure. Lab Invest 46:254, 1982.

15. Matzke GR, Lucarotti RL, Shapiro HS. Controlled comparison of gentamicin and tobramycin nephrotoxicity. Am J Nephrol 3:11, 1983.

16. Eneas JF, Schoenfeld PY, Humphreys MH. The effect of infusion of mannitol-sodium bicarbonate on the clinical course of myoglobinuria. Arch Intern Med 139:801, 1979.

17. Braun SR, Weiss FR, Keller AI, Ciccone JR, Preuss HG. Evaluation of the renal toxicity of hemoproteins and their derivatives: A role in the genesis of acute tubular necrosis. J Exp Med 131:443, 1970.

18. Gardner RJ, Lancaster JR, Tarnay TJ, Warden HE, Currie RA. Five year history of surgically treated abdominal aortic aneurysms. Surg Gynecol Obstet 130:981, 1970.

19. O'Donnell D, Clarke G, Hurst P. Acute renal failure following surgery for abdominal aortic aneurysm. Aust NZ J Surg 59:405, 1989.

20. Thompson JE, Hollier LH, Patman RD, Persson AV. Surgical management of abdominal aortic aneurysms: Factors influencing mortality and morbidity—A 20-year experience. Ann Surg 181:654, 1975.

21. Volpetti G, Barker CF, Berkowitz H, Roberts B. A twenty-two year review of elective resection of abdominal aortic aneurysms. Surg Gynecol Obstet 142:321, 1976.

22. Bergqvist D, Olsson P-O, Takolander R, Almén T, Cederholm C, Jonsson K. Renal failure as a complication to aortoiliac and iliac reconstructive surgery. Acta Chir Scand 149:37-41, 1983.

23. McCombs PR, Roberts B. Acute renal failure following resection of abdominal aortic aneurysm. Surg Gynecol Obstet 148:175, 1979.

24. Diehl JT, Cali RF, Hertzer NR, Beven EG. Complications of abdominal aortic reconstruction, An analysis of perioperative risk factors in 557 patients. Ann Surg 197:49-56, 1983.

25. David JP, Marks C, Bonneval M. A ten year institutional experience with abdominal aneurysms. Surg Gynecol Obstet 138:591, 1974.

26. Hicks GL, Eastland MW, DeWeese JA, Gay AG, Rob CG. Survival improvement following aortic aneurysm resection. Ann Surg 181:863, 1975.

27. Sink JD, Myers RT, James PM. Ruptured abdominal aortic aneurysms: Review of 33 cases treated surgically and discussion of prognostic indicators. Am Surg 42:303, 1976.

28. Gornick CC Jr, Kjellstrand CM. Acute renal failure complicating aortic aneurysm surgery. Nephron 35:145, 1983.

29. Tilney NL, Bailey GL, Morgan AP. Sequential system failure after rupture of abdominal aortic aneurysms: An unsolved problem in postoperative care. Ann Surg 178:117, 1973.

30. Myers BD, Moran SM. Hemodynamically mediated acute renal failure. N Engl J Med 314:97, 1986.

31. Myers BD, Miller DC, Mehigan JT, Olcott C IV, Golbetz H, Robertson CR, Derby G, Spencer R, Freedman S. Nature of the renal injury following total renal ischemia in man. J Clin Invest 73:329, 1984.

32. Moran SM, Myers BD. Course of acute renal failure studied by a model of creatinine kinetics. Kidney Int 27:928, 1985.

33. Hilberman M, Myers BD, Carrie G, Gerby G, Jamison RL, Stinson EB. Acute renal failure following cardiac surgery. J Thorac Cardiovasc Surg 77:880, 1979.

34. Oliver J, MacDowell M, Tracy A. The pathogenesis of acute renal failure associated with traumatic and toxic injury. Renal ischemia, nephrotoxic damage, and the ischemuric episode. J Clin Invest 30:1305, 1951.

35. Miller DC, Myers BD. Pathophysiology and prevention of acute renal failure associated with thoracoabdominal or abdominal aortic surgery. J Vasc Surg 5:518, 1987.

36. Abbott WM, Abel RM, Beck CH. The reversal of renal cortical ischemia during aortic occlusion by mannitol. J Surg Res 16:482, 1974.

37. Hanley MJ, Davidson K. Prior mannitol and furosemide infusion in a model of ischemic acute renal failure. Am J Physiol 241:F556, 1981.

38. Ochsner JL, Mills NL, Gardner PA. A technique for renal preservation during suprarenal abdominal aortic operations. Surg Gynecol Obstet 159:388, 1984.

39. Hilberman M, Maseda J, Stinson EB, Derby GC, Spencer RJ, Miller C, Oyer PE, Myers BD. The diuretic properties of dopamine in patients after open-heart operation. Anesthesiology 61:489, 1984.

40. Lindner A, Cutler RE, Bell AJ. Attenuation of nephrotoxic acute renal failure in the dog with angiotensin-converting enzyme inhibitor (SQ-20, 881). Circ Res 51:216, 1982.

41. Ansell G. Adverse reaction to contrast agents: Scope of problem. Invest Radiol 5:374, 1979.

42. Evans JR, Cutler RE, Pettis JL. Low-osmolar radio-contrast agents and nephrotoxicity. Dialysis Transplant 16:504, 1987.

43. Davidson CJ, Hlatky M, Schwab SJ, Morris K, Skelton T, Bashore T. Nephrotoxicity and nephrotic risk factors: A prospective trial of nonionic contrast media. Ann Intern Med (in press).

44. Miller DL, Chang R, Wells WT, Dowjat BA, Malinosky RM, Doppman JL. Intravascular contrast media: Effect of dose on renal function. Radiology 167:607, 1988.

45. Martin-Paredero V, Dixon SM, Baker JD, Takiff H, Gomes AS, Busuttil RW, Moore WS. Risk of renal failure after major angiography. Arch Surg 118:1417, 1983.

46. Weinrauch LA, Healy RW, Leland OS, Goldstein HH, Kassissieh SD, Libertino JA, Takacs FJ, D'Elia JA. Coronary angiography and acute renal failure in diabetic azotemic nephropathy. Ann Intern Med 86:56, 1977.

47. Harkonen S, Kjellstrand CM. Exacerbation of diabetic renal failure following intravenous pyelography. Am J Med 63:939, 1977.

48. Shieh SD, Hirsch SR, Boshell BR, Pino JA, Alexander LJ, Witten DM, Friedman EA. Low risk of contrast media–induced acute renal failure in nonazotemic type 2 diabetes mellitus. Kidney Int 21:739, 1982.

49. Morris TW, Katzberg RW, Fisher HW. A comparison of the hemodynamic responses to metrizamide and meglumine/sodium diatrizoate in canine renal angiography. Invest Radiol 13:74, 1978.

50. Tejler L, Almen T, Holtas S. Proteinuria following nephroangiography. Acta Radiol (Diagn) 18:634, 1977.

51. Rees ED, Waugh WH. Factors in renal failure in multiple myeloma. Arch Int Med 116:400, 1965.

52. Light JA, Hill GS. Acute tubular necrosis in a renal transplant recipient: Complication from drip-infusion excretory urography. JAMA 232:1267, 1975.

53. Goldstein EJ, Feinfeld DA, Fleischner GM, Elkin M. Enzymatic evidence of renal tubular damage following renal angiography. Radiology 121:617, 1976.

54. Humes HD, Hunt DA, White MD. Direct toxic effect of the radiocontrast agent diatrizoate on renal proximal tubule cells. Am J Physiol 252:F246, 1987.

55. Vari RC, Natarajan LA, Whitescarver SA, Jackson BA, Ott CE. Induction, prevention and mechanisms of contrast media–induced acute renal failure. Kidney Int 33:699, 1988.

56. Parfrey PS, Griffiths SM, Barrett BJ, Paul MD, Genge M, Withers J, Farid N, McManamon PF. Contrast material–induced renal failure in patients with diabetes mellitus, renal insufficiency, or both: A prospective controlled study. N Engl J Med 320:143, 1989.

57. Weaver FA, Pentecost MJ, Yellin AE. Carbon dioxide digital subtraction arteriography: A pilot study. Ann Vasc Surg 4:437, 1990.

58. Kim D, Edelman RR, Kent KC, Porter DH, Skillman JJ. Abdominal aorta and renal artery stenosis: Evaluation with MR angiography. Radiology 174:727, 1990.

III Degeneration

5

Anastomotic Neointimal Hyperplasia and Progression of Atherosclerosis After Arterial Repair

Arkadiusz Jawien   **Alexander W. Clowes**

The treatment of arterial occlusive disease has improved during the last 40 years in part because of the development of vein grafts and synthetic grafts for the reconstruction of diseased vessels. With time some of these grafts develop stenosis, usually followed by spontaneous thrombosis and occlusion. Such lesions frequently occur at the site of the distal anastomosis of the graft to the native artery and are the result of neointimal cellular proliferation and the accumulation of extracellular matrix, hence the use of the term "anastomotic neointimal hyperplasia."

In this chapter, intimal hyperplasia and its role in vein graft or synthetic graft healing are discussed. We attempt to define mechanisms of abnormal neointimal thickening responsible for graft failure and progression of atherosclerosis after arterial repair. We also discuss ways to prevent intimal hyperplasia.

VEIN GRAFT HEALING

For many years autogenous saphenous vein has been recognized as the preferred conduit for aortocoronary and lower limb arterial bypass grafting. Data available on vein graft patency in general show a short-term (within the first year) patency rate of 80% to 90% and a subsequent annual failure of approximately 2.5%.[1] Bourassa et al.,[2] in reviewing the patency rate of saphenous vein aortocoronary bypass grafts in 400 patients, demonstrated that 87% of implanted grafts were patent less then 1 month after surgery, 79% were patent between 6 and 18 months after surgery, and 63% were patent between 10 and 12 years after surgery. They also found that 45% of the grafts patent at 1 year showed angiographic evidence of atherosclerosis between 10 and 12 years after surgery, and 70% of atherosclerotic lesions reduced the graft lumen diameter by 50% or more. In femoropopliteal grafts, Szilagyi and associates[1,3] and Whittemore et al.[4] correlated angiographic changes with subsequent graft failure rates. Stenoses caused by intimal thickening became evident in the interval from 6 to 60 months (mean, 16 months). Progression in 74% of these lesions leading to an eventual 50% closure rate was noted in those grafts that were not repaired.

Thus, despite the obvious advantages of autogenous vein grafts over synthetic conduits, vein grafts still have a significant occlusion rate when used either in aortocoronary or lower extremity revascularization. What, then, are the factors that result in vein graft failure?

The saphenous vein, like any vein, when inserted as a graft into the arterial circulation, undergoes numerous pathologic changes. Under the new hemodynamic conditions it dilates and rapidly develops a thick wall. This process, called "arterialization" by Carrel and Guthrie,[5,6] was described 80 years ago:

The wall of the vein becomes enormously thickened, the muscular and fibrous layer of the middle coat and the inner layer of the outer coat being principally involved. The intima appeared uniform, being very similar to that of the artery in thickness.

They also defined four characteristic features of vein used as artery: adventitial thickening, loss of the inner one third of the media, intimal thickening, and loss of the elasticity, producing a fibrous tube.

Between 6 months and 2 years after vein implantation when the normal thickening process usually stops, focal or diffuse cicatrization associated with a decrease in lumen diameter can be observed. These focal stenoses have a special predilection for sites of vein valves and clamp crush injuries. These luminal stenoses are responsible for reduction in blood flow and eventual graft thrombosis.[7] After 2 years, the pathologic changes of atherosclerosis may develop in vein grafts. These changes are focal necrosis, hemorrhage, calcification, and accumulation of lipids and connective tissue. In some cases, especially in animals fed a high-cholesterol diet, the atherosclerotic changes appear earlier in vein grafts than in adjacent arteries. The changes have been observed frequently in aortocoronary vein bypasses implanted in humans. A study of patients over a 10-year period following surgery at the Montreal Heart Institute demonstrated a significant correlation between elevated plasma low-density lipoprotein (LDL) and apoprotein B levels and graft atherosclerosis. This study also confirmed early findings that an increased high-density lipoprotein (HDL) cholesterol level was associated with reduced atherosclerosis in the grafts and adjacent coronary arteries.[8] Only occasionally, vein grafts become aneurysmal instead of stenotic; this change in structure usually happens when the grafts are placed in arteries subjected to high flow.[9]

Since the histologic evaluation of human vein graft over time is usually impossible, the consequences of different preparative techniques have been defined in experimental models that mimic the clinical situation. Among them, the rabbit or dog models of jugular vein implanted into the carotid circulation are the most common.

Both endothelial cells and smooth muscle cells (SMCs) are damaged to a variable extent depending on the method used to prepare the graft. Such factors as trauma at the time of surgery, rough vein harvesting technique, application of clamps, passage of a balloon embolectomy catheter, or use of different valvulotomes affect the degree to which the vein is damaged.[10] Problems with the method of vein graft preparation, such as excessive vein distention, prolonged ischemia, and use of inappropriate irrigating solutions, can also injure the vein wall.[11-13]

Following implantation, the vein graft is subjected to arterial blood pressure and flow, which might increase the damage incurred during graft preparation.[14] Adcock et al.[15] recently published their data from a canine study in which reversed autogenous jugular vein was implanted into carotid artery. Their findings clearly documented that harvesting veins with standard techniques results in nearly 20% endothelial denudation and widespread adhesion of platelets and leukocytes within the first 30 minutes after vein implantation. What is more, an additional 35% of the remaining endothelial cells are ultrastructurally altered. Graft damage is even more apparent during the next 48 hours as endothelial denudation increases to 40% and ultrastructural alterations rise to more than 50%. Degranulated neutrophils and damaged SMCs are present in the edematous media, whereas macrophages are present only in the intima. In the first week after implantation, all grafts show focal endothelial denudation, resulting in direct exposure of subendothelium to the blood. Platelets and leukocytes readily adhere to subendothelial structures. Some researchers have also reported infiltration of the graft media by thrombus and inflammatory cells.[7] Endothelial regeneration is essentially complete 10 days after vein graft implantation, although macrophages remain underneath the endothelium and intimal thickness is almost five times greater than normal.

Our own study, based on a rabbit model, provides similar data.[16,17] Transplantation of the vein is associated with endothelial denudation and subsequent deposition of platelets, microthrombi, and leukocytes. The endothelial layer is restored by proliferation of the remaining viable endothelial cells and is completed by 2 weeks. Interestingly, the endothelial thymidine labeling index, a measure of cellular proliferation, is still elevated at 4 weeks despite the endothelial layer being complete 2 weeks earlier. This may represent the turnover and replacement of endothelial cells that were exposed to high arterial flow and pressure even though frank denudation is not apparent (nondenuding injury). After 12 weeks, endothelial cells return to a quiescent state, suggesting that a stable environment for them has been established. SMCs, recognized as the predominant cell type in the thickened vein wall, continue to proliferate in this system at a high rate even after the endothelial surface has been reestablished. SMC thymidine labeling index is maximal at 1 week and returns to almost normal levels by 12 weeks. Thus intimal thickness developing within the first 4 weeks is the result of rapid proliferation and accumulation of SMCs. Subsequent wall thickening is caused by continued deposition of extracellular matrix. A similar process of early cellular proliferation and late matrix accumulation has been observed in the thickening intima of injured artery.

The vein wall appears to stop increasing in thickness by 12 weeks after implantation. At this point, the ratio of luminal radius-to-wall thickness equals a relatively universal value for arteries. Since static stress equals the product of pressure and luminal radius divided by wall thickness, these results suggest that wall stress might play a role in regulating wall mass. Recent studies in which stress was relieved by an external support corroborates this hypothesis. Kohler, Kirkman, and Clowes[17] found that a rigid polytetrafluoroethylene (PTFE) wrap surrounding a vein graft reduced not only radius–to–wall thickness ratio but also wall area.

The above data suggest that vein grafts have an initial response to injury similar to that of injured arteries and a more chronic, adaptive response, perhaps caused by increased wall stress. Vein grafts adapt to arterial pressure probably in a manner similar to arteries responding to hypertension. When hypertension is induced by aortic coarctation in rats, aortic medial SMCs start to proliferate and contribute to the wall thickening process.

Another mechanical force that may affect vein grafts is shear stress. Several groups have shown experimentally that there is an inverse correlation between intimal hyperplasia and shear stress.[14,18,19] Their observations provide evidence for a localized autoregulatory mechanism that is capable of sensing changes in shear stress and transducing that information into a message to regulate luminal diameter.

SYNTHETIC GRAFT HEALING

The healing pattern in synthetic grafts differs in important ways from that in vein grafts. Unlike vein grafts, synthetic prostheses lack an endothelium and display a markedly thrombogenic surface to the flowing blood. After a synthetic graft is inserted into an arterial bed, the inner surface of the graft is initially lined with a layer of fibrin, platelets, and other blood elements. In animals, depending on the graft material and structure, mesenchymal cells can migrate in from the outside and form a neointima of connective tissue.[20] This does not occur to any extent in humans. Studies on Dacron grafts have shown that the intima, even at late follow-up, is mainly composed of fibrin and platelets.[21] This finding is also supported by indium-111–labeled platelet studies.[22] McCollum et al.[23] used a gamma camera to examine patients receiving platelets labeled with indium-111 at different points in time following aortofemoral graft implantation. They found that as late as 9 years after graft implantation, uptake of indium-111 was still observed. Since platelets can adhere to the graft or arterial wall only if the endothelial layer is absent, these results document that synthetic grafts in humans remain without endothelium for a long period of time and may never heal. The coverage of the inner surface of synthetic grafts by endothelium and subendothelial connective tissue in humans is probably limited to the first few centimeters at either anastomotic end, with the adjacent artery as a source of endothelial cells and SMCs.[21] Why these cells are unable to migrate along the graft for a greater distance is not known. In synthetic grafts, significant intimal thickening composed of endothelium, SMCs, and matrix develops at the anastomoses or just beyond in the distal vessels.[24]

Despite incomplete healing, most prostheses placed in large arteries appear to function well. The 5-year patency rate for fabric prostheses varies depending on the vascular bed. In the aortofemoral area, patency rates range from 85% to 95%,[25] in the axillobifemoral location the range is 70% to 75%,[26] and femorofemoral bypasses yield patency rates from 80% to 85%.[27] If a synthetic graft is used as a conduit for small vessels (e.g., in the femoropopliteal region), its patency rate decreases rapidly. A prospective, randomized study of PTFE grafts and saphenous vein grafts used as femoropopliteal bypasses indicates that the patency rate is almost the same for both types of grafts up to 2 years after surgery. After that, the failure rate is greater in the PTFE group. The failure rate is highest for PTFE grafts inserted into infrapopliteal vessels.[28]

As with vein grafts, it is extremely difficult in humans to document with time course studies the extent of cellular ingrowth and the sequence of postoperative events in PTFE grafts. Studies of animal models are required to get a perspective on this process. Based on the experimental findings in large animals (dog, pig, baboon), two sources of endothelial coverage of the graft

have been described: (1) migrating endothelial cells derived from the cut edge of the adjacent artery and (2) capillaries migrating from the perigraft tissue through the interstices of the graft[29] (Fig. 5-1). In the baboon, the conventional clinically available, low-porosity (30 mm internodal distance) PTFE graft heals by the first mechanism mentioned above.[30,31] Endothelium and SMCs grow in from the cut edges of the host artery. SMCs appear to migrate and to proliferate only underneath the endothelium and not where endothelium is absent. Once endothelial repair has progressed, SMC proliferation slows, except in the region of the anastomosis. Endothelial ingrowth in this baboon model is limited to 2 to 3 cm, even at 1 year after implantation. Consequently, the intimal thickness is greatest at the anastomosis and decreases or is absent in the midportion of the graft. These anastomotic hyperplastic le-

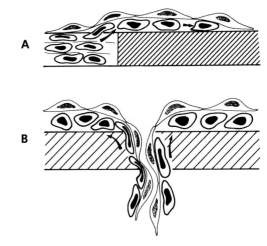

Fig. 5-1. Diagrammatic representation of healing by endothelium (and SMCs) of low-porosity **(A)** and high-porosity **(B)** PTFE grafts. In low-porosity grafts, endothelium is derived from cut edges of adjacent artery and grows as a continuous monolayer toward the center of the graft. In high-porosity grafts, capillaries derived from surrounding granulation tissue penetrate the graft matrix and provide multiple sources of endothelium at the luminal surface. (From Clowes AW, Kirkman TR, Reidy MA. Mechanisms of arterial graft healing. Rapid transmural capillary ingrowth provides a source of intimal endothelium and smooth muscle in porous PTFE prostheses. Am J Pathol 123:220-230, 1986.)

sions are very similar to those seen in vein grafts.

A slight increase in PTFE graft porosity, from 30 to 60 μm internodal distance, dramatically changes the pattern of graft healing.[20,32] Our laboratory has demonstrated that capillaries from granulation tissue surrounding the 60 mm PTFE graft can migrate through the interstices of the graft and provide multiple sources of endothelium at the luminal surface.[20] An endothelial lining is then formed within 2 weeks. SMCs seem to accompany the migrating capillary endothelium, and after reaching the graft surface, they start to proliferate and accumulate to create a thickened intima.

As in the 30 μm PTFE grafts, SMC proliferation and accumulation in the 60 μm grafts occur only under a confluent endothelial layer. This finding is in total opposition to what we have observed in injured arteries. In injured vessels once the endothelium is reestablished, intimal proliferation of SMCs appears to cease.[29]

From the information noted above we might postulate that porosity plays an important role in the completeness of graft healing. Why, then, does the usual, porous, clinical Dacron graft not heal in the same way when used in humans? Zacharias, Kirkman, and Clowes[33] demonstrated that baboon Dacron grafts heal, in fact, by mechanisms similar to those of 60 μm PTFE grafts but at a slower rate; often the coverage is incomplete. Some studies have indicated that Dacron itself has an inhibitory effect on endothelial and SMC proliferation.[34] Higher electronegativity and complement activation by Dacron grafts have been suggested as mechanisms by which Dacron might exert an inhibitory effect on endothelial cell and SMC proliferation and migration, but this process is still unclear.

Why synthetic grafts develop hyperplastic lesions at the anastomotic site continues to be an open question. Some researchers have suggested that a "compliance mismatch" between the mechanical properties of a synthetic graft and host artery is an important factor in the development of subsequent anastomotic intimal hyperplasia.[35] In experimental end-to-end anastomoses, compliance is increased either proximal and distal to the suture line and is decreased at the suture line. However, the peak of the perianastomotic hypercompliant zone is usually located 3.6 mm from the suture line at both sites of anastomosis. Furthermore, it has been proved that the perianastomotic hypercompliant zone corresponds to the region of maximal intimal hyperplasia. Thus compliance mismatch, which creates conditions for greater flow turbulence, may possibly lead to increased endothelial permeability and intimal cell proliferation at the anastomoses.

MECHANISM OF INTIMAL THICKENING

From the observations described above, we can conclude that vascular cell proliferation is an important component in the pathogenesis of the stenosing intimal lesion. Much of our understanding of endothelial cell and SMC growth control in injured arteries and in synthetic and autogenous prostheses comes from studies of animal models as well as from studies of cells in culture.

In normal, undiseased vessels, endothelial cells and SMCs are in a quiescent state, and turnover of these cells is hardly detectable (e.g., in the rat, 0.06%/day).[36] After denudation or when the endothelial layer is disrupted, a stereotyped sequence of events leads to intimal thickening. The denuded surface of the artery is immediately covered by a carpet of platelets and other blood-borne cells. Accumulated platelets release their granules, which contain vasoactive and prothrombotic factors (serotonin, fibrinogen, adenosine diphosphate, von Willebrand factor) as well as growth factors (platelet-derived growth factor [PDGF] and transforming growth factor β [TGF-β]).[37]

Endothelial cells grow from uninjured cells adjacent to the damaged vessel and advance as a broad, growing edge.[38] Migration begins within hours after injury and proliferation starts by 24 hours following injury. When the distance between growing edges is too great, endothelial cells may spontaneously stop migrating and proliferating.[39] In injured rat carotid artery, endothelial regrowth stops within 6 weeks despite the fact that approximately half of the artery is still denuded of endothelium. The factors controlling endothelial growth are being elucidated. It has been recently shown that when replication of endothelial cells is high, the regenerating endothelium is stained strongly with an antibody to basic fibroblast growth factor (bFGF).[40] This finding suggests that bFGF, a major endothelial cell mitogen in vitro, is required for endothelial replication. In fact, the cessation of reendothelialization can be overcome by the systemic administration of bFGF, and total regrowth can be achieved within 10 weeks after arterial injury when bFGF is administered twice a week.[41]

SMCs respond to denudation first by proliferation in the media. About 20% to 40% of SMCs enter the growth fraction by beginning to synthesize DNA (S-phase) approximately 27 hours after injury.[42] These cells continue to proliferate for 7 to 14 days, and after this time they spontaneously stop doing so. Four days after injury, SMCs migrate from the media into the intima and proliferate to form an intimal thickening. In injured rat carotid artery, the midportion of the artery remains without endothelium even at 1 year following injury. SMCs located in this region form a surface that is nonthrombogenic, although it does not look like endothelium. These luminal SMCs continue to proliferate at levels about 10- to 100-

fold higher than SMCs in normal artery.[39] This ongoing proliferation represents cell turnover since the number of SMCs does not change. Intimal thickness doubles between 2 and 12 weeks because of the increase in extracellular matrix (elastin, collagen, proteoglycan).[43,44] SMCs present in intima, which has been covered by regenerating endothelial cells, stop proliferating and become quiescent.

Taken together, these observations support the response-to-injury hypothesis of intimal thickening.[45] This hypothesis proposes that early platelet accumulation on the denuded surface of the artery is followed by the release of growth factors that stimulate proliferation and migration. SMC proliferation is the key event in the development of the intimal lesion. Recent data do not fully support this hypothesis. In some circumstances, especially when endothelial denudation is limited, no SMC proliferation or intimal thickening is observed.[40] On the other hand, the intima is massively thickened despite the absence of platelets and the presence of the endothelium in healing vascular grafts.[29] Moreover, the first wave of medial SMC proliferation occurs in a normal fashion in the injured arteries of rats made thrombocytopenic. The adherence of platelets might not be necessary for early medial SMC prolifera-

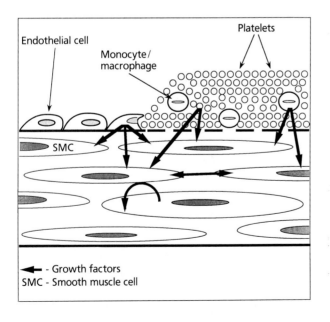

Fig. 5-2. Schematic representation of growth factor expression in developing intimal hyperplastic lesion in injured artery. Platelets, macrophages, injured endothelial cells, and SMCs themselves might release growth factors for SMCs.

tion, but their presence does appear to promote cell migration into the intima and hence strongly influence the formation of the intimal lesion.[46] We still do not know the precise nature of the stimulus that initiates cell growth, but the extent of the trauma to the medial SMCs does correlate with the magnitude of the early proliferative response.

These results bring us to the conclusion that something more than factors from platelets are required for SMC growth. Basic FGF is an important mitogen for SMCs as well as endothelium and is released when cells are disrupted.[47] PDGF and TGF-β are both synthesized by vascular wall cells in culture and potentially could be released at sites of injury.[48,49,49a]

Based on these findings, we have proposed that the factors regulating vascular wall cell growth come from the cells themselves and act in an autocrine or a paracrine manner[29] (Fig. 5-2). We still lack proof of this hypothesis, although recently we have demonstrated that porous PTFE grafts explanted from baboons and perfused ex vivo release PDGF-like mitogen.[50] Furthermore, we have found mRNA for the PDGF genes in the intima of these grafts in the subendothelial regions where SMCs are proliferating.[51] These observations do not prove that the PDGF is actually driving SMC growth. Such proof will depend on a demonstration that proliferation can be blocked with a specific PDGF antagonist. However, preliminary data obtained in studies using pharmacologic doses of recombinant PDGF BB provide evidence that PDGF is probably a SMC growth factor in vivo.[52]

PREVENTION OF INTIMAL HYPERPLASIA

At present, there are three possible ways to prevent intimal hyperplasia: (1) avoid technical errors at the time of surgery, (2) reduce the rate of early thrombosis by using antithrombotic drugs, and (3) employ specific inhibitors of SMC proliferation since, as we have documented, proliferation of SMCs is central to the development of intimal hyperplasia.

Many researchers have demonstrated that intimal hyperplasia can occur despite the best technical effort of surgeons.[3,4,53] Nevertheless,

avoidance of excessive trauma and technical mistakes during surgery will reduce the risk of damage and accumulation of thrombus in the graft. At present, careful follow-up and surgical treatment appear to be extremely important for the prevention of vein graft occlusion. Szilagyi et al.[1] have reported excellent results after surgical repair when graft stenoses were identified and patched before the grafts developed thrombosis. Similarly, Whittemore et al.[4] have demonstrated higher patency rates at 5 years in focally stenotic vein grafts treated surgically with vein patch but without thrombectomy compared with grafts patched after thrombectomy (86% vs. 19%). Hence, a surveillance program should be conducted to identify and to correct stenosing lesions before they cause thrombosis. When this is done assiduously, long-term patency of vein grafts is excellent.

Any form of arterial reconstruction involves some degree of injury. Consequently, platelets and fibrin form at the luminal surface and might play an important role in the development of intimal thickening. Thus it is reasonable to predict that such drugs as aspirin and dipyridamole, which affect cyclooxygenase, prostaglandin synthesis, and platelet aggregation, might also affect graft thrombosis. Aspirin inhibits platelet aggregation by blocking cyclooxygenase and the production of thromboxane A_2 in platelets. Cyclooxygenase has also been found in endothelial cells, where it is responsible for prostacyclin (thromboxane antagonist) generation. Although endothelial cyclooxygenase can be inactivated by aspirin, it is less sensitive than the platelet enzyme and can be rapidly regenerated.[54] Dipyridamole, by inhibiting phosphodiesterase, increases the platelet content of cyclic adenosine monophosphate (cAMP). cAMP appears to stabilize platelets and decrease their adhesion, aggregation, and release of granules.[55]

The available data suggest that if the administration of these drugs is begun just before surgery and continued into the postoperative period, there is an improvement in patency, whereas if the administration of the drugs is delayed, there is no benefit.[56,57] Several clinical studies have proved that aspirin and dipyridamole are very effective in reducing coronary bypass graft failure by approximately 10%.[54] In contrast, clinical and animal studies of the effects of antithrombotic drugs on intimal thickening in either injured arteries or vascular grafts have been inconclusive.[54] These observations suggest that these drugs prevent acute graft occlusion or the early accumulation of thrombus, but their effect on intimal hyperplasia is still uncertain.

Several drugs commonly used for the treatment of other clinical disorders inhibit SMC proliferation. Two of these drugs, heparin and angiotensin-converting enzyme (ACE) inhibitors (e.g., cilazapril), are nearly ready for clinical application. Heparin inhibits SMC proliferation and migration both in vitro and in vivo.[58,59] According to the currently available data, heparin acts to inhibit SMC growth in the prereplicative (G1) phase.[60] What is also interesting is that heparin does not appear to inhibit endothelial cell proliferation and migration; in fact, it may have a stimulatory effect. In animal models of arterial injury, it appears that a short-term heparin treatment produces long-term inhibition of SMC growth. Similar data from human studies are still lacking. In synthetic grafts in which the stimulus for proliferation is of a more chronic nature, heparin might need to be administered over a period of time. Heparin also acts on matrix accumulation in the intima of injured arteries.

Recently, Powell et al.[61] have shown that cilazapril (an ACE inhibitor) inhibits SMC proliferation. They administered cilazapril to normotensive rats in which the carotid artery was injured. Neointimal formation 14 days after denudation was decreased by approximately 80% in treated rats. It is known that the components of the renin-angiotensin system exist in the artery wall and that angiotensin II may be a cofactor for SMC growth.[62,63] It is possible that ACE inhibitors suppress the vascular response to injury by interrupting the conversion of angiotensin I to the active angiotensin II, thus preventing SMC proliferation. This finding supports the hypothesis that the local angiotensin system does have a role in the intimal proliferative response of the vascular wall to injury. Alternatively, the effect of the ACE inhibitor might be caused by some other systemic response. Calcium channel blockers as well as α_1-adrenergic antagonists (e.g., prazosin) can also inhibit SMC proliferation and development of intimal hyperplasia.[64,65]

Finally, gene therapy has been proposed as a radically new approach to the control of intimal hyperplasia.[66] This technique will allow for the introduction of an "inhibitory gene" into vascular wall cells. These transfected cells might then be seeded on grafts or into injured vessels and synthesize and release the product of the inhibitory gene locally. The work of Dichek et al.[67] provides a possible clinical example of gene therapy. They transfected sheep vascular endothelial cells with a gene encoding for human tissue-type plasminogen activator, and subsequently these cells were seeded on an intraarterial stent coated with fibronectin. The transfected cells then expressed significant amounts of plasminogen activator. One could image a similar strategy for the control of intimal SMC hyperplasia in the near future.

REFERENCES

1. Szilagyi DE, Hageman JH, Smith RF, et al. Autogenous vein grafting in femoropopliteal atherosclerosis: The limit of its effectiveness. Surgery 86:836-851, 1979.
2. Bourassa MG, Enjalbert M, Campeau L, et al. Progression of atherosclerosis in coronary arteries and bypass grafts: Ten years later. Am J Cardiol 53:102C-107C, 1984.
3. Szilagyi DE, Elliott JP, Hageman JH, et al. Biologic fate of autogenous vein implants as arterial substitutes. Clinical, angiographic and histopathologic observations in femoro-popliteal operations for atherosclerosis. Ann Surg 178:232-246, 1973.
4. Whittemore AD, Clowes AW, Couch NP, et al. Secondary femoropopliteal reconstruction. Ann Surg 193:35-42, 1981.
5. Carrel A, Guthrie CC. Results of the biterminal transplantation of veins. Am J Med Sci 132:415-422, 1906.
6. Carrel A, Guthrie CC. Uniterminal and biterminal venous transplantations. Surg Gynecol Obstet 2:226-286, 1906.
7. Dilley JR, McGeachie JK, Prendergast FJ. A review of the histologic changes in vein-to-artery grafts, with particular reference to intimal hyperplasia. Arch Surg 123:691-696, 1988.
8. Campeau L, Enjalbert M, Lesperance J, et al. The relation of risk factors to the development of atherosclerosis in saphenous-vein bypass grafts and the progression of disease in the native circulation. N Engl J Med 311:1329-1332, 1984.

9. Stanley JC, Ernst CB, Fry WJ. Fate of 100 aortorenal vein grafts. Characteristics of late graft expansion, aneurysmal dilatation and stenosis. Surgery 74:931-944, 1973.

10. DePalma RG, Chidi CC, Sternfeld WC, et al. Pathogenesis and prevention of trauma provoked atheromas. Surgery 83:429-437, 1977.

11. Abbott WM, Wieland BS, Austen WG. Structural changes during preparation of autogenous venous grafts. Surgery 76:1031-1040, 1974.

12. Bonchek LI. Prevention of endothelial damage during preparation of saphenous veins for bypass grafting. J Thorac Cardiovasc Surg 79:911-915, 1980.

13. Ramos JR, Berger K, Mansfield PB, et al. Histologic fate and endothelial changes of distended vein grafts. Ann Surg 183:205-228, 1976.

14. Faulkner SL, Fisher RD, Conkle DM, et al. Effect of blood flow rate on subendothelial proliferation in venous autografts used as arterial substitutes. Circulation 51/52 (Suppl 1):163-172, 1975.

15. Adcock GD, Adcock OT, Wheeler JR, et al. Arterialization of reversed autogenous vein grafts: Quantitative light and electron microscopy of canine jugular vein grafts harvested and implanted by standard or improved techniques. J Vasc Surg 6:283-295, 1987.

16. Zwolak RM, Adams MC, Clowes AW. Kinetics of vein graft hyperplasia: Association with tangential stress. J Vasc Surg 5:126-136, 1987.

17. Kohler TR, Kirkman TR, Clowes AW. The effect of rigid external support on vein graft adaptation to the arterial circulation. J Vasc Surg 9:277-285, 1989.

18. Karayannacos PE, Rittgers SE, Kakos GS, et al. Potential role of velocity and wall tension in vein graft failure. J Cardiovasc Surg 21:171-178, 1980.

19. Rittgers SE, Karayannacos PE, Guy JR, et al. Velocity distribution and intimal proliferation in autologous vein grafts in dogs. Circ Res 42:792-801, 1978.

20. Clowes AW, Kirkman TR, Reidy MA. Mechanism of arterial graft healing: Rapid transmural capillary ingrowth provides a source of intimal endothelium and smooth muscle in porous PTFE prostheses. Am J Pathol 123:220-230, 1986.

21. Berger K, Sauvage LR, Rao AM, et al. Healing of arterial prostheses in man: Its incompleteness. Ann Surg 175:118-127, 1972.

22. Stratton JR, Thiele BL, Ritchie JL. Platelet deposition on Dacron aortic bifurcation grafts in man. Quantitation with indium 111 platelet imaging. Circulation 66:1287-1296, 1982.

23. McCollum CN, Kester RC, Rajah SM, et al. Arterial graft maturation. The duration of thrombotic activity in Dacron aortofemoral grafts measured by platelet and fibrinogen kinetics. Br J Surg 68:61-64, 1981.

24. LoGerfo FW, Quist WC, Nowak MD, et al. Downstream anastomotic hyperplasia. A mechanism of failure in Dacron arterial grafts. Ann Surg 197:479-485, 1983.

25. Szilagyi DE, Smith RF, Elliot JP, et al. Long-term behavior of a Dacron arterial substitute. Ann Surg 162:453-459, 1965.

26. Johnson WC, LoGerfo FW, Vollman RW, et al. Is axillo-bilateral femoral graft an effective substitute for aortic-bilateral iliac-femoral graft? An analysis of ten years' experience. Ann Surg 186:123-130, 1977.

27. Mannick JA, Maini BS. Femoro-femoral grafting. Indications and late results. Am J Surg 136:190-196, 1978.

28. Veith FJ, Gupta SK, Ascer E, et al. Six year prospective multicenter randomized comparison of autologous saphenous vein and expanded polytetrafluoroethylene grafts in infrainguinal arterial reconstructions. J Vasc Surg 3:104-111, 1986.

29. Clowes AW, Reidy MA. Mechanisms of arterial graft failure: The role of cellular proliferation. Ann NY Acad Sci 516:673-678, 1987.

30. Clowes AW, Gown AM, Hanson SR, et al. Mechanisms of arterial graft failure. I. Role of cellular proliferation in early healing of PTFE prostheses. Am J Pathol 118:43-54, 1985.

31. Clowes AW, Kirkman TR, Clowes MM. Mechanisms of graft failure. II. Chronic endothelial and smooth muscle cell proliferation in healing polytetrafluoroethylene prostheses. J Vasc Surg 3:877-884, 1986.

32. Golden MA, Hanson SR, Kirkman TR, et al. Healing of polytetrafluoroethylene arterial grafts is influenced by graft porosity. J Vasc Surg 11:838-845, 1990.

33. Zacharias RK, Kirkman TR, Clowes AW. Mechanism of healing in synthetic grafts. J Vasc Surg 6:429-436, 1987.

34. Greisler HP, Schwarcz TH, Ellinger J, et al. Dacron inhibition of arterial regenerative activities. J Vasc Surg 3:747-756, 1986.

35. Hasson JE, Megerman J, Abbott WM. Increased compliance near vascular anastomoses. J Vasc Surg 2:419-423, 1985.

36. Clowes AW, Reidy MA, Clowes MM. Kinetics of cellular proliferation after arterial injury. I. Smooth muscle growth in the absence of endothelium. Lab Invest 49:208-216, 1983.

37. Bowen-Pope DF, Ross R, Seifert RA. Locally acting growth factors for vascular smooth muscle cells. Endogenous synthesis and release from platelets. Circulation 72:735-742, 1985.

38. Reidy MA. A reassessment of endothelial injury and arterial lesion formation. Lab Invest 53:513-522, 1985.

39. Clowes AW, Clowes MM, Reidy MA. Kinetics of cellular proliferation after arterial injury. III. Endothelial and smooth muscle growth in chronically denuded vessels. Lab Invest 54:295-304, 1986.

40. Lindner V, Reidy MA, Fingerle J. Regrowth of arterial endothelium. Denudation with minimal trauma leads to complete endothelial cell regrowth. Lab Invest 61:556-563, 1989.

41. Lindner V, Majack RA, Reidy MA. Basic fibroblast factor stimulates endothelial regrowth and proliferation in denuded arteries. J Clin Invest 85:2004-2008, 1990.

42. Clowes AW, Schwartz SM. Significance of quiescent smooth muscle migration in the injured rat carotid artery. Circ Res 56:139-146, 1985.

43. Clowes AW, Reidy MA, Clowes MM. Mechanisms of stenosis after arterial injury. Lab Invest 49:208-218, 1983.

44. Falcone DJ, Hajjar DP, Minick CR. Lipoprotein and albumin accumulation in re-endothelialized and de-endothelialized aorta. Am J Pathol 114:112-117, 1984.

45. Ross R, Glomset J. The pathogenesis of atherosclerosis. N Engl J Med 295:369-377, 1976.

46. Fingerle J, Johnson R, Clowes AW, et al. Role of platelets in smooth muscle cell proliferation and migration after vascular injury in rat carotid artery. Proc Natl Acad Sci USA 86:8412-8416, 1989.

47. Gospodarowicz D, Neufeld G, Schweigerer L. Fibroblast growth factor review. Mol Cell Endocrinol 46:187-195, 1986.

48. DiCorleto PE, Bowen-Pope DF. Cultured endothelial cells produce a platelet-derived growth factor–like protein. Proc Natl Acad Sci USA 80:1919-1923, 1983.

49. Sporn MD, Roberts AB, Wakefield LM, et al. Some recent advances in the chemistry and biology of transforming growth factor-b. J Cell Biol 105:1039-1045, 1987.

49a. Sjolund M, Hedin U, Sejersen T, et al. Arterial smooth muscle cells express platelet-derived growth factor (PDGF), a chain mRNA, secrete a PDGF-like mitogen, and bind exogenous PDGF in a phenotype- and growth state–dependent manner. J Cell Biol 106:403-413, 1988.

50. Zacharias RK, Kirkman TR, Kenagy RD, et al. Growth factor production by polytetrafluoroethylene vascular grafts. J Vasc Surg 7:606-610, 1988.

51. Golden MA, Au YPT, Kenagy RD, et al. Growth factor gene expression by intimal cells in healing polytetrafluoroethylene grafts. J Vasc Surg 11:580-585, 1990.

52. Jawien A, Lindner V, Bowen-Pope DF, et al. Platelet-derived growth factor (PDGF) stimulates arterial smooth muscle cell proliferation in vivo [abstr]. FASEB J 4:A342, 1990.

53. Bandyk DF, Kaebnick HW, Stewart GW, et al. Durability of the in situ saphenous vein arterial bypass: A comparison of primary and secondary patency. J Vasc Surg 5:256-268, 1987.

54. Clowes AW. The role of aspirin in enhancing arterial graft patency. J Vasc Surg 3:381-388, 1986.

55. Fitzgerald GA. Dipyridamole. N Engl J Med 316:1247-1249, 1987.

56. Clyne CAC, Archer TJ, Aterhaire KK, et al. Randomized control of a short course of aspirin and dipyridamole (Persantine) for femorodistal grafts. Br J Surg 74:246-248, 1987.

57. Kohler TR, Kaufman JL, Kacoyanis G, et al. Effect of aspirin and dipyridamole on the patency of lower extremity bypass grafts. Surgery 96:462-466, 1984.

58. Clowes AW, Karnovsky MJ. Suppression by heparin of smooth muscle cell proliferation in injured arteries. Nature 265:625-626, 1977.

59. Clowes AW, Clowes MM. Regulation of smooth muscle proliferation by heparin in vitro and in vivo. Int Angiol 6:45-51, 1987.

60. Clowes AW, Clowes MM. Inhibition of smooth cell proliferation by heparin molecules. Transplant Proc 21:3700-3701, 1989.

61. Powell JS, Clozel JP, Muller RKM, et al. Inhibitors of angiotensin-converting enzyme prevent myointimal proliferation after vascular injury. Science 245:186-188, 1989.

62. Campbell DJ. Circulating and tissue angiotensin systems. J Clin Invest 79:1-6, 1987.

63. Ullian ME, Linas SL. Role of receptor cycling in the regulation of angiotensin II surface receptor number and angiotensin II uptake in rat vascular smooth muscle cells. J Clin Invest 84:840-846, 1989.

64. Jackson CL, Bush RC, Bowyer DE. Inhibitory effect of calcium antagonists on balloon catheter–induced arterial smooth muscle cell proliferation and lesion size. Atherosclerosis 69:115-122, 1988.

65. O'Malley MK, McDermott EWM, Mehigan D, et al. Role for prazosin in reducing the development of rabbit intimal hyperplasia after endothelial denudation. Br J Surg 76:936-938, 1989.

66. Callow AD. The vascular endothelial cell as a vehicle for gene therapy. J Vasc Surg 11:793-798, 1990.

67. Dichek DA, Neville RF, Zwiebel JA, et al. Seeding of intravascular stents with genetically engineered endothelial cells. Circulation 80:1347-1353, 1989.

6

The Healing Characteristics, Durability, and Long-Term Complications of Vascular Prostheses

Glenn C. Hunter   David A. Bull

Arterial and venous autografts remain the materials of choice to replace diseased or damaged blood vessels. However, because of their limited supply, there is an increasing need to develop arterial substitutes that are durable, are readily incorporated by host tissues, possess a non- or hypothrombogenic flow surface, have compliance characteristics that closely approximate the native vessel, are resistant to infection, and are easily sutured.[1,2] Although none of the currently available prostheses manifests all of the desired characteristics of the ideal arterial replacement, large-diameter Dacron grafts used to replace the abdominal aorta have proved adequate, with 5-year cumulative patency rates of 85% to 90%.[3,4] Unfortunately, the longevity of small-diameter prosthetic grafts (6 mm in internal diameter or less) is limited by the development of anastomotic intimal hyperplasia and consequent thromboses of the grafts. When prosthetic grafts such as those fabricated from polytetrafluoroethylene are placed at sites above or below the knee, typical 5-year patency rates are approximately 50% and 30%, respectively.[5-7]

The increasing longevity of the population and the more frequent execution of bypass procedures to the more distal vessels of the extremity have resulted in increases in both the number and complexity of the bypass procedures now performed. It is estimated that approximately one third of patients will require additional surgery related to their bypass graft within 2 years of the initial procedure.[8] Furthermore, complications resulting from errors in technique or deterioration of the graft fabric are not uncommon and the risk of reoperation is increased substantially by the progression of ischemic heart disease and other associated atherosclerotic risk factors in these patients. Reoperative mortality rates of up to 5% and major limb loss rates of 20% recently have been reported.[9] As a consequence patients in whom complications related to their grafts develop may be unable to withstand the secondary operations needed to replace them. These changes in the demographics of the patients requiring repeated arterial reconstructive procedures and the limited supply of autogenous graft material have increased the need for durable arterial substitutes that will continue to function satisfactorily throughout the remaining life span of the patient.

In this chapter we discuss the fabrication, healing characteristics, clinical indications, and complications related to grafts fabricated from polyethylene terephthalate (Dacron), polytetrafluoroethylene (PTFE), and the commonly used biologic grafts—human umbilical vein grafts and bovine xenografts.

DACRON GRAFTS

Dacron is the most common prosthetic material used to replace diseased segments of the aorta and its major branches. Although there are numerous variations in construction, all Dacron grafts can be grouped into several major categories: woven vs. knitted and smooth or veloured surfaces. Woven grafts have functioned satisfactorily when used for repair of thoracic and abdominal aortic aneurysms, aortic replacement in patients with known bleeding diatheses, or in the occasional patient who bleeds through the interstices of a preclotted knitted graft immediately after restoration of flow. Knitted grafts are used to bypass occlusive lesions of the aorta, and the iliac, common femoral, and superficial femoral arteries. They also have been used successfully for axillofemoral or femorofemoral bypass grafting.

Long-term patency rates of 85% to 90% for aortoiliac or aortofemoral bypass grafts and patency rates of 60% to 70% for axillofemoral and above-knee femoropopliteal bypass grafts have been reported.[3-5,10,11]

Fabrication

A knowledge of the fabrication of Dacron grafts is essential for an understanding of the factors that influence healing and/or contribute to the late failure of these grafts.

Woven

Woven grafts constructed by interlacing two sets of yarn at right angles to each other are the strongest prosthetic fabric grafts. About 45% of grafts implanted each year fall into this category.[1,2] Nonveloured woven grafts are dimensionally stable, relatively impervious to blood, noncompliant, and of high tensile strength. However, they are difficult to suture and tend to fray at their cut edges. The velour component, which can be added to woven grafts by incorporating additional nontextured yarns that are interlaced less frequently than the textured ground yarns, permits a reduction in tightness of the weave without altering permeability. This results in a softer graft that is easier to suture.

Knitted

Knitted grafts are of two basic types and are constructed with a set of yarns that are interlooped rather than interlaced. Weft-knitted grafts are formed from one set of yarns interlocked in a circular fashion; warp-knitted grafts are fabricated from several sets of yarns interlooped in a zigzag pattern. Warp-knitted grafts, although more compliant than woven grafts, are less compliant than weft-knitted grafts. Unlike woven grafts they do not run, unravel, or fray at their cut edges.

Even though the walls of knitted grafts are thicker than woven (600 vs. 200 μm), they are more porous because of their construction and as a result readily permit cellular ingrowth through their interstices.[2] The interlooping yarns used in the construction of knitted grafts permit greater expansion of the yarn in the circumferential direction than longitudinally and consequently they have reduced dimensional stability and a tendency to dilate.[1]

Unlike woven grafts the greater porosity of knitted grafts requires that they be made impervious to blood before implantation. This can be achieved either (1) by preclotting the graft with blood[2] or by coating the luminal surface with bovine collagen,[12] gelatin,[13] or albumin,[14] or (2) by autoclaving the graft in albumin or blood (as advocated by Bethea and Reemsta[15] and modified by Cooley et al.[16]). The use of sealant-coated grafts has proved to be particularly advantageous when replacing portions of the thoracic aorta or when repairing ruptured aortic aneurysms in which intraoperative interstitial and anastomotic bleeding are important causes of morbidity and mortality. Although histologically coated grafts appear to have superior healing characteristics compared with noncoated ones, interstitial bleeding occurring immediately after implantation and requiring replacement with an impervious graft has been observed occasionally. The use of albumin-coated grafts also has been associated with inconsistencies in graft porosity and dissection or embolism of the albumin layer.

Healing Characteristics

The body attempts to incorporate the implanted Dacron graft by two distinct cellular processes: (1) *anastomotic pannus ingrowth*, which extends approximately 1 cm from the divided artery and is composed of smooth muscle and endothelial cells derived from components of the arterial wall and (2) *perigraft fibrous tissue*, which encircles the entire external surface of the graft, resulting in encapsulation of the graft. Anastomotic pannus ingrowth, however, does not possess any significant intrinsic tensile strength; hence the anastomotic bond between graft and artery is entirely dependent on the suture material for its integrity. Cells from the outer fibrous capsule readily invade the interstices of the graft but seldom penetrate beyond the midportion of the wall of the prosthesis.[17-19] The addition of a veloured component to these grafts to enhance cellular ingrowth may induce excessive proliferation of perivascular fibrous tissue, which decreases the compliance of the graft or contributes to stenosis of an adjacent structure.

The flow surface of a well-healed patent graft is characterized by a layer of compacted, relatively acellular hypothrombogenic pseudointima, which is uniformly present except in areas adjacent to anastomoses or at bifurcations.[8] If initially a prosthesis of too large a diameter has been used or if the diameter of the prosthesis has increased substantially over time, the thickness of this layer tends to increase so that the lumen of the graft approximates in size that of the outflow vessel. The addition of an internal velour lining may further increase the thickness of this layer and contribute to the ultimate failure of the graft. Poor healing characterized by incomplete covering of the luminal surface has been observed in explants from diabetic patients and those in poor general health.[8]

Guidoin et al.[18] noted that the differences in the healing characteristics among the various types of Dacron prostheses could be related only to the varying thicknesses of the internal fibrous pseudointimal layer and of the external capsule. The thicknesses of the inner and external linings of the grafts were minimal with woven grafts, moderate in knitted grafts, and greatest for grafts with veloured surfaces.[18]

In a histologic evaluation of collagen-coated graft explants in humans, Anderson[19] has observed that the collagen component remains intact for up to 8 days after implantation. Grafts removed beyond 1 year were characterized by a cellular pseudointimal layer with numerous capillary loops and periadventitial infiltration of the graft. Although the number of explants evaluated was not stated, these findings suggest that healing in collagen-coated grafts may be accelerated. However, further long-term studies are necessary to confirm these preliminary observations.

Associated Complications

To date there have been no systematic follow-up studies of all Dacron grafts in otherwise asymptomatic patients; most of the reports in the literature are confined to anecdotal case studies of complications. The noninfectious complications associated with the implantation of these prostheses include (1) dilatation, (2) anastomotic stenosis, (3) ureteric obstruction, and (4) neoplasia. Ninety percent of such failures are believed to occur within the first 3 to 5 years after implantation.

Dilatation

Dilatation, defined as a permanent increase in the diameter of a graft caused by pulsating stresses, has been reported with both arterial homografts and prosthetic grafts used as arterial conduits.[1,20-30] Dilatation may involve the entire length of the graft or be confined to isolated portions, resulting in diffuse or focal aneurysmal change. Significant dilatation of implanted grafts has been documented with all currently available prosthetic materials, including knitted and woven Dacron, nylon, Teflon, Orlon, and PTFE.[22-30] However, dilatation is more commonly observed with knitted Dacron because of its inherent structural properties and its more frequent use as an arterial substitute (Fig. 6-1). Woven grafts have a high initial modulus and therefore are resistant to extension compared with knitted grafts that have very little resistance to extension because of their loop structure. Consequently, their interlocking loops straighten very easily in the direction of greatest stress, resulting in an increase in diameter. The incidence of graft dilatation reported in the literature, ranging from 1% to 3%, probably underestimates the true incidence since only symptomatic patients are likely to undergo imaging.[31,32]

In a 30-year review of 390 cases of graft failure, Pourdeyhimi and Wagner[1] found dilatation in 147 (38%), structural defects in 76 (20%), suture line defects in 56 (14%), and graft infection or bleeding in 30 (8.9%). These complications often are interrelated because graft dilatation may predispose the patient to pseudoaneurysm formation, perforation, or rupture.

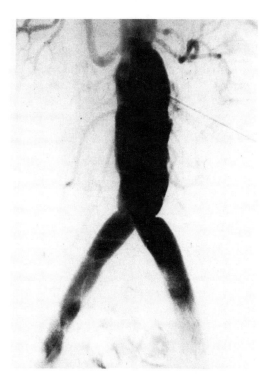

Fig. 6-1. Translumbar aortogram demonstrating a dilated Dacron aortofemoral graft with irregularity of the wall.

Using Doppler ultrasound, Nunn, Freeman, and Hudgins[33] studied 95 Dacron aortic grafts implanted for periods ranging from 2 weeks to 138 months in symptomatic patients. They observed dilatation ranging from 0% to 84% (mean, 17.6%) in 85 of the 95 grafts. Dilatation appeared more pronounced in hypertensive patients (21% vs. 15%). Lundqvist et al.,[34] in a study comparing 36 patients with symptomatic graft dilatation and 65 asymptomatic patients, detected graft dilatation of between 25% and 50% in 42 of 101 patients (42%) evaluated. In 12 patients the diameter of the dilated graft exceeded the preimplantation diameter by more than 50%. Four of these patients had false aneurysms. Furthermore, the incidence of dilatation was greater in symptomatic patients, who also had a higher incidence of false aneurysm formation compared with asymptomatic patients (14% vs. 3%).

Etiology. Permanent deformation of the fabric structure and fatigue of the yarn appear to be important factors in the pathogenesis of graft dilatation. Dilatation of 10% to 22% occurs when knitted grafts are bench tested at static pressures of 120 to 200 mm Hg for 1 minute.[1] This corresponds to the initial dilatation seen when these grafts are exposed to arterial pressure. Whether this increase in diameter reflects restoration of the initial diameter (reduced by chemicals and heat used during the crimping process) or simply represents straightening of the interlacing loop structure is unclear. Although bench testing is a fairly reliable predictor of early dilatation, it does not accurately predict late dilatation related to fiber elongation or yarn fatigue.

A number of factors are believed to contribute to deformation of fabric structure and yarn fatigue of Dacron grafts. They include hypertension,[33] mechanical or chemical degradation of Dacron fibers,[35-38] undetected flaws from the manufacturing process,[32,39] and damage inflicted by the injudicious application of instruments intraoperatively or by repeated sterilization. The contribution of any one of these factors to failure of a given graft often is difficult to ascertain in the individual patient.

In a comprehensive review of Dacron graft explants removed at autopsy or reoperation, the most consistent finding observed by Guidoin[8] was a time-dependent loss of stitch density found in all prostheses examined. The rate of loss of stitch density depends on the type of fabric construction. Weft-knitted fabrics therefore would be less stable than the warp-knitted ones. As a result of this loss of stitch density, the fabric is susceptible to irreversible dilatation when exposed to arterial blood pressure. Clagett et al.[39] observed a similar loss in stitch density in five patients with dilated grafts. Of considerable interest is the size of the grafts implanted in the patients Clagett et al. studied. The diameters of the grafts used were 19 × 9.5 mm (four patients) and 25 × 12.5 mm (one patient), considerably larger than would be chosen today. One can only speculate as to the contribution of initial graft size to eventual failure.

Chemical biodegradation may further exacerbate the dilatation initially induced by a loss of stitch density. King et al.,[37] in a study of 19 explanted Dacron prostheses in residence for

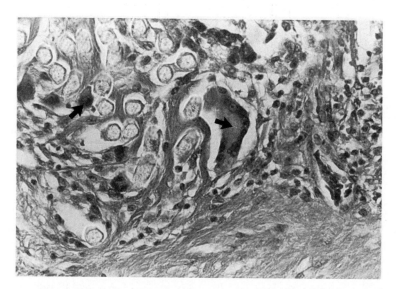

Fig. 6-2. Photomicrograph of the outer surface of a Dacron graft covered with a layer of firmly adherent connective tissue. Foreign body giant cells and macrophages surrounding Dacron fibers are present (original magnification ×50).

intervals ranging from a few hours to 14 years, examined the prostheses using infrared spectroscopy and observed a loss of molecular weight and an increase in the content of carboxyl groups that were proportional to the duration of implantation. It has been postulated that immunologically active macrophages and monocytes that infiltrate the graft as part of the healing process may contribute to chemical deterioration of these grafts by recruitment of biologically active cells that ingest the individual Dacron fibers[38] (Fig. 6-2).

Variations in the fabrication of grafts also have been implicated in cases of late fiber deterioration and graft dilatation. In a study of 493 grafts, Berger and Sauvage[32] found that graft dilatation between 17% and 43% was present in 15 cases that had been implanted for 3 to 15.3 years. The authors postulated that reductions in fiber diameter and/or acute breaks of individual filaments resulting from overheating during the crimping process, frictional wear, or biodegradation were responsible for these changes.

Finally, damage to the graft can occur during implantation from careless handling with instruments or improper resterilization. Isolated areas of damaged fibers suggestive of vascular clamp injury have been observed in graft explants.[8] Thus careful handling during implantation is essential to avoid damage that may increase later susceptibility to deterioration.[32]

Diagnosis. Dilatation of Dacron grafts appears to be a biphasic phenomenon. Early dilatation of approximately 10% to 22%, commencing immediately after the graft is exposed to arterial blood pressure, plateaus within the first year.[1] Late dilatation, caused by yarn slippage or breakage, usually is seen within 2 to 3 years of implantation. Because of the biphasic nature of graft dilatation, evaluation of abnormal dilatation appears unwarranted within the first year after implantation of the graft since this early dilatation is largely attributed to restoration of the initial diameter of the graft. Late graft dilatation, however, is progressive. Once detected, such patients should be carefully monitored for life.

Ultrasound. B-mode ultrasound is widely available, relatively inexpensive, and particularly useful for assessing early and late complications of vascular grafts. Gooding, Effeney, and Goldstone,[40] in a study of 87 patients with aortofemoral grafts, were able to successfully image the anastomotic sites in 84% of the grafts. The authors discovered 23 unsuspected anastomotic aneurysms (2 aortic and 21 femoral) and perigraft accumulation of fluid or blood was observed in 16 patients. In a study of 127 patients with Dacron grafts, Clifford et al.,[41] using Doppler imaging and real-time ultrasound, found graft dilatation of 15% to 70% in five grafts. More recently we have studied patients with dilated grafts using color Doppler imaging and have observed nonlaminar turbulent flow patterns within the grafts reminiscent of those seen in patients with aortic aneurysms. Although this may explain the progressive increase in the neointimal lining in these grafts, to date relatively few patients have been studied and no definitive conclusions can be drawn.

Ideally, follow-up ultrasound scans of all asymptomatic aortofemoral grafts should be performed at 1 year and annually thereafter. If no significant alteration in the diameter of the prosthesis is identified within 5 years of implantation, it seems unlikely that significant dilatation will occur and the frequency of follow-up can be reduced. However, once dilatation has been detected, continuing surveillance is indicated to detect anastomotic aneurysms or an increase in luminal neointima, either of which may threaten the long-term patency of the graft.

Computed tomography. Contrast-enhanced computed tomography (CT) is helpful in accurately assessing the size of anastomotic aneurysms and in excluding other complications such as perigraft collections of fluid or air. Unlike ultrasound, CT can be used to evaluate grafts implanted in the abdomen or chest (Fig. 6-3). Qvarfordt et al.[42] and Brown et al.[43] have described the usefulness of CT scans for detecting early and late complications of prosthetic grafts. However, cost and attendant radiation exposure make CT less desirable for routine follow-up. CT should be limited to the evaluation of symptomatic patients or for those instances in which ultrasound examination fails to adequately delineate the graft.

Complications. Progressive increases in diameter of prosthetic grafts have been implicated in anastomotic aneurysm formation, thrombosis, and rupture of the affected grafts.[34,39,44] Embolization from a dilated graft containing laminated luminal thrombus also must be considered a potential risk; however, the frequency of this event is a matter of speculation since its occurrence has not been well documented in the literature.

Anastomotic aneurysms. Anastomotic aneurysms associated with dilated grafts, which may occur at the artery-graft anastomosis of the aorta or in the groin, may be indicative of true aneurysmal dilatation of the host vessel or, alternatively, pseudoaneurysm formation resulting from partial or complete separation of the graft from the adjacent arterial wall.

The reported incidence of anastomotic aneurysms is about 1% to 2% but the true incidence is more difficult to assess because asymptomatic patients seldom are evaluated.[45] True aortic aneurysms, which occur proximal to prosthetic grafts implanted in the distal aorta, should be distinguished from aneurysms that occur at the site of end-to-side anastomoses between an endarterectomized or unrecognized aneurysmal aorta. Similarly, anastomotic aneurysmal dilatation of the host vessel may occur with end-to-side anastomoses to the iliac or common femoral arteries. In all of these the problem is dilatation of the host vessel and not disruption of the anastomosis. By contrast, anastomotic pseudoaneurysms are far more common. These involve femoral anastomoses in more than 80% of cases. A number of etiologic factors, including weakness of the arterial

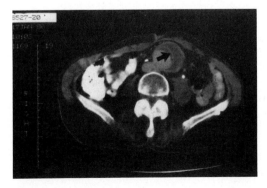

Fig. 6-3. Abdominal CT scan demonstrating a dilated graft (arrow) and the surrounding thrombus from an aortic anastomotic aneurysm.

wall (31%), hypertension (27%), mechanical factors (12%), graft deterioration (12%), impaired wound healing (8%), endarterectomy (7%), and suture failure (3%), have been implicated in a comprehensive study by Szilagyi et al.[45] Here we focus on the contribution of graft dilatation to the development of anastomotic pseudoaneurysms (Figs. 6-4 and 6-5).

How may dilatation of the prosthesis contribute to the development of anastomotic pseudoaneurysms? First, since knitted grafts dilate initially by 10% to 22%, selection of too large a graft may be an important contributing factor. The diameter of the limbs of the graft should approximate that of the outflow vessel. A graft-to-vessel ratio of 1.2 to 1.4:1, as suggested by the experimental studies of Kinley et al.,[46] may be too generous in view of the inherent propensity of knitted grafts to dilate.

The portion of the graft close to the suture line may fail from yarn slippage or breakage. Yarn slippage is common with woven grafts, especially if they are cut on a bias as is commonly done when performing end-to-side anastomoses. Careful placement of sutures and heat sealing of the cut edges may minimize slippage of the yarn. Yarn breakage is associated more commonly with weft-knitted grafts and can be minimized by increasing the number of strands used during fabrication of the graft.

Dilatation and anastomotic aneurysms often occur in association.[39,44] Kim et al.[44] observed significant graft dilatation ranging from 50% to 150% in the patients they studied. Anastomotic aneurysms were present in all instances. Perhaps suture line stress, minimal when the graft-to-artery ratio is 1.4:1 or less, increases progressively as the graft enlarges. Also, as the graft increases in diameter, it has a tendency to shorten in length, thereby increasing suture line tension even further. Courbier and Aboukhater[47] recently have hypothesized that scarring, caused by the graft exiting beneath the inguinal ligament, may be an additional contributing factor. They recommend prophylactic division of the inguinal ligament. We do not concur with this theory. Although the majority of grafts adhere to the inguinal ligament, most do

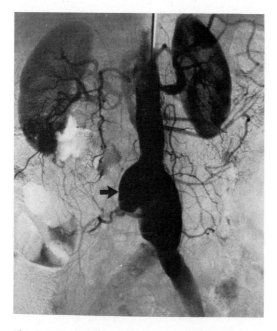

Fig. 6-4. Transaxillary aortogram of a dilated Dacron graft with aortic anastomotic aneurysm (arrow).

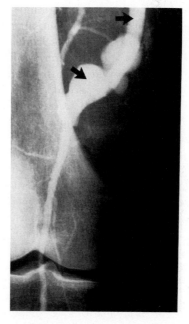

Fig. 6-5. Dilated Dacron femoropopliteal graft (upper arrow) with an anastomotic aneurysm at the popliteal anastomosis (lower arrow).

not exhibit false aneurysm formation. Furthermore, routine division of the inguinal ligament substantially increases the incidence of subsequent inguinal or femoral hernia.

In a series of 42 anastomotic aneurysms, Carson et al.[48] found a significant increase in graft-to-artery ratio in 22 of 42 patients (52%), with a mean increase in diameter of 22%. Dilatation and an increase in graft-to-artery ratio (1.3 to 1.6:1 vs. 1 to 1.3:1) in patients were significant etiologic factors in the recurrence of anastomotic pseudoaneurysms.

Although pseudoaneurysms are subject to the same spectrum of complications as true aneurysms, occlusion of a limb of the graft, especially at the femoral anastomoses, occurs more often than rupture.

Thrombosis. As the diameter of the graft increases, the fibrous, relatively acellular pseudointimal layer lining the luminal surface of the graft likewise progressively increases, resulting in the simultaneous diminution of the diameter of the lumen to approximate that of the outflow vessel. Dislodgment of this material by trauma or during arteriography or the imposition of distal obstruction by progressive atherosclerosis or anastomotic intimal hyperplasia results in occlusion of the limb (Figs. 6-6 and 6-7). The management of limb occlusion secondary to an anastomotic pseudoaneurysm includes thrombectomy and/or the replacement of a segment of the graft.

Rupture. Ruptures of the prosthesis caused by focal defects within the graft or occasionally disruption of the entire prosthesis are rare but devastating complications. Focal rupture caused by fracture and fragmentation of Dacron fibers or longitudinal tears in grafts manufactured with inadequate tensile strength may result in single or multiple areas of false aneurysm formation. These pseudoaneurysms may rupture into a hollow viscus, the retroperitoneum, or freely into the peritoneal cavity.[38,49-53] Rupture of an anastomotic pseudoaneurysm, although uncommon, is a notable cause of morbidity and mortality in patients with prosthetic grafts.

Aortic or iliac anastomotic pseudoaneurysms may rupture into adjacent bowel, most frequently the duodenum. However, other portions of the bowel may be involved also, depending on what portion of the bowel happens

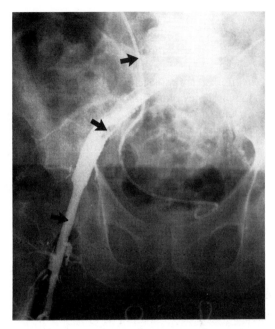

Fig. 6-6. Operative arteriogram demonstrating a dilated Dacron graft with irregular neointimal tissue lining the graft (middle arrow). The nondilated Gore-Tex graft used to repair the anastomotic aneurysm is well demonstrated (lower arrow). A stent to decompress a ureteric obstruction is in place (upper arrow).

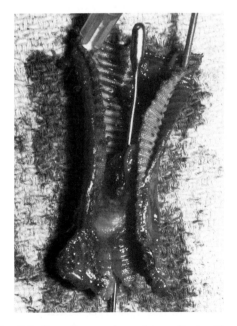

Fig. 6-7. Operative specimen in a patient with an anastomotic stenosis showing the fibrous acellular lining encroaching on the lumen.

to be adjacent to the anastomosis. More rarely these lesions rupture into the peritoneal cavity or the retroperitoneum.

Rarely do femoral anastomotic aneurysms rupture and usually only in patients with very large, long neglected aneurysms.

Management. Asymptomatic dilatation of prosthetic grafts without anastomotic pseudoaneurysm formation seldom is detected clinically unless a complication supervenes. Most often the patient presents with a painless groin swelling (the anastomotic aneurysm) and dilatation of the graft is detected during the ensuing workup. Acute or chronic occlusion of one or both of the limbs of an aortobifemoral graft caused by thrombosis of an anastomotic pseudoaneurysm is a less common mode of presentation.

Patients with significant dilatation of their grafts require careful evaluation before operative intervention is undertaken. Significant risk factors increasing operative morbidity and mortality usually are present and reoperation should be tailored to the individual patient. In addition, careful selection of the prosthesis to be used for the repair is essential if additional complications are to be minimized.

The treatment of graft dilatation may entail (1) local repair of anastomotic aneurysms, (2) thrombectomy and profundaplasty in patients with limb occlusion, or (3) graft replacement if the entire graft is dilated more than 50% of its original diameter or if an aortic anastomotic or para-anastomotic aneurysm is present.

A few salient points must be made about the operative techniques for repair of these aneurysms.

1. When an anastomotic aneurysm or pseudoaneurysm associated with graft dilatation is being repaired, a prosthesis that approximates the diameter of the outflow tract, not the dilated proximal graft, must be selected. We prefer to use PTFE in the repair of noninfected anastomotic femoral aneurysms since this material, as currently manufactured, does not dilate. Use of another Dacron graft approximating the diameter of the dilated primary graft remains a common practice but may further aggravate the problem since the new segment of graft likewise is prone to dilatation (Fig. 6-8).

2. When dilated aortic grafts are being

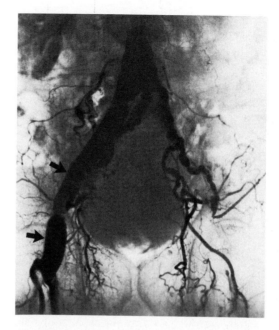

Fig. 6-8. Transaxillary aortogram demonstrating occlusion of the left limb of dilated aortobifemoral graft (upper arrow). The patient previously had repair of a right femoral anastomotic aneurysm with Dacron. The Dacron graft used has subsequently dilated (lower arrow).

replaced, small segments of the old graft adjacent to the proximal anastomosis may be left in place. This allows replacement of the graft without extensive mobilization of aorta, which often is encased in dense fibrous tissue.

3. The risk of injury to distal vessels may be minimized by using balloon catheter occlusion following isolation of the inflow vessel.

It must be remembered that graft dilatation is a problem inherent with knitted Dacron grafts. Although the tendency to yarn slippage can be minimized by increasing the number of yarns used during manufacture, this is limited by the need to preserve the ability to suture.

Anastomotic Stenosis

Stenosis caused by neointimal hyperplasia or progression of atherosclerosis occurs with Dacron aortofemoral grafts but with lesser frequency than with PTFE grafts. Progression of atherosclerosis in the profunda femoris or superficial femoral arteries and neointimal hyperplasia are the most frequent causes of graft anastomotic stenosis[54] (Fig. 6-9). Stenosis occurring at the proximal aortic anastomosis is usually a result of failure to remove residual atherosclerotic plaque or thrombus.

These patients usually present with symptoms of acute or chronic limb ischemia caused by occlusion of one or both limbs of the graft. Arteriography delineates the cause of the obstruction and guides direct repair.

Successful management of stenosis or occlusion at the distal anastomosis can be achieved in approximately 90% of patients.[54] Surgical repair usually includes thrombectomy of the graft plus endarterectomy of the profunda femoris artery with patch angioplasty (using autogenous vein, endarterectomized segments of the occluded superficial femoral artery, or PTFE).[54] Occasionally proximal stenosis may require replacement of the graft after endarterectomy of the severely narrowed aortic segment. In poor-risk patients with progressively increasing proximal aortic stenosis, axillofemoral bypass grafting may be indicated.

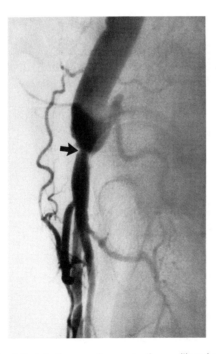

Fig. 6-9. Arteriogram demonstrating a dilated graft with an anastomotic stenosis (arrow) caused by neointimal hyperplasia.

Ureteric Obstruction

Ureteric obstruction is a well-recognized complication of aortic reconstructive procedures. The etiology of hydronephrosis includes ureteric ischemia, kinks, operative trauma, anastomotic aneurysms, graft infection, graft limb thrombosis, and an incidental ureteric tumor. In approximately 1% of patients, dense fibrosis, presumably associated with incorporation of the graft, also encases the ureter and results in hydronephrosis.[55,56]

Ureteric obstruction may be an incidental finding on workup for some other condition or may present as obstructive uropathy or progressive deterioration in renal function. Evaluation should include measures of renal function and delineation of the site and cause of obstruction by intravenous pyelography, CT scanning, ultrasonography, or retrograde pyelography. The position of the ureter relative to the graft is best ascertained by the use of contrast-enhanced CT scanning.

Ureteric obstruction caused by encasement of the ureter by perigraft fibrosis can be avoided by careful positioning of the limbs of the graft posterior to the ureter when performing an aortofemoral bypass. The management of ureteric obstruction depends on the physical condition of the patient and the site and cause of the obstruction. Surgical options include placement of indwelling ureteral stents, division rerouting and reanastomosis of prosthetic graft limbs if anterior to the ureter, or excision and reanastomosis of the ureter for severe segmental fibrotic stenosis.

Neoplasia

There are now a few case reports of angiosarcoma developing in patients with Dacron grafts.[57-59] The possible contribution of Dacron grafts to the development of angiosarcoma is unclear. Although some experimental evidence links plastic materials with neoplastic change, the evidence in humans is less convincing.[60] First, the incidence is extremely low when one compares the number of tumors reported with the number of prosthetic grafts implanted. Second, in the case reported by O'Connell, Fee, and Golding,[58] the tumor was almost certainly incidental to the Dacron graft in view of the short time interval that elapsed between placement of the graft and diagnosis of the angiosarcoma. However, Fehrenbacher et al.[59] reported an angiosarcoma thought to be related to the use of a Dacron graft implanted 12 years previously. Although the time interval between implantation of the graft and the development of the neoplasm is consistent with a possible cause-and-effect relationship, this remains speculative. Nonetheless, although a direct cause-and-effect relationship between the use of Dacron grafts and the development of angiosarcoma cannot be established, continued vigilance seems appropriate.

The diagnosis of angiosarcoma seldom is made antemortem. Progressive stenosis resulting in obstructive or embolic symptoms is the usual clinical presentation. Contrast-enhanced abdominal CT scanning or biplanar arteriography usually will demonstrate an intraluminal filling defect. Excision/grafting and endarterectomy have been advocated for treatment of these lesions. The prognosis is poor: subsequent patient survival usually is only a few months in duration.

EXPANDED PTFE GRAFTS

Expanded polytetrafluoroethylene (PTFE) grafts are used widely as arterial substitutes for axillofemoral and femorofemoral bypasses, dialysis access procedures, and for infrainguinal bypass to the popliteal and tibial vessels when autogenous vein is unavailable. Recently they have been used with increasing frequency in the aortoiliofemoral position because, unlike Dacron grafts, they do not dilate and thrombus is readily removed with a thrombectomy catheter. Moreover, we have found only one report of anastomotic pseudoaneurysm in the absence of infection associated with the use of bifurcation PTFE grafts.[61] However, clinical experience with bifurcation grafts is limited and long-term patency data are not available. It remains to be determined whether these are true advantages or merely reflect the smaller numbers of these grafts that have been implanted for shorter periods of time. In any event these desirable characteristics of PTFE grafts must be balanced against two disadvantages: substan-

tial suture line bleeding sometimes occurs and they are more difficult to handle because of their rigidity.

When used for dialysis access, PTFE grafts have 1-year patency rates of 62% to 93%.[62-65] Primary patency rates for above- and below-knee femoropopliteal bypass grafts range from 46% to 61% and 27% to 39%, respectively, at 8 years.[5-7] Porter[66] recently has reported a 4-year patency rate of 85% for ringed PTFE grafts placed as axillofemoral bypasses.

Fabrication

Manufactured by mechanical extrusion of the chemically inert carbon fluorine–polytetrafluoroethylene polymer, the resulting grafts consist of solid nodes of PTFE interconnected by longitudinally oriented fibrils. The solid-node fibril structure of PTFE comprises only 15% to 20% of the volume of the graft material; the remaining void is filled with air. Thus PTFE is a porous graft that readily accommodates tissue ingrowth.[67]

Continuous deformation, known as "creep," occurs when polymeric materials such as PTFE are subjected to arterial pressure. This is an important factor in aneurysmal dilatation of non-reinforced grafts. Creep occurs in two phases: an initial deformation caused by laxity of the structure is followed by gradual continuous deformation, tending to progress with time.[67] Presently, the commercially available PTFE prostheses are made creep-resistant by increasing wall thickness (0.64 vs. 0.5 mm), by increasing the density of the node fibril structure, or by the application of an external reinforcing sheath also of PTFE.

These prostheses demonstrate very little propensity to dilate, hold sutures well, do not require preclotting, and, because of their smooth luminal surfaces, thrombus is easily removed.

Healing Characteristics

Although the healing characteristics of PTFE grafts have been studied extensively in experimental animals, few studies of explanted grafts in humans are available. Experimentally, PTFE grafts are readily incorporated by dense fibrous tissue. The luminal flow surface is covered first by a layer of protein and cellular elements derived from the blood.[67,68]

Three distinct processes can be observed at both the proximal and distal anastomoses of small-diameter grafts implanted in experimental animals. In animals with patent grafts, pannus ingrowth originates from the host vessel and extends for approximately 1 cm; neointimal hyperplasia also is often seen. In occluded grafts granulation tissue and thrombus are found at the anastomoses. Clowes and associates[69,70] have demonstrated endothelial cell ingrowth extending approximately 1 to 1.25 cm from both proximal and distal anastomoses of 4 mm PTFE grafts implanted into baboons at 1 and 3 months postoperatively. Although the tensile strength at an anastomotic suture line between Dacron and the host vessel is entirely dependent on the suture material for its integrity, there is some evidence that healing may occur at anastomoses constructed with PTFE. Quinones-Baldrich et al.,[71] using polyglycolic acid suture to construct artery-graft anastomoses and artery-artery anastomoses in experimental animals, recently have demonstrated an increase in anastomotic tensile strength with PTFE grafts and double-veloured woven Dacron grafts compared with knitted grafts. These data suggest greater anastomotic healing with these grafts.

Mohring et al.[72] studied explanted PTFE grafts used for dialysis access. They observed distinct differences in the healing between the two commercially available grafts. In nonreinforced grafts, connective tissue ingrowth extending into the interstices of the graft was more pronounced and these grafts had a noticeably increased cellular internal lining in contrast to the relatively cell-free neointimal lining of reinforced grafts.

PTFE grafts explanted from humans are characterized by an external fibrous capsule of varying thickness, which progressively increases in thickness with the length of implantation. Encapsulation, however, is absent in 80% of infected grafts. Cellular invasion arising from the external capsule does not occur to any significant degree. Instead, the luminal surface of PTFE grafts usually is covered with a thin layer of acellular neointima (Figs. 6-10 and 6-11). In a scanning electron microscopic study of 67 human graft explants, Formichi et al.[73] observed bacterial colonization, leukocyte infiltration, and lipid deposition of flow surfaces. Bacterial colonization was present in 31 of 67 specimens (46%) examined, leukocytes in eight (12%), and both bacteria and leukocytes in five (7%). Yet infection was present in only 9 of 31 of the prostheses (29%) with microscopic evidence of colonization. Lipid deposition usually was absent in grafts implanted less than 8 months but was observed with increasing frequency after 1 year.

Complications

Early in their use focal and diffuse dilatation of PTFE grafts was a serious limitation. Although some suggested that hypertension was an important contributing factor, in fact not all patients with dilated grafts were hypertensive. Instead, inherent structural weakness of the prosthesis, related to inadequate wall thickness and creep, was the most likely causative factor.[29,30,67] Modern PTFE prostheses demonstrate very little tendency to dilate (less than 10%).

Late complications of PTFE grafts include anastomotic stenosis or occlusion caused by progression of atherosclerosis or intimal hyperplasia, thrombosis, and, rarely, pseudoaneurysm formation.

Anastomotic Intimal Hyperplasia

The most frequent cause of failure of PTFE grafts is stenosis or occlusion, most frequently involving the distal anastomoses of femoropopliteal grafts.[69,74] A perplexing problem has been the observation that occlusion may occur suddenly without antecedent symptoms.

Anastomotic neointimal hyperplasia and progression of atherosclerosis are the most frequent pathologic findings in occluded grafts (Fig. 6-12). Careful monitoring at regular intervals with Doppler-derived pressure indices, flow velocity measurements, and imaging of anastomoses are essential to detect preocclusive lesions, which are more amenable to correction before thrombosis occurs.

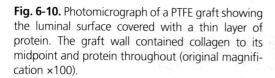

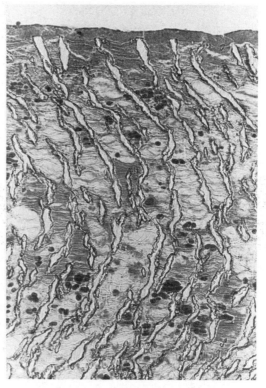

Fig. 6-10. Photomicrograph of a PTFE graft showing the luminal surface covered with a thin layer of protein. The graft wall contained collagen to its midpoint and protein throughout (original magnification ×100).

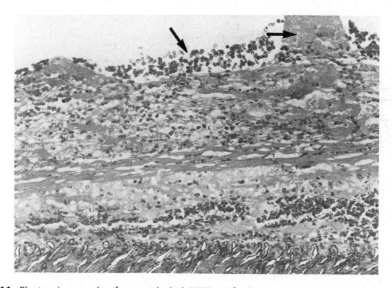

Fig. 6-11. Photomicrograph of an occluded PTFE graft demonstrating thrombus (horizontal arrow) containing neutrophils (oblique arrow) on the luminal surface. No bacteria were observed (original magnification ×100).

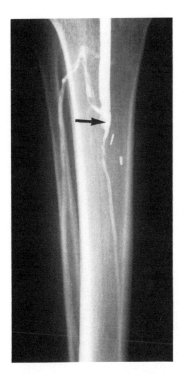

Fig. 6-12. Arteriogram of a PTFE graft implanted 8 months previously. Note the irregularity caused by anastomotic intimal hyperplasia involving the distal anastomosis and the proximal posterotibial artery (arrow).

Once thrombosis has occurred, resolution of this occlusive process is essential. This can be achieved either by lysis of the luminal thrombosis with urokinase or by thrombectomy. Lytic therapy, which successfully delineates the responsible occlusive lesion in approximately 70% of patients with occlusions of less than 14 days' duration, is probably the management of choice in the absence of limb-threatening ischemia.[75] Thrombectomy is preferable if the limb is at risk and when there has been no significant improvement after 24 to 48 hours of lytic therapy.

A number of interventions are available for managing anastomotic stenoses; here the procedure must, however, be tailored to the prevailing circumstances in each patient. Balloon angioplasty and patch angioplasty are the appealing options. However, either procedure is associated with significant reocclusion rates at 3 months. Consequently, our preference is to extend the anastomosis to an uninvolved segment of the vein (for stenosis at the venous end of grafts used for dialysis access) or an uninvolved segment of artery (in patients with occlusion of a femoropopliteal PTFE bypass graft). Construction of an autogenous vein bypass using the saphenous vein or a vein from the arm may be indicated in patients who require a bypass to the tibial vessels.

Anastomotic Pseudoaneurysm

Anastomotic aneurysms associated with the use of PTFE grafts are quite uncommon in the absence of infection. We have identified just one case of an anastomotic aneurysm associated with the use of a bifurcation graft.[61] However, recently we have observed several dialysis patients with pseudoaneurysm formation along the course of PTFE dialysis access fistulas resulting from inadequate compression of needle puncture sites.

Retained pieces of PTFE grafts in patients with failed dialysis access procedures or following above- or below-knee amputation are important reservoirs for bacteria. Nonhealing wounds and infected anastomotic aneurysms, which present with local and systemic signs and symptoms of infection, are not infrequent consequences of this practice. If possible, all residual prosthetic material should be removed from patients with infective lesions in the involved extremity.[76]

The principles of evaluation and management of pseudoaneurysm related to the use of PTFE grafts are similar to those for anastomotic aneurysms occurring with the use of fabric or biologic grafts.

PERIGRAFT SEROMA

The accumulation of fluid around knitted Dacron double-veloured or PTFE grafts first described by Kaupp et al.[77] is a rare complication of vascular bypass procedures. The incidence of perigraft seroma ranges from 0.2% to 1% of major vascular reconstructions.[78] The perigraft reaction is characterized by painless, fluctuant swelling surrounding a portion of or the entire prosthesis, often with erythema of the overlying skin. Grafts placed in extra-anatomic locations (i.e., axillofemoral, femorofemoral, axilloaxillary, or subclavian pulmonary bypass grafts) seem particularly prone to this complication and account for 60% to 75% of cases. Grafts in anatomic positions (aortofemoral, femoropopliteal) account for the remainder.[77-84] Ahn et al.[83] documented perigraft seromas in 4.2% of patients with extra-anatomic bypasses, 1.2% with aortofemoral bypasses, and 0.3% with femoropopliteal bypass procedures.

The interval from graft insertion to the clinical presentation of the seroma typically ranges from 1 to 45 months, with a mean of approximately 25 months.[78] Systemic signs of infection invariably are absent and the straw-colored fluid (unless contaminated by repeated attempts at aspiration) usually is bacteriologically sterile. The fluid that resides within a fibrous capsule investing a portion of or the entire graft is biochemically a transudate of serum. In a survey of the members of the North American Chapter of the International Society for Cardiovascular Surgery, Blumenberg, Gelfand, and Dale[79] noted that knitted Dacron (54%) and PTFE (34%) grafts were the prosthetic grafts most frequently involved.

Histologically, the tissues surrounding Dacron grafts demonstrate a gradation of changes ranging from an acute inflammatory cell infiltrate at 1 week to mature granulation tissue at 4 to 6 weeks. Foreign body giant cells attached to the Dacron fibers frequently are observed. By contrast, the reaction to PTFE grafts is characterized by fibrin deposition with scant giant cell reaction confined almost entirely to the outer surface of the graft.[79]

The precise cause of perigraft fluid accumulation is unknown. However, the fundamental abnormality appears to be failure of incorporation of the graft by the host tissues. Fluid transport through the interstices of the graft, fluid exudation from surrounding tissues, an allergic or immune response, mechanical irritation of the host tissue by repeated motion of the prosthesis, impaired fibrin formation in the graft interstices caused by the use of heparin, and the presence of a fibroblast inhibitory factor in the serum are among the many etiologic factors advanced.[77-84]

Although observation or repeated aspiration to control fluid accumulation is successful in approximately two thirds of patients with perigraft fluid collections, secondary infection or graft thrombosis, reported to occur in 5% to 8% of patients, remains a serious concern.[79] Therefore, except in poor-risk patients, removal of the graft and replacement with a prosthesis of different material is recommended. This will result in cure of more than 90% of patients. The technique of Lowery et al.[85] in which a communication lined with omentum is fashioned between the graft capsule and the peritoneal cavity seems a reasonable alternative when the fluid is sterile.

SUTURE LINE FAILURE

The tensile strength of a prosthetic graft–artery anastomosis is dependent entirely on the suture material for its structural integrity. Healing of this site is limited to pannus ingrowth, which consists of smooth muscle and endothelial cells from the arterial wall adjacent to the anastomosis. Although this may extend for approximately 1 cm onto the prosthetic graft, it constitutes little, if any, tensile strength. Because silk, nylon, and polyethylene sutures lose tensile strength with time, they should not be used with prosthetic grafts.

Silk sutures were the first used in vascular anastomoses. Moore and Hall[86] reported 25 anastomotic aneurysms associated with the use of silk sutures that were found to be either fractured or absent in their cases. This finding was not surprising since Cutler and Dunphy[87] had demonstrated deterioration of silk within 2 years of implantation. Anastomotic aneurysms caused by dissolution of silk sutures still may occasionally be encountered in patients who underwent bypass procedures in the early 1960s (Fig. 6-13).

Braided Dacron and monofilament sutures, such as polypropylene, which do not deteriorate over time, are presently the sutures most often used in constructing vascular anastomoses. However, they will fracture if carelessly handled with instruments.[88] Dissolution or fracture of a monofilament suture results in variable disruption of the anastomosis and

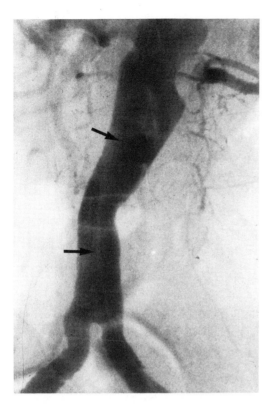

Fig. 6-13. Transfemoral aortogram demonstrating a dilated graft (lower arrow) and an anastomotic aneurysm (upper arrow) in a patient whose anastomosis was constructed using silk sutures in 1966.

consequent false aneurysm formation. The latter may rupture or erode into adjacent bowel, causing graft enteric fistula. Although a polypropylene suture may fracture, this has been extremely rare in our experience.[89-92] Careful selection of sutures of appropriate composition and with sufficient tensile strength is an essential first step in ensuring the integrity of an anastomosis.

Polypropylene, the suture material most commonly used to perform vascular prosthetic anastomoses, demonstrates no decrease in tensile strength when subjected to load or exposed to body tissue fluids for prolonged periods of time.[88] However, excessive manipulation of the suture with surgical instruments or inadvertent knotting may weaken the suture mechanically and lead to breakage. Indeed, few complications are ascribable to the failure of modern sutures.

UMBILICAL VEIN GRAFTS

Glutaraldehyde-stabilized human umbilical vein (HUV) grafts presently are used as alternatives to PTFE grafts for femoropopliteal or tibial bypasses and for dialysis access.

Preparation

These grafts are prepared from umbilical cords harvested in the delivery room, which are manually cleaned and stripped. The collagen of cords with acceptable diameter and quality is then cross-linked with glutaraldehyde, and soluble proteins and excess Wharton's gel are extracted with ethanol.[93] The external surface is covered with a supporting Dacron mesh. Glutaraldehyde starch has been shown to be superior to dialydehyde starch as a cross-linking agent. This results in a more stable graft that is less prone to biodegradation. Five-year primary patency rates of 83% for above knee and 57% for bypasses to the crural vessels have been reported.[94,95]

Healing Characteristics

The healing characteristics of these grafts in humans have been described by Guidoin et al.[96] and more recently by Julien et al.[97] in a study of 80 explants. Macroscopically, they demonstrated irregular thickening of their walls. Folds of varying depths involved the luminal surface. The external surfaces of the grafts were covered by fibrous capsules of variable thicknesses, increasing proportionately with the duration of implantation.[96,97]

Histologically, 29 prostheses demonstrated evidence on lipid deposition, and in 26% of the grafts bacteria were present even though clinical infection was not diagnosed. Cellular infiltrates, most severe when clinical infection was present, were readily demonstrable. Also seen was delamination of the luminal surface.[97]

Complications
Dilatation

The incidence of aneurysmal dilatation, a not infrequent complication of HUV grafts, increases progressively beyond 5 years. Dilatation of HUV grafts is biphasic: early enlargement of grafts from 4 to 6 mm at the time of implantation to approximately 9 mm in diameter is the norm. Using B-mode ultrasound, Dardik et al.[95] have demonstrated a 21% incidence of dilatation and 36% incidence of focal aneurysms in patients studied beyond 5 years. Cranley et al.[98] found discrete aneurysms (diameter greater than 20 mm) in 11 of 25 patients (44%) surviving with patent grafts for 5 years.

Two morphologic variants of aneurysms have been described by Dardik et al.[94] in association with HUV grafts: uniform diffuse dilatation of both the graft and its Dacron mesh or erosion of the graft with rupture of the mesh, resulting in multiple false aneurysms.

The progressive increase in diameter of these grafts beyond 5 years is not entirely unexpected. Reversal of glutaraldehyde-induced cross-linking and immunologic mechanisms have been proposed to explain aneurysm formation in these grafts.[95] The frequent observation of bacteria within these grafts in the absence of overt infection is intriguing and deserves further study. It may play a role in aneurysm formation.

The guidelines for excision and grafting of aneurysmal HUV grafts are not clear. Dardik et al.[94] state that approximately 6% of these aneurysms in grafts implanted more than 5 years previously are of sufficient size to require surgical excision and repair. However, it appears prudent from the studies of Cranley et al.[98] to consider resection if the dilated segment exceeds 20 to 30 mm in size. Excision and grafting of segmental aneurysmal change or replacement of the entire graft if diffusely dilated may be necessary.

Anastomotic Aneurysms

Anastomotic aneurysms have been reported infrequently (1.4%) with the use of HUV grafts and appear to develop more often at anastomotic sites between HUV and Dacron grafts (9%) than between HUV host arteries (0.6%).[95] Serial monitoring with duplex imaging, with examinations increasing in frequency beyond the 5-year mark, is essential if significant complications are to be avoided.

Anastomotic Stenosis

Late thrombosis of HUV grafts caused by anastomotic stenosis (in 2.1% of the patients reported by Dardik et al.[95]) usually is associated with neointimal hyperplasia or progression of atherosclerosis at the distal anastomosis. Dissection of these grafts often may be extremely difficult because of the dense fibrous reaction that frequently envelops them. If the distal anastomosis can be exposed, a longitudinal arteriotomy is made and extended onto the native vessel beyond the occlusive lesion. Adherent thrombus is removed carefully and the arteriotomy and graftotomy closed with a vein patch. Thrombus within the grafts should be flushed out with heparinized saline solution rather than extracted with a thrombectomy catheter since these often fracture the luminal surface, thus predisposing the patient to secondary thrombosis. Using these techniques to restore patency to popliteal and crural vessels, Dardik et al.[94] have reported early secondary patency rates of 44% to 56%.

Although bacteria can be demonstrated in significant numbers of HUV graft explants, the incidence of clinical infection nonetheless remains low. In a series of 907 patients, Dardik et al.[94] reported an overall infection rate of 4.3%. The incidence was 0.6% in patients undergoing primary revascularization and 3.7% after reoperation. The clinical presentation, evaluation, and management of infection involving HUV grafts are similar to those seen with other prosthetic and biologic grafts and are fully discussed elsewhere.[94]

BOVINE XENOGRAFTS

When first introduced, bovine xenografts were used for dialysis access and for femoropopliteal bypass grafting. However, poor long-term patency rates of 50% at 5 years, a 3% to 6% incidence of aneurysmal dilatation, and a 6% to 7% incidence of infection when used for infrainguinal bypass grafting have limited their use to dialysis access fistulas.[99] There are several advantages to their use for that purpose, including availability, ease of implantation, and immediate use following insertion.

Preparation

These grafts were first processed by ficin digestion of bovine carotid arteries in an attempt to remove the antigenic smooth muscle.

However, the use of enzymes to prepare the artery dissolved elastic tissue and smooth muscle, resulting in a mushy collagen tube. This tube was then placed over a mandrel and tanned with dialydehyde starch to cross-link the collagen. It soon became apparent that the resultant heterograft readily elongated and had a tendency to dilate to approximately 130% to 135% of its original diameter.[99] More recently the grafts have been processed by tanning the intact vessel with dialydehyde starch or glutaraldehyde without prior digestion of the fibrous proteins. A Dacron mesh wrap has been added to promote tissue ingrowth and provide reinforcement. When implanted, the modified bovine xenograft evokes a fibroblastic response that invades the outer half of the wall as opposed to the intense inflammatory infiltrate evoked by the untreated xenograft.[2,99]

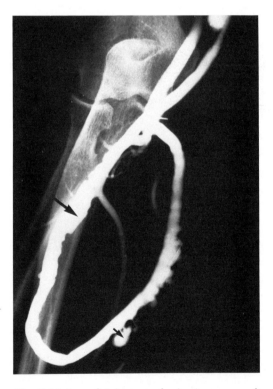

Fig. 6-14. Loop fistulogram of a bovine xenograft demonstrating an area of dilatation (large arrow) and multiple pseudoaneurysms at needle puncture sites (small arrow).

The late complications of bovine xenografts used for dialysis access include thrombosis caused by hyperplasia at the venous anastomosis, pseudoaneurysm formation at needle puncture sites, infection that may result in dissolution of segments of the graft, and dilatation of the entire graft (Fig. 6-14). In a comprehensive retrospective analysis of 385 bovine heterografts, Brems, Castaneda, and Garvin[100] reported 160 episodes of thrombosis, 18 cases of dilatation, 18 cases of puncture site pseudoaneurysms, and eight wound infections.

When used for dialysis access procedures, bovine xenografts have a 1-year patency of 26% to 91% and a 2-year patency between 42% and 83%[64,65,100-102] compared with patency rates of 62% to 93% and 57% to 85% at 1 and 2 years, respectively, for PTFE grafts.[63-65,101] Hurt et al.,[103] in a study of 140 grafts comparing PTFE grafts and bovine xenografts, were unable to demonstrate any significant difference between the two.

Thrombosis of bovine heterografts usually necessitates thrombectomy and revision of the venous outflow tract.

Infection occurring within the first month of implantation almost invariably involves the anastomoses, requiring removal of the prosthesis. Since late infection usually occurs at needle puncture sites, replacement of segments of the graft may be undertaken. Dilatation of the entire prosthesis or diffuse pseudoaneurysm may require complete removal of the graft. Focal pseudoaneurysms in the absence of infection can be managed by local excision and placement of an interposition graft to bypass the involved segment.

CONCLUSION

The introduction of prosthetic and biologic grafts into clinical practice has substantially improved the survival of patients with peripheral vascular disease. However, vascular surgeons generally have not been critical in their evaluation of prostheses used to bypass or replace diseased vessels. The more frequent implantation of grafts into younger patients and the extension of surgical techniques to distal, small-vessel bypasses have heightened the need for durable prostheses and an improved understanding of interactions at the blood surface interface. It is evident that large-diameter grafts (greater than 8 mm internal diameter), although they generally function well, are nevertheless subject to complications that may lead to loss of life or limb. The long-term patency of small-diameter grafts (less than 6 mm) remains considerably lower than that of their larger diameter counterparts. Anastomotic intimal hyperplasia and thrombosis of these grafts have not been significantly reduced by the use of antiplatelet agents. Concerted efforts by graft manufacturers to produce durable nonthrombogenic grafts along with careful patient selection, operative technique, modification of risk factors, improvement in our understanding of the interaction between the graft and the host tissues, and continued surveillance are essential if we are to improve the long-term survival and function.

REFERENCES

1. Pourdeyhimi B, Wagner D. On the correlation between the failure of vascular grafts and their structural and material properties: A critical analysis. J Biomed Mater Res 20:375-409, 1986.

2. Sauvage LR. Biologic behavior of grafts in arterial system. In Haimovici H, ed. Vascular Surgery, 3rd ed. East Norwalk, Conn.: Appleton & Lange, 1989, pp 136-160.

3. Malone JM, Moore WS, Goldstone J. The natural history of bilateral aortofemoral bypass grafts for ischemia of the lower extremities. Arch Surg 110:1300-1306, 1975.

4. Szilagyi DE, Elliot JP, Smith RF, Reddy DJ, McPharlin M. A thirty-year survey of the reconstructive surgical treatment of aortoiliac occlusive disease. J Vasc Surg 3:421-436, 1986.

5. Prendiville EJ, Yeager A, O'Donnell RG, Coleman JC, Jaworek A, Callow AD, Mackey WC, Deterling RA. Long-term results with the above-knee popliteal expanded polytetrafluoroethylene graft. J Vasc Surg 11:517-524, 1990.

6. Moore WS. Late results of infrainguinal revascularization with PTFE grafts: A ten-year experience with a modern series. Presented at the Seventeenth Annual Symposium of Current Critical Problems and New Horizons in Vascular Surgery. New York: Nov. 16-18, 1990.

7. Raithel D. Role of grafts in infrainguinal arterial reconstructions: A ten-year experience. Presented at the Seventeenth Annual Symposium on Current Critical Problems and New Horizons in Vascular Surgery. New York: Nov. 16-18, 1990.

8. Guidoin R. A biological and structural evaluation of retrieved Dacron arterial prostheses. U.S. Department of Commerce/National Bureau of Standards Implant Retrieval: Material and Biological Analysis. Washington, D.C.: Jan. 1981.

9. Harris PL. Aortoiliac femoral reoperative surgery. Supplementary surgery at secondary operations. Acta Chir Scand 538:51-55, 1987.

10. Rutherford RB, Patt A, Pearce WH. Extraanatomic bypass: A closer view. J Vasc Surg 6:437-446, 1987.

11. Schultz GA, Sauvage LR, Mathisen SR, Mansfield PB, Smith JC, Davis CC, Hall DG, Rittenhouse EA, Kowalsky TE. A five- to seven-year experience with externally supported Dacron prostheses in axillofemoral and femoropopliteal bypass. Ann Vasc Surg 1:214-224, 1986.

12. Jonas RA, Schoen FJ, Levy RJ, Castaneda AR. Biological sealants and knitted Dacron: Porosity and histological comparisons of vascular graft materials with and without collagen and fibrin glue pretreatments. Ann Thorac Surg 41:657-663, 1986.

13. Jonas RA, Ziemer G, Schoen FJ, Britton L, Castaneda AR. A new sealant for knitted Dacron prostheses: Minimally cross-linked gelatin. J Vasc Surg 7:414-419, 1988.

14. McGee GS, Shuman TA, Atkinson JB, Weaver FA, Edwards WH. Experimental evaluation of a new albumin-impregnated knitted Dacron prosthesis. Am Surg 53:695-701, 1987.

15. Bethea MC, Reemsta K. Graft hemostasis: An alternative to preclotting. Ann Thorac Surg 27:374, 1979.

16. Cooley DA, Ramagnoli A, Nilam JD, Bossort MI. A method of predisposing woven Dacron grafts to prevent interstitial hemorrhage. Cardiovasc Dis (Bulletin of Texas Heart Institute) 8:48,1981.

17. Wesolow A. The healing of arterial prostheses—The state of the art. Thorac Cardiovasc Surg 30:196-208, 1982.

18. Guidoin R, Cosselin C, Martin L, Marois M, Laroche F. Polyester prostheses as substitutes in the thoracic aorta of dogs. I. Evaluation of commercial prostheses. J Biomed Mater Res 17:1049-1077, 1983.

19. Anderson JM. Microvel with hemashield vascular grafts. A preliminary report of the healing response in humans. Angiol Arch Bd 9:73-77, 1985.

20. Knox WG, Miller RE. Long-term appraisal of aortic and arterial homografts implanted in years 1954-1957. Ann Surg 172:1076-1078, 1970.

21. Humphries AW, Hawk WA, DeWolfe VG, Le Fevre FA. Clinicopathologic observations on the fate of arterial freeze-dried homografts. Surgery 45:59-71, 1959.

22. Cooke PA, Nobis PA, Stoney RJ. Dacron aortic graft failure. Arch Surg 108:101-103, 1974.

23. Perry MO. Early failure of Dacron prosthetic grafts. J Cardiovasc Surg 16:318-321, 1975.

24. Blumenberg RM, Gelfand ML. Failure of knitted Dacron as an arterial prosthesis. Surgery 81:493-496, 1977.

25. Nucho RC, Gryboski WA. Aneurysms of a double velour aortic graft. Arch Surg 119:1182-1184, 1984.

26. Creech OJ, Deterling RA, Edwards S, Julian OC, Linton RR, Shumacker H. Vascular prostheses: Report of the Committee for the Study of Vascular Prostheses of the Society for Vascular Surgery. Surgery 41:62-80, 1957.

27. Eastcott HHG. Rupture of Orlon aortic graft after six years. Lancet 2:75-76, 1962.

28. Hayward RH, White RR. Aneurysm in a woven Teflon graft. Angiology 22:188-190, 1971.

29. Campbell CD, Brooks DH, Webster MW, Bondi RP, Lloyd JC, Hynes MF, Bahnson HT. Aneurysm formation in expanded polytetrafluoroethylene prostheses. Surgery 79:493-496, 1976.

30. Roberts AK, Johnson N. Aneurysm formation in an expanded microporous polytetrafluoroethylene graft. Arch Surg 113:211-213, 1978.

31. Trippestad A. Dilatation and rupture of Dacron arterial grafts. Acta Chir Scand 529:77-79, 1985.

32. Berger K, Sauvage LR. Late fiber deterioration in Dacron arterial grafts. Ann Surg 193:477-491, 1980.

33. Nunn DB, Freeman MH, Hudgins PC. Postoperative alterations in size of Dacron aortic grafts. Ann Surg 189:741-745, 1979.

34. Lundqvist B, Almgren B, Bowald S, Lorelius LE, Eriksson I. Deterioration and dilatation of Dacron prosthetic grafts. Acta Chir Scand 529:81-85, 1985.

35. Yashar JJ, Richman MH, Dyckman J, Witoszka M, Burnard RJ, Weyman AK, Yashar J. Failure of Dacron prostheses caused by structural defect. Surgery 84:659-663, 1978.

36. Ratto GB, Truini M, Sacco A, Canepa G, Badini A, Motta G. Multiple aneurysmal dilatations in a knitted Dacron velour graft. J Cardiovasc Surg 26:589-591, 1985.

37. King MW, Guidoin R, Blais P, Gayton A, Cunasekera KR. Degradation of polyester arterial prostheses: A physical or chemical mechanism? In Fraker AC, Griffen CD, eds. Corrosion and Degradation of Implant Materials. Second Symposium, ASTM STP 859, American Society for Testing and Materials. Philadelphia: 1985, pp 294-307.

38. Lundstrom OR, Angquist KA, Hallmans G. Bilateral aneurysm of Dacron graft following aortofemoral graft operation. Acta Chir Scand 142:479-482, 1976.

39. Clagett GP, Salander JM, Eddleman WL, Cabellon S, Youkey JR, Olson DW, Hutton JE, Rich NM. Dilatation of knitted Dacron aortic prostheses and anastomotic false aneurysms: Etiologic considerations. Surgery 93:9-16, 1983.

40. Gooding GAW, Effeney DJ, Goldstone J. The aortofemoral graft: Detection and identification of healing complications by ultrasonography. Surgery 89:94-101, 1981.

41. Clifford PC, Skidmore R, Woodcock JP, Bird DR, Lusby RJ, Baird RN. Arterial grafts imaged using Doppler and real-time ultrasound. Vasc Diag Ther 2:43-58, 1981.

42. Qvarfordt PG, Reilly LM, Mark AS, Goldstone J, Wall SD, Ehrenfeld WK, Stoney RJ. Computerized tomographic assessment of graft incorporation after aortic reconstruction. Am J Surg 150:227-231, 1985.

43. Brown OW, Stanson AW, Pairolero PC, Hollier LH. Computerized tomography following abdominal aortic surgery. Surgery 91:716-721, 1982.

44. Kim GE, Imparato AM, Nathan I, Riles TS. Dilatation of synthetic grafts and junctional aneurysms. Arch Surg 114:1296-1303, 1979.

45. Szilagyi DE, Smith RF, Elliott JP, Hageman JH, Dali'Olmo CA. Anastomotic aneurysms after vascular reconstruction: Problems of incidence, etiology, and treatment. Surgery 78:800-816, 1975.

46. Kinley CE, Paasche PE, MacDonald AS, Marble AE. Stress at vascular anastomosis in relation to hose artery: Synthetic graft diameter. Surgery 75:28-30, 1974.

47. Courbier R, Aboukhater R. Progress in treatment of anastomotic aneurysms. World J Surg 12:742-749, 1988.

48. Carson SN, Hunter GC, Palmaz J, Guernsey JM. Recurrence of femoral anastomotic aneurysms. Am J Surg 146:744-778, 1983.

49. Biedermann H, Flora G. Fatigue problems in Dacron vascular grafts. Artif Organs 32:205-206, 1982.

50. Orringer MB, Rutherford RB, Skinner DB. An unusual complication of axillofemoral artery bypass. Surgery 72:769-771, 1972.

51. Lantsberg L, Khodadadi J, Goleman L, Hertzanu Y, Szendro G. Unusual pseudoaneurysm of Dacron femoro-popliteal graft shaft. J Cardiovasc Surg 29:320-321, 1988.

52. Sladen JG, Gerein AN, Miyagishima RT. Late rupture of prosthetic aortic grafts. Am J Surg 153:453-458, 1987.

53. Watanabe T, Kusaba A, Kuma H, Kina M, Okadome K, Inokuchi K. Failure of Dacron arterial prostheses caused by structural defects. J Cardiovasc Surg 24:95-100, 1983.

54. Goldstone J. Management of late failures of aortofemoral reconstructions. Acta Chir Scand 555:149-153, 1990.

55. Johnston KW. Nonvascular complications of vascular surgery. Presented at the Seventeenth Annual Symposium on Current Critical Problems and New Horizons in Vascular Surgery. New York: Nov. 16-18, 1990.

56. Wright DJ, Ernst CB, Evans JR, Smith RF, Reddy DJ, Shepard AD, Elliott JP. Ureteral complications and aortoiliac reconstruction. J Vasc Surg 11:29-37, 1990.

57. Burns WA, Kanhouwa S, Tillman L, Saini N, Herrmann JB. Fibrosarcoma occurring at the site of a plastic vascular graft. Cancer 29:66-83, 1972.

58. O'Connell TX, Fee JH, Golding A. Sarcoma associated with Dacron prosthetic material. J Thorac Cardiovasc Surg 72:94-96, 1976.

59. Fehrenbacher JW, Bowers W, Strate R, Pittman J. Angiosarcoma of the aorta associated with a Dacron graft. Ann Thorac Surg 32:297-301, 1980.

60. Brand KC. Foreign body tumorogenesis, timing and location of preneoplastic events. J Natl Cancer Inst 47:829, 1971.

61. Cintora I, Pearce D, Cannon JA. A clinical survey of aortobifemoral bypass using two inherently different graft types. Ann Surg 208:625-630, 1988.

62. Tilney NL, Kirkman RL, Whittemore AD, Osteen RT. Vascular access for dialysis and cancer chemotherapy. In Mannick JA, Camon JL, Jordan GL, et al., eds. Advances in Surgery. Chicago: Year Book, 1986, pp 221-268.

63. Tellis VA, Kohlbert WI, Bhat DJ, Driscoll B, Veith FJ. Expanded polytetrafluoroethylene graft fistula for chronic hemodialysis. Ann Surg 189:101-105, 1979.

64. Raju S. PTFE grafts for hemodialysis access. Ann Surg 206:666-673, 1987.

65. Sicard G, Allen BT, Anderson CB. Polytetrafluoroethylene grafts for vascular access. In Sommer BF, Henry ML, eds, Vascular Access for Hemodialysis. Chicago: Pluribus Press, 1989.

66. Porter JM. Is axillofemoral bypass as poor an operation as we think: Factors contributing to improved results. Presented at the Seventeenth Annual Symposium on Current Critical Problems and New Horizons in Vascular Surgery. New York: Nov. 16-18, 1990.

67. Boyce B. Physical characteristics of expanded polytetrafluoroethylene grafts. In Stanley JC, ed. Biologic and Synthetic Vascular Prostheses. New York: Grune & Stratton, 1982, pp 553-561.

68. Graham LM, Bergan JJ. Expanded polytetrafluoroethylene vascular grafts: Clinical and experimental observation. In Stanley JC, ed. Biologic and Synthetic Vascular Prostheses. New York: Grune & Stratton, 1982, pp 536-586.

69. Clowes AW, Gown AM, Hanson SR, Reidy MA. Mechanisms of arterial graft failure: Role of cellular proliferation in early healing of PTFE prostheses. Am J Pathol 118:43-54, 1985.

70. Clowes AW, Kirkman TR, Clowes MM. Mechanisms of arterial graft failure. II. Chronic endothelial and smooth muscle cell proliferation in healing polytetrafluoroethylene prostheses. J Vasc Surg 3:877-884, 1986.

71. Quinones-Baldrich WJ, Ziomek S, Henderson T, Moore WS. Primary anastomotic bonding in polytetrafluoroethylene grafts? J Vasc Surg 5:311-318, 1987.

72. Mohring K, Osbach HW, Bersch W, Ikinger U, Schüler PJ. Clinical implications of pathomorphological findings in vascular prostheses. In Robinson BHB, Hawkins JB, eds. Dialysis, Transplantation Nephrology. London: Pitman, 1978, pp 582-583.

73. Formichi MJ, Guidoin RG, Jausseran JM, Awad JA, Johnston W, King MW, Eng P, Courbier R, Marois M, Rouleau C, Batt M, Girard JF, Gosselin C. Expanded PTFE prostheses as arterial substitutes in humans: Late pathological findings in 73 excised grafts. Ann Vasc Surg 2:14-27, 1988.

74. Echave V, Koornick AR, Haimov M, Jacobson JH. Intimal hyperplasia as a complication of the use of the polytetrafluoroethylene graft for femoral-popliteal bypass. Surgery 86:791-798, 1979.

75. Graor RA, Risius B, Denny KM, Young JR, Beven EG, Hertzer NR, Ruschhaupt WF, O'Hara PJ, Geisinger MA, Zelch MG. Local thrombolysis in the treatment of thrombosed arteries, bypass grafts, and arteriovenous fistulas. J Vasc Surg 2:406-414, 1985.

76. Rubin JR, Yao JST, Thompson RG, Bergan JJ. Management of infection of major amputation stumps after failed femorodistal grafts. Surgery 93:810-815, 1985.

77. Kaupp HA, Matulewicz TJ, Lattimer GL, Kremen JE, Celani VJ. Graft infection or graft reaction? Arch Surg 114:1419-1422, 1979.

78. Paes E, Vollmar JF, Mohr W, Hamann H, Brecht-Krauss D. Perigraft reaction: Incompatibility of synthetic vascular grafts? New aspects on clinical manifestation, pathogenesis, and therapy. World J Surg 12:750-755, 1988.

79. Blumenberg RM, Gelfand ML, Dale WA. Perigraft seromas complicating arterial grafts. Surgery 97:194-203, 1985.

80. Amato JJ, Marbey ML, Bush C, Galdieri RJ, Cotroneo JV, Bushong J. Systemic-pulmonary polytetrafluoroethylene shunts in palliative operations for congenital heart disease. J Thorac Cardiovasc Surg 95:62-69, 1988.

81. Buche M, Schoevaerdts JC, Jaumin P, Ponlot R, Chalant CH. Perigraft seroma following axillofemoral bypass: Report of three cases. Ann Vasc Surg 1:374-377, 1986.

82. Bhuta I, Dorrough R. Noninfectious fluid collection around velour Dacron graft: Possible allergic reaction. South Med J 74:870-872, 1981.

83. Ahn SS, Machleder HI, Gupta R, Moore WS. Perigraft seroma: Clinical, histologic, and serologic correlates. Am J Surg 154:173-178, 1987.

84. Bolton W, Cannon JA. Seroma formation associated with PTFE vascular grafts used as arteriovenous fistulae. Dialysis Transplant 10:60-64, 1981.

85. Lowery RC, Wicker HS, Sanders K, Peniston RL. Management of recalcitrant periprosthetic fluid collection. J Vasc Surg 6:77-80, 1987.

86. Moore WS, Hall AD. Late suture failure in the pathogenesis of anastomotic false aneurysms. Ann Surg 172:1064-1068, 1970.

87. Cutler EC, Dunphy JE. The use of silk in infected wounds. N Engl J Med 224:101-107, 1941.

88. Dobrin PB. Surgical manipulation and the tensile strength of polypropylene sutures. Arch Surg 124: 665-668, 1989.

89. Calhoun TR, Kitten CM. Polypropylene suture—Is it safe? J Vasc Surg 4:98-100, 1986.

90. Myhre OA. Breakage of prolene suture. Ann Thorac Surg 36:121, 1983.

91. Szarnicki RJ. Polypropylene suture fracture. Ann Thorac Surg 35:222, 1983.

92. Aldrete V. Polypropylene suture fracture. Ann Thorac Surg 37:264, 1984.

93. Stanley JC, Lindenauer SM, Graham LM, Zelenock GB, Wakefield TW, Cronenwett JL. Biologic and synthetic vascular grafts. In Moore WS, ed. Vascular Surgery: A Comprehensive Review. Orlando, Fla.: WB Saunders, 1990, pp 275-294.

94. Dardik H, Miller N, Dardik A, Ibrahim IM, Sussman B, Berry SM, Wolodiger F, Kahn M, Dardik I. A decade of experience with the glutaraldehyde-tanned human umbilical cord vein graft for revascularization of the lower limb. J Vasc Surg 7:336-346, 1988.

95. Dardik H, Ibrahim IM, Sussman B, Kahn M, Sanchez M, Klausner S, Baier RE, Meyer AE, Dardik II. Biodegradation and aneurysm formation in umbilical vein grafts. Ann Surg 199:61-68, 1984.

96. Guidoin R, Gagnon Y, Roy PE, Marois M, Johnston W, Batt M. Pathologic features of surgically excised human umbilical vein grafts. J Vasc Surg 3:146-154, 1986.

97. Julien S, Gill F, Guidoin R, Guzman R, Charara J, Roy PE, Marois M, Laroche G, Batt M, Roy P, Serise JM, Marois D. Biologic and structural evaluation of 80 surgically excised human umbilical vein grafts. Can J Surg 32:101-108, 1989.

98. Cranley JJ, Karkow WS, Hafner CD, Flanagan LD. Aneurysmal dilatation in umbilical vein grafts. In Yao JST, Bergan JJ, eds. Reoperative Arterial Surgery. New York: Grune & Stratton, 1986, pp 343-358.

99. Rosenberg N. Dialdehyde starch tanned bovine heterografts. In Sawyer PN, Kaplitt MJ, eds. Vascular Grafts. New York: Appleton-Century-Crofts, 1978, pp 261-270.

100. Brems J, Castaneda M, Garvin PJ. A five-year experience with the bovine heterograft for vascular access. Arch Surg 121:941-944, 1986.

101. Andersen RC, Ney AL, Madden MC, LaCombe MJ. Biologic conduits for vascular access: Saphenous veins, umbilical veins, bovine carotid arteries. In Sommer BG, Henry ML, eds. Vascular Access for Hemodialysis. Chicago: Pluribus Press, 1989, pp 65-83.

102. Sabanayagam P, Schwartz AB, Soricelli RR, et al. A comparative study of 402 bovine heterografts and 225 reinforced expanded PTFE grafts as AVF in the ESRD patient. Trans Am Soc Artif Intern Organs 26:88-91, 1980.

103. Hurt AV, Batello-Cruz M, Skipper BJ, Teaf SR, Sterling WA. Bovine carotid artery heterografts versus polytetrafluoroethylene grafts. Am J Surg 146:844-847, 1983.

7

Anastomotic Aneurysms

Jerry Goldstone

One of the late complications of arterial reconstructive surgical procedures is the development of an anastomotic aneurysm.[1-3] Although development of an aneurysm at the site of an arterial anastomosis is an infrequent occurrence, it is important nevertheless because of its potential for significant morbidity. True aneurysmal degeneration can occur in arterial (or arterialized vein) segments that include an anastomosis or suture line, but the vast majority of anastomotic aneurysms are *false aneurysms*, also referred to as pseudo, junctional, or suture line aneurysms. As such, histopathologic examination of the aneurysm wall shows primarily fibrous connective tissue without the normal layers and components of an arterial wall, thereby distinguishing it from a true aneurysm. In simplest terms an anastomotic aneurysm is nothing more than a pulsating hematoma.

INCIDENCE

Although the incidence of anastomotic aneurysms ranges from about 1.4% to 4%, it varies substantially depending on the type of operation that preceded the formation of the aneurysm, its anatomic location, and the time interval from the original procedure. Furthermore, the incidence varies with the method of reporting. Some authors report incidence rates according to number of patients or operations; others use a ratio that includes the number of anastomoses at risk. Since every anastomosis and suture line constitute a potential site of aneurysm formation, it is more accurate to express incidence in terms of number of anastomoses. For example, Szilagyi et al.[1] reported a 3.9% incidence (by patient) of anastomotic an-

eurysms after 4214 arterial reconstructive operations. On the other hand, when computed per anastomosis, the incidence was 1.7% (205 of 9561 anastomoses). Of these, the incidence was 3% for anastomoses involving the common femoral artery, 1.2% for the iliac artery, 1.1% for the popliteal artery, and 0.2% for the aorta. Overall, however, 80% of the anastomotic aneurysms involved the common femoral artery. At the other extreme, Stoney, Albo, and Wylie[4] reported a per patient incidence of 23.7% in 145 patients with femoral or popliteal artery anastomoses—an extremely high incidence by contemporary standards. However, in this series most of the aneurysms were caused by the use of silk sutures for the primary arterial repairs. Silk sutures have since been uniformly abandoned for arterial anastomoses involving prosthetic grafts. This emphasizes the effects of improvements in surgical technique and reconstructive materials over time on the incidence of this complication. Haimovici[5] compiled five large series that included 308 anastomotic aneurysms that occurred in 249 patients after 7366 surgical procedures. The incidence of anastomotic aneurysms was 3.4% per patient and 4.1% per procedure. No data were supplied in this review on the incidence per anastomosis at risk.

Another factor that affects the incidence of anastomotic aneurysms is length of follow-up after the surgical procedure. Wandschneider and Denck's review[6] of 119 anastomotic aneurysms showed a bimodal incidence: the first peak occurred within the first year after the primary arterial reconstruction and a second, larger peak occurred after about 5 years. Courbier and Larranaga[7] reported a similar distribution with a mean interval of 50 months between initial operation and diagnosis of anastomotic aneurysm but with two distinct peaks at about 8 and 30 months. These incidence distributions over time may reflect the influence of different etiologic factors. Since most anastomotic aneurysms are now caused by deterioration of the arterial wall to which a prosthetic graft is attached, it is not surprising that the incidence of anastomotic aneurysms increases with the duration of follow-up.

LOCATION

Obviously any site of anastomosis between two vascular structures can become aneurysmal, but this is extremely rare when completely autogenous repairs are performed. Indeed, aneurysm formation at the site of endarterectomy alone is rare, occurring only three times (incidence 0.4%) in Szilagyi's review.[8] Similarly, aneurysms involving saphenous vein anastomoses to the femoral or popliteal arteries occurred only six times (incidence 0.9%) in this same series. It has been a very rare complication in the large endarterectomy experience extending over nearly 40 years at the University of California, San Francisco. Perhaps of most current interest and concern in this regard is the occasional disruption of a saphenous vein patch used for closure of the carotid artery following endarterectomy.[9-11] This type of acute anastomotic aneurysm almost always occurs within the first 3 to 4 postoperative days and produces acute hemorrhage and a high rate of serious neurologic complications and death.

Almost all clinically significant anastomotic aneurysms occur at sites of prosthetic–to–native vessel anastomoses, and by far the most common location is the common femoral artery at the distal end of an aortofemoral bypass. A review of eight published series that includes 584 anastomotic aneurysms in which prosthetic material was used indicates that 78.6% occurred at the femoral artery in the groin (Table 7-1). Intra-abdominal sites are the next most frequent: aortic and iliac sites combined account for nearly 15% of all such lesions (Figs. 7-1 and 7-2). When only those operations performed in the past few years are considered, the

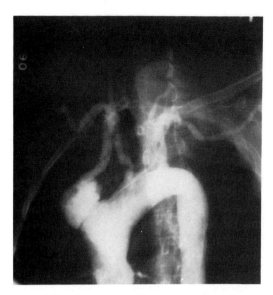

Fig. 7-1. Arch aortogram showing anastomotic aneurysm at site of origin of aortoinnominate and left common carotid bypass graft. No suture material was found during repair of the anastomotic aneurysm and it is assumed that silk sutures were used in the original procedure, which was performed about 30 years before aortogram was made.

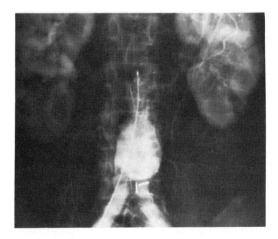

Fig. 7-2. Abdominal aortogram showing infrarenal aortic anastomotic aneurysm at the site of end-to-side anastomosis of aortobifemoral bypass graft. No evidence of infection or suture failure was identified at the time of repair although there was moderate dilation of the graft.

Table 7-1. Anatomic Locations of Anastomotic Aneurysms*

Author	Aortic No. (%)	Iliac No. (%)	Femoral No. (%)	Extremities No. (%)	Carotid No. (%)	Other No. (%)	Total No.
Szilagyi et al.[1] (1975)	4 (2.5)	19 (11.7)	129 (79.1)	9 (5.5)	2 (1.2)	—	163
Nichols et al.[12] (1980)	3 (7)	3 (7)	36 (83.7)	—	—	1 (2.3)	43
Satiani et al.[13] (1980)	2 (6.9)	1 (3.4)	22 (75.9)	2 (6.9)	1 (3.4)	1 (3.4)	29
Briggs et al.[14] (1983)	5 (15.2)	1 (3)	27 (81.8)	—	—	—	33
Mehigan et al.[15] (1985)	1 (4.3)	3 (13)	19 (82.6)	—	—	—	23
Sedwitz et al.[16] (1988)	12[†] (14.8)	—	61 (75.3)	8 (9.9)	—	—	81
Wandschneider and Denck[6] (1988)	6 (5)	—	99 (83.1)	3 (2.5)	2 (1.7)	9 (7.6)	119
Gaylis and Dewar[3] (1990)	17 (18.2)	7 (7.5)	66 (70.9)	3 (3.2)	—	—	93
TOTAL	50 (8.6)	34 (5.8)	459 (78.6)	25 (4.3)	5 (0.9)	11 (1.9)	584

*Includes only anastomoses that involve prosthetic material.
†Includes iliac.

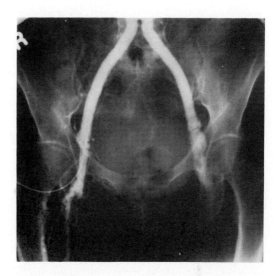

Fig. 7-3. Bilateral femoral anastomotic aneurysms, left larger than right, in same patient as shown in Fig. 7-2. As with proximal anastomosis, deterioration of arterial wall and graft dilation were believed to be etiologic factors.

prevalence of anastomotic aneurysms at the common femoral location is probably even higher, perhaps in excess of 90% as suggested by at least one author.[8] To place this in proper perspective, when anastomotic aneurysms occur after aortobifemoral bypass grafting, the femoral area is ten times more frequently involved than the aorta.[7] Aneurysms involving the femoral artery obviously are detected easier than those that arise retroperitoneally, but this factor alone does not account for the extremely high proportion of these lesions occurring in the groin. Furthermore, approximately 30% of patients who have one anastomotic aneurysm will have at least one other such lesion simultaneously (Fig. 7-3).

PATHOGENESIS

Anastomotic pseudoaneurysms involve a defect in the suture line holding two vascular conduits together. This defect, usually small to begin with, permits blood to escape, creating a hematoma that is in continuity with the arterial lumen. Varying amounts of mural thrombus line the aneurysm cavity surrounding the unclotted blood lining. Fibroblastic organization of the hematoma leads to formation of a connective tissue capsule or wall surrounding the central cavity. The arterial pressure constantly exerted within this cavity is responsible for the tendency for these lesions to enlarge.

Several factors have been implicated in the causation of anastomotic aneurysms; different authors implicate different factors as being of primary importance. It is well known that the strength of any arterial anastomosis involving a prosthesis is forever dependent on the integrity of the suture line because permanent healing (i.e., a stable fibrous union) of the prosthetic-arterial junction never occurs. Since the existence of an anastomotic false aneurysm implies at least partial disruption of the involved anastomosis, one or more of the following must occur for an anastomotic aneurysm to develop: suture failure, weakening and loss of holding power of the arterial wall, weakening or disruption of the prosthesis, and impaired wound healing.

Suture Failure

Historically, suture breakage was among the earliest recognized factors leading to anastomotic aneurysm formation. In the early days of arterial reconstructive surgery, silk was considered a permanent suture and was the suture most frequently used. Its weakening, dissolution, and breakage were implicated as the major factor in the formation of anastomotic aneurysms in several reports from the 1960s and early 1970s. For example, deterioration of silk sutures was the most important causative factor in the series reported by Stoney, Albo, and Wylie[4] in 1965. Similarly, Moore et al.[17] determined that silk suture failure was responsible for all 25 of the femoral anastomotic aneurysms they reported in 1968. As synthetic sutures became available, silk was abandoned for use with vascular prostheses. But other suture types also have been implicated in false aneurysm formation, including monofilament polyethylene, which is thought to become brittle, weak, and subject to fracture. Braided polyester has been the suture preferred by most vascular surgeons for many years, although monofilament polypropylene is also widely used and expanded polytetrafluoroethylene (PTFE) is gaining in popularity. Fears that the monofilament polypropylene would be associated with the same anastomotic aneurysm frequency as polyethylene have not been substantiated, although it is well known that this type of suture is particularly vulnerable to damage by inappropriate handling with surgical instruments. No suture type is exempt from breakage and subsequent anastomotic aneurysm formation, and none of those commonly used today is associated with a higher incidence of this complication than the others. Despite the virtual universal use of permanent synthetic sutures, the incidence of anastomotic aneurysms has remained more or less constant in recent years, making other causative factors more important.

Almost all anastomotic aneurysms occur in vascular operations in which prosthetic materials are used. Anastomotic aneurysms are rare after artery-artery or even artery-vein anastomoses, even when infection is present. Although aneurysms involving anastomoses between an artery and vein have been reported, most of these represent true aneurysmal degeneration of the venous component of the anastomotic site. These observations have focused attention on the prosthesis itself as a major factor in anastomotic aneurysm formation.

Weakening, dilation, and disruption of the arterial prosthesis have been found in some anastomotic aneurysms.[18-20] A number of design and manufacturing imperfections can lead to weakening of the graft fabric, with subsequent rupture or pulling out of the sutures. This is probably a rare problem today but Dacron grafts have been shown to dilate by as much as 15% to 20% of their original diameters. Knitted grafts tend to dilate more than woven ones.[12] Nunn, Freeman, and Hudgins[21] reported a mean diameter dilation, determined by ultrasound, of 17.6% in Dacron grafts within 33 months of implantation. This probably does not represent deterioration of fiber strength but a loss of compactness of the knit, which is attributed to the application of heat during the manufacturing process. The resulting luminal enlargement leads to hydrodynamic stresses on the anastomosis, as predicted by Laplace's law. In addition, implanted prostheses become less compliant over time, leading to compliance mismatch between host artery and prosthesis. These latter two factors probably are important in anastomotic aneurysm formation and are discussed in more detail later in this chapter.

One other prosthesis-related problem that can contribute to the development of anastomotic aneurysms is the tendency for woven grafts to fray at the cut edges, which facilitates the pulling out of sutures. Despite these considerations, woven grafts have not been associated with a higher incidence of anastomotic aneurysm than knitted grafts. Relatively few anastomotic aneurysms involving expanded PTFE grafts have been reported. In a series of recurrent anastomotic aneurysms (all involving Dacron grafts) reported by Carson et al.,[20] none occurred in patients in whom expanded PTFE grafts were used for repair of the first anastomotic aneurysm. However, it should be emphasized that the total number of Dacron grafts used for aortofemoral reconstructions far exceeds the number constructed with expanded PTFE, which has only been available relatively recently in a bifurcated configuration. Design and manufacturing improvements continue to be introduced and contemporary polyester prosthetic materials are extremely durable and maintain their tensile strength for many years.

Arterial Wall Failure

Weakness of the arterial wall is now the defect thought to be responsible for most anastomotic aneurysms. This has been confirmed in several series in which anastomotic aneurysms were carefully inspected at the time of their surgical repair.[18,22,23] In these studies the sutures were found to have pulled out of the host artery, creating the disruption in the anastomosis that defines an anastomotic aneurysm (Fig. 7-4). This could be caused by insufficiently large suture bites of arterial wall taken during construction of the anastomosis or by excessive tension placed on the graft (e.g., graft too short, joint flexion), but the influence of both of these factors is augmented by an arterial wall with reduced tensile strength. Weakening of the host artery can result from several causes. Progressive atherosclerosis may be responsible for further deterioration of the arterial wall and

probably plays a role in most cases. The histologic appearance of the arteries involved in anastomotic aneurysms shows considerable thinning of the elastic fibers in the media, fibrinohyalinosis of the intima, and frequently the presence of a monocytic reaction with foreign body giant cells. In about 20% of cases, a chronic inflammatory reaction is the predominant pathologic abnormality in addition to the underlying atherosclerosis. Excessive mobilization of the vessels during the original arterial reconstruction further damages the arterial wall by interfering with its blood supply (vasa vasora). This is the mechanism proposed for the relationship between anastomotic aneurysms and repeat operations (dissections) on the same artery. The concomitant performance of endarterectomy also has been mentioned by some authors as an important causative factor, but this has been disputed by others, including Szilagyi and associates,[1,8] who reported an incidence of anastomotic aneurysm after endarterectomy of only 0.4%.

It is well known that the arterial wall also can be weakened by infection and anastomotic aneurysms are a well-recognized complication of prosthetic graft infection. The bacteria do not

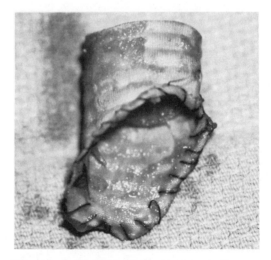

Fig. 7-4. Graft specimen from abdominal aortic anastomotic aneurysm showing intact suture line on prosthesis. In this case the sutures were pulled through an aortic wall that was degenerated but not infected.

affect the integrity of the prosthesis but instead produce weakening and destruction of the adjacent arterial wall. For this reason any anastomotic aneurysm must be considered as possibly infectious in origin and appropriate surgical plans should deal with this problem. This includes the careful evaluation of the aneurysm wall and contents by the microbiology laboratory. Kaebnick et al.,[24] using special culture techniques, recovered microorganisms from 19 of 21 clinically uninfected femoral anastomotic aneurysms. Slime-producing *Staphylococcus epidermidis* was isolated from most of these aneurysms. Data such as these suggest an important role for subclinical infection in the pathogenesis of anastomotic aneurysms, although in most series there is a very low incidence of clinically detectable infection.

Mechanical Factors

Several mechanical factors may play an important role in the development of anastomotic aneurysms. These are greatly influenced by the location and type of anastomosis. Most anastomotic aneurysms involve the femoral anastomoses of aortofemoral bypass grafts and most of these anastomoses are constructed in an end-to-side configuration. This results in a much larger effective radius at the anastomotic site, which, by application of Laplace's law, is associated with a considerable increase in the tangential tension in the wall of the vessels. The effects of hypertension also are exerted through this mechanism. The resulting increase in tangential wall tension may contribute to the pulling out of sutures or disruption of the arterial wall if it is weakened, as described previously.

Another local mechanical factor is excessive tension on the anastomosis. This can occur by pulling the graft too tight in an effort to completely flatten out the crimps of woven and knitted Dacron grafts. This should be less of a problem for noncrimped prostheses such as expanded PTFE grafts although anastomotic aneurysms have occurred with grafts of this type. Excessive tension also has been assumed to occur in the femoral region with hip flexion. This has led some surgeons to temporarily restrict patient activity following aortofemoral

bypass. However, Szilagyi et al.[1] have shown that these bending forces are not likely to have a significant effect on a common femoral anastomosis until the thigh is put into a position of flexion of about 70 degrees. Courbier and Larranaga[7] have suggested that the normal slippage of the external iliac/common femoral artery under the inguinal ligament may be replaced by fibrous fixation of a prosthetic graft limb to the ligament. When this occurs, flexion of the hip may place linear tension on the distal anastomotic site.

Still another local mechanical factor that contributes to anastomotic aneurysm formation is too short a bevel cut into the graft limb. This creates uneven tension around the anastomosis, with the maximum at the apex of the bevel where contact between the graft and the artery is least and suture bites are typically smaller. This represents the weakest point of a distal anastomosis and has been a frequent site of the anastomotic disruption responsible for anastomotic aneurysms.

Compliance mismatch, highly regarded as a major contributor to anastomotic neointimal hyperplasia, also is believed to play a role in the formation of anastomotic aneurysms.[15] Prosthetic grafts become stiffer (less compliant) after implantation because of fibrous tissue ingrowth. This stiffness can become three to five times that of even an atherosclerotic artery, resulting in greater expansion of the host artery with each pulse than of the prosthesis. This causes permanent abnormal suture line stresses acting longitudinally along the artery (axial stress) and circumferentially (hoop stress) as well as a shearing stress acting both longitudinally and radially. All of these stresses are maximal at the suture line and may contribute to anastomotic rupture.

When a graft-artery anastomosis is constructed in an end-to-side fashion, the resulting geometry favors turbulence, which produces vibrations of the vessel wall. It has been suggested that these vibrations not only increase the shear stress, but also have a deleterious effect on the elastic tissue of the arterial wall, leading to loss of tensile strength and subsequent suture line disruption.[12]

Some authors have implicated impedance

mismatch at the level of the femoral artery bifurcation as another mechanical factor that increases stress on anastomoses at that level. Impedance mismatch is said to occur when the ratio of graft diameter to host artery diameter is less than the ideal of 1.4 to 1.5 : 1. In addition, the angle of the graft-artery anastomosis may cause increased turbulence, mechanical stresses, and eventual anastomotic weakening. Whereas an end-to-end anastomosis between vessels of equal size transmits energy as efficiently as a normal artery, in an end-to-side anastomosis the larger the angle between the vessels, the less the rate of flow. The energy liberated by this loss of flow is distributed, at least in part, to the anastomotic site.

Miscellaneous Factors

Unrecognized host factors, such as enhanced collagenase activity as reported in some patients with abdominal aortic aneurysms, may be present in some patients with anastomotic aneurysms but the significance of these findings has not been determined.[14]

Systemic factors also have been implicated in the causation of anastomotic aneurysms The findings of multiple anastomotic aneurysms in up to 60% of patients and associated aortic anastomotic aneurysms in some series support the concept of systemic factors that predispose some patients to formation of these lesions. Among these factors are hyperlipidemia, continued tobacco use, and hypertension. Each of these also is associated with progressive atherosclerosis.

Other causes of anastomotic aneurysms have been demonstrated. Infection, through its effect on the arterial wall, has been mentioned earlier.[25] The incidence of anastomotic aneurysms is increased, at least in the femoral region, when wound healing problems occur after the primary arterial reconstruction. Among these are perigraft serum, lymph, or blood collections. Such fluid collections impair fibrous tissue ingrowth into the prosthesis and may result in deficient fibrous bonding at the anastomotic site. They also may contribute to subsequent infection of the graft.

Faulty surgical technique plays an important role in many anastomotic aneurysms. Inade-quate or improperly placed sutures, both in the graft and the host artery, can cause suture line disruption. Enough sutures must be placed far enough away from the cut edge so they will not pull out of the artery wall. Endarterectomy, if performed properly, leaves the adventitia and external elastic lamina as the major structural components of the arterial wall. An endarterectomy plane improperly developed too deeply in the arterial wall will leave a wall incapable of withstanding the many stresses normally exerted on the anastomosis.

Now that nonbiodegradable synthetic sutures are used universally for prosthetic graft–artery anastomoses, it usually is difficult to determine a single factor responsible for any anastomotic aneurysm. Most of these aneurysms probably are caused by multiple factors acting together. Nevertheless, infection, imperfections in surgical technique, and host vessel weakness with aseptic suture line disruption are probably the most important and common causes.

The average interval between the original arterial operation and the detection of an anastomotic aneurysm varies from a few weeks to 10 to 15 years. The average interval in most large series has ranged from 44.5 to 70 months.[26-29] In some respects the etiologic factors involved in the formation of an anastomotic aneurysm influence the length of time it takes for the aneurysm to develop. Technical errors, healing complications, and mechanical factors have been associated with anastomotic aneurysms that occur early, within the first 6 to 12 months after the index arterial reconstruction. The mechanical factors and the effects of hypertension appear to be more important in late years of postoperative observation.[1] Other factors, including deterioration of the arterial wall, probably exert their influence evenly throughout the period of follow-up.

Any discussion of the cause of anastomotic aneurysms must take into account the following factors: the nearly universal involvement of a prosthetic component in the involved anastomosis; the very high percentage that occur at the distal anastomoses of reconstructions terminating at the common femoral artery; the high percentage of end-to-side type of anastomosis; and the virtual universal use of modern synthetic sutures for the original vascular repair. The fact remains that anastomotic aneurysms are very uncommon lesions and many of the contributing factors leading to their development are present as frequently in patients who do not develop them as in those who do.

CLINICAL MANIFESTATIONS

The clinical manifestations of anastomotic aneurysms are determined in large part by their location. Since a large percentage of these lesions occur in the inguinal area where they are close to the skin, detection of swelling and the presence of local pain are common. The appearance of a pulsatile and enlarging mass in the groin or thigh is hard to overlook, but unless the mass is large, its presence in the abdomen may escape detection by even a careful examiner. In Gaylis' series[18] of 93 prosthesis-related anastomotic aneurysms, 59% presented with swelling and 39% with pain in the groin. Only 20% were asymptomatic. Rupture was the presenting manifestation in 13% of the cases in this series but it occurred in 23.5% of the aortic anastomotic aneurysms. In the report by Briggs, Jarstfer, and Collins,[14] of 33 anastomotic aneurysms, the diagnosis was established by the presence of a palpable groin mass that occurred in 88.9% of the anastomotic aneurysms in the femoral area. Three of five aortic anastomotic aneurysms were palpable but only two presented with abdominal pain. Similar findings have been reported by others, including Sedwitz, Hye, and Stabile.[16] The most common clinical presentation in their series was pain and a palpable, pulsatile mass that occurred in 51 of 81 lesions (63%). Signs and symptoms of systemic or localized infection were the presenting manifestations of 11 aneurysms (13.6%). More important, rupture occurred in eight (9.9%). Rupture also was an important and relatively frequent occurrence in Courbier and Larranaga's series,[7] occurring in 15 of 103 cases (14.6%). This complication is especially dangerous when aortic anastomoses are involved because of the aforementioned difficulty of detecting small anastomotic aneurysms in that location, the relatively poor tissue support to prevent or contain the rupture, and the magni-

tude of the bleeding that usually occurs. Aortic anastomotic aneurysms often go unnoticed until they become large enough to produce discomfort by pressure on adjacent organs or structures or by rupture. Erosion into an adherent segment of bowel can create an aortoenteric fistula with resultant sepsis and/or gastrointestinal bleeding. Ureteral obstruction also has occurred as a result of compression of iliac anastomotic aneurysms (Fig. 7-5), as has massive melena caused by rupture into the colon. Thus anastomotic aneurysms are not harmless. Hemorrhage, graft thrombosis, and embolization are not uncommon. These life- and limb-threatening complications are the presenting manifestations in about 15% of patients.

The continuous potential for development of anastomotic aneurysms, their predilection for occurring in the groin, and the ease of detection in this location all emphasize the importance of repeated careful physical examination during lifelong follow-up of these patients.

Many anastomotic aneurysms, especially those that are small and asymptomatic or located in locations inaccessible by physical examinations (chest, abdomen), can be detected only by special imaging studies, including ultrasound, computed tomography (CT), and magnetic resonance imaging (MRI) (Figs. 7-5 and 7-6). A recent report by Lacy et al.[30] suggests that color Doppler imaging can enhance the diagnostic accuracy of duplex ultrasound for these lesions, especially those located peripherally. Arteriography, like CT and MRI, has the same advantages and limitations in the evaluation of anastomotic aneurysms as it does for the evaluation of true aneurysms. It frequently fails to show the true extent of extraluminal contrast accumulation (Figs. 7-7 and 7-8). Nevertheless, arteriography is essential for planning the repair of an anastomotic aneurysm. It usually is not possible to distinguish true from false aneurysms by these methods, but knowledge of the patient's medical history should allow the clinician to make the correct diagnosis.

The detection of an anastomotic aneurysm, especially if it involves one or both femoral anastomoses of an aortofemoral graft, is an indication for imaging the remaining anastomoses since the presence of multiple anastomotic aneurysms is not uncommon.

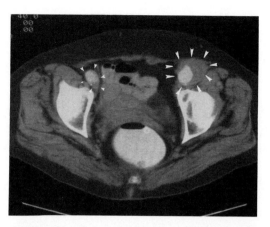

Fig. 7-5. CT scan of same patient as in Figs. 7-2 and 7-3. Note large size of aneurysm on left relative to angiographic appearance.

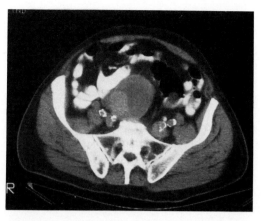

Fig. 7-6. CT scan of patient with left iliac aneurysm. Again, note underestimation of aneurysm size by angiogram (see Fig. 7-7).

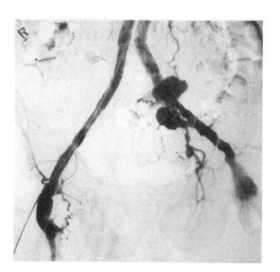

Fig. 7-7. Abdominal angiogram of same patient as in Fig. 7-6 showing left iliac aneurysm at site of distal anastomosis of aortobi-iliac graft implanted for aortic aneurysm. Bilateral femoral true aneurysms also are obvious.

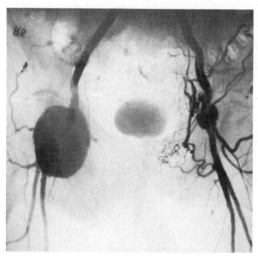

Fig. 7-8. Angiogram showing large right femoral and smaller left femoral anastomotic aneurysms. This patient had an anastomotic aneurysm previously at the site of a right common iliac anastomosis. These aneurysms were caused by arterial wall weakness.

TREATMENT

Indications for treatment and the type of treatment for anastomotic aneurysms depend on several factors, including the location, size, presumed etiology, and clinical manifestations. For example, most authors agree that asymptomatic femoral anastomotic aneurysms smaller than 2 cm in diameter can safely be observed without surgical intervention until they reach 2 cm in size or produce symptoms. The same criteria can be applied to similar-sized anastomotic aneurysms in other superficial locations, with the possible exception of those involving the carotid artery because of the hazard of distal embolization into the brain. In contrast, aortic false aneurysms, because of the difficulty in maintaining accurate assessment of their size and the seriousness of their complications, probably should be repaired as soon as they are identified, regardless of size. Intrathoracic anastomotic aneurysms also can be placed in the same treatment category. In this regard anastomotic aortic aneurysms differ from their non-anastomotic counterparts in which size is usually the single most important factor leading to operation. Urgent operations are indicated for the acute complications of anastomotic aneurysms, including hemorrhage, graft occlusion, and distal embolization.

The cause of an anastomotic aneurysm, which usually cannot be determined without operation and often not even then, will greatly influence the method of repair. Anastomotic aneurysms caused by infection involving either prosthetic material or autogenous tissue require complex repairs that are discussed in detail elsewhere (see Ch. 18). Nevertheless, all anastomotic aneurysms should be considered as possibly infected until proven otherwise and appropriate plans should be made for dealing with this problem. Fortunately, infection is an uncommon cause of anastomotic aneurysm even though anastomotic aneurysm is a common manifestation of prosthetic graft infection.

In each case the basic principles of management of anastomotic aneurysms are the same: proximal and distal control of the aneurysm's inflow and outflow vessels must be obtained by careful dissection. Until this is accomplished, it is best to avoid the aneurysm itself, mobilization of which is often very difficult because of the fibrosis resulting from prior operations. Recall that the performance of multiple operations in the same location (e.g., groin) is one of the factors frequently associated with the development of anastomotic aneurysms. Extreme care must be exercised during this dissection (which often is tedious and bloody) to avoid injuring important arterial branches, débridement of the adventitia (so-called exarterectomy), or disruption of the aneurysm prematurely, which can cause serious hemorrhage. Gentle handling of the aneurysm is also important to avoid dislodgment and distal embolization of mural thrombus. Sometimes it is easier

and safer to use intraluminal balloon catheters to occlude the outflow vessels rather than to persist in mobilizing a densely adherent femoral bifurcation (or other vessel) and its branches, especially the posterior aspect. This technique also may be useful for the proximal inflow vessel. For large femoral anastomotic aneurysms, proximal inflow control is best achieved through a small suprainguinal incision.

As noted, specific technical details for the repair of an anastomotic aneurysm will depend on the etiology and local anatomic factors. One very important component of these operations is a careful inspection of the anastomotic site in an effort to determine the cause of the suture line disruption. Special attention should be paid to determine the presence or absence of prosthetic graft infection. Although this is usually obvious because of the presence of perianastomotic fluid and poor fibrous tissue incorporation of the graft, it is unusual for this fluid to reveal organisms on Gram's stain and, since culture results are not available for at least 1 or 2 days, a clinical decision must be made based on the gross appearance. Nevertheless, specimens should be submitted for thorough microbiologic analysis as an aid to postoperative antibiotic therapy.

Careful dissection and exposure of an anastomotic aneurysm are important not only for determination of its cause, but also for enabling the surgeon to perform a secure, uncompromised repair. If the cause of the aneurysm is found to be a broken suture, the anastomosis can simply be redone. Occasionally repair of the defect is all that is required. If deterioration or fraying of the prosthetic graft is evident, a new segment of graft should be used to reconstruct the anastomosis. Careful attention must be paid to selecting the correct size of graft appropriate to both the inflow and outflow vessels. Use of a new segment of graft as an interposition graft between the host artery and the old graft is the most frequent method of repair of the most common type of anastomotic aneurysm—that is, the femoral portion of aortofemoral bypass.[2,31] This method was used in 71% of the femoral anastomotic aneurysm repairs reported by Satiani, Kazmers, and Evans.[13]

Since most anastomotic aneurysms are attributed to progressive deterioration of the arterial wall, exposure must be adequate to débride the vessel sufficiently for the construction of a new and secure anastomosis. Conversion of end-to-side into end-to-end anastomoses is believed to be important by some, although this should not be done if it will exclude perfusion of important collateral branches. These vessels are frequently the source of troublesome backbleeding if not controlled and, since many of them are small, this is not often possible with intraluminal catheters. End-to-end anastomoses theoretically are superior to end-to-side anastomoses because they result in a smaller diameter, thereby reducing the lateral wall tension on the vessels. In addition, with the proper size match between graft and artery, there will be less turbulence and therefore less stress on the newly created suture line. Use of an interposition graft also facilitates creation of a tension-free anastomosis.

The same general principles can be applied to the treatment of anastomotic aneurysms at other locations. For proximal aortic lesions of this kind, supraceliac aortic control is useful. Since a substantial percentage of these will be associated with prosthetic graft infection, reconstruction usually will include oversewing of the infrarenal aorta and lower extremity revascularization via an alternate route (i.e., axillofemoral). Débridement of the aorta to healthy appearing tissue and a double-layered closure without tension are important technical maneuvers. If the aortic anastomosis was originally end to side, the aortotomy sometimes can be closed with an autogenous patch and perfusion maintained in the native circulation.

RESULTS OF ANASTOMOTIC ANEURYSM REPAIR

Although generally excellent and durable results are reported, the repair of anastomotic aneurysms can be difficult and significant morbidity and mortality can occur. Satiani, Kazmers, and Evans[13] summarized the results of the operative treatment of 411 anastomotic aneurysms in 350 patients. Overall there was an 8.5% procedure-related mortality rate, an 8% amputation rate, and a 7.2% recurrence rate.

Recurrence rates higher than this have been reported in several series.[12,20,28,31,32] The nature and location of the lesion greatly influence the results. For example, aortic anastomotic aneurysms, particularly if they are infectious in origin, are associated with the highest mortality. In Satiani, Kazmers, and Evans' series,[13] 3 of 24 patients died (patient mortality, 12%), but two of the deaths occurred in the two patients with aortoenteric fistulas. The results of anastomotic aneurysm repair are worse when the operations are performed urgently for acute complications. In the series of Szilagyi,[8] long-term patency was lower and operative mortality and recurrence rates were higher in emergency surgical patients compared with that in those patients operated on electively.

Some authors believe that the incidence of recurrence is higher when anastomotic aneurysms are repaired by direct suture only rather than by complete anastomotic revision, but firm conclusions cannot be made from the available data. Carson et al.[20] reviewed 20 recurrent femoral anastomotic aneurysms, all involving end-to-end anastomoses between a Dacron interposition prosthesis and the femoral artery. They suggested that mismatch in diameter between the graft and host artery was the most important causative factor and attributed this to gradual dilation of the graft. Thus, although the incidence of anastomotic aneurysms is low and the results of their surgical treatment are generally excellent, it is probable that with better and longer follow-up assessment, recurrent anastomotic aneurysms will increase in incidence.

PREVENTION

Knowledge of the causes of anastomotic aneurysms and use of careful surgical technique are the most important factors for preventing this complication of arterial reconstruction. Permanent synthetic sutures should be used whenever a prosthetic graft is implanted. At the present time the available suture types appropriate for this purpose are braided polyester, PTFE, and monofilament polypropylene. Others will certainly be introduced into clinical practice in the future.

Arterial anastomoses should be constructed

without excessive tension. The crimps in woven and knitted Dacron prostheses make it difficult to determine the proper amount of tension on a graft limb. Noncrimped grafts such as those of expanded PTFE may be advantageous in this regard. Adequately large suture bites in the artery will help minimize the pulling out of sutures. An appropriately sized graft attached at an acute angle (for end-to-side anastomoses) will limit shearing and hoop stresses. Barker[33] has advocated the use of a T-shaped arteriotomy (with the horizontal portion of the T at the distal or apical end) and suggested that this technical modification allows placement of generous suture bites in this critical area of an end-to-side anastomosis. Local thromboendarterectomy may play a small role in reducing an artery's suture-holding strength but this can be compensated for by taking larger suture bites of the artery; endarterectomy should not be omitted when its use is required to ensure adequate lumen size. Meticulous technique should be used to minimize postoperative blood and lymph collections and wound infections since these wound complications are common in patients in whom anastomotic aneurysms later develop and they may play a role in the development of prosthetic infection. Because anastomotic aneurysm is one of the most common manifestations of prosthetic graft infection, all of the usual measures to prevent this complication should be used.

As noted earlier, multiple factors probably are involved in the formation of most anastomotic aneurysms. Many of these are beyond the control of the surgeon and therefore it is unlikely that all anastomotic aneurysms can be prevented. However, by observing the general principles described herein, surgeons should be able to maintain the incidence at an acceptable minimum.

REFERENCES

1. Szilagyi DE, Smith RF, Elliott JP, Hageman JH, Dall'Olmo CA. Anastomotic aneurysms after vascular reconstruction: Problems of incidence, etiology, and treatment. Surgery 78:800-816, 1975.
2. Evans WE, Hayes JP, Vermilion B. Anastomotic femoral false aneurysms. In Bernhard VM, Towne JB, eds. Complications in Vascular Surgery, 2nd ed. New York: Grune & Stratton, 1985, pp 205-211.
3. Gaylis H, Dewar G. Anastomotic aneurysms: Facts and fancy. Surg Annu 22:317-341, 1990.
4. Stoney RJ, Albo RJ, Wylie EJ. False aneurysms occurring after arterial grafting operations. Am J Surg 110:153-161, 1965.
5. Haimovici H. Extrafemoral anastomotic aneurysms: General considerations and techniques. In Haimovici H, ed. Vascular Surgery Principles and Techniques, 3rd ed. East Norwalk, Conn.: Appleton & Lange, 1989, pp 691-697.
6. Wandschneider W, Denck H. Anastomotic aneurysms—An unsolvable problem. Eur J Vasc Surg 2:115-119, 1988.
7. Courbier R, Larranaga J. Natural history and management of anastomotic aneurysms. In Bergan JJ, Yao JST, eds. Aneurysms: Diagnosis and Treatment. New York: Grune & Stratton, 1982, pp 567-580.
8. Szilagyi DE. Common femoral anastomotic aneurysms. In Haimovici H, ed. Vascular Surgery Principles and Techniques, 3rd ed. East Norwalk, Conn.: Appleton & Lange, 1989, pp 685-690.
9. Hertzer NR, Bevan EF, O'Hara PJ, Krajewski LP. A prospective study of vein patch angioplasty during carotid endarterectomy. Ann Surg 206:628-635, 1987.
10. Rosenthal D, Archie JP Jr, Garcia-Rinaldi R, Seagraves MA, Baird DN, McKinsey JF, Lamis PA, Clark MD, Erdoes LS, Whitehead T, Pallos LL. Carotid patch angioplasty: Immediate and long-term results. J Vasc Surg 12:326-333, 1990.
11. Archie JP Jr. Saphenous vein rupture pressure, rupture stress, and carotid endarterectomy patch reconstruction. Surgery 107:389-396, 1990.
12. Nichols WK, Stanton M, Silver D, Keitzer WF. Anastomotic aneurysms following lower extremity revascularization. Surgery 88:366-374, 1980.
13. Satiani B, Kazmers M, Evans W. Anastomotic arterial aneurysms: A continuing challenge. Ann Surg 192:674-682, 1980.
14. Briggs RM, Jarstfer BS, Collins GJ. Anastomotic aneurysms. Am J Surg 146:770-773, 1983.
15. Mehigan DG, Fitzpatrick B, Browne HI, Bouchier-Hayes DJ. Is compliance mismatch the major cause of anastomotic arterial aneurysms?: Analysis of 42 cases. J Cardiovasc Surg 26:147-150, 1985.
16. Sedwitz MM, Hye RJ, Stabile BE. The changing epidemiology of pseudoaneurysm: Therapeutic implications. Arch Surg 123:473-476, 1988.
17. Moore WS, Cafferata HT, Hall AD, Blaisdell FW. In defense of grafts across the inguinal ligament: An evaluation of early and late results of aorto-femoral bypass grafts. Ann Surg 168:207-214, 1968.
18. Gaylis H. Pathogenesis of anastomotic aneurysms. Surgery 90:509-515, 1981.
19. Ochsner JL. Management of femoral pseudoaneurysms. Surg Clin North Am 62:431-440, 1982.
20. Carson SN, Hunter GC, Palmaz J, Guernsey JM. Recurrence of femoral anastomotic aneurysms. Am J Surg 146:774-778, 1983.
21. Nunn DB, Freeman MH, Hudgins PC. Postoperative alterations in size of Dacron aortic grafts: An ultrasonic evaluation. Ann Surg 189:741-745, 1979.

22. McCabe CJ, Ashby CM, Malt RA. Host-artery weakness in the etiology of femoral anastomotic false aneurysms. Surgery 95:150-153, 1984.

23. Dennis JW, Littooy FN, Greisler HP, Baker WH. Anastomotic pseudoaneurysms: A continuing late complication of vascular reconstructive procedures. Arch Surg 121:314-317, 1986.

24. Kaebnick HW, Bandyk DF, Bergamini TM, Towne JB. The microbiology of explanted vascular prostheses. Surgery 102:756-762, 1987.

25. Nussaume O, Elzaabi M, Icard P, Branger C, Bouttier S, Andreassian B. False aneurysm infected by *Aspergillus fumigatus*: An unusual complication of aortofemoral bypass graft. Ann Surg 4:388-392, 1990.

26. Agrifoglio G, Costantini A, Lorenzi G, Agus GB, Castelli PM, Zaretti D. Femoral noninfected anastomotic aneurysms: A report of 56 cases. J Cardiovasc Surg 31:453-456, 1990.

27. Christensen RD, Bernatz PE. Anastomotic aneurysms involving the femoral artery. Mayo Clin Proc 47:313-317, 1972.

28. Schellack J, Salam A, Abouzeid MA, Smith RB, Stewart MT, Perdue GD. Femoral anastomotic aneurysms: A continuing challenge. J Vasc Surg 6:308-317, 1987.

29. Youkey JR, Clagett GP, Rich NM, Brigham RA, Orecchia PM, Salander JM. Femoral anastomotic false aneurysms: An 11-year experience analyzed with a case control study. Ann Surg 199:703-709, 1984.

30. Lacy JH, Box JM, Connors O, Penney L, Wright CB. Pseudoaneurysm diagnosis with color Doppler ultrasound. J Cardiovasc Surg 31:727-730, 1990.

31. Hollier LH, Batson RC, Cohn I. Femoral anastomotic aneurysms. Ann Surg 191:715-720, 1980.

32. DiMarzo L, Strandness EL, Schultz RD, Feldhaus RJ. Reoperation for femoral anastomotic false aneurysm. Ann Surg 206:168-172, 1987.

33. Barker W. Anastomotic aneurysms: Etiology, diagnosis, prevention, and treatment. Surg Rounds Sept.:43-56, 1988.

IV Coagulation

8

Hypercoagulable States and Unexplained Vascular Graft Thrombosis

Jonathan B. Towne

Hypercoagulable states as a cause of unexplained vascular thrombosis present a difficult clinical problem. Most graft failures in the perioperative period are presumed to occur because of technical errors in the construction of the anastomosis, problems with the conduit, or poor patient selection. The diagnosis of an abnormal hypercoagulable state is often made only after all of these other factors have been excluded. Although failure of heparin to prevent clotting in the operative field or immediate thrombosis of a vascular repair suggests abnormal coagulation, the diagnosis can be confirmed only by the blood coagulation laboratory. The clotting disorder must be detected early in the course of the disease to obtain a favorable outcome. Abnormal thrombosis falls into five general categories: (1) heparin-induced platelet aggregation, (2) abnormalities in the antithrombin system, (3) abnormalities of the fibrinolytic system, (4) thrombosis caused by lupus-like anticoagulant, and (5) a miscellaneous category consisting primarily of abnormal platelet aggregation and protein C and protein S defi-

HEPARIN-INDUCED THROMBOSIS

Paradoxical thrombotic complications of heparin sodium anticoagulant therapy are uncommon but potentially limb threatening and occasionally fatal. Several investigators have identified a chemically induced, immune thrombocytopenia as the cause of heparin-induced intravascular thrombosis, which usually occurs after 4 to 10 days of continued exposure to the drug.[1-5] The immune factor that triggers the thrombocytopenia has been identified as an IgG antibody, which produced agglutination of normal platelets when either porcine gut or beef lung heparin is added. The thrombi that occur with heparin-induced thrombosis have an unusual grayish white appearance in contradistinction to the red color of most thrombi. The white color is secondary to the creation of fibrin-platelet aggregates, which can be clearly identified on electron microscopy.[6]

Rhodes, Dixon, and Silver[7] found a heparin-dependent IgG antibody in the serum of several patients by means of the complement lysis inhibitions test. They also demonstrated a residual heparin-platelet aggregating effect 12 days to 2 months after patient recovery from the initial exposure to heparin. In these patients a 24-hour infusion of heparin caused a mean reduction of platelet count of 197,000/mm³. Since heparin preparations are not pure substances, it is also possible that a high-molecular contaminant not eliminated by the extraction procedure may cause the antiplatelet effect.

Clinical Presentation

Heparin-induced intravascular thrombosis can occur following a wide variety of indications for heparin administration, including thrombophlebitis with and without pulmonary embolus, perioperative heparin prophylaxis in patients at risk for thrombophlebitis, cardiac surgery, and vascular reconstruction. Platelet aggregation induced by heparin can result from both porcine gut and bovine lung heparin and can affect either the arterial or venous circulation. Both subcutaneous and intravenous heparin administration can produce this phenomenon.[8] Even heparin-coated catheters can cause heparin-induced thrombocytopenia. Laster and Silver[9] reported the development of heparin-induced thrombocytopenia in ten patients in whom heparin-coated pulmonary artery catheters were inserted. Despite discontinuation of all other sources of heparin, the thrombocytopenia persisted. Although all of the patients also were given heparin, it is theoretically possible that heparin-coated catheters alone could have caused abnormal platelet aggregation.

The clinical features of this syndrome are often dramatic. In any patient who has had thrombotic complications while receiving heparin therapy, heparin-induced aggregation of platelets should be considered. This is especially important in patients with arterial occlusions who do not have any other evidence of atherosclerotic vascular disease. At operation, the finding of a white clot at thrombectomy should alert the surgeon to the possibility of a heparin-induced thrombosis. In contrast to several reports in the literature, increased heparin sensitivity rather than increased heparin resistance was noted in several of our patients.[6] The cause of this is uncertain, but it is presently believed that it is unrelated to the heparin-induced aggregative immunoglobulin.

Diagnosis

Definitive diagnosis of heparin-induced intravascular thrombosis is obtained by performing platelet aggregation tests. Two patterns of response have been noted. The more common pattern is for the patient's platelet-poor plasma to aggregate donor platelets on the addition of heparin, indicating the presence of a relatively nonspecific platelet-aggregating factor in the patient's plasma. The less common pattern is for the patient's plasma to be active against only the patient's platelets and have no effect on donor platelets.

Other clotting factors are usually normal: fibrinogen level is normal, fibrin split products level may be mildly elevated but not in the range seen with intravascular coagulation, and prothrombin time is normal or slightly prolonged. All patients have a marked reduction in platelet count of less than 100,000/mm³ or a 50% decrease from admission level. In our series,[6] the platelet count averaged 37,500/mm³, with a range of 6000 to 73,000/mm³.

Patients with arterial thromboses often present with unique angiographic findings. These lesions consist of broad-based, isolated, lobulated excrescences that produce a variable amount of narrowing of the arterial lumen. Usually these findings have an abrupt appearance, with prominent luminal contour deformities in arterial segments that are otherwise normal. This distribution of disease is unusual and distinct from findings commonly seen with atherosclerosis. These changes occur in both the suprarenal and infrarenal portions of the abdominal aorta and represent adherent mural thrombi composed of aggregates of platelets and fibrin incorporating varying amounts of leukocytes and erythrocytes. Platelet aggregation tests also should be performed on any patient in whom recurrent pulmonary embolism developed while receiving adequate heparin therapy.

Treatment

When heparin-induced thrombocytopenia is diagnosed, heparin treatment should be reversed immediately with protamine sulfate, and dextran 40 should be administered for its antiaggregating and rheologic effects. Warfarin therapy also should be initiated and continued for several months. In patients with arterial occlusive manifestations of heparin-induced thrombosis, long-term warfarin therapy is recommended because of the possibility of coexisting latent venous occlusive disease.

The response of the platelet count to discontinuation of heparin therapy is usually prompt, often resulting in thrombocytosis, with a platelet count of 500,000 to 600,000/mm^3 being achieved in several days.

Coagulation tests distinguish heparin-induced platelet aggregation from other clotting disorders. The fibrinogen level and prothrombin time are usually normal. The fibrin split products level and prothrombin time are normal or slightly elevated. The sole patient in our series with a noticeable elevated fibrin split products level was the initial patient, in whom the diagnosis was not made antemortem. Heparin therapy was not stopped, and before her death (caused by an intracerebral hemorrhage), she had massive venous thrombosis involving both upper and lower extremities, which resulted in an elevated fibrin split products level. Early identification of heparin-induced thrombosis is necessary to minimize the catastrophic complications of major limb amputation and death.

This experience suggests that it is imperative that all patients receiving heparin therapy have serial platelet counts done from the fourth day of heparin therapy onward. It is our policy to perform platelet counts every other day starting on the fourth day of heparin therapy. If thrombocytopenia develops, platelet aggregation studies should be performed immediately. With early recognition of complications, the mortality and morbidity of major amputation can be prevented. Morbidity and mortality rates reported in the literature vary from 22% to 61% and 12% to 33%, respectively.[10,11]

Strategies for Patients With Heparin-Induced Platelet Aggregation

Patients who require subsequent heparin therapy for other vascular or cardiac surgery procedures require special management. In patients in whom heparin-induced platelet aggregation develops, the platelet aggregation tests usually revert to normal from 6 weeks to 3

months. Preferably vascular or cardiac surgery procedures are delayed until these tests revert to normal. We test the patient at 6 weeks and then every 2 weeks thereafter to determine when the platelet aggregation tests are negative. When they are negative, the patient is then admitted to the hospital for surgery. Cardiac catheterization or angiography is done as required without the use of heparin flush solutions, since even small amounts of heparin in the flush solutions can stimulate the development of heparin-induced antiplatelet antibodies. The vascular or cardiac surgery procedure is then performed with the usual administration of heparin. At the conclusion of the procedure, the heparin is reversed with protamine and care is taken during the postoperative period to ensure the patient does not receive heparin inadvertently through the flushing of either central venous catheters or arterial lines. By using this procedure, we have not had any difficulty with reexposure to heparin.

However, for those patients who require an additional vascular or cardiac surgery procedure and who cannot wait until the results from heparin-induced platelet aggregation tests are negative, a different strategy is necessary. In patients requiring procedures that can be done without the use of heparin, such as resection of abdominal aortic aneurysms, heparin is not used. However, in patients who require complex lower extremity revascularization or cardiopulmonary bypass, some sort of anticoagulation is necessary. There are basically two approaches. The approach favored by Laster, Elfrink, and Silver[12] involves administering aspirin and dipyridamole (Persantine) preoperatively and then using heparin for the operative procedure as is customary. In addition to aspirin and dipyridamole, we prefer to also use low-molecular-weight dextran, which, in addition to its rheologic properties, coats the platelets and interferes with platelet adhesion. In some patients, however, as noted by Kappa et al.,[13] the administration of aspirin has no effect on heparin-induced platelet aggregation. Makhoul, Greenberg, and McCann[14] noted that although aspirin abolished platelet aggregation in 9 of 16 patients with heparin-induced platelet aggregation, it only decreased platelet aggregation in the remaining seven, suggesting that aspirin is not able to reverse abnormal platelet aggregation in all patients. Based on these reports, our procedure is to administer aspirin and dipyridamole for several days before the operative procedure. On the day of operation, platelet aggregation tests are performed with the addition of heparin. If the heparin causes abnormal platelet aggregation, iloprost is then used to prevent heparin-induced platelet aggregation during the procedure. The use of iloprost can be complicated, particularly since it is a very potent vasodilator, and rather large doses of α-adrenergic agents are often required to support blood pressure.

Sobel et al.[15] reported an alternate technique in which patients receive warfarin anticoagulation combined with dextran as a means of preventing intraoperative thrombosis during reconstruction. This is a reasonable alternative for peripheral vascular reconstructions but is not possible for cardiopulmonary bypass. In the future, different substances may be available to allow for adequate anticoagulation. Makhoul, Greenberg, and McCann[14] noted in vitro that heparinoids did not cause platelet aggregation in patients with heparin-induced platelet aggregation. These new anticoagulant agents are being developed in Europe and may in the future be available for anticoagulant therapy in the United States.

Cole and Bormanis[16] have reported the use of ancrod, which is made from the venom of the Malaysian pit viper *(Agkistrodon rhodostoma)*, as an anticoagulant in patients who have heparin-induced platelet aggregation. Ancrod acts enzymatically on the fibrinogen molecule to form a product that cannot be clotted by physiologic thrombin. At the present time this medication is in the investigational phase and like heparinoids may be cleared by the Food and Drug Administration (FDA) in the not too distant future.

ANTITHROMBIN DEFICIENCY

Antithrombin III (AT III) is an α-globulin manufactured in the liver and perhaps by vascular endothelium, with a molecular weight of approximately 60,000 d and a half-life of 2.8 days.[17] It is a serine proteinase inhibitor that binds in equimolar ratios to several enzymes participating in the intrinsic pathway of blood coagulation including thrombin and factors IXa, Xa, and XIa.[18] Heparin significantly accelerates the rate at which AT III neutralizes these enzymes, limiting sequential clotting reactions and preventing fibrin formation. In 1965, Egeberg[19] described a family with an inborn defect of AT III. Subsequent research has confirmed the genetic transmission of this deficiency.[20-23] The frequency of this defect is approximately 1 in 2000 to 1 in 5000 in the general population.[24,25] There are probably at least two types of AT III deficiency. In the classic form both the protein level of AT III (as determined by measurement of its protein concentration) and its activity level are reduced in the patient's plasma.[26] However, there are other patients in whom the concentration of AT III is normal or even slightly elevated as measured by protein level, but the biologic function as measured by activity level tests is abnormal.[27] This suggests that these patients are manufacturing a defective antithrombin molecule. Acquired AT III deficiency can occur in patients with severe liver disease, nephrotic syndrome, hypoalbuminemia, malnutrition, and disseminated intravascular coagulation, and in some patients taking oral contraceptives. AT III deficiency may be an indicator of significant protein catabolism. Flinn et al.[28] noted low AT III activity in 16% of patients undergoing vascular surgery. There was low serum albumin (<3 mg/dl) in 48% of these patients, which was associated with an increased incidence of early graft failure.

Clinical Presentation

Although AT III deficiency is inherited, it is rare for episodes of thrombosis to be clinically manifested before the second decade of life. Despite continuously depressed levels of AT III in these patients, thrombotic episodes are often related to predisposing factors such as surgery, childbirth, and infection and rarely occurs spontaneously. This deficiency can cause venous thrombosis, pulmonary embolism, dialysis fistula failure, arterial graft occlusion, and spontaneous arterial occlusion. In our initial report, we identified seven patients (five men, two women; age range, 21 to 65 years) with antithrombin deficiencies as a cause of thrombosis.[29] Three presented with early thrombosis of femorodistal grafts (Fig. 8-1). In two of these patients the grafts became occluded shortly after surgery in the brief interval between completion of the anastomoses and performance of an operative angiogram. Despite repeated thrombectomies, graft patency could not be maintained for longer than 5 minutes. Two patients presented with spontaneous arterial thrombosis. One had acute ischemia of the right lower extremity with angiographic demonstration of multiple areas of thrombosis of the distal superficial femoral, popliteal, and

tibial systems. The other presented with ischemia of one arm and both legs secondary to extensive thromboses of the brachial artery and its branches of one arm and the femoral, popliteal, and tibial systems of both legs. Extensive angiography of the entire aorta and cardiac evaluation failed to reveal a proximal origin of embolic material. Another patient had spontaneous thrombosis of the tibial outflow vessels to the foot while undergoing an extended profundaplasty. What distinguishes these patients from those with thrombotic occlusive disease secondary to atherosclerotic disease is the unique history, distribution of occluded vessels, unusual angiographic findings, and absence of any proximal source of embolic material. Often clot formation in the operative field despite heparin administration is the first clue that the patient may have an AT III deficiency. The presence of multiple thrombi on operative angiograms is suggestive of a clotting abnormality.

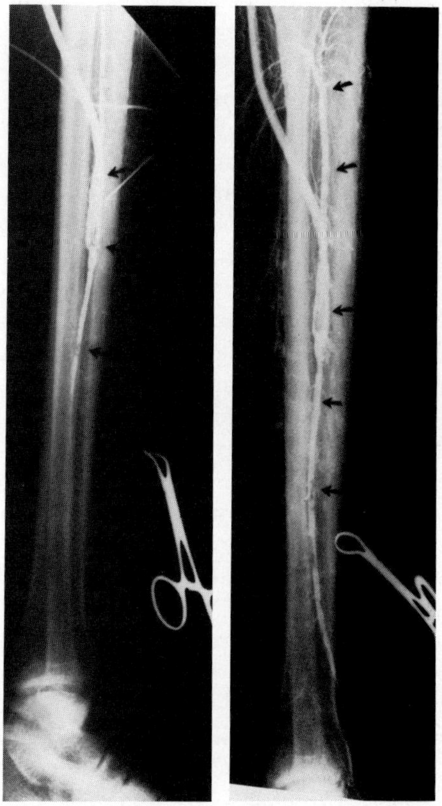

Fig. 8-1. A, Patient with thrombosed femoroperoneal graft the night following surgery. Following graft thrombectomy, patient had evidence of residual thrombi as noted by arrows. **B,** Rethrombosis of graft. More widespread residual thrombi is evident. AT III deficiency was diagnosed and treated, resulting in long-term (>24 months) patency.

Diagnosis

Results of routine coagulation tests are normal in patients with AT III deficiency. Generally reductions in AT III are measured by both immunologic (tests that measure the total amount of the protein) and functional (tests that measure the activity of the AT III molecules) assays.

Initially, patients with repeated episodes of venous thrombosis were identified because of the reduction of AT III to levels 50% to 60% of normal values. Subsequent research identified patients with arterial thrombosis secondary to low AT III levels. Lynch, Leff, and Howe[30] demonstrated a correlation between low preoperative plasma functional AT III levels and the occurrence of postoperative thrombotic complications following cardiac and vascular surgery. Thrombotic complications included arterial thrombosis, graft thrombosis, deep vein thrombosis (DVT), cerebral vascular thrombosis, spinal infarction, and embolic cortical blindness.

A decrease in AT III levels causes the increased thrombotic tendency in patients taking oral contraceptives. Sagar et al.[31] demonstrated that AT III activity was significantly lower in patients taking oral contraceptives than in control patients. During surgery, AT III activity fell in both the contraceptive and control groups, but the decline was greater in patients taking oral contraceptives. The only patients in whom DVT developed postoperatively as determined by the ^{125}I fibrinogen test were those taking oral contraceptives. Five of the 31 patients taking oral contraceptives had an AT III activity level below 50%, and in three of these patients DVT developed.

More recent study has demonstrated that the administration of heparin tends to lower the AT III level. Conrad et al.[32] demonstrated that it is the presence of heparin and not the rate of administration that determines the decrease in AT III; he noted that both subcutaneous and intravenous heparin causes AT III levels to drop the same amount. Since heparin is dependent on AT III for its antithrombotic action, the AT III–lowering effect of heparin in patients with an already low AT III concentration probably indicates that patients are at risk of thrombosis for two reasons. First, heparin is relatively ineffective in patients with low levels of AT III. Second, because heparin binds with AT III, the already low level is decreased even further, possibly to dangerous levels. This is the theoretical basis of paradoxical thrombotic episodes occasionally seen in patients following cessation of heparin. Since heparin administration decreases the level of AT III, sometimes to significantly dangerous levels, cessation of heparin is followed by a period when the patient is hypercoagulable because the lower AT III level is not counteracted by the heparin. This is why warfarin administration should be overlapped with heparin cessation when treating thrombotic problems. Patients with a congenital AT III deficiency should receive chronic long-term warfarin therapy because of the risk of recurrent thrombotic episodes. In addition to its anticoagulant effect, warfarin increases the level of AT III by an as yet undetermined mechanism. More recently, purified AT III can be obtained by recombinant techniques, which will in the future change the treatment of this deficiency. AT III concentrate was used as factor-specific replacement by Tengborn and Bergqvist[33] in patients with AT III deficiency.

DEFECTS IN THE FIBRINOLYTIC SYSTEM

The fibrinolytic system has become better understood in recent years and has been found to be the source of coagulation abnormalities. The components of the fibrinolytic system include plasminogen; plasminogen activators, including human tissue-type plasminogen activator (t-PA) and urokinase; and inhibitors directed against plasminogen activators, plasmin inhibitors (the most important of which is α_2-antiplasmin), and cellular plasmin inhibitors, which have been identified in platelets and endothelial cells and are very poorly characterized at the present time.[34,35] The degradation of fibrin is normally carried out by the proteolytic enzyme plasmin, which is formed from the proenzyme plasminogen by the activation action of plasminogen activators such as t-PA or urokinase. The process is regulated at many different levels, resulting in localized plasmin formation at the fibrin surface. t-PA is the most important activator and is produced and released from vascular endothelium.[36]

Plasminogen is a normal plasma protein consisting of a single polypeptide chain, with a molecular weight of 90,000 to 94,000 d.[37] Thin-layer–gel electrofocusing, coupled with immunofixation, can demonstrate up to ten different forms of plasminogen, with each variant having a glutamic acid as its terminal amino acid. Plasminogen is converted to plasmin by activators, many of which are released from endothelial cells. Plasmin, a serine proteinase, is an important member of the fibrinolytic system that acts by cleaving fibrinogen and fibrin.[38-40]

The biosynthesis of plasminogen and fibrinolytic inhibitors is probably under genetic control. In 1978, Aoki et al.[41] reported a patient with recurrent thrombosis who had a hereditary molecular defect of plasminogen. This was followed by similar reports by Kazama et al.[42] in 1981 and Soria et al.[43] in 1983. These authors demonstrated that abnormal plasminogen does not have the functional ability of normal plasminogen, resulting in a discrepancy between the biologic activity and the amount of plasminogen detected in the serum by radioimmunoassay. These patients had normal concentrations of plasminogen antigen, with approximately one half of the activity of normal plasminogen. Using electrofocusing techniques coupled with immunofixation and zymograms, they were able to identify ten additional bands, each of which was located on the basic side in close proximity to the corresponding normal band.

Determination of amino acid sequence has demonstrated defects in the arginine 516–valine bond and the substitution of alanine 600 by threonine.[44] The major function of the fibrinolytic system in vivo is the limitation of fibrin deposition. A reduction of fibrinolytic activity may provoke a thrombotic tendency by allowing the growth and development of thrombi after the initiating thrombotic event. Most patients with abnormal plasminogen are characterized by a normal antigen concentration and decreased functional activity. Liu, Lyons, and McDonagh[45] reported a plasminogen characterized by both low functional activity and low antigen concentration and called it plasminogen San Antonio.

In a study of patients with unusual and unexplained thromboses who had an abnormal plasminogen band detected on immunoelectrophoresis, we noted that only one of the initial eight patients in the study demonstrated a decreased functional level of plasminogen compared with antigenic levels.[46] We believed that this may be related to the assay of functional activity used in the study or may represent a different form of abnormality than previously reported in the literature. One patient had a low functional plasminogen level at the time of thrombotic activity, but when studied 4 months after the institution of warfarin therapy, the patient demonstrated an increase in functional plasminogen to 70% the normal level. One year later he had normal plasminogen activity. The patient continued to show an abnormal band of plasminogen in the electrophoretic pattern, demonstrating persistence of an abnormal plasminogen molecule in the plasma. This patient has had two episodes of pulmonary emboli.

Ikemoto, Sakata, and Aoki[47] reported that the genetic characteristics of this disorder follow an autosomal codominant inheritance pattern, with both alleles being completely expressed. The results of the study of two families in our series concur with these findings. The clinical history of recurrent phlebitis in one of our patients and his sister supports the genetic aspect of this disease.

The immunoelectrophoresis technique used in our study is quicker, simpler, and less costly than isoelectric focusing and is more applicable to the screening of large groups of patients. The significance of abnormal plasminogen is uncertain. It is present in 10% of the normal population and its presence does not ensure that a patient will experience thrombotic complications. More likely, the presence of abnormal plasminogen results in the relative defect of the fibrinolytic system, which places the patient at increased risk should he be in a thrombosis-prone situation. Our data suggest, however, that once a thrombotic episode occurs, it is likely to recur, emphasizing the need to identify and treat these patients with long-term warfarin therapy.

Clinical Presentation

We have noted thrombosis occurring on both the arterial and venous sides of the circulation in patients with abnormal plasminogen. In our initial report of eight patients, the age of onset of the first thrombotic episode ranged from 21 to 57 years. Three patients had venous thrombosis, two had spontaneous arterial thrombosis, two had occlusion of an arterial reconstruction in the early postoperative period, and one patient had separate episodes of both arterial and venous occlusions.

Thrombosis involving the venous system occurred in four patients: two had complete obstruction of the iliofemoral venous segment and inferior vena cava, one had primarily popliteal vein thrombosis, and the remaining patient had axillary and subclavian vein thrombosis. Two of these patients had concomitant pulmonary emboli, which occurred in one patient 4 months after the thrombotic event. Arterial thrombosis occurred in five patients; two patients presented with spontaneous thrombosis of the iliofemoral segment. Following thrombectomy with Fogarty catheters, there was no evidence of inflow obstruction, and a complete evaluation for the proximal source of the emboli was negative (Fig. 8-2). Postoperative occlusions of arterial reconstructions occurred in two patients. In the first patient, the site of Dacron patch angioplasty of the vertebral artery orifice became occluded the night following surgery. At reexploration no stricture of the repair was found, and the thrombosis was limited to the area of the patch angioplasty without distal propagation. In the second patient, thrombosis occurred in a saphenous vein femoral–posterior tibial graft the night following surgery. At reexploration the thrombus formation was limited to the graft and did not extend to the runoff vessels. Complete angiograms following both initial surgery and reoperation demonstrated technically satisfactory anastomoses. Postoperatively the graft remained patent for 34 months. We noted one patient with chronic progressive thrombosis of

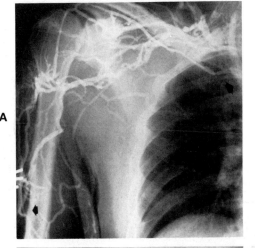

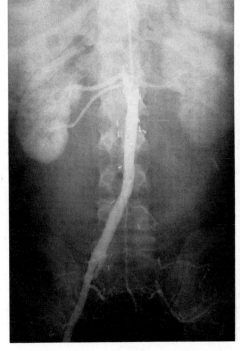

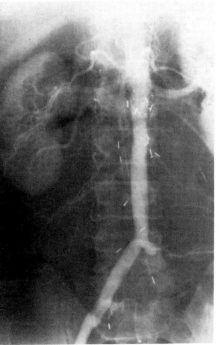

Fig. 8-2. A, Venogram demonstrating subclavian and axillary vein thrombosis in patient who had separate episodes of arterial and venous thrombosis. **B,** Angiogram of patient 9 months later, demonstrating occlusion of the left common iliac artery. **C,** Angiogram obtained 37 months later, showing reocclusion of common iliac artery. (From Towne JB, Bandyk DF, Hussey CV, et al. Abnormal plasminogen: A genetically determined cause of hypercoagulability. J Vasc Surg 1:896-902, 1984.)

the runoff vessel in both legs. This patient was not diabetic and initially presented with a 6-month history of rest pain in both feet that progressed to digital gangrene. The ankle/brachial index (ABI) of the right lower extremity was 0.95 with a toe pressure of 40 mm Hg. The ABI of the left leg was 0.65 with a toe pressure of 10 mm Hg. Arteriography demonstrated a normal aortoiliac system, a 50% stenosis of the left superficial femoral artery, and patent tibial vessels to the ankle bilaterally, but occlusion of the pedal and metatarsal arteries was present.

Six patients had recurrent thrombosis. Two patients had three recurrences and four patients had two recurrences. The interval between thrombotic episodes ranged from 4 to 36 months. Significantly, five patients who had recurrent thrombosis were treated with warfarin following the first episode. Recurrent episodes of thrombosis occurred 2 weeks to several months following cessation of warfarin therapy,

and recurrent thrombosis did not develop in any patient while receiving anticoagulant therapy. We subsequently identified four patients who had abnormal plasminogen as detected by an abnormal arc on immunoelectrophoresis in whom severe thrombosis in the upper extremities developed (Fig. 8-3).[48] The lack of atherosclerosis in the upper extremities as well as the absence of any proximal embolic source further points out the sometimes catastrophic consequences that can occur in patients with abnormal plasminogen. In our experience of over 30 patients in whom we have detected abnormal plasminogen over the last 5 years, recurrent thrombosis has developed in only one patient while receiving warfarin therapy.

Methods of Testing

A complete coagulation profile on each patient should be performed, including tests of platelet aggregation, prothrombin time, partial thromboplastin time, fibrinogen level, and

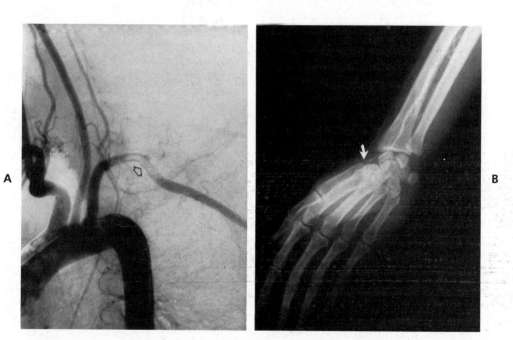

Fig. 8-3. A, Nonoccluding thrombi of subclavian artery occurring several days after carotid angiography from a femoral approach. **B,** Evidence of distal embolization of the distal radial artery and palmar arch in same patient. (From Towne JB, Hussey CV, Bandyk DF. Abnormalities of the fibrinolytic system as a cause of upper extremity ischemia: A preliminary report. J Vasc Surg 7:661-666, 1988.)

platelet count. Functional assays of AT III and plasminogen α_2-antiplasmin should be performed. Measurements of antigenic activity levels of AT III, plasminogen, α_1-antitrypsin, and α_2-macroglobulins likewise should be obtained. With immunoelectrophoresis, abnormal plasminogen presents as an abnormal band that is separate on the electrophoretic pattern located nearer the anode and distinct from the normal band. We have also noted one patient in whom plasminogen was demonstrated as separate from the main band but was not confined to a distinct band. Indeed this may represent still another species. Several investigators are involved in ongoing studies to further characterize the molecular defect in these plasminogens and to assess the functional impairment. This research requires rather sophisticated techniques to determine amino acid sequencing and to test the functional ability of the various components of the plasminogen molecule.

t-PA and Anti–t-PA

With the development of a method to measure t-PA, investigators have discovered that levels of t-PA can vary in relation to the occurrence of thrombotic disease.[49] Also, the presence of an anti–t-PA that counteracts the effects of t-PA has been detected.[50,51] Several studies have identified patients who are thrombosis prone because of increased levels of anti–t-PA.[52-54] Both the mechanisms and the effect of alterations of these mechanisms are poorly understood at the present time. Wiman[49] first developed the test to measure t-PA. In a study of patients with DVT, he found that 40% of his patients had a reduced fibrinolytic potential, which was found to be caused by a reduced capacity to release t-PA or an increased plasma level of an anti–t-PA, or a combination of these two.[53] He also noted a significant correlation between plasma anti–t-PA and the levels of serum triglycerides in patients below the age of 45 with myocardial infarction. Obviously these are preliminary data, but they emphasize the need for ongoing investigation to determine more precisely the role of the fibrinolytic system in the pathogenesis of thrombotic disorders.

PROTEIN C DEFICIENCY

Protein C is a vitamin K–dependent proenzyme that is involved in the control of clotting and fibrinolysis. Protein C itself is activated by thrombin but slowly. This activation is increased up to 20,000-fold when thrombin forms a complex with an endothelial cell membrane called thrombomodulin (Fig. 8-4). Activated protein C, when combined with phospholipids, calcium, and protein S, inactivates the cofactors of the two rate-limiting steps of coagulation, factors Va and VIIIa.[55-57]

Protein S is likewise a vitamin K–dependent factor. It acts as a cofactor for the anticoagulant activity of activated protein C by promoting its binding to lipid and platelet surfaces, thus localizing protein C activity.[58,59] Protein C, in conjunction with protein S, also acts as a profibrinolytic agent by increasing plasmin activity through the inactivation of the major inhibitor of t-PA.[55,56]

Heterozygous protein C deficiency is inherited in an autosomal dominant fashion. In hereditary protein C deficiency, the homozygous state is associated with a very high risk of thrombosis.[60,61] It usually presents as massive venous thrombosis in the neonatal period, which is often fatal. The in utero survival of affected infants may reflect the protection afforded by maternal transfer of protein C or the reduced synthesis of other procoagulants by the fetal liver, which thus compensates for the deficiency of protein C.

In the heterozygous form of the deficiency, a protein C level of 50% is sufficient to predispose individuals to venous thrombosis.[61] The incidence of thrombophlebitis in patients who are heterozygous for this deficiency is uncertain. Some kindreds have been identified in which there is a very high incidence of venous thrombosis (up to 80%) by the age of 40, and there are others in which the occurrence of thrombosis is sporadic.[62,63] Acquired protein C deficiency can be observed in patients in the acute phase of thrombosis, in patients with disseminating intervascular coagulation, in patients with liver disease, and in postoperative patients.

Protein C deficiency generally manifests with

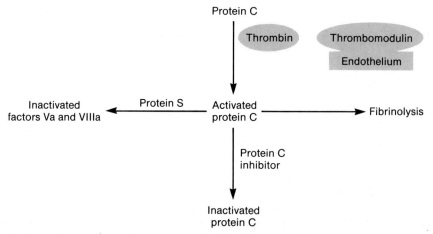

Fig. 8-4. Protein C is produced in liver and circulates in blood in inactive form. When thrombin becomes bound to endothelial cofactor (thrombomodulin), the complex formed rapidly activates protein C. Activated protein C is a potent plasma anticoagulant. It inactivates cofactors of two rate-limiting steps of coagulation (factors Va and VIIIa) and enhances fibrinolysis. These processes require the presence of protein S. Protein C is inactivated by protein C inhibitor in a one-to-one fashion. (From Tollefson DFJ, Friedman KD, Marlar RA, et al. Protein C deficiency: A cause of unusual or unexplained thrombosis. Arch Surg 123:881-884, 1988. Copyright 1988. American Medical Association.)

venous thrombosis, either as lower extremity DVT, oftentimes accompanied by pulmonary embolism, or as mesenteric venous thrombosis. We recently reported five patients (age range, 28 to 41 years) with protein C deficiency: four had DVT of the lower extremity as the initial thrombotic event and one had mesenteric venous thrombosis with small bowel necrosis.[64] Two patients had recurrent lower extremity thrombosis, which was bilateral in one. One patient experienced only one clinical episode of DVT, but venous stasis ulceration developed, suggesting multiple episodes of subclinical phlebitis. One patient had a pulmonary embolus. Green, Ganger, and Blei[65] evaluated eight consecutive patients with splanchnic venous thrombosis and demonstrated decreases in the levels of AT III and protein C in all. They were unable to document whether the low levels of protein C and AT III were a result or cause of the thrombosis. Two patients had had a history of venous thrombotic problems and evaluation of six patients following a period of 1 to 6 months revealed a persistent low level of pro-

tein C, which would certainly suggest a congenital etiology. The only case of arterial thrombosis secondary to protein C reduction was reported by Coller et al.,[66] who treated a patient who experienced the onset of the first of three episodes of thrombophlebitis at age 23. At 27 the patient had a pulmonary embolus, at 28 he had a myocardial infarction and superficial femoral artery thrombosis, and at age 31 simultaneous radial and ulnar artery occlusions developed, followed shortly by the development of left ventricular thrombus, which caused embolus to the leg.

Methods of Testing

Standard testing includes a radiolabeled Laurell electroimmunoassay to determine human protein C antigen in plasma samples. Normal values should be between 70% and 130% of normal activity. In our patients with venous thrombosis, the level of protein C ranged from 34% to 67%.[64] As with the evaluation of all patients with unusual or unexplained thrombosis, measurement of AT III and protein S and routine coagulation studies should be performed simultaneously. We evaluated the family of our patient with mesenteric venous occlusion for protein C deficiency and found the results to indicate an autosomal dominant–type of transmission. No thrombotic episodes have been reported by other family members with low protein C levels. Since thrombosis does not develop in all family members with low protein C levels, asymptomatic patients with low levels of protein C should be monitored closely and not receive prophylactic anticoagulant therapy. However, they should receive prophylactic anticoagulants preoperatively if major surgery or prolonged immobilization is required. In those in whom thrombotic events develop, the onset typically occurs between 15 to 30 years of age. This delay in onset of the first thrombotic episode and the fact that protein C rarely causes arterial thrombosis, as contrasted with our experiences with either abnormal plasminogen or AT III abnormalities, are not well understood. It may be that protein C deficiency requires slower moving blood and increased endothelial surface area found in the venous system to manifest. However, when protein C deficiency is homozygous, thrombosis is widespread, resulting in death in infancy unless treated.

Because of the risk of recurrent thrombotic events with the possible sequelae of pulmonary emboli and venous stasis disease, long-term warfarin therapy is recommended. No loading dose should be administered, as this could precipitate warfarin-associated skin necrosis.[58,59] Such necrosis occurs 2 to 5 days following the initiation of warfarin therapy and presents as an erythematous patch on the skin that rapidly progresses to a hemorrhagic area that can become gangrenous. There is a propensity for involvement of the breasts, abdomen, buttocks, and thighs. The proposed mechanism is one of a transient hypercoagulable state that is created by bolus loading doses of warfarin given to initiate anticoagulation. Because of it short half-life, protein C levels fall faster than factor X and prothrombin levels, and thus the inhibitory effect of protein C on the coagulation cascade is further diminished. If these levels fall below a critical level, the procoagulant effects of the coagulation cascade proceed unabated and thrombosis ensues. Administration of oral warfarin 5 mg daily should be started to gradually attain a prothrombin time of 1.5 to 2 times the control value. Heparin therapy and warfarin therapy should overlap by 4 to 5 days.

PROTEIN S DEFICIENCY

Protein S is a vitamin K–dependent protein that functions as a cofactor of anticoagulant activity of activated protein C. The liver is the major location of synthesis, although more recently the endothelial cells and megakaryocyte were identified as other sites of synthesis. Protein S functions by expediting the binding of activated protein C to lipid and platelet surfaces. To date, only patients with heterozygous protein S deficiency have been reported.[61] Symptomatic patients often have protein S levels 50% of the normal value, and like protein C deficiency, protein S deficiency primarily causes venous thrombosis.[67-69] It has been estimated by some to be the cause of approximately 10% of cases of spontaneous venous thrombosis. Coller et al.[66] also reported the only known case history of a protein S–deficient patient having arterial occlusive problems. This patient had had recurrent episodes of thrombophlebitis over several years, resulting in venous stasis disease. At age 21, he experienced thrombotic problems in the legs, which resulted in a below-knee amputation. As with patients with protein C problems, patients with protein S deficiency have clotting abnormalities that tend to be recurrent and therefore it is essential that they remain on long-term warfarin therapy. The association of deficiencies in protein C and its cofactor protein S with hypercoagulable states has only been recently appreciated. Data now suggest that the incidence of protein C and protein S deficiencies is more common than either AT III or plasminogen abnormalities. In a recent report evaluating 139 individuals who had at least one major venous thrombotic event, 7% were protein C deficient, 5% were protein S deficient, 2% were deficient in plasminogen, and 3% were deficient in AT III.[70] A majority (79%), however, had no coagulopathy detectable with current testing methods.

LUPUSLIKE ANTICOAGULANT

Lupuslike anticoagulants are IgG or IgM antibodies that are directed against phospholipids that participate in coagulation disorders. They are present in 16% to 33% of patients with lupus erythematosus, but they are also associated with a variety of other disorders and are even found in normal individuals.[71-73] These antibodies belong to a family of antiphospholipid antibodies, which were initially detected because of their effect in vitro on the prolongation of plasma coagulation times. Most commonly, there is a prolongation of activated partial thromboplastin time and in some patients also a prolongation of prothrombin time. There have been only rare reports of bleeding tendencies related to the demonstration of a lupuslike anticoagulant; however, in the last decade there has been an increasing number of reports of the presence of lupuslike anticoagulants associated with abnormal thrombosis in both the arterial and venous systems, spontaneous abortion secondary to placental thrombosis, cerebrovascular accidents, and thrombocytopenia. Lupuslike anticoagulants also cause false-positive tests for syphilis. On occasion, lupuslike anticoagulants can develop after administration of phenothiazines, procainamide, or penicillin; following viral infections in children; and in patients with AIDS suffering from *Pneumocystis carinii* pneumonia.

Clinical Presentation

Recurrent thromboses have been reported in about one third of patients with lupuslike anticoagulant.[74] The most common manifestation is venous thromboses, usually involving the lower extremities. Pulmonary hypertension caused by recurrent pulmonary emboli or intrapulmonary thrombosis may develop. Repeated strokes have been reported in 15% to 55% of the patients. Obstetric complications (e.g., spontaneous abortions, intrauterine growth retardation, fetal death) occurring in the second and third trimester have been reported in 25% to 35% of the women with lupuslike anticoagulant.[71-73] Ahn et al.,[75] in a study of patients with lupuslike anticoagulant who were undergoing surgery, noted that 9 of 18 vascular surgery

procedures were complicated by thrombosis. Seven of these patients suffered multiple postoperative thrombotic complications, resulting in amputation in three.

The mechanism of action of lupuslike anticoagulants is not known. Several theories have been suggested, including an inhibitory activity on prostacyclin (PGI_2), which is a potent in vivo inhibitor of platelet aggregation. IgG fractions with lupuslike anticoagulant activity have been shown experimentally to block the production of prostacyclin in rat aortic endothelial cells.[76] Other investigators suggest that lupuslike anticoagulant inhibits protein C activation, which is important in preventing thrombosis. Tsakiris et al.[77] believe that the inhibition of the catalytic activity of thrombomodulin might be explained by the direct attachment of lupuslike anticoagulant to thrombomodulin or to adjacent phospholipids of the cell membrane, preventing thrombin and/or protein C from binding to thrombomodulin.

Diagnosis

Often the only indication that a patient has lupuslike anticoagulant is an abnormally prolonged activated partial thromboplastin time. On occasion, such a patient can also have a prolonged prothrombin time. An abnormal rabbit brain neutralization procedure and an enzyme-linked immunosorbent assay for the presence of anticardiolipin antibodies can more precisely identify lupuslike anticoagulant.[75]

Treatment

Because the precise mechanism by which lupuslike anticoagulant causes intravascular thrombosis is not known, treatment has varied from administration of antiplatelet medications (aspirin and dipyridamole), anticoagulation with warfarin and heparin, and the administration of steroids. The basis for treatment with antiplatelet medication is that some researchers believe that the lupuslike anticoagulant causes a decrease in the availability of arachidonic acid, which is necessary for the synthesis of prostacyclin inhibitor and platelet aggregation in vessel walls. In obstetric patients it has been reported that steroid and aspirin administration is effective in preventing spontaneous abortion. Prednisone has been shown to suppress production and/or activity of lupuslike anticoagulant, as measured by lessened prolongation of the activated partial thromboplastin time. Until more information is available, we prefer to initiate antiplatelet therapy with aspirin and dipyridamole before surgical procedures. We administer dextran routinely in all vascular reconstructions, and patients are given heparin perioperatively. Postoperatively heparin therapy is converted to warfarin therapy.

UNEXPLAINED THROMBOSIS
Guidelines for Identifying Hypercoagulable Patients

A thorough patient history remains the most important means of identifying patients with potential hypercoagulable disorders. Patients should be asked about previously unexplained thromboses experienced by themselves or family members. Patients with hypercoagulable syndromes will often report episodes of thrombophlebitis as a young adult. Of particular importance are those episodes of thrombophlebitis without any contributing factors for their development (e.g., long leg fractures, prolonged immobilization, bed rest because of illness). Hypercoagulable disorders become even more significant in patients with recurrent episodes of thrombophlebitis. Likewise, a history of arterial thrombosis, especially if the episodes occurred at a young age, is an indicator of a coagulation disorder. Eldrup-Jorgensen et al.[78] found a 30% incidence of coagulation abnormalities in patients younger than 51 years undergoing vascular reconstruction. Abnormal clotting syndromes noted were protein S deficiency, protein C deficiency, presence of lupuslike anticoagulants, and plasminogen deficiency. The incidence of arterial graft thrombosis in hypercoagulable patients was 20% at 30 days, which is markedly increased from what one would expect from this type of vascular reconstruction.

Clinical Presentation

With experience one has a sense for what kinds of reconstructions should work and has some expectations concerning the types of problems that can occur. Likewise, one develops a feel for what are typical presentations of atherosclerotic occlusive disease. Unusual or unexplained thromboses (e.g., a thrombosed suprarenal aorta, upper extremity thrombosis, or total tibial artery occlusion in a patient who is neither diabetic nor has any evidence of atherosclerotic occlusive disease elsewhere) should alert the surgeon to consider hypercoagulable disorders as the cause. Unusual x-ray findings—in particular, occlusions seen in young patients or in one extremity when the other extremity has no evidence of any disease—should trigger an investigation of the coagulation system.

The role of screening vascular surgery patients for hypercoagulable states is difficult to ascertain. Donaldson et al.[79] found a 9.5% overall incidence of vascular surgery patients with abnormal test results indicating potential hypercoagulability. The three most common entities demonstrated were heparin-induced platelet aggregation, lupuslike anticoagulants, and protein C deficiency. The incidence of infrainguinal graft occlusion within 30 days was 27% in the hypercoagulable group compared with 1.6% in the noncoagulable group. Currently we do not perform routine screening to detect patients with hypercoagulable states. We depend on patient history and clinical evaluation to identify those patients who may be hypercoagulable, which is probably more cost effective and efficient than routine screening.

The most difficult experience for a vascular surgeon is dealing with unexplained thrombosis that occurs intraoperatively. Often this situation occurs during late evening or nighttime hours when support from the coagulation laboratory is not available. The first step, if indeed heparin has been given, is to determine if there is any clotting in the operative field, which would indicate an AT III deficiency, since AT III is essential for heparin's anticoagulant effect. The anesthesiologist should then test the heparin effect by determining partial thromboplastin time or by performing one of the other variety of tests to measure heparin anticoagulation. The next step is to obtain a platelet count. If it is higher than 100,000/mm^3 and the activated clotting time (ACT) is not prolonged, the problem is presumed to be the antithrombin system. The patient is then given 2 units of fresh frozen plasma, with 2 units given every 12 hours for 5 days. AT III deficiency is confirmed usually the next day with tests done on blood drawn before the next administration of fresh frozen plasma. Patients with AT III deficiency are maintained on long-term warfarin therapy. If the platelet count is less than 100,000/mm^3, we presume heparin-induced platelet aggregation has developed. The patient's history should be carefully examined to try to document the prior administration of heparin. At this time we administer a 50 ml bolus dose of dextran and continue dextran therapy at 25 ml/hr. The heparin is reversed with protamine, and platelet aggregation abnormality is confirmed in the morning. Warfarin treatment is continued for 3 weeks to 6 months.

If the platelet count is greater than 100,000/mm^3 and the ACT is prolonged, we presume the patient has some other sort of hypercoagulable state, which includes fibrinolytic abnormalities as well as potential problems with protein C, protein S, or lupuslike anticoagulants. In these patients we institute continuous heparin therapy both intraoperatively and postoperatively and give the patient 2 units of fresh frozen plasma. Fresh frozen plasma is shotgun therapy for a wide variety of coagulation abnormalities.

In the operating room, before the institution of any therapy, blood should be drawn for coagulation tests; it should be kept in mind that many of these tests (e.g., plasminogen electrophoresis; determination of protein C, protein S, and lupuslike anticoagulant) are quite involved, sometimes taking days to a week at some centers. However, if the blood is properly handled spun down, and frozen, the tests can be done routinely. Our policy is to repeat all abnormal tests in 5 days. One of the problems in accurately diagnosing coagulation abnormalities is that in the process of clotting, clotting factors can be consumed and abnormalities may be the result of clotting and not the cause of it. For all factors that still demonstrate abnormal values at 5 to 7 days, tests are repeated at 1 month. Patients who have persistently abnormal values are then labeled truly hypercoagulable.

McDaniel et al.[80] have noted the change in coagulation factors with operation. They determined that AT III levels fell on the third postoperative day and subsequently returned to normal by 1 week postoperatively. AT III declined from a mean preoperative level of 110% to 71% on the third postoperative day. This value returned to normal by the seventh postoperative day, when it was 95% or at the normal activity level. This variablity demonstrates the dynamic aspect of the clotting system and points to the danger of attaching significance to just one isolated laboratory finding. In most patients who sustain complications because of hypercoagulable states, warfarin therapy is instituted in the perioperative and postoperative period. In patients with heparin-induced platelet aggregation, therapy can usually be stopped after 3 months; however, we have recommended prolonged administration in patients with protein C or S deficiency, AT III deficiency, and plasminogen abnormalities because of the risk of recurrent thrombosis.

REFERENCES

1. Babcock RB, Dumper CW, Scharfman WB. Heparin-induced immune thrombocytopenia. N Engl J Med 295:237-241, 1976.
2. Baird RA, Convery RF. Arterial thromboembolism in patients receiving systemic heparin therapy. J Bone Joint Surg 59:1061-1064, 1977.
3. Bell WR, Romasulo PA, Alving BM, et al. Thrombocytopenia occurring during the administration of heparin. Ann Intern Med 87:155-160, 1976.
4. Fratantoni JC, Pollet R, Gralnick HR. Heparin-induced thrombocytopenia: Confirmation of diagnosis with in vitro methods. Blood 45:395-401, 1975.
5. Nelson JC, Lerner RG, Goldstein R, et al. Heparin-induced thrombocytopenia. Arch Intern Med 138:548-552,1978.
6. Towne JB, Bernhard VM, Hussey C, et al. White clot syndrome. Arch Surg 114:372-377, 1979.
7. Rhodes GR, Dixon RH, Silver D. Heparin-induced thrombocytopenia. Ann Surg 186:752-758, 1977.
8. Kapsch DN, Adelstein EH, Rhodes GR, et al. Heparin-induced thrombocytopenia, thrombosis, and hemorrhage. Surgery 86:148-154, 1979.
9. Laster J, Silver D. Heparin-coated catheters and heparin-induced thrombocytopenia. J Vasc Surg 7:667-672, 1988.
10. Silver D, Kapsch DN, Tsoi EKM. Heparin-induced thrombocytopenia, thrombosis, and hemorrhage. Ann Surg 198:301-306, 1983.

11. Laster J, Cikrit D, Walker N, et al. The heparin-induced thrombocytopenia syndrome: An update. Surgery 102:763-770, 1987.

12. Laster J, Elfrink R, Silver D. Reexposure to heparin of patients with heparin-associated antibodies. J Vasc Surg 9:677-682, 1989.

13. Kappa JR, Fisher CA, Berkowitz HD, et al. Heparin-induced platelet activation in sixteen surgical patients: Diagnosis and management. J Vasc Surg 5:101-109, 1987.

14. Makhoul RG, Greenberg CS, McCann RL. Heparin-associated thrombocytopenia and thrombosis: A serious clinical problem and potential solution. J Vasc Surg 4:522-528, 1986.

15. Sobel M, Adelman B, Szaboles S, et al. Surgical management of heparin-associated thrombocytopenia. J Vasc Surg 8:395-401, 1988.

16. Cole CW, Bormanis J. Ancrod: A practical alternative to heparin. J Vasc Surg 8:59-63, 1988.

17. Abildgaard U, Fagerhol MK, Egeberg O. Comparison of progressive antithrombin activity and the concentration of three thrombin inhibitors in human plasma. Scand J Clin Lab Invest 26:349-354, 1970.

18. Seegers WH. Antithrombin III: Theory and clinical applications. Am J Clin Pathol 69:367-374, 1978.

19. Egeberg O. Inherited antithrombin deficiency causing thrombophilia. Thromb Diath Haemorrh 13:516-530, 1965.

20. Brozovic M, Stirling Y, Hamlyn AN. Thrombotic tendency and probable antithrombin III deficiency. Thromb Haemost 39:778-779, 1978.

21. Mackie M, Bennett B, Ogston D, et al. Familial thrombosis: Inherited deficiency of antithrombin III. Br Med J 1:136-138, 1978.

22. Marciniak E, Farley CH, DeSimone PA. Familial thrombosis due to antithrombin III deficiency. Blood 43:219-231, 1974.

23. Sorensen PJ, Dyerburg J, Stotterson E, et al. Familial functional antithrombin III deficiency. Scand J Haematol 24:105-109, 1980.

24. Collen D, Schetz J, DeCock F, et al. Metabolism of antithrombin III (heparin cofactor) in man: Effects of venous thrombosis and of heparin administration. Eur J Clin Invest 7:27-35, 1977.

25. Ødegaard OR, Abildgaard U. Antithrombin III: Critical review of assay methods. Significance of variations in health and disease. Haemostasis 7:127-134, 1978.

26. Chan V, Chan TK, Wong V, et al. The determination of antithrombin III by radioimmunoassay and its clinical application. Br J Haematol 41:563-572, 1979.

27. Sas G, Blasko G, Banghogyi D, et al. Abnormal antithrombin III (antithrombin Budapest) as a cause of familial thrombophilia. Thromb Diath Haemorrh 32:105-115, 1974.

28. Flinn WR, McDaniel MD, Yao JST, et al. Antithrombin III deficiency as a reflection of dynamic protein metabolism in patients undergoing vascular reconstruction. J Vasc Surg 1:888-895, 1984.

29. Towne JB, Bernhard VM, Hussey C, et al. Antithrombin deficiency—A cause of unexplained thrombosis in vascular surgery. Surgery 89:735-742, 1981.

30. Lynch DM, Leff LK, Howe SE. Preoperative AT-III values and clinical postoperative thrombosis: A comparison of three antithrombin III assays. Thromb Haemost 52:42-44, 1984.

31. Sagar S, Stamatakis JD, Thomas DP, et al. Oral contraceptives, antithrombin III activity, and postoperative deep vein thrombosis. Lancet 1:509-511, 1976.

32. Conrad J, Lecompte T, Horellou MH, et al. Antithrombin III in patients treated with subcutaneous or intravenous heparin. Thromb Res 22:507-511, 1981.

33. Tengborn L, Bergqvist D. Surgery in patients with congenital antithrombin III deficiency. Acta Chir Scand 154:179-188, 1988.

34. Salem HH, Mitchell CA, Firkin BG. Current views on the pathophysiology and investigations of thrombotic disorders. Am J Haematol 25:463-474, 1987.

35. Towne JB. Hypercoagulable states. Semin Vasc Surg 1(4):201-215, 1988.

36. Wiman B, Ljungberg B, Chmielewska J, et al. The role of the fibrinolytic system in deep vein thrombosis. J Lab Clin Med 105:265-270, 1985.

37. Castellino FJ, Powell JR. Human plasminogen. Methods Enzymol 80:365-378, 1981.

38. Wallen P, Wiman B. Characterization of human plasminogen. Biochem Biophys Acta 257:122-134, 1972.

39. Mullertz S. Fibrinolysis: An overview. Semin Thromb Hemost 10:1-5, 1988.

40. Summaria L, Arzadon P, Bernabe P, et al. Studies on the isolation of the multiple molecular forms of human plasminogen and plasmin by isoelectric focusing methods. J Biol Chem 247:4691-4702, 1972.

41. Aoki N, Moroi M, Sakata Y, et al. Abnormal plasminogen: A hereditary molecular abnormality found in patients with recurrent thrombosis. J Clin Invest 61:1186-1195, 1978.

42. Kazama M, Tohura C, Suzuki Z, et al. Abnormal plasminogen—A cause of recurrent thrombosis. Thromb Res 21:517-522, 1981.

43. Soria J, Soria C, Bertrand O, et al. Plasminogen Paris I: Congenital abnormal plasminogen and its incidence in thrombosis. Thromb Res 32:229-238, 1983.

44. Scharrer IM, Wohl RC, Hach V, et al. Investigation of a congenital abnormal plasminogen, Frankfurt I, and its relationship to thrombosis. Thromb Haemost 55:396-401, 1986.

45. Liu Y, Lyons RM, McDonagh J. Plasminogen San Antonio: An abnormal plasminogen with a more cathodic migration, decreased activation, and associated thrombosis. Thromb Haemost 59:49-53, 1988.

46. Towne JB, Bandyk DF, Hussey CV, et al. Abnormal plasminogen: A genetically determined cause of hypercoagulability. J Vasc Surg 1:896-902, 1984.

47. Ikemoto S, Sakata Y, Aoki N. Genetic polymorphism of human plasminogen in a human population. Hum Hered 32:296-297, 1982.

48. Towne JB, Hussey CV, Bandyk DF. Abnormalities of the fibrinolytic system as a cause of upper extremity ischemia. J Vasc Surg 7:661-666, 1988.

49. Wiman B. The role of the fibrinolytic system in thrombotic disease. Acta Med Scand (Suppl) 715:169-171, 1986.

50. Chmielewska J, Ranby M, Wiman B. Evidence of a rapid inhibitor to tissue plasminogen activator in plasma. Thromb Res 31:427-436, 1983.

51. Kruithof EKO, Tran-Thang C, Ransijn A, et al. Demonstration of a fast-acting inhibitor of plasminogen activators in human plasma. Blood 64:907-913, 1984.

52. Hamsten A, Wiman B, deFaire U, et al. Increased plasma levels of a rapid inhibitor of tissue plasminogen activator in young survivors of myocardial infarction. N Engl J Med 313:1557-1563, 1985.

53. Wiman B, Ljungberg B, Chmielewska J, et al. The role of the fibrinolytic system in deep venous thrombosis. J Lab Clin Med 105:265-270, 1985.

54. Wiman B, Chmielewska J, Ranby M. Inactivation of tissue plasminogen activator in plasma. J Biol Chem 259:3644-3647, 1984.

55. Marlar RA. Protein C in thromboembolic disease. Semin Thromb Hemost 11:387-393, 1985.

56. Clouse LH, Comp PC. The regulation of hemostasis: The protein C system. N Engl J Med 314:1298-1303, 1986.

57. Stenflo J. Structure and function of protein C. Semin Thromb Hemost 10:109-121, 1984.

58. Kazmier FJ. Thromboembolism, coumarin necrosis, and protein C. Mayo Clin Proc 60:673-674, 1985.

59. Peterson CE, Kwaan HC. Current concepts of warfarin therapy. Arch Intern Med 146:581-584, 1986.

60. Branson HE, Kate J, Marble R, et al. Inherited protein C deficiency and coumarin-responsive chronic relapsing purpura fulminans in a newborn infant. Lancet 2:1165-1168, 1983.

61. Salem HH, Mitchell CH, Firkin BG. Current views on the pathophysiology and investigations of thrombotic disorders. Am J Hematol 25:463-474, 1987.

62. Broekmans AW, Veltkamp JJ, Bertina RM. Congenital protein C deficiency and venous thromboembolism: A study of three Dutch families. N Engl J Med 390:340-344, 1983.

63. Griffen JG, Evatt B, Zimmerman TS, et al. Deficiency of protein C in congenital thrombotic disease. J Clin Invest 68:1370-1373, 1981.

64. Tollefson DFJ, Friedman KD, Marlar RA, et al. Protein C deficiency: A cause of unusual or unexplained thrombosis. Arch Surg 123:881-884, 1988.

65. Green D, Ganger DR, Blei AT. Protein C deficiency in splanchnic venous thrombosis. Am J Med 82:1171-1173, 1987.

66. Coller BS, Owen J, Jesty J, et al. Deficiency of plasma protein S, protein C, or antithrombin III and arterial thrombosis. Atherosclerosis 7:456-462, 1987.

67. Comp PC, Esmon CT. Recurrent venous thromboembolism in patients with a partial deficiency of protein S. N Engl J Med 311:1526-1528, 1984.

68. Schwarz HP, Fischer M, Hopmeier P, et al. Plasma protein S deficiency in familial thrombotic disease. Blood 64:1297-1300, 1984.

69. Rodgers GM, Shuman MA. Congenital thrombotic disorders. Am J Hematol 21:419-430, 1986.

70. Gladson CL, Griffen JH, Hach V, et al. The incidence of protein C and protein S deficiency in 139 young thrombotic patients. Thrombosis 66:350a, 1985.

71. Espinoza LR, Hartmann RC. Significance of the lupus anticoagulant. Am J Hematol 22:331-337, 1986.

72. Tabechnik-Schor NF, Lipton SA. Association of lupus-like anticoagulant and nonvasculitic cerebral infarction. Arch Neurol 43:851-852, 1986.

73. Shi W, Krilis SA, Chong BH, et al. Prevalence of lupus anticoagulant and anticardiolipin antibodies in a healthy population. Aust NZ J Med 20:231-236, 1990.

74. Dührsen U, Brittinger G. Lupus anticoagulant associated syndrome in benign and malignant systemic disease. Klin Wochenschr 65:818-822, 1987.

75. Ahn SS, Kalunian K, Rosove M, et al. Postoperative thrombotic complications in patients with the lupus anticoagulant: Increased risk after vascular procedure. J Vasc Surg 7:749-756, 1988.

76. Greenfield LJ. Lupus-like anticoagulants and thrombosis. J Vasc Surg 7:818-819, 1988.

77. Tsakiris DA, Settas L, Makris PE, et al. Lupus anticoagulant-antiphospholipid antibodies and thrombophilia: Relation to protein-C and protein-S thrombomodulin. J Rheumatol 17:785-789, 1990.

78. Eldrup-Jorgensen J, Flanigan DP, Brace L, et al. Hypercoagulable states and lower limb ischemia in young adults. J Vasc Surg 9:334-341, 1989.

79. Donaldson MC, Weinberg DS, Belkin M, et al. Screening for hypercoagulable states in a vascular surgery practice: A preliminary study. J Vasc Surg 11:825-831, 1990.

80. McDaniel MD, Pearce WH, Yao JST, et al. Sequential changes in coagulation and platelet function following femoro-tibial bypass. J Vasc Surg 1:261-268, 1984.

9

Complications and Failures of Anticoagulant Therapy

John R. Hoch   Donald Silver

Anticoagulants have played a major role in the development of vascular surgery and are important in the prophylaxis and treatment of most thromboembolic disorders. Vascular surgeons must be knowledgeable about the pharmacology of each agent, indications for use, and the means by which the effect of the agent is monitored. Most failures of anticoagulant therapy arise from improper choice of agent or administration of insufficient or excessive amounts of the anticoagulant. The major complication of anticoagulant therapy is hemorrhage; however, other, less common adverse effects may affect the survival of life and/or limb.

Today, there are many drugs available to the vascular surgeon that act as anticoagulant or antithrombotic agents. Major classes of anticoagulants include (1) heparins, which induce inhibition of activated coagulation proteins by their interaction with the natural anticoagulant antithrombin III (AT III); (2) prothrombinopenic agents such as warfarin (Coumadin); (3) fibrinogenopenic agents such as ancrod; (4) platelet-function inhibitors, which include aspirin, dipyridamole, sulfinpyrazone, iloprost, and other prostaglandin synthetase and phosphodiesterase inhibitors; and (5) agents such as dextran whose anticoagulant effect is the result of a combination of platelet-function inhibition, decreased concentrations of coagulation proteins, and rheologic factors. Each class has a different mode of action and indication for use in the treatment or prophylaxis of thromboembolic disease.

HEPARIN

Heparin is the anticoagulant of choice for the management of most acute thromboembolic disorders. It is also an effective prophylaxis for patients at risk for deep vein thrombosis (DVT).

Pharmacology

Standard or unfractionated heparin (UH) is a mixture of straight-chain glycosaminoglycuronan sulfate esters with molecular weights ranging from 4000 to 40,000 d. UH has a mean molecular weight of 15,000 d and contains 10 to 90 saccharides per molecule.[1] Studies of commercial heparin preparations have demonstrated that up to 70% of the preparation by weight has less than 15% of the anticoagulant activity.[2] Beef lung and porcine intestinal mucosa have traditionally been the primary sources for commercial heparin and have different ratios of high- and low-molecular-weight fractions with differing anticoagulant activities. Because of this variation in activity, heparin is dispensed in international units rather than by weight.

Heparin's anticoagulant effect is dependent on normal concentrations of the plasma proteinase inhibitor AT III. Heparin potentiates the activity of AT III, the most physiologically important natural anticoagulant, in neutralizing the activated coagulation proteins thrombin (factor IIa), factor IXa, factor Xa, factor XIa, and factor XIIa. The interaction between heparin and AT III requires a unique sequence of monosaccharides, the AT III–binding site.[3] Only one third of the molecules in commercially prepared UH contain the AT III–binding site. Heparin combines with AT III in a 1:1 stoichiometric ratio and produces a conformational change in AT III that fully activates its serine proteinase–inhibitory site. Two different mechanisms are involved between the heparin molecules and AT III–binding sites. Heparin molecules with molecular weights less than 5000 d composed of sequences less than 18 saccharides long form a binary complex with AT III capable of inactivating factor Xa and factor XIIa.[3] Heparin molecules with molecular weights greater than 5000 d composed of sequences at least 18 saccharides long form a ternary complex composed of heparin, AT III, and an activated coagulation factor (thrombin, factor IXa, or factor XIa).[3] Heparin may dissociate from the complex and catalyze other thrombin–AT III interactions once the AT III has neutralized an activated coagulation factor.[2]

The success of low-dose heparin for venous thromboembolic prophylaxis has been attributed to the inhibition of thrombin production by the heparin–AT III complex inhibition of factor Xa. One microgram of the binary heparin–AT III complex is able to inhibit 32 units of factor Xa, which is equivalent to the inhibition of 1600 units of thrombin. In contrast, 1000 µg of AT III would be required to directly inactivate a similar amount of thrombin.[1]

Individual responses to heparin administration vary according to AT III concentrations, the presence of antiheparin substances such as platelet factor IV, and the level of coagulant activity. Heparin has limited anticoagulant activity in patients with congenital or acquired AT III deficiencies. AT III concentrations may decrease during heparin therapy, with up to a 12% decrease at 4 hours after initiation of therapy and a 33% decrease with continued therapy. Patients with preexisting AT III deficiencies may experience even greater decreases in circulating AT III concentrations with prolonged heparin administration.[4]

After intravenous injection, heparin rapidly binds to plasma proteins. It is not excreted by the kidney nor does there appear to be an enzymatic pathway for degradation in the liver or plasma. The half-life of circulating heparin is about 90 minutes, with the most likely mechanism for its clearance being the reticuloendothelial system. Heparin binds to arterial and venous endothelium and may be concentrated there up to 7500 times its concentration in plasma. The clearance of heparin is dose dependent and is prolonged with higher doses.[2]

Both the molecular weight and the cation to which the heparin is bound affect its absorption from the subcutaneous tissues. Higher molecular-weight fractions and calcium preparations are more slowly absorbed than the sodium preparations or lower molecular-weight fractions.[5]

Renal failure does not affect the anticoagulant half-life or clearance of heparin. Hepatic insufficiency has no significant effect on heparin clearance but may affect anticoagulant activity by reducing the availability of AT III and other clotting factors. "Standard" amounts of heparin are not effective in patients with pulmonary embolism and extensive DVT because of the presence of large quantities of activated clotting factors.

Clinical Application

Multiple studies have documented the effectiveness of low-dose heparin (5000 units subcutaneously 2 hours before surgery and every 8 to 12 hours postoperatively until the patient is ambulatory) in reducing the incidence of postoperative DVT and fatal pulmonary embolism.[6-12] In high-risk patients (i.e., patients with a past history of DVT or malignant disease or patients undergoing major abdominal, thoracic, gynecologic, or orthopedic procedures), the incidence of postoperative DVT has been reduced from 30% to 50% in untreated patients to 6% to 12% in treated patients.[10,11] The protective effect was less marked for those patients undergoing total hip and knee replacement or open prostatectomy; however, it was noted that when DVT did occur in treated patients, there was a lower incidence of bilateral involvement and the thrombotic process usually remained below the popliteal vein.[10]

DVT and acute pulmonary embolism are treated with large initial doses of heparin followed by continuous infusion to stop the coagulation process and prevent thrombus propagation. In the absence of contraindications to the use of heparin, treatment may be initiated when acute thromboembolism is suspected, before confirmation by angiography and/or ventilation-perfusion scanning. Patients at increased risk for hemorrhagic complications should not be given heparin (or should receive smaller amounts) until after the diagnosis of thromboembolism has been confirmed.

Patients with DVT or acute pulmonary embolism initially receive as a bolus, heparin 200 to 300 U/kg of body weight. The heparin bolus is followed by a continuous intravenous infusion of heparin that is adjusted frequently to maintain the activated partial thromboplastin time (APTT) at twice the control value. The continuous intravenous infusion method is preferred because it has been associated with a lesser incidence of hemorrhagic complications, it is easier and more accurate to monitor, and it usually requires smaller amounts of heparin to achieve an adequate level of anticoagulation.[13] Continuous infusion may also avoid the swings of coagulability associated with intermittent intravenous or subcutaneous administration of heparin.

Several methods are available to monitor the anticoagulant effect of heparin. The APTT is most widely used, with maintenance of the APTT in the range of 1.5 to 2 times the control values associated with inhibition of intravascular coagulation without excessive risk of hemorrhage.[14] The activated clotting time (ACT) may also be used and has the advantage of a linear response to increasing doses of heparin.[15] Maintenance of the ACT in the range of 150 to 200 seconds provides adequate levels of anticoagulation in the treatment of DVT or acute pulmonary embolism.[15] The APTT or ACT must be determined several times a day during the initial stages of therapy because the heparin requirements for maintenance of safe and effective levels of anticoagulation will change as the thrombotic process and coagulation mechanism are brought under control.

Continuous intravenous heparin infusion is maintained at therapeutic levels for 7 to 10 days, after which many patients receive 5000 units of heparin subcutaneously every 8 hours for the remainder of their hospital stay and for 3 months following discharge. For those patients who cannot be managed with subcutaneous heparin, oral anticoagulant therapy is begun on the fifth day of intravenous heparin therapy. Continuous intravenous heparin infusion is maintained at therapeutic levels until a satisfactory state of hypoprothrombinemia is achieved with oral anticoagulant therapy.

During revascularization procedures 5000 to 7000 units of heparin is administered intravenously immediately before application of vascular clamps to prevent clotting in vessel segments. If necessary, an additional 1000 to 2000 units is given after each hour of vascular occlusion. When good hemostasis is achieved, heparin reversal is rarely required. Postoperatively, patients at high risk for DVT (e.g., after femoropopliteal or femorotibial bypass) are maintained on continuous low-dose heparin infusions (400 to 600 U/hr) or subcutaneous heparin (5000 U/8 hr) until they are ambulatory.

Heparin is used in the management of acute arterial thromboembolic disease to prevent thrombus propagation and to permit collaterals to develop. To reduce or prevent clot propagation while appropriate diagnostic and therapeutic measures are instituted, patients with an acute peripheral arterial embolus are given a bolus of 10,000 units of heparin, which is followed by continuous infusion of heparin to maintain the APTT at 1.5 to 2 times the control value. Following thromboembolectomy, the continuous infusion is maintained for 3 to 4 days to reduce coagulability while endothelial healing occurs. Postoperative hemorrhage is rare if adequate hemostasis is obtained intraoperatively and the APTT is not allowed to exceed twice the control value.

Complications

The most common complication of heparin therapy is hemorrhage, which may vary from mild mucosal oozing or hematuria to extensive intracranial, intrathoracic, gastrointestinal, or urinary bleeding. The risk of hemorrhage from prophylactic low-dose subcutaneous heparin therapy is negligible. The incidence of wound hematomas in patients placed on prophylactic heparin therapy postoperatively is less than 15% if 15,000 units or less of heparin is administered daily.[8,10] The incidence of hemorrhage requiring transfusion in this patient group is less than 4%.[10]

The risk of bleeding with therapeutic doses of heparin is 6% to 10% and is increased in groups such as postmenopausal women and patients with preexisting abnormalities of the coagulation mechanism, thrombocytopenia, or uremia. In this patient group the risk of significant hemorrhage may approach 50% and heparin must be administered advisedly and with careful monitoring. Hemorrhage is rarely experienced with continuous intravenous infusions of heparin when the APTT remains less than twice the control value.

Cerebral axial tomographic scans should be obtained before heparin therapy is initiated in a patient with an acute stroke. Heparin administration is contraindicated if there is evidence of a hemorrhagic infarct because it may contribute to additional bleeding with expansion of the infarct.

Non–life-threatening hemorrhage is best managed by discontinuation of heparin therapy. If bleeding continues or threatens life, heparin may be neutralized with protamine sulfate. The amount of protamine sulfate required can be calculated from the results of a protamine titration test or the ACT. If the tests cannot be done, 1 to 1.5 mg of protamine are usually required to neutralize 100 units of heparin. Portions of the calculated dose, 30% to 50%, are given slowly intravenously to reduce the risk of hypotension, bradycardia, and peripheral vasodilatation. Excess administration of protamine should be avoided as protamine may also act as an anticoagulant. If the bleeding continues and the APTT remains prolonged, additional small amounts of protamine may be given with caution until the bleeding ceases or the APTT returns towards normal.

An infrequent, but potentially life- and limb-threatening complication of heparin therapy is the development of thrombocytopenia with thrombosis and hemorrhage. This heparin-induced thrombocytopenia has occurred with a frequency of 0.6% to 30% (mean, 6%) in patients receiving heparin and appears to be independent of the source or amount of heparin administered.[16-18] Thrombocytopenia, which is progressive, usually develops after 6 to 8 days of therapy but may occur within 48 hours of therapy initiation in patients who have received heparin previously. Thrombocytopenia may be preceded by increasing heparin requirements to maintain adequate levels of anticoagulation. This complication is best detected before the onset of thrombohemorrhagic sequelae with platelet-count monitoring.

Heparin-induced thrombocytopenia has been associated with 23% mortality and 61% morbidity.[18] However, with early recognition and treatment, mortality and morbidity can be reduced to 12% and 22.5%, respectively.[19] In patients receiving heparin in whom thrombocytopenia (platelet count <100,000/mm^3) or new or progressive thromboembolic events develop, platelet aggregation studies should be performed and heparin administration should be discontinued. An increase in platelet count following cessation of heparin, and/or positive aggregation studies, confirms the diagnosis. If patients with this syndrome continue to receive heparin, they will be at high risk for thromboembolic complications. This disorder appears to be caused by the development of a heparin-dependent platelet membrane antibody that is capable of inducing platelet aggregation in the presence of heparin. Thrombocytopenia improves and thromboembolic complications remit when heparin therapy is discontinued. Patients with this disorder are given aspirin and warfarin if continued inhibition of the coagulation process is required.[18,19]

Sensitivity reactions consisting of bronchiole constriction, lacrimation, or urticaria may occur in 2% to 5% of patients receiving heparin. Anaphylaxis with circulatory collapse is a rare complication of heparin administration.

Long-term administration of heparin may be associated with alopecia and osteoporosis. The incidence of alopecia is higher in patients who are also receiving oral anticoagulants. Hair growth usually resumes once heparin administration is discontinued. Osteoporosis and pathologic fractures of the vertebral column and long bones have been reported in patients receiving heparin for more than 6 months in dosages exceeding 10,000 U/day.[20,21]

Failures

Most failures of heparin therapy are iatrogenic and are related to (1) the use of heparin in patients with contraindications, (2) the administration of insufficient amounts of heparin, (3) not beginning the prophylactic heparin regimen early enough, and (4) on rare occasions, the development of sensitivities to heparin or a congenital or acquired AT III deficiency. Prophylactic regimens must be initiated either before or concomitant with the event placing the patient at risk for thromboembolic complications. Once thrombosis of the deep venous system or pulmonary embolism has occurred, prophylactic regimens are inadequate and large amounts of heparin are required. Blaisdell, Graziano, and Effeney[22] have noted that local thrombus propagation, as demonstrated by fibrinogen consumption studies, may occur in the presence of "adequate" levels of systemic anticoagulation and that additional heparin, up to 4000 U/hr, may be required to control the local thrombotic process.

Failure to achieve therapeutic levels of anticoagulation with increasing amounts of heparin suggests the presence of an AT III deficiency, excessive concentrations of circulating procoagulants, or the development of heparin-induced thrombocytopenia. If the platelet count is greater than 100,000/mm³, assays of factor VIII and AT III should be obtained. If factor VIII and AT III assays are not available, the response of the ACT to an intravenous heparin infusion should be determined. A normal response, with prolongation of the ACT, suggests the presence of elevated concentrations of factor VIII, which can produce a falsely shortened APTT and a picture of heparin resistance.[17] Failure of the ACT to respond to the administered heparin often indicates the presence of an acquired or congenital AT III deficiency. A platelet count less than 100,000/mm³ suggests the possibility of heparin-induced thrombocytopenia.

Patients with a congenital or acquired AT III deficiency are treated with oral anticoagulants unless immediate anticoagulation is necessary. When immediate anticoagulation is required, the patient may be given fresh frozen plasma or cryoprecipitate (to replenish deficient levels of AT III) and heparin while oral anticoagulant therapy is initiated.

Heparin remains the agent of choice for the treatment of pulmonary embolism. Most often new filling defects are demonstrated by perfusion scan or angiogram during the first few days of therapy. These new emboli are frequently attributed to failure of heparin therapy. However, they usually are an indication of the effectiveness of heparin—an adequate amount of circulating heparin inhibits clotting and permits thrombolysis to occur. As the embolus in the pulmonary arteries or the thrombus in the pelvis or leg veins begins to lyse, it frequently fragments and produces new emboli that are rapidly lysed in the pulmonary arteries.

LOW-MOLECULAR-WEIGHT HEPARINS

Heparin derivatives with even higher anti–factor Xa and lower anti–factor IIa activity have been developed and are the so-called low-molecular-weight heparins (LMWHs). LMWH fractions may be separated from unfractionated heparin (UH) by gel filtration or ultrafiltration. Commercial LMWHs are prepared by acidic hydrolysis, esterification, enzymatic depolymerization, or fractionation of UH.[23] Most LMWHs currently undergoing clinical trials have molecular weights between 4000 and 6000 d and are composed of chains with a length of 2 to 30 saccharides.[1] LMWHs require AT III just like UH but possess relatively greater anti–factor Xa (antithrombotic) activity and less anti–factor IIa (anticoagulation) activity compared with UH. The half-life clearance for anti–factor Xa activity of LMWHs is much longer (two to four times) than that of UH and the anti–factor Xa activity may persist after the LMWH has been cleared from the circulation.[24]

Clinical trials with LMWH have demonstrated that a single daily injection of LMWH is as effective as twice-daily doses of UH in preventing venous thromboembolism in surgical patients.[25,26] Theoretically, LMWHs might prevent thrombosis with a lower incidence of hemorrhagic complications than UH. Some studies have suggested that intraoperative bleeding is less when LMWH is used preoperatively and postoperatively for DVT prophylaxis, whereas other studies have noted no differences in blood loss.[27,28] LMWH has not been released for use in the United States; however, several preparations are being investigated in clinical trials. Although the early results suggest that LMWHs will be useful in deep venous thromboembolic prophylaxis, additional studies are needed to determine their effectiveness and their complication rates.

The risk for hemorrhagic complications associated with the use of LMWH has not been adequately defined. Sensitivity and anaphylactic reactions to LMWH are said to be low. Patients receiving LMWH are also susceptible to the development of heparin-induced thrombocytopenia.

ORAL ANTICOAGULANTS
Pharmacology

Warfarin, first synthesized in 1944, is the most popular oral anticoagulant. Gastrointestinal absorption of warfarin is complete with peak plasma concentrations being reached 2 to 12 hours after a single oral dose. Warfarin is bound (97%) to albumin and has a circulating half-life of 36 to 40 hours. Oral anticoagulants are principally metabolized by the microsomal fraction of the hepatocyte. The metabolites are water soluble and are excreted in the urine.[29,30]

A genetically determined resistance to the effects of the oral anticoagulants is encountered in a small number of patients. One autosomal dominant trait produces an abnormal vitamin K sensitivity and another produces enhanced metabolism of the drug.[29,30] Patients' responses to the oral anticoagulants vary (and may change from one of hyperresponsiveness to one of relative resistance during therapy) and frequent drug adjustment may be needed to achieve safe anticoagulation.

Warfarin and the other oral anticoagulants interfere with the action of vitamin K in the synthesis of clotting factors II, VI, IX, and X by the liver. Vitamin K is a cofactor in the reaction that converts glutamyl residues of clotting factor precursors to the carboxyglutamyl residues necessary for the binding of calcium. Patients receiving oral anticoagulants produce antigenically similar clotting factors that do not have procoagulant activity because of their abnormal calcium binding characteristics.[31] This effect on the vitamin K–carboxylase reaction is reversible and can be blocked by the administration of vitamin K.

Anticoagulation with oral anticoagulant administration is dependent on the reduction of the concentrations of all affected clotting factors and may take 3 to 5 days to achieve. The administration of large loading doses of the oral anticoagulant does little more than severely depress concentrations of factor VII, which has been associated with the risk of hemorrhage.[29,30] The time required to reach therapeutic levels of anticoagulation is affected by the rate of "turnover" of the clotting factors. Ninety percent of the total change occurs within 20 hours for factor VII, 65 hours for factor IX, 130 hours for factor X, and 8 days for factor II.[29,30] A new steady state concentration will be achieved for each affected factor following a change in the maintenance dose of oral anticoagulant. Factor X activity depression is the most common cause of hemorrhage resulting from chronic excesses of the oral anticoagulants.[30] Following discontinuation of oral anticoagulant therapy, the return to normal clotting factor concentrations follows a similar time course.

Warfarin also alters the synthesis of the vitamin K–dependent natural anticoagulant proteins C and S. Protein C is a vitamin K–dependent proenzyme that, when converted to its active serine proteinase form (protein Ca), becomes a potent anticoagulant.[32] This anticoagulation pathway is activated by the generation of thrombin. Thrombin binds to an endothelial cell surface glycoprotein, thrombomodulin, which then initiates the activation of protein C. Protein C then complexes with another vitamin K–dependent protein, protein S, on the surface of either platelets or endothelial cells. These complexes catalyze the proteolytic inactivation of factors Va and VIIIa, destroying the cofactors of the two rate-limiting steps of coagulation.[32] Protein C's half-life is only 4 to 6 hours; thus levels are reduced early in warfarin therapy, creating the potential for a transient procoagulant state, especially in patients with preexisting protein C deficiencies. Therapeutic anticoagulation with heparin should therefore be obtained before warfarin administration and must be continued for 3 to 5 days until low steady states for coagulation factors II, VII, IX, and X are achieved.

The biologic effects of the oral anticoagulants may be potentiated by certain disease states (primarily those that produce hyperca-

Table 9-1. Factors Affecting the Anticoagulant Activity of Vitamin K Antagonists

Factor	Effect	Mechanism
Hepatic insufficiency	Potentiation	Decreased clotting factor synthesis
Malnutrition	Potentiation	Decreased vitamin K stores
Hypermetabolic states (e.g., fever, hyperthyroidism)	Potentiation	Increased clotting factor "turnover"
Hypometabolic states (e.g., hypothyroidism)	Antagonism	Decreased clotting factor "turnover"
Drugs	Potentiation	See Table 9-2
	Antagonism	See Table 9-3

Table 9-2. Drug Interactions Producing Potentiation of Oral Anticoagulant Activity

Drugs	Mechanism of action
Chloramphenicol	Inhibition of enzyme activity
Ethanol Diazoxide Ethacrynic acid Indomethacin Mefenamic acid Oxyphenbutazone Phenylbutazone Salicylates Sulfonamides Tolbutamide	Responsible for drug degradation
Clofibrate D-Thyroxine Antibiotics*	Reduced availability of vitamin K
Anabolic steroids Quinidine	Reduced clotting factor synthesis

*Especially moxalactam and other second- and third-generation cephalosporins.

Table 9-3. Drug Interactions Producing Antagonism of Oral Anticoagulant Activity

Drugs	Mechanism of action
Barbiturates Meprobamate Griseofulvin	Induction of enzymes responsible for oral anticoagulant metabolism
Cholestyramine	Decreased intestinal absorption of the oral anticoagulants
Oral contraceptives Vitamin K (pregnancy)	Increased synthesis of clotting factors

tabolism, hypocatabolism, or hepatic insufficiency) or vitamin K deficiency states (Table 9-1). In addition, many common therapeutic agents may alter the response of the coagulation system to regularly administered doses of the oral anticoagulant through decreased absorption from the gastrointestinal tract, displacement of the drug from its binding site on albumin, increases in the rate at which it is metabolized by the liver, decreased vitamin K availability, or decreases or increases in the plasma half-life of the affected clotting factors (Tables 9-2 and 9-3).

Clinical Application

Oral anticoagulants have been demonstrated to be effective in the prophylaxis of postoperative DVT and the prevention of recurrent thromboembolism. These agents have also been found to reduce the risk of embolism arising from prosthetic heart valves, the enlarged left atria of patients with mitral stenosis, or chronic atrial fibrillation.[29,30] The use of oral anticoagulants in ischemic cerebrovascular disease has been supplanted by platelet function–inhibiting agents. The oral anticoagulants have no established role in the treatment of chronic peripheral arterial disease.

For postoperative venous thromboembolism prophylaxis, oral anticoagulants must be started 3 to 4 days before surgery to achieve a prothrombin time 1.5 times the control value on the day of surgery. The prophylaxis may be initiated with warfarin at doses of 5 to 10 mg daily; the dose is then adjusted to maintain the prothrombin time at 1.5 to 2 times the control value postoperatively.[33] We recommend therapeutic anticoagulation administration with heparin for at least 3 to 4 days for all patients beginning warfarin therapy unless heparin therapy is contraindicated. Lower initial doses (i.e., 2 to 5 mg daily) should be used in elderly patients and in those receiving parenteral nutrition or recovering from surgery because these individuals are more responsive to the prothrombinopenic effects of oral anticoagulants.

After a massive thromboembolic event, long-term anticoagulation therapy with warfarin is usually begun after 5 to 7 days of intravenous heparin therapy. However, recent data suggest earlier administration of warfarin is safe following submassive thromboembolism.[34] The initial warfarin dose is 7.5 to 10 mg daily; subsequent daily doses are adjusted to maintain a prothrombin time at 1.5 to 2 times the control value. Recent prospective data suggest that maintaining a prothrombin time ratio as low as 1.25, compared to 1.5 to 2 times the control value, provides similar protection against recurrent thromboembolism (2% incidence of both groups) while being associated with a lower incidence of hemorrhagic complications (4% vs. 22%).[35] The heparin infusion is discontinued when the prothrombin ratio reaches 1.5 times the control value. Patients who are elderly, have hepatic insufficiency, or have vitamin K deficiencies should receive reduced initial doses of warfarin. Anticoagulant therapy is continued for at least 3 months following an acute thromboembolic event in order to reduce the incidence of recurrent thromboembolism.[35] After 3 to 4 months of anticoagulant administration, the risk of hemorrhage may exceed the potential beneficial effect of continued therapy. However, we recommend 6 months of warfarin therapy following major pulmonary embolism or recurrent DVT.

Recent retrospective reviews have indicated that systemic anticoagulation therapy with heparin and warfarin following femorodistal bypass with polytetrafluoroethylene (PTFE) grafts may extend graft patency compared with historical controls.[36] A multicenter comparative study of PTFE and saphenous vein grafts used for infrapopliteal bypass has demonstrated only a 12% 4-year graft patency rate.[37] Flinn et al.[36] reviewed a similar cohort of patients who un-derwent femorotibial or femoroperoneal bypass with PTFE grafts (97% for limb salvage) but who received perioperative heparin and long-term anticoagulation with warfarin and found a significant increase in graft patency rates (37% 4-year graft patency). Prothrombin times were maintained at twice the control values. Warfarin may prevent PTFE graft occlusion caused by the graft's inherent thrombogenicity or caused by the low flow states secondary to tibial or peroneal anastomotic narrowing.

Complications

Hemorrhage is the most common complication of anticoagulant therapy. Oral anticoagulant therapy should be avoided or used with extreme caution in patients with defects in the hemostatic mechanism, limited hepatic reserve, active ulcer disease, and other disease processes predisposing to hemorrhage. In addition, patients receiving oral anticoagulants must possess sufficient reliability and intelligence to administer the drug, return for regular follow-up laboratory testing, and recognize the symptoms and signs of excessive anticoagulation.

The frequency of hemorrhage with oral anticoagulants varies widely and is a function of the level of anticoagulation. Forfar[38] reported an incidence of 4.3% of clinically significant hemorrhage per treatment year in patients maintained within the therapeutic range. Severe hemorrhage is more common when the prothrombin time exceeds the therapeutic range (greater than twice the control value). The risk of hemorrhage is increased in patients in whom control has proved to be unreliable, in men with an aortic valve prosthesis, and in patients who have received anticoagulant therapy for more than 3 years. Advanced age, urologic and gynecologic disorders, postpartum state, and initiation of therapy with a large loading dose also increase the risk of hemorrhage.[29,30]

The nose, skin, and gastrointestinal and urinary tracts are the most common sites of hemorrhage. Intracerebral or gastrointestinal hemorrhage cause the majority of bleeding-related fatalities. Forfar[38] reported that nearly 20% of the hemorrhagic complications occurred in the retroperitoneal or perinephric spaces and are associated with a very high mortality. When the prothrombin time is within the therapeutic range and gastrointestinal or urinary tract bleeding occurs, the source of this bleeding should be evaluated, as an unsuspected colon or renal carcinoma may have been "unmasked."

When a patient receiving oral anticoagulant therapy bleeds, therapy should be discontinued. If the bleeding is excessive, anticoagulation may be reversed within 24 hours by intravenous administration of 20 mg of vitamin K_1. Life-threatening hemorrhage is best managed with replacement therapy using infusions of fresh frozen plasma in addition to administration of vitamin K_1.

The adverse effects of oral anticoagulants, other than hemorrhage, are rare and include alopecia, dermatitis, fever, nausea, diarrhea, abdominal cramping, and hypersensitivity reactions. An interesting syndrome of "purple toes" occurs in a few patients. These patients present with toes that have an appearance similar to that seen after frostbite or with ischemic changes. The condition is usually reversible. A rare complication of oral anticoagulant therapy is extensive dermal gangrene, the risk of which is increased with loading dose regimens for initiating therapy. Its etiology, as well as the etiology of "purple toes," has been attributed to dermal microvascular thrombosis. This occurs early after warfarin administration when protein C levels are decreased while the intrinsic coagulation pathway remains intact; patients with congenital or acquired protein C deficiency are at greater risk for this complication. Women appear to be more at risk for this complication than men. The skin of the thigh, breasts, and buttocks is involved most often. Some of these cases resolve spontaneously, whereas others require débridement, grafting, or even amputation. Simultaneous heparin administration at the beginning of warfarin therapy prevents this complication.[17]

Oral anticoagulants should not be given during the first trimester of pregnancy because of the teratogenicity related to their interference with the vitamin K–mediated carboxylation reactions necessary for the calcification of bone. These drugs have also been shown to cause nervous system abnormalities. Oral anticoagulants also should not be administered to lactating women because the anticoagulants are secreted in the breast milk and could lead to hemorrhagic problems in the nursing infant.[29]

Failures

Failure that occurs with oral anticoagulant therapy, that is, the inability to inhibit coagulation, is most frequently caused by the use of insufficient amounts of the agent. Individuals with genetically determined resistance to the oral anticoagulant may require up to 80 mg of warfarin daily to achieve an acceptable level of anticoagulation.

The laboratory method for monitoring the anticoagulant effect may affect the therapeutic efficacy of the drug. The thromboplastin reagents have differing sensitivities to the clotting factor changes produced by oral anticoagulants. Therapeutic prothrombin time ratios (patient: control), may range from 2 to 4 for the British comparative thromboplastin to 2 to 3.5 for the thrombotest reagent and 1.4 to 1.8 for the Ortho reagent.[30] It is imperative therefore to consult with the laboratory responsible for monitoring the anticoagulant effect so that appropriate therapeutic prolongations of the prothrombin time are maintained. Recently, the World Health Organization (WHO) noted that the different commercial thromboplastin preparations used by American and European clinical laboratories produced different prothrombin times for the same level of warfarin anticoagulant intensity. The WHO has recommended that prothrombin ratios be normalized to an international ratio (International Normalized Ratio or INR). Most coagulation laboratories now are reporting prothrombin ratios for the specific laboratory and an INR.

Several drugs interfere with the response to, or action of, the oral anticoagulants and thus reduce their anticoagulant effect. Drug interactions and their mechanism of action are listed in Tables 9-2 and 9-3.

Patients receiving oral anticoagulants who are scheduled for surgery and who will continue oral anticoagulant therapy postoperatively are best treated with subcutaneous heparin therapy instituted perioperatively and continued until satisfactory anticoagulation with the oral anticoagulants is achieved again postoperatively. If there is a need to reverse the anticoagulant effect rapidly, fresh frozen plasma should be administered in amounts sufficient to reduce the patient's prothrombin ratio to less than 1.4. Administration of vitamin K makes these patients more resistant to the oral anticoagulants and delays the establishment of therapeutic anticoagulation levels postoperatively.

DEXTRAN
Pharmacology

Dextran is a branched polysaccharide produced by the bacterium *Leuconostoc mesenteroides* by fermentation of saccharose. Dextran was first used clinically in 1944 as a plasma volume expander. Two dextran preparations are available: high-molecular-weight dextran (dextran 70), with an average molecular weight of 70,000 d, and low-molecular-weight dextran (dextran 40), with an average molecular weight of 40,000 d. The circulating half-life for dextran 70 is 24 hours, whereas that for dextran 40 is 6 hours. Although most clinical trials investigating dextran's antithrombotic effect have used dextran 70, their antithrombotic effect appears equivalent.[39]

Dextran exhibits both rheologic and antithrombotic properties. The first clinical study of dextran for venous thromboembolism prophylaxis was published in 1962 by Koekenberg.[40] Dextran's osmotic effect causes plasma volume expansion, hemodilution and improvement of blood flow, and reduction of venostasis. These rheologic factors may be of greater importance in exerting an antithrombotic effect in the arterial circulation than in the venous circulation. Dextran's antithrombotic effects are caused by its interaction with both platelets and the coagulation system.[41] Dextran appears to decrease platelet adhesiveness while also reducing platelet aggregation by altering the platelet granule–release reaction. These effects on platelets are maximal after 4 to 6 hours of dextran infusion. Dextran also has been found to complex with the von Willebrand factor, de-

creasing its plasma concentration. Dextran increases endothelial cell and blood cell electronegativity. Finally, dextran appears to interfere with fibrin polymerization, thus increasing fibrin's susceptibility to lysis by plasmin.[41]

Clinical Application

Dextran has been used prophylactically to prevent both venous and arterial thromboses. Clagett and Reisch,[42] using meta-analysis, pooled the results of randomized clinical trials using dextran as a prophylactic agent for DVT. DVT developed in 15.6% (115 of 738) of patients receiving dextran and 24.2% (193 of 799) of control patients. Dextran also significantly decreased the incidence of pulmonary embolism (1.2%) compared with controls (2.8%). Dextran has been reported to reduce by half the incidence of DVT in patients with malignancies and femur fractures and those undergoing hip surgery.

The amount of dextran proven effective in clinical trials has varied between 500 ml of a 6% solution of dextran 70 to 1000 ml of a 10% solution of dextran 40 over 24 hours.

Dextran is indicated in the management of thromboembolism in patients who cannot receive heparin because of heparin-induced thrombocytopenia or in patients with an increased risk of hemorrhage. A slow infusion of dextran, 25 to 40 ml/hr, is recommended for the management of venous thromboembolism. Total infusion volume should not exceed 10% of the patient's blood volume during a 24-hour period in order to avoid volume overload and an increased risk of hemorrhage.

The role of dextran in preventing arterial thrombosis has recently been studied. A clinical trial of dextran 40 in patients undergoing "difficult" lower extremity bypass procedures decreased the early postoperative occlusion rate by more than threefold.[43] Rutherford et al.[43] recommended a 4-day regimen, consisting of five 500 ml units of dextran 40, the first administered with induction of anesthesia at 100 ml/hr, a second unit administered on the day of operation, and an additional unit administered on each of the first 3 postoperative days. Further clinical trials of dextran, however, are necessary before its role as an arterial antithrombotic, prophylactic agent can be defined.

Complications

Total infusion volume of either dextran preparation should not exceed 10% of the patient's blood volume during a 24-hour period in order to avoid volume overload as well as increased hemorrhagic risk. Large doses of dextran should be used with caution in patients treated concomitantly with anticoagulant or platelet-inhibiting medications. Pulmonary edema secondary to plasma volume expansion in patients with cardiac compromise is a major complication of dextran therapy. Although dextran is nonimmunogenic, allergic reactions are not infrequent and range from skin rashes to anaphylactoid reactions. When anaphylaxis occurs, it is usually at the beginning of the dextran infusion and is secondary to preformed dextran-reactive antibodies.[44] It is possible to prevent these reactions by blocking the reactive sites of these antibodies with the prior infusion of short-chain (3000 to 6000 d) dextrans in patients known to be sensitive. A further complication of dextran therapy is the development of renal failure. Patients must be closely monitored to prevent dehydration to ensure that an adequate urine output is maintained at a low specific gravity. Dextran is contraindicated in patients with active bleeding, coagulopathy, congestive heart failure, impaired renal function, or a history of hypersensitivity to the drug.

Failures

Dextran should probably be given as early as possible in connection with surgery. The majority of dextran failures are associated with surgical complications, causing the surgeon to order the cessation of dextran therapy. No formal study on different dosages of dextran has been published. Appropriate laboratory testing for the antithrombotic effects of dextran therapy has not been defined.

ANCROD
Pharmacology

Ancrod, the venom of the Malayan pit viper (*Agkistrodon rhodostoma*), achieves its anticoagulant effect by cleaving the A-fibrinopeptides (A, AY, and AP) but not fibrinopeptide B from the fibrinogen molecule to yield a viable, unstable non–cross-linked fibrin that is incapable of clot formation.[45] This imperfectly polymerized fibrin is rapidly removed from the circulation by fibrinolysis with the formation of fibrin split products and by the reticuloendothelial system. Ancrod appears to deplete circulating fibrinogen selectively; it has little direct effect on formed thromboses. However, ancrod may stimulate fibrinolytic activity in established thrombi by initiating a release of tissue plasminogen activator from endothelial cells. Platelet counts and coagulation proteins are unaffected by ancrod. Blood viscosity is lowered because of the hypofibrinogenemia, thus improving blood flow and reducing venous stasis.

Circulating ancrod has a half-life of 3 to 5 hours and is excreted largely unchanged in the urine and cleared by the reticuloendothelial system. Serum fibrinogen levels return to hemostatic levels (50 mg/100 ml) within several hours after the cessation of ancrod therapy; however, it may take several weeks before pretreatment fibrinogen levels are reached.

Clinical Application

Ancrod is ideally suited for use in patients in whom heparin-induced thrombocytopenia develops and who continue to require systemic anticoagulation for treatment of thromboembolism. Alternatively, patients with a history of heparin-induced thrombocytopenia who subsequently require anticoagulation for recurrent thromboembolism or coronary artery bypass surgery can be safely treated with ancrod.[45,46] Patients with AT III deficiency who require anticoagulation for thromboembolism and in whom heparin is ineffective may be effectively managed with ancrod.

Although ancrod can be administered subcutaneously, the intravenous route is preferred for easier titration of the induced hypofibrinogenemia. Infusion of 70 units (one ampule) over 2 to 4 hours results in fibrinogen levels less than 40 mg/ml within 6 to 12 hours. Slower infusion of 70 units over 18 to 36 hours should produce similar reduction in fibrinogen levels. A continuous infusion of 70 units every 24 to 36 hours is recommended to maintain anticoagulation. Serum fibrinogen levels should be determined frequently (every 12 hours) at the start of therapy and the rate of infusion should be adjusted to maintain levels between 20 mg/100 ml and 40 mg/100 ml.

Complications

Complications including fever and minor allergic reactions have been reported following subcutaneous administration. Hemorrhagic complications have been reported, but patients have safely undergone surgery while receiving ancrod. If hemorrhage does occur, rapid reversal of ancrod is achieved by administering cryoprecipitate to restore hemostatic levels of fibrinogen ($\geq$50 mg/100 ml). An ancrod antidote capable of restoring plasma fibrinogen levels to normal within 1 hour is available; however, this antidote may be associated with a foreign protein–type allergic reaction and administration of cryoprecipitate is therefore preferred.

Failures

The efficacy of ancrod in producing systemic anticoagulation has been demonstrated in several clinical trials. Failure of ancrod therapy is associated with inadequate monitoring of fibrinogen levels. Patients who have been treated with ancrod for more than 4 to 6 weeks may develop resistance to ancrod because of the appearance of serum proteinase inhibitors that bind and inactivate ancrod. Therefore ancrod use is recommended for short-term anticoagulation in patients who cannot receive heparin. If long-term anticoagulation is dictated by the clinical circumstance, warfarin therapy is recommended after short-term anticoagulation with ancrod.

PLATELET FUNCTION–INHIBITING AGENTS
Pharmacology

Platelets participate in or initiate all in vivo thrombotic processes and are the initial defense against excessive hemorrhage following a break in vascular integrity. Platelet-derived growth factors may have a role in the development and progression of atherosclerosis and perianastomotic pseudointimal hyperplasia.[47-50] The basement membrane of injured vessels may become exposed to platelets, which induces the platelets to undergo a variety of changes that produce the "hemostatic plug." The aggregating platelets also release vasoactive substances such as serotonin, adenosine diphosphate (ADP), and platelet factors III and IV. Platelet factor III provides the lipid cofactor requirement for the activation of factor X, and platelet factor IV has heparin-neutralizing activity. The platelet membrane serves as a reactive surface for many coagulation interactions. Many of the coagulation factors are bound to the platelet's surface. Platelet aggregation may be induced by other stimuli such as thrombin, ADP, epinephrine, viruses, prostaglandins, and immune complexes. These stimuli appear to induce platelet aggregation by reducing intracellular concentrations of adenosine 3':5'-cyclic phosphate (cAMP). Drugs and conditions that increase intracellular concentrations of cAMP inhibit platelet aggregation.

The platelet function–inhibiting agents primarily interfere with platelet aggregation by inhibiting the production of thromboxane A_2, a powerful proaggregatory prostaglandin metabolite, or by increasing intracellular concentrations of cAMP through inhibition of phosphodiesterase. Aspirin, indomethacin, and ibuprofen inhibit the generation of thromboxane A_2 by interfering with the action of cyclooxygenase. Aspirin produces an irreversible inhibition of cyclooxygenase as it acetylates the active center of the enzyme. The inhibitory effects of the other agents are transient and reversible.[48,50]

Dipyridamole inhibits platelet phosphodiesterase and increases intracellular cAMP concentrations by reducing the rate of degradation of cAMP. The inhibitory action of dipyridamole on phosphodiesterase is transitory. Sulfinpyrazone inhibits the platelet release reaction and interferes with platelet adhesion to subendothelial tissues.[47]

Prostacyclin (PGI_2) is the most potent naturally occurring platelet inhibitor identified. Its clinical use is limited by its profound vasodilating effects and its extreme instability at neutral pH. Currently three prostanoids have been evaluated for clinical use: PGI_2, PGE_1, and the prostacyclin analogue iloprost.[51] The proposed mechanism of action of these prostanoids is the activation of adenylate cyclase, which causes increased intracellular levels of cAMP. All three prostanoids effectively inhibit platelet aggregation induced by ADP, epinephrine, and thrombin in a dose-dependent fashion. However, at equimolar concentrations, iloprost is at least tenfold more potent than PGI_2 and 100-fold more potent than PGE_1.[51] Iloprost is stable at neutral pH, with an elimination half-life of 15 to 30 minutes. Its effect is immediate at the start of infusion and lasts up to 3 hours after its cessation. The vasodilatory effect of iloprost has been reported to be less severe compared with the other prostanoids.

Clinical Application

The platelet function–inhibiting agents are ineffective in the treatment of active thrombosis because they have no direct effect on the coagulation cascade. Their major indication has been for the prophylaxis of DVT and the prophylaxis and management of patients with cerebral transient ischemic attacks (TIAs) arising from microemboli.

Some of the platelet function–inhibiting agents are now being evaluated as agents for maintaining vascular graft patency and reducing the myointimal hyperplasia that occurs after bypass grafting. Chesebro et al.[52] randomized patients to receive dipyridamole for 48 hours preoperatively and aspirin daily beginning 7 hours after aortocoronary artery bypass. Thrombosis occurred in grafts of 10% of patients receiving placebo but in grafts of only 3% of the treated patients. One-year follow-up revealed a 25% occlusion rate among the placebo group and only an 11% occlusion rate in the treated group. Aspirin alone has now proved to be as effective as the combination of aspirin and dipyridamole.[53] Whether the potential benefits of graft patency outweigh the hemorrhagic risk of preoperative aspirin therapy is currently under investigation.

Numerous investigators, using animal models, have demonstrated the efficacy of perioperative platelet inhibitory therapy in the prevention of thromboembolic complications in small-diameter PTFE bypass grafts. Two randomized clinical trials have demonstrated significant improvement in early patency of both saphenous and PTFE grafts when patients were administered aspirin and dipyridamole preoperatively.[54,55] However, Kohler et al.[56] reported a large prospective trial in which no proven difference in femoropopliteal bypass graft patency occurred when aspirin and dipyridamole therapy was initiated 24 hours postoperatively. We recommend that aspirin administration, 325 mg daily, begin several days before a planned femorodistal bypass procedure and that it be continued indefinitely.

Dipyridamole, used alone, has not been demonstrated to have a significant effect on the incidence of recurrent myocardial infarction or the progression of peripheral arterial occlusive disease.[47,50] When combined with aspirin, dipyridamole has been shown to reduce the incidence of recurrent myocardial infarction when therapy is begun within 6 months of the initial infarct.[57-59] Aspirin, alone or in combination with sulfinpyrazone, has decreased the incidence of recurrent myocardial infarction and thromboses associated with peripheral arterial disease; however, the difference between treated and nontreated groups was not statistically significant.[49,59] The use of sulfinpyrazone has been demonstrated to decrease the incidence of hemodialysis access shunt thrombosis and may be useful in reducing cardiac deaths after myocardial infarction.[50]

Iloprost has been shown to inhibit heparin-induced aggregation of platelets in patients with heparin-induced thrombocytopenia syndrome. Iloprost has been used successfully to prevent heparin-induced platelet aggregation in patients undergoing carotid endarterectomy, hemodialysis, and open heart surgery.[60-62]

The U.S. cooperative study evaluating the effect of 650 mg of aspirin twice a day on the incidence of TIAs, cerebral infarction, and death found that the treated group had fewer TIAs, but there was a statistically insignificant reduction in the incidence of stroke in patients treated operatively or nonoperatively.[63,64] The Canadian cooperative study involving the administration of 325 mg of aspirin four times daily, alone or in combination with sulfinpyrazone, demonstrated a significant reduction in the incidence of TIAs, stroke, and death in men only.[65] Additional multicenter randomized clinical trials of aspirin or aspirin in combination with dipyridamole have demonstrated beneficial trends with reduction of the incidence of stroke and death in treated patients vs. those receiving a placebo.[50,57,66] In addition, most of these studies have demonstrated a statistically significant decrease in the incidence of fatal myocardial infarction in the aspirin- or aspirin and dipyridamole–treated groups.[57,67] Physicians' Health Study was a randomized, double-blind, placebo-controlled trial designed to determine whether a low-dose aspirin regimen (325 mg every other day) decreases cardiovascular mortality.[68] This study demonstrated a 44% reduction in the risk of myocardial infarction in the aspirin group. A slightly increased risk of stroke among those taking aspirin was not statistically significant. No reduction in mortality from all cardiovascular causes was associated with aspirin ingestion. Further analysis demonstrated that the reduction in the risk of myocardial infarction was apparent only among those physicians who were 50 years of age or older.[68]

Several clinical studies have evaluated dosages ranging from 80 mg once daily to 625 mg twice daily to reduce the incidence of graft thrombosis, TIAs and stroke, recurrent or initial myocardial infarction, and the progression of atherosclerotic occlusive disease.[48,59,66,69,70]

We currently administer 325 mg of aspirin daily to patients with peripheral arterial occlusive disease and to patients with TIAs during and subsequent to their evaluation. Patients who experience gastric irritation from aspirin are given enteric-coated aspirin or, at times, 80 mg aspirin tablets twice a day with meals. We administer dipyridamole (25 to 200 mg two to four times a day) only when the patient cannot take aspirin or other nonsteroidal anti-inflammatory agents. Sulfinpyrazone is administered 200 mg four times daily.

Complications

In contradistinction to heparin and oral anticoagulants, the use of the platelet function–inhibiting agents is rarely associated with clini-cally significant hemorrhage. In patients maintained on 1.2 gm of aspirin daily, gastrointestinal upset developed in 20% and 7% had bleeding, predominantly from the gastrointestinal tract, requiring hospitalization.[47] The incidence of complication associated with aspirin can be reduced by administering the drug at mealtime or by using the enteric-coated form of the drug. Dipyridamole causes temporary epigastric discomfort in 10% of patients; however, it is rarely associated with clinically significant hemorrhage. Sulfinpyrazone causes few gastrointestinal side effects, and bleeding complications are rare.

Chronic aspirin administration may be associated with elevation of blood urea and uric acid concentrations; however, it rarely causes gout. Headache is the major side effect of dipyridamole administration and may occur in 10% of patients receiving this drug. Sulfinpyrazone may potentiate the action of oral hypoglycemic agents. It is also a powerful uricosuric agent and may precipitate the formation of uric acid renal stones. Patients receiving prolonged therapy with sulfinpyrazone should have periodic monitoring of bone marrow function because of the potential for bone marrow suppression.

Failures

Most failures of therapy with the platelet function–inhibiting agents are related to their inappropriate application, delayed initiation of therapy, or incorrect dosage. Platelet function–inhibiting agents are ineffective in the control of active thrombosis and should not be used as the single therapeutic agent in the therapy of acute thrombotic disease. They may be used in combination with heparin or oral anticoagulants; however, their concomitant administration may increase the risk of hemorrhage.

The timing of the initiation of therapy appears to be important. Patients receiving antiplatelet agent therapy soon after myocardial infarction had a lower incidence of reinfarction than those in whom therapy was initiated more than 6 months after the initial acute event. This effect, however, was not statistically significant in the small groups of patients studied to date.[59]

REFERENCES

1. Haas S, Bluemel G. An objective evaluation of the clinical potential of low molecular weight heparins in the prevention of thromboembolism. Semin Thromb Hemost 15:424-434, 1989.
2. Estes JW. Clinical pharmacokinetics of heparin. Clin Pharmacokinet 5:204-220, 1980.
3. Choay J. Structure and activity of heparin and its fragments: An overview. Semin Thromb Hemost 15:359-364, 1989.
4. Thomas DP. Heparin. Clin Hematol 1:443-458, 1981.
5. Thomas DP, Sagar S, Stomatakis JD, et al. Plasma heparin levels after administration of calcium and sodium salts of heparin. Thromb Res 9:241-248, 1976.
6. Borow M, Goldson H. Postoperative venous thrombosis: Evaluation of five methods of treatment. Am J Surg 141:245-251, 1981.
7. Coon WW. Management of anticoagulant and thrombolytic agents in deep venous thrombosis. Vasc Surg 15:1-7, 1982.
8. Council on Thrombosis of the American Heart Association. Prevention of venous thromboembolism in surgical patients by low-dose heparin. Circulation 55: 423A-426A, 1977.
9. Kakkar VV, Corrigan TP, Fossard DP. Prevention of fatal postoperative pulmonary embolism by low doses of heparin. Lancet 1:45-51, 1975.
10. Kakkar VV. Prevention of venous thromboembolism. Clin Hematol 10:543-583, 1981.
11. Rosenow EC III, Osmundson PJ, Brown M. Pulmonary embolism. Mayo Clin Proc 56:161-178, 1981.
12. Wessler S, Gitel SN. Low-dose heparin. In Lundblad RL, Brown WV, Mann KG, et al., eds. Chemistry and Biology of Heparin. New York: Elsevier/Holland, 1981, pp 503-512.
13. Ware JA, Lewis J, Salzman EW. Antithrombotic therapy. In Rutherford RB, et al., eds. Vascular Surgery. Philadelphia: WB Saunders, 1989.
14. Hull R, Raskob G, Hirsh J, et al. Continuous intravenous heparin compared with intermittent subcutaneous heparin in the initial treatment of proximal-vein thrombosis. N Engl J Med 315:1109-1114, 1986.
15. Hattersley PG, Mitsuoka JC, King JH. The use of the activated coagulation time (ACT) as a monitor of heparin therapy. In Lundblad RL, Brown WV, Mann KG, et al., eds. Chemistry and Biology of Heparin. New York: Elsevier/Holland, 1981, pp 659-664.
16. Ansell J, Slepchuk N Jr, Raminder K, et al. Heparin induced thrombocytopenia: A prospective study. Thromb Haemost 43:61-65, 1980.
17. Kapsch DN, Kasulke RJ, Silver D. Anticoagulant therapy: Pharmacology, clinical uses and complications. Vasc Diagn Ther 2:19-33, 1981.
18. Silver D, Kapsch DN, Tsoi EKM. Heparin-induced thrombocytopenia, thrombosis and hemorrhage. Ann Surg 198:301-306, 1983.
19. Laster J, Cikrit D, Walker N, et al. The heparin-induced thrombocytopenia syndrome: An update. Surgery 102:763-770, 1987.

20. Griffith GC, Nichols G Jr, Asher J, et al. Heparin osteoporosis. JAMA 193:91-94, 1965.
21. Jaffe MD, Willis PW III. Multiple fractures associated with long-term sodium heparin therapy. JAMA 193: 152-154, 1965.
22. Blaisdell FW, Graziano CJ, Effeney DJ. In vivo assessment of anticoagulation. Surgery 82:827-839, 1977.
23. Nielsen JI, Ostergaard P. Chemistry of heparin and low molecular weight heparin. Acta Chir Scand Suppl 534:52-56, 1988.
24. Bara L, Samara M. Pharmacokinetics of low molecular weight heparins. Acta Chir Scand Suppl 543:65-72, 1988.
25. Bergquist D, Burmark US, Frisell J, et al. Low molecular weight heparin once daily compared with conventional low dose heparin twice daily. A prospective double-blind multicentre trial on prevention of postoperative thrombosis. Br J Surg 73:304-308, 1986.
26. Holm HA, Ly B, Handeland GF, et al. Subcutaneous heparin treatment of deep vein thrombosis: A comparison of unfractionated and low molecular weight heparin. Haemostasis 16(Suppl):30-37, 1986.
27. Kakkar VV, Murray WHG. Efficacy and safety of low molecular weight heparin (CY216) in preventing postoperative venous thromboembolism: A cooperative study. Br J Surg 72:786-791, 1985.
28. Koller M, Schoch U, Buchmann P, et al. Low molecular weight heparin (KABI-2165) as thromboprophylaxis in elective visceral surgery. Thromb Haemost 56: 243-246, 1986.
29. Walsh PN. Oral anticoagulant therapy. Hosp Pract 18: 101-120, 1983.
30. Winter JH, Douglass AS. Oral anticoagulants. Clin Hematol 10:459-480, 1981.
31. Suttie JW. Oral anticoagulant therapy: The biosynthetic basis. Semin Hematol 14:365-374, 1977.
32. Esmon CT. The roles of protein C and thrombomodulin in the regulation of blood coagulation. J Biol Chem 264:4743-4746, 1989.
33. Salzman EW. Prevention of venous thromboembolism by oral anticoagulants and drugs affecting platelet function. In Bergan JJ, Yao JST, eds. Venous Problems. Chicago: Year Book, 1978, pp 515-551.
34. Gallus A, Jackman J, Tillet J, et al. Safety and efficacy of warfarin started early after submassive venous thrombosis or pulmonary embolism. Lancet 2:1293-1296, 1986.
35. Hull R, Hirsh J, Jay R, et al. Different intensities of oral anticoagulation therapy in the treatment of proximal vein thrombosis. N Engl J Med 307:1676-1681, 1982.
36. Flinn WR, Rohrer MJ, Yao JST, et al. Improved long-term patency of infragenicular polytetrafluoroethylene grafts. J Vasc Surg 7:685-690, 1988.
37. Veith FJ, Gupta SK, Ascer E, et al. Six-year prospective multicenter randomized comparison of autologous saphenous vein and expanded polytetrafluoroethylene grafts in infrainguinal arterial reconstruction. J Vasc Surg 3:104-114, 1986.

38. Forfar JC. A seven-year analysis of haemorrhage in patients on long-term anticoagulant treatment. Br Heart J 42:128-132, 1979.

39. Ring J, Messmer K. Incidence and severity of anaphylactoid reactions to colloid volume substitutes. Lancet 1:466-469, 1977.

40. Koekenberg LJL. Experimental use of macrodex as a prophylaxis against post-operative thrombo-embolism. Bull Soc Int Chir 21:501-512, 1962.

41. Aberg M, Hedner U, Bergentz SE. The antithrombotic effect of dextran. Scand J Haematol 34 (Suppl):61-68, 1979.

42. Clagett GP, Reisch JS. Prevention of venous thromboembolism in general surgical patients. Ann Surg 208:227-240, 1988.

43. Rutherford RB, Jones DN, Bergenz SE, et al. The efficacy of dextran 40 in preventing early postoperative thrombosis following difficult lower extremity bypass. J Vasc Surg 1:765-773, 1984.

44. Ljungstrom KG. The antithrombotic efficacy of dextran. Acta Chir Scand Suppl 543:26-30, 1988.

45. Cole CW, Bormanis J. Ancrod: A practical alternative to heparin. J Vasc Surg 8:59-63, 1988.

46. Zulys V, Teasdale S, Michel E, et al. Ancrod anticoagulation for cardiopulmonary bypass [abstr]. Clin Invest Med 10:C44, 1987.

47. Fuster V, Chesebro JH. Antithrombotic therapy: Role of platelet inhibitor drugs. II. Pharmacologic effects of platelet-inhibitor drugs. Mayo Clin Proc 56:185-195, 1981.

48. Harlan JM, Harker LA. Hemostasis, thrombosis, and thromboembolic disorders: The role of arachidonic acid metabolites in platelet-vessel wall interactions. Med Clin North Am 65:855-880, 1981.

49. Preston FE. Aspirin, prostaglandins, and peripheral gangrene. Am J Med 74:55-60, 1983.

50. Turpie AGG. Antiplatelet therapy. Clin Hematol 10:497-520, 1981.

51. Fisher CA, Kappa JR, Sinha AK, et al. Comparison of equimolar concentrations of iloprost, prostacyclin, and prostaglandin E$_1$ on human platelet function. J Lab Clin Med 109:184-190, 1987.

52. Chesebro JH, Fuster V, Elvback LR, et al. Effect of dipyridamole and aspirin on late vein-graft patency after coronary bypass operation. N Engl J Med 310:209-214, 1984.

53. Lorenz RL, Weber M, Lotzur J, et al. Improved aortocoronary bypass patency by low-dose aspirin (100 mg daily). Lancet 1:1261-1264, 1984.

54. Goldman M, Hall C, Dykes J, et al. Does 111-indium-platelet deposition predict patency in prosthetic arterial grafts? Br J Surg 70:635-638, 1983.

55. Green RM, Roedersheimer R, DeWeese JA. Effects of aspirin and dipyridamole on expanded PTFE graft patency. Surgery 92:1016-1026, 1982.

56. Kohler TR, Kaufman JL, Kacoyanis G, et al. Effect of aspirin and dipyridamole on the patency of lower extremity bypass grafts. Surgery 96:462-466, 1984.

57. Bousser MG, Eschwege E, Haguenau M, et al. "AICLA" controlled trial of aspirin and dipyridamole in the secondary prevention of athero-thrombotic cerebral ischemia. Stroke 14:5-14, 1983.

58. Elwood PC. British studies of aspirin and myocardial infarction. Am J Med 74:50-54, 1983.

59. Mustard JF, Kinlough-Rathbone RL, Packham MA. Aspirin in the treatment of cardiovascular disease: A review. Am J Med 74:43-49, 1983.

60. Kappa JR, Cottrell ED, Berkowitz HD, et al. Carotid endarterectomy in patients with heparin-induced platelet activation: Comparative efficacy of aspirin and iloprost (2K36374). J Vasc Surg 5:693-701, 1987.

61. Kappa JR, Fisher CA, Berkowitz HE, et al. Heparin-induced platelet activation in sixteen surgical patients: Diagnosis and management. J Vasc Surg 5:101-107, 1985.

62. Kraenzler EJ, Starr NJ. Heparin-associated thrombocytopenia: Management of patients for open heart surgery. Case reports describing the use of iloprost. Anesthesiology 69:964-967, 1988.

63. Fields WS. Aspirin for the prevention of stroke. Am J Med 74:61-65, 1983.

64. Fields WS, Lemah NA, Frankowski RF, et al. Controlled trial of aspirin in cerebral ischemia. Stroke 8:301-316, 1977.

65. Canadian Cooperative Study Group. A randomized trial of aspirin and sulfinpyrazone in threatened stroke. N Engl J Med 299:53-59, 1978.

66. Ramirez-Lassipas M. Platelet inhibitors for TIAs: A review of prospective drug trial results. Postgrad Med 75:52-62, 1984.

67. Sorensen PS, Pedersen H, Marquardsen J. Acetylsalicylic acid in the prevention of stroke in patients with reversible cerebral ischemic attacks. A Danish cooperative study. Stroke 14:15-22, 1983.

68. Steering Committee of the Physicians' Health Study Research Group. Final report of the aspirin component of the ongoing physicians' health study. N Engl J Med 321:129-135, 1989.

69. Green RM, Roedersheimer LR, DeWeese JA. Effects of aspirin and dipyridamole on expanded polytetrafluoroethylene graft patency. Surgery 92:1016-1026, 1982.

70. Lewis HD Jr, Davis JW, Archibald DG, et al. Protective effects of aspirin against acute myocardial infarction and death in men with unstable angina. N Engl J Med 309:396-403, 1983.

V Aortic Surgery

10

Gastrointestinal and Visceral Ischemic Complications of Aortic Reconstruction

David F.J. Tollefson   Calvin B. Ernst

The progressive decline of mortality and morbidity rates for abdominal aortic reconstruction has been achieved as a result of improvements in operative techniques and refinements in preoperative and postoperative care. Despite these advances gastrointestinal (GI) complications continue to occur. However, early identification of patients at high risk for GI complications and institution of preventive measures to preclude their development will minimize mortality and morbidity following such events. The purpose of this chapter is to provide guidelines for diagnosis and therapy of GI problems associated with aortic reconstruction and to offer principles for their prevention. These complications include intestinal ischemia, cholecystitis, pancreatitis, peptic ulcer disease, and problems concerning intra-abdominal malignancy.

INTESTINAL ISCHEMIA
Magnitude of the Problem

Intestinal ischemia following aortic reconstruction was first reported by Moore[1] in 1954 when a rectal stricture developed after ligation of the inferior mesenteric artery and both hypogastric arteries. Intestinal ischemia can follow abdominal aortic reconstruction for either aneurysmal or occlusive disease, with aneurysmal disease predominating.[2-9] Although intestinal ischemia reportedly has occurred after aortoiliac endarterectomy, it most commonly follows aortic replacement or bypass with prosthetic grafts.[2,8] Both small and large bowel ischemia may develop, but small bowel involvement is uncommon: the reported incidence is 0.15%.[6] The incidence of ischemic colitis, based largely on retrospective studies, has ranged from 0.2% to 10%; 2% is the commonly accepted frequency.[2-15]

In a prospective study in which colonoscopic examinations were performed following abdominal aortic reconstruction, the overall incidence of ischemic colitis was 6%, 4.3% for occlusive disease and 7.4% for aneurysmal disease.[4,5] Following repair of a ruptured abdominal aortic aneurysm, the incidence of ischemic colitis can be as high as 60%.

Morbidity and mortality rates parallel the

severity of bowel ischemia with mortalities of 50% to 90% for transmural involvement.* No deaths have been reported when the ischemia has been limited to the mucosa. Although death is rare with muscularis involvement, morbidity results from subsequent stricture formation. When small bowel ischemia occurs, usually it is so extensive that death is almost universal.[17]

Conservative estimates of the number of aortic reconstructions for aneurysmal disease performed in 1985 in the United States approached 33,000.[18] The number of other forms of aortic reconstruction totaled 41,000. Based on these estimates and an incidence of 2% to 6%, one can conclude that approximately 1500 to 4500 patients annually could develop clinical or subclinical ischemic colitis following aortic reconstruction. Thus prevention of this complication should decrease both morbidity and mortality following aortic reconstruction.

Anatomy

Intestinal ischemia is caused by a watershed perfusion phenomenon of the circulation to the colon. The superior mesenteric artery (SMA), inferior mesenteric artery (IMA), and hypogastric arteries and their respective branches supply the intestine (Fig. 10-1). The IMA arises from the left anterolateral aspect of the aorta; 3 to 4 cm from its aortic origin, it branches into the left colic, sigmoid, and superior rectal arteries and is the chief blood supply to the left colon. The marginal artery of Drummond, originally described by Von Haller in 1786, and the meandering mesenteric artery are connecting links between the SMA and IMA systems. However, Griffiths[19] and others[20] noted that in the area of the splenic flexure, the normal anastomosis of the left colic branch of the SMA and ascending branch of the left colic artery from the IMA—necessary to provide continuity of the marginal artery of Drummond—was lacking in 5% of individuals (Fig. 10-2). Griffiths[19] also noted an absence of the middle colic artery in 20% of the population, emphasizing the importance of both the right colic branch from the SMA and the hypogastric arteries when ligating the IMA. It has also been

*References 3, 6, 8, 9, 15, 16.

noted that the marginal artery of Drummond may be lacking in the region of the ascending colon in 5% of the population, in the area of the sigmoid colon in 20%, and even more frequently at the rectosigmoid junction.[21]

The meandering mesenteric artery, which is a large, continuous, and direct communication between the left branch of the middle colic artery (SMA circulation) and the left colic artery (IMA circulation), has also been termed the central anastomotic artery of the colon, the marginal artery, the mesomesenteric artery, the middle-left colic collateral, the artery of Drummond, the arch of Riolan, and the arch of Treves[22] (Fig. 10-3). This profusion of names has confused the literature regarding colon circulation. The preferred term for this important communication between the SMA and IMA circuits is the meandering mesenteric artery.[22] The meandering mesenteric artery is potentially present in about two thirds of the population

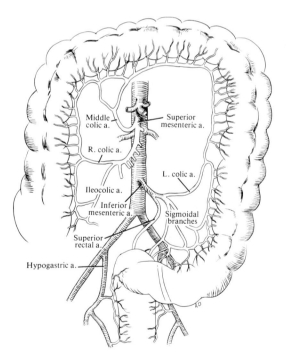

Fig. 10-1. Normal arterial circulation of colon and rectum. (From Ernst CB. Intestinal ischemia following abdominal aortic reconstruction. In Bernhard VM, Towne JB, eds. Complications in Vascular Surgery, 2nd ed. Philadelphia: WB Saunders, 1985.)

and has been identified on routine abdominal aortograms in 27% and 35% of patients with aneurysmal and occlusive diseases, respectively.[16]

The hypogastric circulation connects to the IMA system through the middle and inferior rectal branches by a superior rectal branch of the IMA. The major collateral circulation to the distal sigmoid colon and rectum is provided by these circuits. In 1907 Sudek[23] drew attention to what he believed was a critical point of blood supply between the last sigmoid artery and superior rectal artery in the collateral blood supply to the sigmoid colon. However, the studies of Griffiths[19] later pointed out that Sudek drew incorrect conclusions and that this

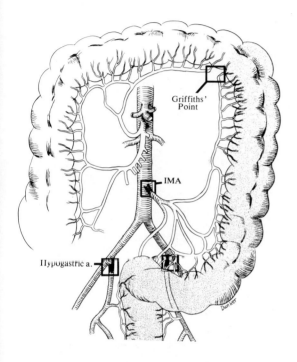

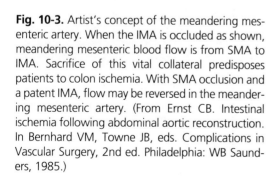

Fig. 10-2. Lack of marginal artery continuity at splenic flexure (Griffiths' point) along with inferior mesenteric and hypogastric arterial occlusion predispose patients to left colon ischemia. (From Ernst CB. Intestinal ischemia following abdominal aortic reconstruction. In Bernhard VM, Towne JB, eds. Complications in Vascular Surgery, 2nd ed. Philadelphia: WB Saunders, 1985.)

Fig. 10-3. Artist's concept of the meandering mesenteric artery. When the IMA is occluded as shown, meandering mesenteric blood flow is from SMA to IMA. Sacrifice of this vital collateral predisposes patients to colon ischemia. With SMA occlusion and a patent IMA, flow may be reversed in the meandering mesenteric artery. (From Ernst CB. Intestinal ischemia following abdominal aortic reconstruction. In Bernhard VM, Towne JB, eds. Complications in Vascular Surgery, 2nd ed. Philadelphia: WB Saunders, 1985.)

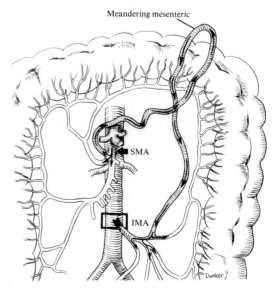

area actually was supplied quite well with collateral vessels.

SMA occlusion is compensated by collateral circulation from the celiac artery via pancreaticoduodenal arcades and by the meandering mesenteric artery from the IMA. Should the small bowel derive a significant amount of blood from the IMA via the meandering mesenteric artery, interruption of this vital collateral may cause gangrene of the entire midgut.[6,11,24-27] Additional SMA collateral circuits pass through the splenic and left colic arteries, iliolumbar artery, and superior and inferior epigastric arteries through the circumflex iliac and femoral arteries.

Detailed knowledge of the anatomic pathways of collateral circulation to the colon is required to preserve critical segments of blood supply to the colon. Clearly, preservation of as many collateral circuits as possible and restoration of blood flow to as many vital arterial branches as possible are important to prevent intestinal ischemia following aortic reconstructions.

Pathophysiology

Bowel ischemia following aortic construction almost always is caused by arterial compromise. Venous ischemic injury is rare.[8,28] Factors predisposing the patient to the development of ischemic colitis include improper IMA ligation, failure to restore IMA or hypogastric arterial blood flow, ruptured aneurysm with mesenteric compression, manipulative trauma to the colon by retractors, persistent hypotension and hypoperfusion, congenitally inadequate collateral communications between mesenteric circulations, and injury to major collateral vessels such as the meandering mesenteric artery. Superior mesenteric occlusion with abdominal angina may result in postoperative small bowel ischemia unless mesenteric arterial reconstruction is performed during aortic reconstruction. When the superior mesenteric and celiac arteries are occluded, compensatory meandering mesenteric blood flow is from the IMA system to the SMA system. Meandering mesenteric arterial injury under these conditions predisposes the patient to small bowel and colon ischemia.[24,25]

The clinical manifestations of colon ischemia are variable and relate to the degree of ischemia. Predisposing the colon to ischemia is its inherent low blood flow in addition to interruption of IMA blood flow. Most investigators agree that the large bowel has lower blood flow than other segments of the GI tract.[29-32]

Boley, Brandt, and Veith[33] have classified colon ischemia into three levels of involvement. In type I ischemia, injury is limited to the mucosa and is transient and reversible. Mucosal ischemia may lead to submucosal edema and hemorrhage. The mucosa becomes friable and an inflammatory reaction develops in response to the injury. Bacterial invasion of the colonic submucosa follows loss of the mucosal barrier. Mucosal slough with ulceration may follow, exposing the underlying mucosa or muscularis. Such changes are transient and reversible and typically proceed to heal in days to weeks with no residual sequelae. Type II ischemic injury penetrates deeper to involve the muscularis. It usually heals satisfactorily but there may be residual stricture formation, depending on the severity of the ischemic insult (Fig. 10-4). Type III ischemic injury is transmural, with the de-

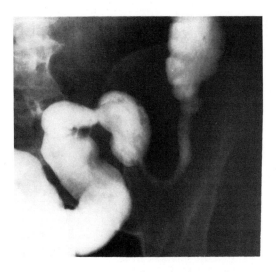

Fig. 10-4. Barium enema documenting a stricture at the junction of the descending colon and sigmoid colon following an acute episode of ischemic colitis. (From Ernst CB. Intestinal ischemia following abdominal aortic reconstruction. In Bernhard VM, Towne JB, eds. Complications in Vascular Surgery, 2nd ed. Philadelphia: WB Saunders, 1985.)

velopment of gangrene. With type III injury profound physiologic changes develop as reflected by acidosis, sepsis, and cardiovascular collapse. Generalized feculent peritonitis may occur or a delayed fecal fistula may develop.

Most reports, retrospective in nature, suggest that type III ischemic injury occurs in 60% of cases and types I and II each occur in 20%. However, this may reflect overlooked instances of milder injuries wherein symptoms are obscured in the postoperative period.

Classification of bowel ischemia following aortic reconstruction relates to the type of aortic operation performed (aneurysm repair, aortofemoral bypass, or aortoiliac endarterectomy), segment of intestine involved (left colon, rectum, or small bowel), and thickness of bowel wall compromised (mucosa, mucosa and muscularis, or transmural). The most common intestinal ischemia following aortic reconstruction is type I involving the left colon after abdominal aortic aneurysmectomy with IMA ligation.*

Clinical Manifestations and Diagnosis

Clinical manifestations vary depending on the degree of bowel ischemia. Some cases of minor degrees of ischemia probably go unrecognized and the patients recover uneventfully.[8,13,16,34] However, some minor and all major degrees of ischemia produce symptoms, but these may be masked, confused, and complicated by the systemic responses and altered abdominal findings that normally occur after a major abdominal operation.

Diarrhea, with or without blood, is the most common symptom of ischemic colitis. Although diarrhea may occur as long as 14 days after operation, it occurs within 24 to 48 hours of aortic reconstruction in 75% of patients with ischemic colitis.[†] Some investigators have reported bloody diarrhea to be a more ominous prognostic sign than nonbloody diarrhea; others find no correlation.[8,34] Nevertheless, bloody diarrhea should alert the surgeon to perform immediate flexible colonoscopy.

Other symptoms include extraordinary postoperative pain, especially in the left abdomen,

progressive abdominal distention not relieved by gastric decompression, and signs of peritoneal irritation. Signs of sepsis such as unexplained leukocytosis in the range of 20,000 to 30,000 mm³, severe or refractory acidosis, progressive oliguria, and elevated temperatures should alert the surgeon to colon ischemia, usually severe. Severe thrombocytopenia, less than 90,000 platelets /mm³, has been suggested as a marker of bowel necrosis and should also arouse suspicion of ischemic colitis.[38]

A high index of suspicion and liberal use of flexible colonoscopy are essential to make an early diagnosis. The reported high mortality rates from ischemic colitis suggest that the delay in diagnosis may preclude effective therapy.[6] Ottinger et al.[8] noted that among 13 patients suffering from transmural ischemic colitis, the diagnosis was made from 6 to 13 days following aortic reconstruction.

Flexible sigmoidoscopy, performed at the bedside, is essential to detect early ischemic involvement.* Early changes include circumferential petechial hemorrhages and edema. Advanced lesions will exhibit pseudomembranes, erosions, and ulcers. Transmural involvement is suggested by a yellowish green necrotic noncontractile surface. Flexible sigmoidoscopy needs to be performed only to 40 cm or until the first lesion is noted. It is unusual to have more proximal colonic involvement without distal colitis unless rare focal lesions develop in the splenic flexure or transverse colon.[5]

Early recognition requires flexible sigmoidoscopy within 48 hours of aortic reconstruction. Although identification of ischemic colitis can be made on a single examination, the extent and clinical course require repeated examinations by the same examiner to determine resolution or progression of the ischemic process.[4] When ischemic colitis is identified, the endoscopic study should be terminated. Passage of the endoscope beyond the involved bowel segment should be avoided lest perforation occur.

Although barium contrast studies are helpful in diagnosing late sequelae of ischemic colitis, they are not indicated in the immediate postop-

---

*References 2, 3, 6, 8-11, 13, 15, 19, 34-36.
†References 6, 8-10, 13, 15, 34, 37.

*References 4, 5, 9, 10, 16, 37, 39.

erative period. The inability of barium contrast studies to identify early ischemic changes and the hazards of barium peritonitis preclude their use. Likewise, arteriography has no role in the diagnosis of ischemic colitis following aortic reconstruction since it can provide only indirect evidence of ischemic colitis by the presence or absence of collateral circulation.

The keys to early diagnosis of intestinal ischemia are a high degree of awareness of the possibility of ischemic colitis and early diagnostic flexible sigmoidoscopy in persons who are at high risk.

Medical Treatment

Treatment is dictated by the clinical situation. Nonoperative therapy is preferred in early mild ischemic colitis. Optimal fluid and electrolyte balance is obtained and broad-spectrum antibiotic therapy is instituted and continued until the ischemic process resolves. Progression of the ischemia documented by deteriorating clinical signs, worsening of symptoms, and advancing endoscopic findings requires prompt operative intervention. Increasing abdominal tenderness, fever and leukocytosis, and worsening diarrhea that may evolve from nonbloody to bloody all suggest progression. Diarrhea persisting for more than 2 weeks probably reflects a walled-off perforation with local peritonitis.

Conversely, resolution suggested by subsidence of diarrhea, improvement in vital signs and laboratory parameters, and endoscopic resolution of the ischemic process justifies continued nonoperative therapy. Bowel rest with GI decompression by nasogastric intubation along with hyperalimentation supplying needed nutrition are important components of therapy.

Reversible lesions generally improve within 7 to 10 days. Late ischemic stricture is treated nonoperatively unless clinically significant.

Operative Treatment

Prompt operative intervention is required for transmural bowel involvement with or without peritonitis. Fluid and electrolyte abnormalities should be corrected as quickly as possible with the aid of a central venous line and Swan-Ganz catheter monitoring. Nonviable bowel should be resected by colostomy and either Hartmann's pouch or mucous fistula construction. Primary bowel anastomosis is contraindicated. The aortic graft must be protected from contamination by appropriate packing that isolates it from the operative field.

Rectal necrosis requires removal of the rectum with perineal drainage, but wide excision of the rectal segment is not necessary. Removal of only the necrotic muscle and mucosa may be all that is necessary to achieve pelvic débridement. During reperitonealization of the pelvic floor, the area of prosthesis must be isolated. An omental graft sutured into the pelvis may be required to achieve this isolation.

Prevention

Prevention of intestinal ischemia is more successful in minimizing mortality and morbidity than in treating clinically manifest cases. Mortality from all forms of ischemic colitis averages 40%. Morbidity from prolonged hospitalization following an acute event and late stricture of bowel segments with chronic diarrhea may be disabling. The complicated and lengthy postoperative course of transmural colitis in patients who survive with a colostomy, which often is permanent, adds further morbidity from this preventable complication.

Prevention requires identification of individuals who are at risk for development of ischemic colitis by appropriate preoperative and operative assessments. Prophylactic and therapeutic maneuvers may then be taken to minimize the risk of development of bowel ischemia.

Clinical findings that identify persons at risk for colon ischemia following aortic reconstruction include the symptoms of intestinal angina. In these persons SMA and celiac occlusive disease may be present and the meandering mesenteric artery may supply the entire gut. Likewise, patients with a ruptured abdominal aortic aneurysm have an increased risk of developing postoperative intestinal ischemia.[5]

Preoperative aortography has proved useful in identifying patients at risk for developing intestinal ischemia.* Although preoperative aortography is universally accepted for the

---

*References 2, 4, 6, 16, 24, 40, 41.

management of aortoiliac occlusive disease, its use in management of aneurysmal disease remains controversial. Nonetheless, valuable information concerning gut blood supply and collateral circulation is obtained.[40] Arteriographic documentation of a meandering mesenteric artery signifies SMA or IMA atherosclerosis.[4,6] Opacification of the IMA from the SMA via the meandering mesenteric artery is predictive of minimal risk of ischemic colitis following aortic reconstruction[4] (Fig. 10-5). Conversely, documentation of reversal of blood flow in the meandering mesenteric artery, from the IMA to the SMA, on serial radiographs demands lateral filming following a second contrast injection to document SMA ostial disease. Under these circumstances SMA or IMA reconstruction or both are required to prevent catastrophic postoperative small bowel ischemia.[6,24] If a large IMA or IMA-to-SMA meandering mesenteric blood flow is documented by preoperative aortography in patients with occlusive disease, an end-to-side aortic anastomosis, preserving IMA blood flow, may be preferred over an end-to-end anastomosis.[42] Such reconstruction is preferred particularly if it appears by means of preoperative aortographic study that retrograde femoro-ilio-aorto–inferior mesenteric blood flow is not likely.

Documentation of presence or absence of hypogastric artery patency by aortography has proved useful in preserving or restoring pelvic blood flow. When the IMA is ligated, the hypogastric arteries assume importance in providing collateral circulation to the rectum. In almost 90% of patients with aneurysmal disease and 70% with occlusive disease, preoperative hypogastric opacification has been noted on aortographic studies.[4]

Bowel Preparation and Protection

Comparison of the course of intestinal infarction in the fetus with that of intestinal infarction after birth suggests that intestinal flora play an adverse role in the latter. In utero, full-thickness infarction of sterile intestine does not lead to perforation, whereas full-thickness infarction in the adult does. This is particularly true of the bacterial-laden colon. Prophylactic antibiotic bowel preparation has been suggested as an adjunct to reduce the incidence of infarction.[2,9-11,32] Whereas bowel sterilization reduces the incidence of gut infarction in laboratory animals, its efficacy in humans requires documentation. Although preoperative antibiotic bowel preparation may be controversial, mechanical bowel preparation with enemas and cathartics may be helpful not only to decrease intestinal flora, but also to avoid problems of retracting and packing the fecal-laden colon during operation. Systemic antibiotics, which are used prophylactically by all vascular surgeons when implanting prostheses, may afford some protection in preventing ischemic colitis or blunting its clinical severity.

Prevention of bowel distention by nasogastric GI decompression before, during, and after aortic reconstruction may influence development of ischemic colitis. Increases in intraluminal pressure may cause decreased nutrient blood flow and measures to avoid colonic distention may be beneficial.

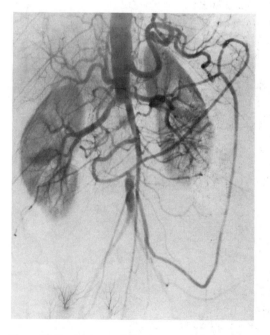

Fig. 10-5. Aortographic demonstration of the meandering mesenteric artery. Flow is from SMA to IMA.

Technical Maneuvers

Strict attention to operative technical details is mandatory to avoid the development of ischemic colitis after aortic reconstruction. Gentle technique is essential. Dislodging of debris from the aorta can lead to embolization of such material to peripheral vessels or the hypogastric and IMA circuits, resulting in colon ischemia.[15,37] Just as such embolic debris to the legs has been termed "trash foot," "trash colon" similarly follows manipulative trauma of the abdominal aorta. Likewise, trauma from overly vigorous retraction may occlude mesenteric collateral channels, particularly in the left colon mesentery and mesosigmoid. The mesenteric hematoma from a ruptured aneurysm should not be evacuated lest vital collateral channels be damaged. Administration of heparin sodium during elective aortic reconstruction, although not primarily used for preservation of colon collateral blood flow, may be helpful in maintaining critical collateral circulation during required packing and retraction of abdominal viscera.

Common to all instances of ischemic colitis following aortic aneurysmectomy is ligation of the IMA. The IMA bifurcates 3 to 4 cm from its aortic origin into ascending and descending branches, and improper ligation can injure these collateral vessels. Occasionally, when the IMA is not dissected to its aortic origin, one of its ascending or descending branches may be mistaken for the main IMA and ligated, thereby interrupting the ascending-descending collateral pathway (Fig. 10-6). Such collateral branches are particularly vulnerable during the management of large aneurysms when one of the IMA branches, draped over the aneurysm, is mistaken for the main IMA. Consequently, control of IMA back-bleeding is best achieved by oversewing the IMA ostium from inside the aneurysmal sac.

Restoration of blood flow to the IMA should prevent the development of bowel ischemia. Although a patent IMA could be reconstructed in all aortic operations, this policy would unnecessarily prolong and complicate most procedures. Therefore selective IMA reconstruction seems appropriate. To determine the need for reimplantation of the IMA or the time when it may be safely ligated, two techniques have been commonly used. Doppler ultrasound is used to confirm arterial flow in the IMA, in the bowel mesentery, and on the surface of the left colon before and after IMA occlusion[42-44] (Fig. 10-7). The other technique uses measurement of IMA stump pressure as an index for safe ligation of the IMA during aortic aneurysmal repair[3,16] (Fig. 10-8).

Hobson and associates[42,43] concluded that the presence of audible Doppler flow signals over the base of the mesentery and surface of the colon may correlate with bowel viability. In their studies clinically manifest ischemic colitis did not develop, but since routine postoperative colonoscopy was not performed, the incidence of subclinical ischemic colitis was not determined. Nonetheless, it was concluded that the

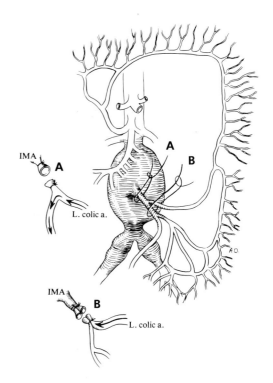

Fig. 10-6. A, Correct method of IMA ligation, which preserves continuity of the ascending and descending branches. **B,** Incorrect ligation of IMA interrupts continuity of the ascending and descending branches and predisposes patients to colon ischemia. (From Ernst CB. Intestinal ischemia following abdominal aortic reconstruction. In Bernhard VM, Towne JB, eds. Complications in Vascular Surgery, 2nd ed. Philadelphia: WB Saunders, 1985.)

presence of arterial flow, determined by Doppler insonation along the left colon, confirmed the presence of collateral flow; absence of flow during temporary IMA occlusion suggested potential colon ischemia. However, because control data were not obtained, the need for IMA reconstruction when Doppler signals are lost can only be implied.

The need for objectively determining when the IMA may be safely ligated after abdominal aortic aneurysmectomy led to the development and description of the technique of IMA stump pressure measurement.[16] Since both prereconstruction (before interrupting aortic flow) and postreconstruction IMA stump pressure data were gathered for evaluation during the original study, the IMA had to be divided to be cannulated with the 18-gauge Teflon catheter attached to a pressure transducer. At the present time, only postreconstruction measurements are obtained. Thus, division of the IMA is no longer required and its orifice is cannulated through the opened aneurysm sac (Fig. 10-8).[3] Of 64 patients, all of whom underwent postoperative colonoscopy, there were three in whom pelvic blood flow could not be restored. In two, the IMA stump mean blood pressure measured more than 40 mm Hg and the IMA

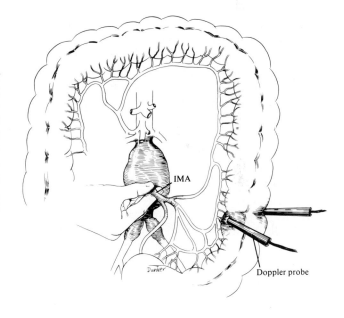

Fig. 10-7. Application of sterile Doppler probe to antimesenteric and mesenteric borders of left colon during digital compression of the IMA documents the presence or absence of collateral blood flow. Vascular clamp or torceps also may be used to occlude the IMA origin. (From Ernst CB. Intestinal ischemia following abdominal aortic reconstruction. In Bernhard VM, Towne JB, eds. Complications in Vascular Surgery, 2nd ed. Philadelphia: WB Saunders, 1985.)

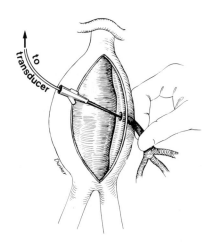

Fig. 10-8. Method of IMA stump blood pressure measurement. The cannula is threaded into the IMA orifice through the opened aneurysm sac and is secured by compression of the IMA and adjacent mesentery between thumb and forefinger. (From Ernst CB. Prevention of intestinal ischemia following abdominal aortic reconstruction. Surgery 93:104, 1983.)

was ligated. Ischemic colitis developed in neither patient. In the other patient, IMA mean blood pressure was less than 40 mm Hg; IMA reconstruction was not performed and postoperative ischemic colitis occurred. In two additional patients, postreconstruction IMA stump mean blood pressure measured less than 40 mm Hg. In one, IMA reconstruction was not performed and ischemic colitis developed. In the other, the IMA was implanted into the prosthesis and postoperative ischemic colitis did not develop.

Since ischemic colitis is an unusual complication, acquisition of objective data by a prospective randomized study to determine statistical significance would seem to be beyond practicality. Nonetheless, it appears that if IMA stump mean blood pressure measures more than 40 mm Hg, the IMA orifice may be oversewn from within the aneurysm sac or ligated with impunity. Conversely, if the mean stump pressure is less than 40 mm Hg, the IMA should be reconstructed. However, reliance on IMA stump pressure measurements assumes that systemic blood pressure and regional perfusion are maintained during the postoperative period at least at the same levels as when operative measurements were taken.

The use of IMA stump pressure measurements to determine bowel viability may offer advantages over the hearing of Doppler flow signals because Doppler-audible flow may be present even though perfusion pressure, less than the critical closing pressure of the nutrient bed vessels, is low. Critical closing pressure is approximately 40 mm Hg.[45] A false sense of security may accompany the hearing of Doppler flow signals if the perfusion pressure is less than 40 mm Hg. However, complete cessation of flow appears to be a discriminatory endpoint with Doppler evaluation.

It must be recognized that the IMA stump blood pressure technique may not be applicable when aortoiliac occlusive disease is being managed since the IMA orifice is not available for cannulation as it is when aneurysmal disease is being treated. Under these circumstances Doppler evaluation is suggested.

Recently two additional methods for predicting colon viability have been described and include measurement of colonic intramural pH by silicone balloon tonometry and operative photoplethysmography combined with transcolonic oxygen saturation measurements.[46,47]

Measurement of colon pH is performed by the placement of a gas-permeable silicone balloon into the sigmoid colon. This tonometer measures colonic intramural pH indirectly. Saline solution injected into the gas-permeable silicone balloon equilibrates with the P_{CO_2} of the mucosa of the sigmoid colon. The simultaneous measurement of the P_{CO_2} in the balloon saline solution and HCO_3 in arterial blood allows one to determine the pH of the mucosa of the sigmoid colon using the Henderson-Hasselbalch equation. Preliminary studies suggest that a pH below 6.86 may be indicative of colon ischemia.[47]

Loss of arterial pulsations measured by the pulse oximeter probe along with unmeasurable transcolonic oxygen saturations also suggests colonic ischemia.[46]

It is clear that there is a set of circumstances that places a patient at greater or lower risk for postoperative ischemic colitis (see box). Patients who are at greatest risk for postoperative ischemic colitis include those with preoperative symptoms of visceral ischemia. Likewise, if the

---

RISK PREDICTION FOR ISCHEMIC BOWEL FOLLOWING ABDOMINAL AORTIC RECONSTRUCTION

Greatest risk

Symptoms of visceral ischemia
Aortic aneurysm (ruptured)
Patent IMA
Operative Doppler flow absent
IMA stump pressure less than 40 mm Hg
IMA-to-SMA flow in meandering mesenteric
  artery

Least risk

Thrombosed IMA
SMA-to-IMA flow in meandering mesenteric
  artery
Operative Doppler flow present
IMA stump pressure greater than 40 mm Hg
Reconstruction for occlusive disease

IMA is patent and flow in the meandering mesenteric artery is from the IMA to SMA, there is also an increased risk. An absence of operative Doppler flow or an IMA stump pressure of less than 40 mm Hg also places the patient at greater risk, as does treatment for a ruptured abdominal aortic aneurysm.

Conversely, patients at the least risk for postoperative ischemic colitis include those with a thrombosed IMA or those with SMA-to-IMA flow in the meandering mesenteric artery. Likewise, the presence of operative Doppler flow, IMA stump pressure greater than 40 mm Hg, or reconstruction for occlusive disease places the patient at a lower risk for ischemic colitis.

MESENTERIC ARTERIAL RECONSTRUCTIVE TECHNIQUES

Colonic circulation relying on collateral blood flow following IMA ligation may be more susceptible to hypotension and hypoperfusion than when the IMA is intact. Therefore, hypotension and hypoperfusion must be avoided by the proper administration of blood and crystalloid. It has been documented that intact collateral circuits maintain IMA blood pressure near preligation levels.[16] Likewise, preservation of vital collateral circulation by restoring pulsatile blood flow to one or both hypogastric arteries is recommended to avoid or minimize development of ischemic colitis and proctitis.[10,15,16,48] Retrograde perfusion of at least one internal iliac artery may be accomplished in more than 90% of patients.[16] Following aneurysmectomy, hypogastric perfusion is usually maintained because distal anastomoses are to the aorta or the common iliac arteries. When aneurysmal disease of the common iliac arteries precludes common iliac anastomoses, end-to-side distal anastomoses to the external iliac arteries may be used. The common iliac vessels are stapled and retrograde internal iliac perfusion is maintained. If hypogastric blood flow cannot be restored without resorting to complex reconstructive techniques, IMA stump pressure measurements may document when hypogastric reconstruction is not required.[16]

When IMA reconstruction is required, several techniques are possible. The IMA origin as an excised button from the host aorta may be anastomosed onto the side of the body of the aortic prosthesis.* This technique uses the terminolateral principle originally described by Carrel[52] in 1912 (Fig. 10-9). Alternative techniques include reimplantation of the IMA without an aortic button and interposition grafts from the prosthesis to the end of the IMA (Fig. 10-10). Reimplantation of a small IMA (less than 3 mm in diameter) into the prosthesis may prove difficult. Under such circumstances interposition grafting may be required. Both autogenous saphenous vein and prosthetic limbs attached to the graft are acceptable as interposition grafts. Saphenous vein, because of its pliability, facilitates precise suturing and is preferred. Both distal and proximal ends of the vein must be spatulated to provide patulous

---

*References 6, 8, 26, 42, 49-51.

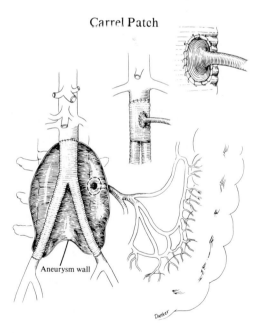

Carrel Patch

Aneurysm wall

Dunker

Fig. 10-9. Carrel patch technique of IMA reconstruction. Excision of the button of aneurysm wall surrounding the IMA orifice facilitates repair. (From Ernst CB. Intestinal ischemia following abdominal aortic reconstruction. In Bernhard VM, Towne JB, eds. Complications in Vascular Surgery, 2nd ed. Philadelphia: WB Saunders, 1985.)

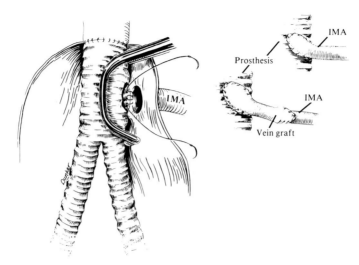

Fig. 10-10. Reconstruction of the IMA by anastomosing a rim of aneurysmal sac, including the IMA orifice, to the prosthesis. Reconstruction is accomplished with autogenous saphenous vein graft. The large IMA is implanted into the side of the prosthesis. A button of the prosthesis must be excised to ensure patulous anastomoses. (From Ernst CB. Postoperative intestinal ischemia. In Haimovici H, ed. Vascular Emergencies. East Norwalk, Conn.: Appleton-Century-Crofts, 1982, p 511.)

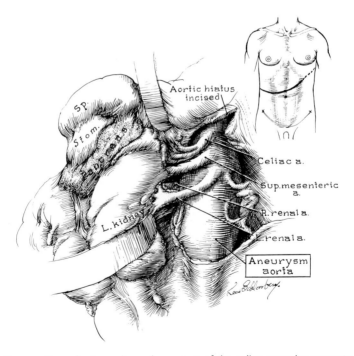

Fig. 10-11. Transperitoneal-retroperitoneal exposure of the celiac, superior mesenteric, and left renal arterial origins. Descending colon, spleen, stomach, pancreas, and kidney are mobilized to the right. Incision of median arcuate ligament and diaphragmatic crura opens the aortic hiatus and facilitates proximal exposure for concomitant SMA reconstruction. (From Ernst CB. Exposure of inaccessible arteries. Part II. Abdomen and leg exposure. Surgical Rounds 8:28, 1985.)

anastomoses to the prosthesis and the IMA. An alternative to anastomosis of the divided IMA to the prosthesis is anastomosis of a portion of the aneurysmal sac, including the rim of the IMA orifice, to the prosthesis; this is the inclusion technique popularized by Crawford (Fig. 10-10).

Techniques to reconstruct the SMA include endarterectomy and aortomesenteric bypass. Because the origin of the SMA is obscured by the pancreas, SMA endarterectomy may prove challenging through the usual transabdominal approach used for aortic reconstruction. The retroperitoneal approach for aortic reconstruction may facilitate SMA reconstruction when such reconstruction is anticipated from preoperative arteriographic studies. However, the retroperitoneal approach precludes thorough examination of the bowel. Under such circum-

stances, the transperitoneal-retroperitoneal approach may prove useful[53] (Fig. 10-11).

The preferred method of small bowel revascularization is autogenous saphenous vein–aorto-SMA bypass (Fig. 10-12). The aortic end of the vein graft is anastomosed to the left anterolateral aspect of the prosthesis. The vein graft assumes a reversed C configuration in the retroperitoneum after it is anastomosed to the SMA. A short, straight transperitoneal graft from the anterior aspect of the aortic prosthesis is not recommended because such a graft configuration may kink after the viscera are replaced into the abdomen.

INTRA-ABDOMINAL DISEASES COMPLICATING AORTIC RECONSTRUCTION

Although nonvascular procedures have occasionally been performed with aortic reconstruction, contemporary standards dictate a conservative approach and most surgeons are reluctant to perform other intra-abdominal procedures that may increase the risk of aortic graft contamination.[54] Nonetheless, Ochsner, Cooley, and DeBakey[55] reported in 1960 that 69% of 931 patients undergoing abdominal aortic aneurysmectomy underwent an associated abdominal or pelvic operation. These associated procedures included appendectomy, which accounted for the majority, cholecystectomy, and partial colon or gastric resections. However, because of anecdotal reports recounting catastrophic infectious complications following concomitant procedures, simultaneous management of intra-abdominal lesions requires a thorough knowledge of the natural history of the associated disease to balance the risk of performing simultaneous intra-abdominal procedures against the risk of aortic reconstruction alone.

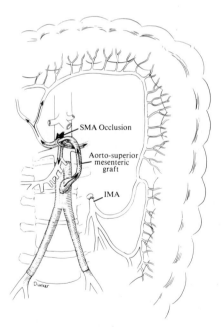

Fig. 10-12. Autogenous saphenous vein–aorto-SMA reconstruction. The vein graft lies in retroperitoneal position, assuming a gentle reversed "C" configuration. Spatulation of the ends of the graft ensures patulous anastomoses. A button of prosthesis must be excised. (From Ernst CB. Postoperative intestinal ischemia. In Haimovici H, ed. Vascular Emergencies. East Norwalk, Conn.: Appleton-Century-Crofts, 1982, p 501.)

Biliary Tract Disease

The natural history of cholelithiasis has been documented by several reports.[56-60] Comfort, Gray, and Wilson[56] noted development of biliary symptoms among 50% of patients initially found to have asymptomatic gallstones. Wenckert and Robertson[60] followed up 781 patients with known cholelithiasis for up to 11 years. In

35% of patients, symptoms or complications of the gallstones developed over the 11-year follow-up interval. In 1960 Lund[58] reported a 70% incidence of complicated biliary tract disease developing among asymptomatic patients when followed up for as long as 20 years. In contrast to these reports, recent studies document a low incidence of complicated biliary tract disease among patients with asymptomatic cholelithiasis. Gracie and Ransohoff[57] reported that biliary symptoms developed in only 15% of asymptomatic patients followed up for 10 years. Similarly, McSherry et al.[59] noted a low complication rate of 10.4% in 135 asymptomatic patients followed up over a 49-month interval. Of these patients, only 7.4% required operative intervention.

Biliary tract disease complicates aortic reconstruction only occasionally. The incidence of cholecystitis following aortic reconstruction is variable and it often develops without gallstones. Devine, Farnell, and Mucha[61] reported a frequency of postoperative cholecystitis of 1.2 episodes/10,000 operations following trauma or any operative procedure. Acalculous cholecystitis accounted for 25% of cases. Ottinger[62] noted that 35% of postoperative cholecystitis cases were caused by acalculous disease and 81% of his patients with postoperative cholecystitis had no preoperative symptoms of biliary tract disease.

Ouriel et al.[63] recorded a 1% incidence of cholecystitis following aortic aneurysm repair. In three fourths of patients, acalculous cholecystitis was found. The 50% mortality they reported confirmed other reports of postoperative cholecystitis. Fry and Fry[64] reported three patients in whom biliary symptoms developed after aortic reconstruction for occlusive disease. Two had acalculous cholecystitis and the third had no evidence of biliary disease at reoperation. Therefore it appears that prediction of postoperative cholecystitis, based on the presence of gallstones, is difficult since most episodes of postoperative cholecystitis are acalculous.

The need to perform concomitant cholecystectomy and aortic reconstruction mandates that both diseases require correction at one operation and that to defer correction of either problem would be detrimental. However, natural history data of asymptomatic cholelithiasis suggest that most patients will not require cholecystectomy. Furthermore, the incidence of postoperative cholecystitis is very low and when it does occur, more often than not, it is acalculous.

Reports of concomitant cholecystectomy and aortic reconstruction rarely include the duration of follow-up and are anecdotal.[55,65,66] To justify cholecystectomy during aortic reconstruction on the basis of such reports seems unwarranted, particularly when one considers that the risk of contamination of the aortic prosthesis is real. The frequency of positive bile cultures during cholecystectomy ranges from 15% to 61%.[61,63] Ouriel et al.[66] noted that a graft infection developed in one of 18 patients (5.5%) after aortic resection and cholecystectomy. Becker and Blundell,[67] reporting on 14 infected aortic grafts, suggested that concomitant cholecystectomy contributed to two of these infections. Bickerstaff et al.[68] have reported an increase in complications when cholecystectomy was performed with aortic reconstruction, but their data were not statistically significant because of the small number of patients.

Based on the low incidence of postoperative cholecystitis, the natural history of asymptomatic gallstones, the high frequency of acalculous cholecystitis, and the limited number of reports available from which to draw objective conclusions, the following guidelines are suggested:

1. Prophylactic cholecystectomy during aortic reconstruction is not recommended.

2. When unsuspected acute cholecystitis is encountered during aortic reconstruction, cholecystectomy should be performed and aortic reconstruction deferred.

3. If both a symptomatic or large aneurysm and acute cholecystitis are encountered, aortic reconstruction should be performed, followed by cholecystectomy after secure closure of the retroperitoneum. However, if the aneurysm is small (less than 6 cm) and asymptomatic, aortic reconstruction should follow cholecystectomy by several weeks.

Pancreatitis

Pancreatitis following abdominal aortic reconstruction is unusual. Most reported episodes have followed repair of ruptured abdominal aortic aneurysms complicated by large retroperitoneal hematomas, vigorous retraction or dissection of the pancreas, and hypotension and hypoperfusion.[69-71] Along with severe upper abdominal tenderness, shoulder pain, extraordinary requirements for postoperative intravenous crystalloid and colloid administration, and a markedly elevated white blood cell count, pancreatitis also can present as a prolonged gastroduodenal ileus or duodenal obstruction.[69] The lethality of postoperative pancreatitis following any intra-abdominal or extra-abdominal operative procedure has been adequately documented. Consequently, vigorous and aggressive therapy is required using nasogastric decompression, fluid replacement, antibiotic therapy, and long-term nutritional support, often with parenteral nutrition methods.

Except for previous episodes of pancreatitis secondary to biliary tract disease or chronic alcoholism, there are no predictors for the development of pancreatitis following abdominal aortic reconstruction; as a consequence, prevention of this complication may prove difficult.

Peptic Ulcer Disease

With the advent of histamine H_2 receptor antagonists in 1977, there has been a steady decline in the frequency of operation for peptic ulcer disease.[72] Before widespread use of effective acid inhibition therapy, Bouhoutsos, Barabas, and Martin[73] reported 51 consecutive patients undergoing abdominal aortic aneurysm repairs, 12 of whom had peptic ulcers. Perforation or bleeding of the ulcer developed in 7 of these 12 in the immediate postoperative period. Eight of the 51 patients died and complications from peptic ulcer disease accounted for five of the deaths. On the basis of this experience, it was recommended that in persons with both an aortic aneurysm and peptic ulcer, concomitant aortic reconstruction, vagotomy, and pyloroplasty should be performed. However, contemporary experience suggests that for most elective aortic reconstructions, thorough preoperative assessment will identify patients with peptic ulcer disease and allow successful medical therapy before aortic repair. Even following emergent aortic reconstruction, bleeding caused by stress ulceration or peptic ulcer disease can be controlled with H_2 blocking agents and antacids.[74] Acute gastric outlet obstruction caused by peptic ulcer disease is best managed with nasogastric decompression. Parenteral hyperalimentation and antacid therapy usually provide short-term resolution during which time elective aortic reconstruction may be performed. Patients who do not respond to conservative therapy may be treated surgically before aortic reconstruction. If aortic reconstruction is emergent or urgent, vagotomy and pyloroplasty may be performed after the aortic graft has been protected by reperitonealization.

Malignant Disease

Despite the prevalence of malignant intra-abdominal disease in the elderly, the frequency with which it is encountered among patients with aortic aneurysms is surprisingly low. In a 1967 report from the Henry Ford Hospital, only 31 of 803 patients (3.8%) were found to have coincidental intra-abdominal malignancies during aortic aneurysm repair.[75] When a coincidental malignant lesion, most commonly involving the colon, is encountered in patients with abdominal aortic aneurysmal disease, the lesion that has the greatest potential for causing death assumes the highest priority for treatment. This is usually the aneurysm.

Concern has been expressed that if the malignant lesion is treated first, the aneurysm may rupture while the patient is convalescing from the operation for the malignancy. It has been suggested that celiotomy may be a factor in precipitating aneurysm rupture by activation of the collagenolytic system.[76,77] Szilagyi, Elliott, and Berguer[75] noted that of 12 patients with known abdominal aortic aneurysms and coincidental malignancies who did not undergo treatment for the abdominal aortic aneurysm, five died from rupture of the aneurysm. In addition, Nora et al.[78] reported 17 patients who had abdominal aortic aneurysms and intra-abdominal malignancies. Of eight patients who underwent only resection of the cancer, three died from complications of the abdominal aortic aneurysm (two ruptured and one thrombosed). Therefore, although supported only by anecdotal data, it appears that other intra-abdominal operations may precipitate aneurysmal rupture.

Simultaneous repair of a GI neoplasm and abdominal aortic aneurysm is not recommended. The potential for prosthetic contamination under such circumstances precludes such operations. If possible, treatment should be staged, with the lethal lesion—namely, the abdominal aortic aneurysm—taking precedence. However, if the bowel malignancy is obstructing or bleeding, it must be managed first. Unless there are compelling indications such as obstruction or bleeding, the GI malignancy can be successfully treated within 6 to 8 weeks of aneurysm repair without compromising patient survival. Among patients with proved metastatic intra-abdominal disease, aneurysm repair is indicated only if the aneurysm is symptomatic or ruptured.

Other Inflammatory Lesions

When acute inflammatory processes such as diverticulitis or appendicitis are encountered during celiotomy for aortic reconstruction, the inflammatory process should be treated first to resolve the infectious process and minimize the potential for contamination of the prosthesis. Aneurysm repair then follows several weeks later. In the unlikely event that an acute purulent process is encountered along with a ruptured abdominal aortic aneurysm, there is no alternative but to treat both at the same time, making efforts to minimize contamination. The inflammatory lesion should be treated after securely closing the retroperitoneum over the aortic graft. Ligation of the infrarenal aorta followed by axillofemoral bypass after the management of the purulent process is an option, but only when there is a strong likelihood of aortic graft contamination and if the patient's condition does not preclude extending the operating time required for immediate extra-anatomic reconstruction.

REFERENCES

1. Moore SW. Resection of the abdominal aorta with defect replaced by homologous graft. Surg Gynecol Obstet 99:745, 1954.
2. Birnbaum W, Rudy L, Wylie EJ. Colonic and rectal ischemia following abdominal aneurysmectomy. Dis Colon Rectum 7:293, 1964.
3. Ernst CB. Prevention of intestinal ischemia following abdominal aortic reconstruction. Surgery 93:102, 1983.
4. Ernst CB, Hagihara PF, Daugherty ME, et al. Ischemic colitis incidence following abdominal aortic reconstruction: A prospective study. Surgery 80:417, 1976.
5. Hagihara PF, Ernst CB, Griffen WO Jr. Incidence of ischemic colitis following abdominal aortic reconstruction. Surg Gynecol Obstet 149:571, 1979.
6. Johnson WC, Nabseth DC. Visceral infarction following aortic surgery. Ann Surg 180:312, 1974.
7. Miller RE, Know WG. Colon ischemia following infrarenal aorta surgery: Report of four cases. Ann Surg 163:639, 1966.
8. Ottinger LW, Darling RC, Nathan MJ, et al. Left colon ischemia complicating aorto-iliac reconstruction. Arch Surg 105:481, 1972.
9. Young JR, Humphries AW, deWolfe VG, et al. Complications of aortic surgery. Part II: Intestinal ischemia. Arch Surg 86:85, 1963.
10. Bernatz PE. Necrosis of the colon following resection for abdominal aortic aneurysms. Arch Surg 81:373, 1960.
11. Bernstein WC, Bernstein EF. Ischemic ulcerative colitis following inferior mesenteric arterial ligation. Dis Colon Rectum 6:54, 1963.
12. Javid H, Julian OC, Dye WS, et al. Complications of abdominal aortic grafts. Arch Surg 85:142, 1962.
13. Perdue GD, Lowry K. Arterial insufficiency to the colon following resection of abdominal aortic aneurysms. Surg Gynecol Obstet 115:39, 1962.
14. Rob C, Snyder M. Chronic intestinal ischemia: A complication of surgery of the abdominal aorta. Surgery 60:1141, 1966.
15. Smith RF, Szilagyi DE. Ischemia of the colon as a complication in the surgery of the abdominal aorta. Arch Surg 80:806, 1960.
16. Ernst CB, Hagihara PF, Daugherty ME, et al. Inferior mesenteric artery stump pressure. A reliable index for safe IMA ligation during abdominal aortic aneurysmectomy. Ann Surg 187:641, 1978.
17. Rogers DM, Thompson JE, Garrett WV, et al. Mesenteric vascular problems: A 26-year experience. Ann Surg 195:554, 1982.
18. Ernst CB, Rutkow IM, Cleveland RJ, et al. Vascular surgery in the United States. J Vasc Surg 6:611, 1987.
19. Griffiths JD. Surgical anatomy of the blood supply of the distal colon. Ann R Coll Surg Engl 19:241, 1956.
20. Gibson WE III, Pearce CW, Creech O Jr. Infarction of the left hemicolon due to primary vascular occlusion. Dis Colon Rectum 12:323, 1969.

21. Steward JA, Rankin FW. Blood supply of large intestine: Its surgical considerations. Arch Surg 26:843, 1933.
22. Moskowitz M, Zimmerman H, Felson B. The meandering mesenteric artery of the colon. Am J Roentgenol 92:1088, 1964.
23. Sudek P. Ueber die Gefassversorgung des Mastdarmes in Hinsicht auf die operative Gangran. Munch Med Wochenschr 54:1314, 1907.
24. Connolly JE, Kwaan JHM. Prophylactic revascularization of the gut. Ann Surg 190:514, 1979.
25. Connolly JE, Stemmer EA. Intestinal gangrene as a result of mesenteric arterial steal. Am J Surg 126:197, 1973.
26. Gonzalez LL, Jaffe MS. Mesenteric arterial insufficiency following abdominal aortic resection. Arch Surg 93:10, 1966.
27. Shaw RS, Green TH. Massive mesenteric infarction following inferior mesenteric artery ligation in resection of the colon for carcinoma. N Engl J Med 248:890, 1963.
28. Case records of the Massachusetts General Hospital. N Engl J Med 172:254, 1964.
29. Delaney JP, Custer J. Gastrointestinal blood flow in the dog. Circ Res 7:394, 1965.
30. Geber WF. Quantitative measurement of blood flow in various areas of small and large intestine. Am J Physiol 198:985, 1960.
31. Goodhead B. Distribution of blood flow in various selected areas of small and large intestine in the dog. Am J Physiol 217:835, 1969.
32. Steiner SH, Mueller GCE. Distribution of blood flow in the digestive tract of the rat. Circ Res 9:99, 1961.
33. Boley SJ, Brandt LJ, Veith FJ. Ischemic disorders of the intestines. Curr Probl Surg 15:1, 1978.
34. Bicks RO, Bale GF, Howard H, et al. Acute and delayed colon ischemia after aortic aneurysm surgery. Arch Intern Med 122:249, 1968.
35. Movius HJ II. Resection of abdominal arteriosclerotic aneurysm. Am J Surg 90:298, 1955.
36. Papadopoulos CD, Mancini HW, Marino AWM Jr. Ischemic necrosis of the colon following aortic aneurysmectomy. J Cardiovasc Surg 15:494, 1974.
37. McBurney RP, Howard H, Bicks RO, et al. Ischemia and gangrene of the colon following abdominal aortic resection. Ann Surg 36:205, 1970.
38. Lannerstad L, Bergentz SE, Berquist D, et al. Ischemic intestinal complications after aortic surgery. Acta Chir Scand 151:599, 1985.
39. Carter R, Vannix R, Hinshaw DB, et al. Inferior mesenteric vascular occlusion. Sigmoidoscopic diagnosis. Surgery 45:845, 1959.
40. Brewster DC, Retana A, Waltman AC, et al. Angiography in the management of aneurysm of the abdominal aorta. N Engl J Med 292:822, 1975.
41. Robicsek F. Discussion of Ottinger LW, Darling RC, Nathan MJ, et al. Left colon ischemia complicating aorto-iliac reconstruction. Arch Surg 105:841, 1972.
42. Hobson RW II, Wright CB, Rich NM, et al. Assessment of colon ischemia during aortic surgery by Doppler ultrasound. J Surg Res 20:231, 1976.
43. Hobson RW II, Wright CB, O'Donnell JA, et al. Determination of intestinal viability by Doppler ultrasound. Arch Surg 114:165, 1979.
44. Lee BY, Trainor FS, Kavner D, et al. Intraoperative assessment of intestinal viability with Doppler ultrasound. Surg Gynecol Obstet 149:671, 1979.
45. Folkow B, Neil E. Gastrointestinal and liver circulations. In Folkow B, Neil E, eds. Circulation. New York: Oxford University Press, 1971.
46. Ouriel K, Fiore WM, Geary JE. Detection of occult colonic ischemia during aortic procedures: Use of an intraoperative photoplethysmographic technique. J Vasc Surg 7:5, 1988.
47. Fiddian-Greene RG, Amelin PM, Hermann JB, et al. Prediction of the development of sigmoid ischemia on the day of aortic operations. Arch Surg 121:654, 1986.
48. Launer DP, Miscall BG, Beil AR Jr. Colorectal infarctions following resection of abdominal aortic aneurysms. Dis Colon Rectum 21:613, 1978.
49. Hardy JD. Preservation of accessory arterial supply in abdominal aneurysm resection. Surg Gynecol Obstet 123:1318, 1966.
50. Hardy JD, Timmis HH. Abdominal aortic aneurysms: Special problems. Ann Surg 173:945, 1971.
51. Morris GC Jr. Discussion of Ernst CB, Hagihara PF, Daugherty ME, et al. Inferior mesenteric artery stump pressure; A reliable index for safe IMA ligation during abdominal aortic aneurysmectomy. Ann Surg 187:641, 1978.
52. Carrel A. Technique and remote results of vascular anastomoses. Surg Gynecol Obstet 14:246, 1912.
53. Ernst CB. Exposure of inaccessible arteries. Part II. Surgical Rounds 8:26, 1985.
54. Thomas SH, McCroskey BL, Iliopoulos JI, et al. Aortoiliac reconstruction combined with nonvascular operations. Am J Surg 146:784, 1983.
55. Ochsner JL, Cooley DA, DeBakey ME. Associated intraabdominal lesions encountered during resection of aortic aneurysm. Dis Colon Rectum 3:485, 1960.
56. Comfort MW, Gray HK, Wilson JM. The silent gallstone: A ten to twenty year follow-up study of 112 cases. Ann Surg 128:931, 1948.
57. Gracie WA, Ransohoff DF. The natural history of silent gallstones: The innocent gallstone is not a myth. N Engl J Med 307:798, 1982.
58. Lund J. Surgical indications in cholelithiasis. Ann Surg 151:153, 1960.
59. McSherry CT, Ferstenberg H, Calhoun WF, et al. The natural history of diagnosed gallstone disease in symptomatic and asymptomatic patients. Ann Surg 202:59, 1986.
60. Wenckert A, Robertson B. The natural course of gallstone disease: Eleven year review of 781 nonoperated cases. Gastroenterology 50:376, 1966.

61. Devine RM, Farnell MB, Mucha P. Acute cholecystitis as a complication in surgical patients. Arch Surg 119:1389, 1984.

62. Ottinger LW. Acute cholecystitis as a postoperative complication. Ann Surg 184:162, 1976.

63. Ouriel K, Green RM, Ricotta JJ, et al. Acute acalculous cholecystitis complicating abdominal aortic aneurysm resection. J Vasc Surg 1:646, 1984.

64. Fry RE, Fry WJ. Cholelithiasis and aortic reconstruction: The problem of simultaneous surgical therapy. J Vasc Surg 4:345, 1986.

65. Ameli FM, Weiss M, Provan JL. Safety of cholecystectomy with abdominal aortic surgery. Can J Surg 30:170, 1987.

66. Ouriel K, Ricotta JJ, Adams JT, et al. Management of cholelithiasis in patients with abdominal aortic aneurysm. Ann Surg 198:717, 1983.

67. Becker RM, Blundell PE. Infected aortic bifurcation grafts: Experience with fourteen patients. Surgery 80:544, 1976.

68. Bickerstaff LK, Hollier LH, Van Peenen HJ, et al. Abdominal aortic aneurysm repair combined with a second surgical procedure: Morbidity and mortality. Surgery 95:487, 1984.

69. Aldridge MC, Eastcott HG. Prolonged gastroduodenal ileus, complicating aortic aneurysm surgery. J R Coll Surg Edinb 29:310, 1984.

70. Hans SS. Pancreatitis and duodenal obstruction after aortic surgery. Am Surg 56:177, 1989.

71. Warshaw A, O'Hara PJ. Susceptibility of the pancreas to ischemic injury in shock. Ann Surg 188:197, 1978.

72. Fineberg HV, Pearlman LA. Surgical treatment of peptic ulcer in the United States. Lancet 1:1305, 1981.

73. Bouhoutsos J, Barabas A, Martin P. The association of peptic ulcer and abdominal aortic aneurysm and its significance. Br J Surg 60:302, 1973.

74. Fromm D. Duodenal ulcer. In Moody FG, ed. Surgical Treatment of Digestive Disease, 2nd ed. St. Louis: Mosby-Year Book, 1990.

75. Szilagyi DE, Elliot JP, Berguer R. Coincidental malignancy and abdominal aortic aneurysm. Arch Surg 95:402, 1967.

76. Busuttil RW, Abou-Zamzam AM, Machleder HI. Collagenase activity of the human aorta: A comparison of patients with and without abdominal aortic aneurysms. Arch Surg 115:1373, 1980.

77. Swanson RJ, Littooy FN, Hunt TK, et al. Laparotomy as a precipitating factor in the rupture of intraabdominal aneurysms. Arch Surg 115:299, 1980.

78. Nora JD, Pairolero PC, Nivatvongs S, et al. Concomitant abdominal aortic aneurysm and colorectal carcinoma: Priority of resection. J Vasc Surg 9:630, 1989.

11

Spinal Cord Ischemia

Larry H. Hollier   **Charles D. Procter, Sr.**   **Thomas C. Naslund**

Paraplegia following aortic surgery has been unpredictable and, in general, unpreventable. The functional, social, and emotional consequences of this complication are devastating for the patient, family, and surgeon. Economically it is a burden of great magnitude that can deplete the financial resources of most of these unfortunate patients.

At the present time we are unable to reliably prevent paraplegia. Despite the use of adjunctive maneuvers and despite a technically perfect operative procedure, paraplegia or paraparesis can still occur. Nonetheless, a thorough knowledge of the pathophysiology of paraplegia, the clinical variables that predispose to paraplegia, and the techniques that can ameliorate adverse influences on spinal cord perfusion may help the surgeon minimize, as much as possible, the risk of neurologic deficit.

SPINAL CORD BLOOD SUPPLY

The spinal cord lies within the vertebral canal and extends for a length of approximately 45 cm from its continuation with the medulla oblongata of the brain to its termination at the level of the second lumbar vertebrae, tapering to the conus medullaris. Distally the lumbar and sacral nerves pass almost vertically downward within the dura, forming the cauda equina before the nerves reach their exit foramina.

Embryologically the spinal cord receives 62 radicular arteries, most of which degenerate during fetal development. Usually six to eight radicular arteries remain and fuse centrally along the anterior surface of the spinal cord to form the anterior spinal artery. More numerous radicular arteries (10 to 23) fuse to form the

paired posterior spinal arteries, which supply blood to the posterior one third of the spinal cord.[1] The anterior spinal artery supplies blood to the anterior two thirds of the spinal cord; the anterior spinal artery, however, is not always intact throughout the length of the spinal cord.

The anterior radicular arteries in the adult usually arise as branches of the vertebral, thyrocervical trunk, intercostal, and lateral sacral arteries (branches of the posterior division of the hypogastric arteries). A major radicular branch often arises from intercostal arteries around the level of T5 and another branch, the commonly known artery of Adamkiewicz, arises at T10; both are highly variable in origin[2] (Fig. 11-1).

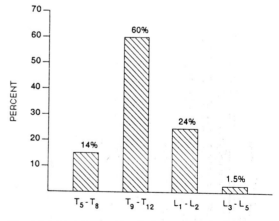

Fig. 11-1. Variability of level of origin of the artery of Adamkiewicz in relation to the vertebrae. (From Hollier LH. Causes and prevention of spinal cord ischemia. In Veith FJ, ed. Current Critical Problems in Vascular Surgery, vol. 2. St. Louis: Quality Medical Publishing, 1990.)

Although the anterior spinal artery may be continuous and of adequate size throughout its length in some individuals, it is important to recognize that in others it may be inadequate to supply blood to segments of the spinal cord if one or more of these critical feeding arteries is temporarily or permanently interrupted. It is also noteworthy that interconnections between the anterior and posterior spinal arteries do not exist within the spinal cord.[2]

INCIDENCE OF PARAPLEGIA
Infrarenal Aortic Surgery

Fortunately paraplegia following surgery of the infrarenal aorta is rare. When it does occur, it is often associated with catastrophic events such as ruptured abdominal aortic aneurysm, prolonged episodes of hypotension, aortic thrombosis, or thrombosis of an aortic graft in the early postoperative period.

Szilagyi et al.[3] reported a 0.25% incidence of paraplegia in 3164 operations on the infrarenal aorta. The incidence of neurologic deficit was 0.2% following nonruptured abdominal aortic aneurysm repair and 2% following repair of ruptured abdominal aortic aneurysms. Suprarenal aortic clamping and hypotension increased the probability of neurologic injury. Neurologic deficit did not occur after aortic procedures for occlusive disease. Since the degree to which hypogastric blood flow was restored is unclear, we cannot tell whether the neurologic complication was caused by the interruption of a very low-lying artery of Adamkiewicz or by inadequate revascularization of critical spinal artery collaterals from the hypogastric artery.

Picone et al.[4] reported seven cases (0.94%) of lower extremity neurologic deficit in a series of 744 patients undergoing infrarenal aortic reconstruction. In that report, bilateral and unilateral hypogastric interruption occurred in three and two cases, respectively. All seven patients had bifurcated aortic grafts and two patients apparently had atheromatous embolization into the hypogastric arteries.

In most other large series of infrarenal aortic reconstructions paraplegia is a very rare occurrence, and the actual risk of paraplegia following elective infrarenal aortic reconstruction is

negligible. In our personal experience with over 1000 infrarenal aortic reconstructions, transient paraparesis occurred only once, in a patient who underwent repair of a ruptured abdominal aortic aneurysm. We are aware of two patients in whom paraplegia developed at our institution; both cases occurred in association with graft limb occlusion or hypogastric artery occlusion in the immediate postoperative period.

Thoracic and Thoracoabdominal Aortic Surgery

The incidence of paraplegia/paraparesis following thoracic or thoracoabdominal aortic surgery appears to be directly related to the duration of aortic occlusion, presence of aortic dissection, and extent of aortic replacement (Fig. 11-2). Jex et al.[5] reported an overall incidence of 19.6% following repair of thoracic aortic dissections. Risk of paraplegia increased significantly with increasing cross-clamp time in patients without protection of the distal circulation, but when a bypass or shunt was used, cross-clamp time did not adversely affect the incidence of paraplegia.[5] Livesay et al.[6] reported a 6.5% incidence of paraplegia in 360 patients with thoracic aneurysmectomy, but a shunt or bypass did not reduce paraplegia risk. Cross-clamp time greater than 30 minutes increased the risk from 3% to 11%; however,

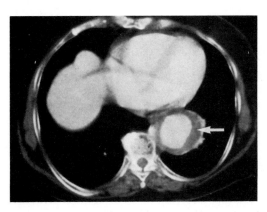

Fig. 11-2. CT scan of a patient with a large thoracoabdominal aneurysm. Note extensive thrombus within the aneurysm sac (arrow).

increased cross-clamp time was also indicative of more extensive aortic replacement.

A low paraplegia rate without bypass or shunting (0.9%) was reported by Crawford et al.[7] in 112 patients with descending thoracic aortic aneurysms. The one case of paraplegia occurred in a patient with a 32-minute clamp time and a ruptured aneurysm. However, paraplegia or paraparesis is reported to occur in approximately 30% of patients when extensive graft replacement of the descending thoracic and abdominal aorta is required[8] or when clamp time exceeds 60 minutes.[6]

In addition to the extent of aortic replacement, etiology of the pathologic process is also important. Patients with aortic dissection are clearly at greater risk of paraplegia than patients undergoing aortic replacement for atherosclerotic aneurysmal disease. Crawford et al.[8] noted a 21% incidence of paraplegia following repair of type II thoracoabdominal aortic aneurysms vs. a 40% incidence in patients with aortic dissection.

The risk of paraplegia/paraparesis in elective repair of nondissecting thoracoabdominal aortic aneurysm has generally been in the range of 5% to 11%.[8-10] However, the risk of paraplegia developing is clearly related to the extent of aortic replacement. In a series of 605 thoracoabdominal aortic aneurysms, Crawford et al.[8] noted an 11% overall incidence of paraplegia/paraparesis; however, neurologic deficit varied by extent of aneurysm replaced: type I, 8%; type II, 21%; type III, 2%; and type IV, 1%.

In our experience with 130 nondissecting thoracoabdominal aortic aneurysms, we have seen an overall neurologic deficit of 4.6% (1.5% paraplegia, 3.1% paraparesis) with a variable risk related to extent of aortic replacement: type I, 7.7% (2 of 26 patients); type II, 9.9% (2 of 22 patients); type III, 6.3% (2 of 32 patients); and type IV, 0% (0 of 50 patients).

PATHOPHYSIOLOGY OF PARAPLEGIA

It must be understood that the precise mechanism of paraplegia and paraparesis, both acute and delayed, is not clearly defined. However, multiple studies on the various aspects of neuronal injury provide sufficient data to allow a reasonable construct of the pathophysiology of paraplegia.

Paraplegia/paraparesis is a consequence of the interaction of the interdependent variables of (1) severity of neuronal ischemia, (2) the rate of neuronal metabolism during ischemic periods, and (3) the extent of postischemic reperfusion by oxygen-derived free radicals and by both direct and complement-mediated leukocyte injury; other cellular mechanisms undoubtedly also play a role in late neuronal injury.

Occlusion of the thoracic aorta results in decreased distal aortic pressure and thus decreased flow through the distal intercostal arteries and recipient anterior spinal artery. Perfusion pressure to the spinal cord is therefore decreased. Concomitantly, clamping of the proximal thoracic aorta increases cerebrospinal fluid (CSF) production and CSF pressure.[11-13] The combined effect of a decrease in anterior spinal artery pressure and an increase in CSF pressure is a decrease in spinal cord perfusion pressure and resultant spinal cord ischemia.

This spinal cord ischemia is termed "incomplete" since blood flow persists, though in an amount insufficient to maintain normal aerobic metabolism.[14,15] Continued metabolism under such hypoxic conditions results in the production of noxious metabolic by-products, such as oxygen-derived free radicals, and acidosis, which is aggravated by high glucose loads, which in turn increases metabolic activity in the hypoxic state.[14,15]

Studies on cerebral ischemia have documented that the level of neuronal activity can influence the degree of injury induced by ischemia. Steen and Mitchenfelder[16] and Arnfred and Secher[17] have demonstrated that barbiturate-induced coma is protective against ischemic injury. Similarly, cooling, corticosteroids, calcium channel blockers, free radical scavengers, and other pharmacologic interventions have all been shown to beneficially influence neurologic function during experimental neuronal ischemia.[15-22] Unfortunately, such beneficial effects have not been proved following spinal cord ischemia in humans. Nonetheless, these studies support the concept that the rate of neuronal activity during ischemia is a factor in the severity of neuronal injury during ischemia and following reperfusion. The relative influence of ischemic injury itself vs. injury following reperfusion needs further clarification.

PREVENTION OF PARAPLEGIA
Infrarenal Aortic Surgery

Although paraplegia/paraparesis is rare following infrarenal aortic surgery, it is a complication that should be considered. Patients who present with shock and a ruptured aneurysm are at particular risk for this complication. Every effort should be made to promptly restore not only an adequate systemic blood pressure, but also adequate perfusion of the vessels to the pelvis and lower extremities. Although an exceptionally rare case of paraplegia following elective infrarenal aortic replacement may be caused by an atypically low-lying artery of Adamkiewicz, we believe that most cases of paraplegia following infrarenal aortic surgery are the result of inadequate perfusion through branches of the hypogastric arteries. It is unwise to attempt any reimplantation of lumbar arteries into the aortic graft; any possible theoretical benefits are very likely to be greatly outweighed by potential complications associated with such surgical exuberance. It is far more realistic and prudent to conscientiously revascularize at least

one of the hypogastric arteries in every case of aortic reconstruction. This is most likely to significantly reduce any risk of neurologic injury to the spinal cord and, at the same time, minimize the risk of colon ischemia.

Thoracic and Thoracoabdominal Aortic Surgery

As stated previously, paraplegia/paraparesis is not entirely preventable following thoracic and thoracoabdominal aortic replacement. Nonetheless, one would hope to be able to decrease the risk of neurologic injury by appropriate ancillary measures. Since paraplegia appears to result from the interaction of the interdependent variables of severity of neuronal ischemia, metabolic activity of the spinal cord neurons, and the degree of reperfusion and postischemic injury (Figs. 11-3 and 11-4), any attempt to improve results should be directed toward all of these areas of influence.[21] The severity of ischemia theoretically may be reduced in several ways: use of a shunt or bypass (heparin-bonded shunt; femorofemoral, atriofemoral, or axillofemoral bypass), elevation of systolic blood pressure, and/or reduction of CSF pressure. Reimplantation of intercostal arteries also falls into this category since some patients clearly will become paraplegic if critical

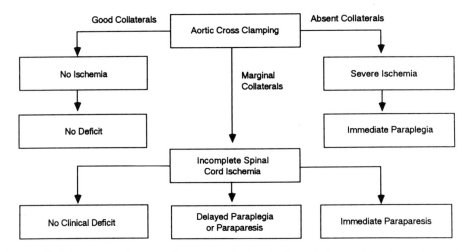

Fig. 11-3. Mechanism of progressive neuronal injury in the spinal cord following spinal cord ischemia. Severe ischemia may cause immediate infarction. Incomplete ischemia may lead to progression of ischemia following reperfusion.

intercostal arteries are not reimplanted. To accomplish intercostal revascularization one may choose to do preoperative angiographic visualization of the spinal arteries, perform routine intercostal reimplantation, or use motor or somatosensory-evoked potential monitoring to select patients for intercostal reimplantation. CSF drainage has been shown experimentally to allow a longer safe clamp time,[12,13] which theoretically may improve perfusion pressure of the spinal cord and may thus reduce cord ischemia to some extent. Although Crawford et al.[23] did not show any benefit of CSF drainage in 46 patients with type I and type II thoracoabdominal aneurysms (33% were dissections), these patients clearly represented those at greater risk for paraplegia and thus may not demonstrate any benefit of CSF drainage; the same may not be true of patients with

aneurysms at lesser risk. Thus, despite their findings, we continue to use routine CSF drainage as an integral part of perioperative management of thoracoabdominal aortic aneurysm patients.

Experimental evidence clearly suggests that reduction of the neuronal metabolic rate has a protective effect on the brain during periods of incomplete ischemia.[15-22] Metabolic rate can be simply and safely reduced by mild to moderate cooling and by administration of large doses of intravenous thiopental (Pentothal) before aortic clamping. Although profound cooling without bypass may result in unacceptable cardiac dysfunction, cooling to a core temperature of 32° to 34°C has appeared to us to be relatively safe and readily reversible. We have similarly noted no deleterious effects from the administration of large doses of intravenous thiopental.

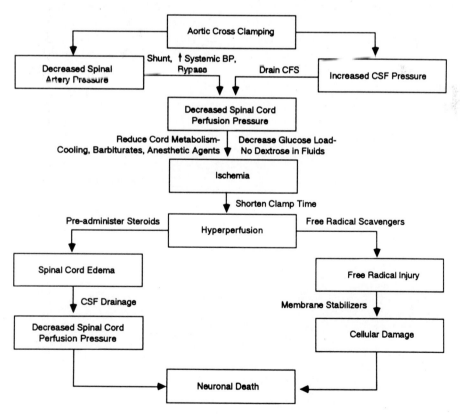

Fig. 11-4. Ischemic neurologic injury cascade and possible methods of intervention at various stages. (From Hollier LH, Marino RJ. Thoracoabdominal aortic aneurysms. In Moore WS, ed. Vascular Surgery: A Comprehensive Review, 3rd ed. Philadelphia: WB Saunders, 1990, pp 295-303.)

Clinical prevention of reperfusion injury is poorly understood and undocumented. The most potent free radical scavengers are not yet available for generalized use.[22] However, we have adopted the routine use of intravenous mannitol infusion before aortic declamping; mannitol does seem to have some ability to modify free radical injury and thus may be of some clinical benefit. Similarly, allopurinol, because it inhibits xanthine oxidase and thus theoretically reduces production of oxygen-derived free radicals, may be of some benefit, but we have not yet adopted its use clinically for thoracoabdominal aortic aneurysm repair.

Stabilization of neuronal and lysosomal membranes and prevention of leukocyte-induced neuronal injury may offer an opportunity for further protection. However, at this time the mechanisms of injury are poorly understood. Additional research is clearly needed in this area.

Operative Procedure: Thoracoabdominal Aortic Aneurysm

Any attempt to significantly reduce paraplegia should include a multifactorial approach. We have instituted such a protocol as outlined in Fig. 11-4.[9,21] After general anesthesia is induced in the patient, a soft Silastic intrathecal catheter is placed through the second or third lumbar space, which permits aspiration of CSF and allows continuous monitoring of CSF pressure throughout the operative and postoperative periods. Fifteen milliliters of CSF is initial-ly withdrawn. The CSF pressure is maintained at or below 10 mm Hg by intermittent CSF drainage in 10 to 15 ml increments. Peripheral arterial pressure is maintained slightly higher (15 to 20 mm Hg) than normal for that patient. Administration of intravenous nitroprusside is started when the surgical incision is made, and the patient is volume-loaded with crystalloid solution containing no dextrose.[21,24,25]

The room temperature is reduced moderately and intravenous fluids and inhalation agents are not warmed, allowing the patient's temperature to fall to about 33° to 34°C. Dramatic cooling of the patient is not performed because of the increased risks of hemorrhagic and cardiac complications. Methylprednisolone (Solu-Medrol; 30 mg/kg) and hydrocortisone (100 mg) are administered intravenously at the beginning of the operation. A large intravenous bolus of barbiturate (thiopental sodium, 20 mg/kg) is administered approximately 15 minutes before aortic occlusion, and mannitol (12.5 gm) is administered 15 minutes before clamping and again just before unclamping. Expeditious surgical technique is of the utmost importance in this situation. Attempts are made to restore flow to as many intercostal arteries as possible by incorporation into the anastomosis, direct reimplantation, or use of a separate interposition graft (Fig. 11-5).

Postoperatively meticulous care is mandatory. Careful control of all hemodynamic parameters is necessary to avoid any episodes of hy-

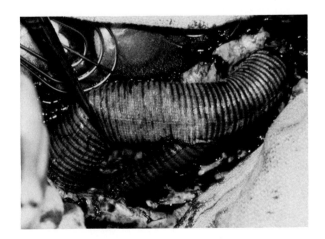

Fig. 11-5. Operative view of an additional use of an interposition Dacron graft to revascularize multiple pairs of intercostal arteries.

potension or reduced tissue perfusion. CSF pressures are carefully monitored for an additional 1 to 3 days, depending on the extent of aneurysm repair performed.

CONCLUSION

At present there are no reliable methods of completely eliminating the risk of spinal cord injury associated with aortic surgery. The severity of spinal cord injury appears to be related to the interdependent variables of duration of ischemia of the spinal cord, rate of neuronal metabolism, and the extent of cellular injury following reperfusion of the cord. However, various technical and pharmacologic interventions may help to minimize neurologic injury associated with complex aortic surgery.

REFERENCES

1. Djindjian R, Hurth RM, Houdart M, et al. Arterial supply of the spinal cord. In Djindjian R, Hurth RM, Houdart M, et al., eds. Angiography of the Spinal Cord. Baltimore: University Park Press, 1970, pp 3-13.
2. Gray H, Clemente CD, eds. Gray's Anatomy of the Human Body, 30th ed. Philadelphia: Lea & Febiger, 1985, pp 964-976.
3. Szilagyi DE, Hageman JH, Smith RF, et al. Spinal cord damage in surgery of the abdominal aorta. Surgery 83:38-56, 1978.
4. Picone AL, Green RM, Ricotta JR, et al. Spinal cord ischemia following operations on the abdominal aorta. J Vasc Surg 3:94-103, 1986.
5. Jex RK, Schaff HV, Piehler JM, et al. Early and late results following repair of dissection of the descending thoracic aorta. J Vasc Surg 3:226-237, 1986.
6. Livesay JJ, Couley DA, Ventimiglia RA, et al. Surgical experience in descending thoracic aneurysmectomy with and without adjuncts to avoid ischemia. Ann Thorac Surg 39:37-46, 1985.
7. Crawford ES, Walker HS, Saleh SA, et al. Graft replacement of aneurysm in the descending thoracic aorta: Results without bypass or shunting. Surgery 89:73-85, 1981.
8. Crawford ES, Crawford JL, Safi HJ, et al. Thoracoabdominal aortic aneurysms: Preoperative and intraoperative factors determining immediate and long-term results of operations in 605 patients. J Vasc Surg 3:389-404, 1986.
9. Hollier LH, Moore WM. Avoidance of renal and neurologic complications following thoracoabdominal aortic aneurysm repair. Acta Chir Scand Suppl 555:129-135, 1990.
10. Hollier LH, Symmonds JB, Pairolero PC, et al. Thoracoabdominal aortic aneurysm repair: Analysis of postoperative morbidity. Arch Surg 123:871-875, 1988.
11. Blaisdell FW, Cooley DA. The mechanism of paraplegia after temporary thoracic aortic occlusion and its relationship to spinal fluid pressure. Surgery 51:351-355, 1963.
12. McCullough JL, Hollier LH, Nugent M. Paraplegia after thoracic aortic occlusion: Influence of cerebrospinal fluid drainage. J Vasc Surg 7:153-160, 1988.
13. Bower TC, Murray MJ, Gloviczki P, et al. Effects of thoracic aortic occlusion and cerebrospinal fluid drainage on regional blood flow in dogs: Correlation with neurologic outcome. J Vasc Surg 9:135-144, 1988.
14. Lundy EF, Ball TD, Mandell MA, et al. Dextrose administration increases sensory/motor impairment and paraplegia after infrarenal aortic occlusion in the rabbit. Surgery 102:737-742, 1987.
15. Hollier LH. Protecting the brain and spinal cord. J Vasc Surg 5:524-528, 1987.
16. Steen PA, Mitchenfelder JD. Cerebral protection with barbiturates: Relation to anesthetic effect. Stroke 9:140-142, 1978.
17. Arnfred I, Secher O. Anoxia and barbiturates: Tolerance to anoxia in mice influenced by barbiturates. Arch Int Pharmacodyn Ther 139:67-74, 1962.
18. Vacanti FX, Ames AA. Mild hypothermia and Mg^{++} protects against irreversible damage during CNS ischemia. Stroke 15:695-698, 1984.
19. Laschinger JC, Cunningham JN, Cooper MM, et al. Prevention of ischemic spinal cord injury following aortic cross-clamping: Use of corticosteroids. Ann Thorac Surg 38:500-507, 1984.
20. Steen PA, Newberg LA, Milde JH, et al. Nimodipine improves cerebral blood flow and neurologic recovery after complete cerebral ischemia in the dog. J Cereb Blood Flow Metab 3:38-43, 1983.
21. Hollier LH, Marino RJ. Thoracoabdominal aortic aneurysms. In Moore WS, ed. Vascular Surgery: A Comprehensive Review, 3rd ed. Philadelphia: WB Saunders, 1990, pp 295-303.
22. Granke K, Hollier LH, Moore WM, et al. Paraplegia following thoracic aortic cross-clamping in the canine model: Effect of interventional therapy. J Vasc Surg (submitted for publication).
23. Crawford ES, Svensson LG, Hess KR, et al. A prospective study of cerebrospinal fluid drainage to prevent paraplegia after high risk surgery on the thoracoabdominal aorta. J Vasc Surg (in press).
24. Bunt TJ, Manczuk M, Varley KV. Nitroglycerin induced volume loading. Surgery 103:513-519, 1988.
25. Bush HL. Aortic surgery: Volume loading and vasodilation. In Bergan JJ, Yao JST, eds. Aortic Surgery. Philadelphia: WB Saunders, 1989, pp 59-73.

12

Impotence Following Aortic Surgery

Richard F. Kempczinski

Although Leriche and Morel[1] first described the association between impotence and distal aortic occlusion, Harris and Jepson[2] were the first to report erectile dysfunction as a complication of aortic surgery. These studies first called our attention to vasculogenic impotence, but a true appreciation of the magnitude of this problem awaited more refined diagnostic techniques and a better understanding of the mechanism of erection.

Impotence, the inability to achieve or maintain an erection adequate for satisfactory coitus, must be distinguished from *retrograde ejaculation,* which is primarily a neurogenic disorder in which bladder neck closure does not occur and semen is deposited into the bladder. In such cases the patient is still able to complete coitus and achieve an orgasm. Although impotence, by the above definition, appears to be a disorder limited to men, women with aortoiliac arterial obstructive disease may complain of insufficient vaginal lubrication and loss of orgasm.[3] However, this is a much less common problem because female genital sensation depends in great part on the integrity of the somatic pudendal nerves and their efferent sensory fibers. These are situated deep within the pelvis and are protected by the thick layer of endopelvic fascia. Furthermore, collateral arterial blood supply to the female sexual organs is quite extensive. As a result female organic "impotence" is extremely uncommon.[4]

This chapter describes the physiology of erection as we currently understand it and explores how the normal interplay of neural and vascular elements can be disturbed by the development of arterial occlusive disease or by

surgical attempts to correct it. Because vascular surgeons are often consulted by patients with erectile dysfunction, the various diagnostic techniques that may be necessary in these patients are emphasized. Finally, those technical modifications that should be employed during aortic surgery to prevent iatrogenic impotence, as well as the most effective current treatment for established impotence, are discussed.

PHYSIOLOGY OF ERECTION

In the 40 years since Leriche and Morel[1] first described the association between aortoiliac arterial occlusive disease and impotence, medical research has broadened our understanding of the complex interplay between psychologic, hormonal, neurologic, and vascular elements that is required to achieve an adequate erection.

Satisfactory male sexual function presupposes anatomically normal male genitalia, an appropriate hormonal milieu, intact nerve and blood supply to the genitalia, and appropriate physical and/or psychic stimulation. Absence of any one of these elements or moderate dysfunction in several of them may result in impotence.

Neurophysiology

The precise neurophysiologic basis for erection remains unknown. The afferent and efferent neural pathways that appear to be involved in erection are depicted in Fig. 12-1. Thoracolumbar sympathetic nerves (T12-L4) are believed to be important in mediating psychogenic erections, which can occur even in patients with complete sacral cord destruction.[5] However, younger individuals undergoing bilateral radical retroperitoneal node dissection in which both sympathetic nerve chains are usually removed rarely become impotent.[6] Therefore sacral efferent (parasympathetic) outflow appears capable of mediating both psychogenic and reflex erections. Clearly, bilateral resection of the T12-L1 sympathetic ganglia can result in retrograde ejaculation. However, this should not be confused with erectile dysfunction.

Based on current neurophysiologic research, erection appears to develop as a result of neural transmissions that reach the genitalia via the pelvic parasympathetic nerves. Destruction of the parasympathetic outflow from the sacral cord will cause impotence. Pelvic operations, such as radical prostatectomy or abdominal perineal resection of the rectum in which parasympathetic nerve damage often occurs, have been associated with postoperative impo-

tence in 70% to 100% of cases.[7] The final common pathway for this hemodynamic control appears to be short adrenergic nerves within the penis.

The CNS loci that initiate erection have not been precisely identified. However, since these signals must reach the genitalia via the spinal cord, injury or transection of the cord may result in impotence. Reflex erections are possible in a high percentage of patients with lesions of the upper spinal cord, but the level of injury largely determines the preservation of erectile potency. These reflex erections appear to require the integrity of the afferent pudendal nerves since pudendal neurectomies in such patients result in impotence.

Most drugs that produce impotence do so by their actions on these neurophysiologic pathways. However, it is difficult to determine

NEUROPHYSIOLOGY OF ERECTION

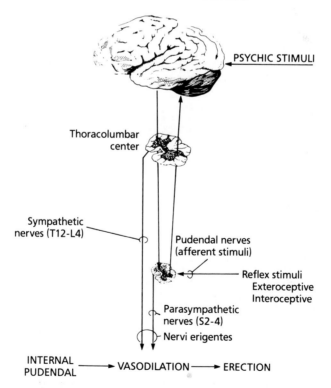

Fig. 12-1. Diagrammatic representation of the neural pathways involved in penile erection. (From Kempczinski RF, Birinyi LK. Impotence following aortic surgery. In Bernhard VM, Towne JB, eds. Complications in Vascular Surgery, 2nd ed. Philadelphia: WB Saunders, 1985, pp 311-324.)

whether their actions are peripheral or central. Ganglion-blocking agents, such as hexamethonium, are a well-known cause of impotence and ejaculation disturbances. Propranolol frequently causes impotence when administered in doses greater than 200 mg/day. Drugs such as reserpine, α-methyldopa, and tricyclic antidepressants probably produce impotence by their action on the CNS.

In summary, normal erectile function appears to involve both pelvic parasympathetic nerves and penile corporal short adrenergic receptors. Although both α-adrenergic and β-adrenergic receptors are present within the penis, α-adrenergic receptors are believed to predominate in a 10:1 ratio. In addition, recent studies have suggested that vasoactive intestinal polypeptide, either alone[8] or in synergy with α-adrenergic blockade[9] or acetylcholine,[10] may be responsible for erection. Thus erection can no longer be considered to be a purely cholinergic event and acetylcholine is not the final neural transmitter. Nevertheless, many questions remain regarding the neurophysiology of erection.

Penile Blood Supply

When neural pathways are intact, the ability to achieve an erection is largely determined by the adequacy of arterial inflow. The blood supply of the penis arises from the internal pudendal artery, which is one of the terminal branches of the internal iliac artery. The paired internal pudendal arteries enter the male perineum through the lesser sciatic foramina. Each of the internal pudendal arteries in turn gives rise to a dorsal penile artery, a more laterally placed deep artery of the penis, which supplies the corpus cavernosum, and a bulbourethral artery, which supplies the corpus spongiosum (Fig. 12-2). Terminal branches of the penile arteries and the penile vessels themselves appear to communicate with the cavernous spaces

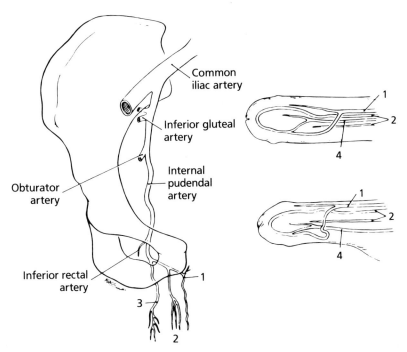

Fig. 12-2. Major blood supply to the penis is from the deep and dorsal penile arteries and the urethral artery. These are branches of the internal pudendal artery, which in turn is a branch of the internal iliac artery. *1,* Dorsal artery of the penis; *2,* deep artery of the penis; *3,* perineal artery; *4,* urethral artery. (From Queral LA, Flinn WR, Bergan JJ, Yao JST. Sexual function and aortic surgery. In Bergan JJ, Yao JST, eds. Surgery of the Aorta and Its Body Branches. Orlando, Fla.: Grune & Stratton, 1979.)

via structures previously called polsters, Ebner pads, or coussinets.[11]

Recent investigations in animal models and human volunteers have settled some of the long-standing controversies regarding the precise sequence of events in erection.[12] In the flaccid state the arterioles are constricted and the venous sinusoids are contracted. Together they exert maximal resistance against arterial flow, thus allowing only a small amount of nutrient blood to enter the corpora. The venules in the periphery of the corpora run between the adjacent sinusoidal wall, whereas the larger intermediary venules traverse the sinusoidal wall and tunica albuginea for some distance before exiting as the emissary veins. While the sinusoids are contracted, these venules drain freely to extrapenile veins.

During erection the smooth muscles of the sinusoids and arterioles relax, which in turn increases sinusoidal compliance and causes a maximal decrease in the peripheral resistance. This results in an immediate increase in arterial flow and filling of the sinusoids. The resulting dilation of the arterial tree not only allows blood to enter rapidly, but also permits transmission of approximately 80% of the arterial systolic pressure to the sinusoidal spaces (*vascular* or *full erection phase*). Subsequent contraction of the bulbocavernous and ischiocavernous muscles either spontaneously or reflexly compresses the proximal corpora and culminates in cavernosal rigidity, with further engorgement of the glans penis as seen during intercourse (*skeletal muscle* or *rigid erection phase*). In the full erection phase mean pressure in the corpora cavernosa is approximately 90 to 100 mm Hg. In the rigid erection phase compression of the blood-distended corpora can increase the intracavernous pressure well above arterial systolic pressure.

This proposed sequence of events is further supported by the work of Newman, Northrup, and Devlin,[13] who infused the pudendal arteries of human cadavers at a pressure of 200 mm Hg but were unable to produce a normal erection. Subsequently, direct infusion of the corpora cavernosa at rates ranging from 20 to 50 ml/min resulted in a normal erection. Once an erection was obtained, it was possible to maintain turgidity with decreased infusion rates. These results are similar to those of studies by Michal and Pospichal,[14] who demonstrated that a mean infusion rate of 90 ml/min directly into the corpora was initially necessary to produce erections in normal human subjects, but once an erection was achieved, a maintenance flow rate of 62 ml/min was satisfactory to maintain erection.

By injecting microspheres into the internal pudendal arteries in cadavers, investigators have confirmed the presence of arteriovenous shunts measuring 100 millimicra in diameter.[13] They also noted that occlusion of the dorsal vein of the penis failed to result in an erection. Thus erection appears to occur as the result of preferential redirection of increased arterial flow into the corporal spaces and active venoconstriction is apparently unnecessary.

Psychic Influences

Although recent work has emphasized the frequent organic nature of postoperative impotence, the contribution of psychogenic factors should not be lightly dismissed. Following major surgical procedures, the patient and his sexual partner may be concerned that resumption of normal sexual activity could be potentially harmful, thus resulting in decreased libido and functional impotence. Even if such subconscious fears alone may be inadequate to cause erectile dysfunction, they may be contributory in the presence of marginal penile perfusion. When initial attempts at resumption of normal sexual activity in the postoperative period meet with failure, a reactive depression may result, which can prolong the problem. If appropriate neurologic and vascular causes of impotence have been excluded postoperatively, complete evaluation of the patient, and if possible, his sexual partner, by a concerned and knowledgeable psychiatrist may be helpful.

DIAGNOSIS

Since so many factors can result in erectile dysfunction, a multimodal diagnostic approach to the problem is essential (Fig. 12-3). Even in those cases in which the underlying defect cannot be directly corrected, confirmation of the organic nature of the patient's impotence is vital in preventing the emotional havoc that this problem can wreak on his personal life. Fur-

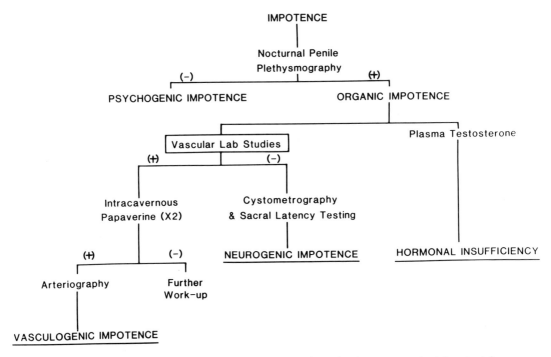

Fig. 12-3. Algorithm suggesting a diagnostic approach to the impotent patient (see text for details). (From Kempczinski RF, Birinyi LK. Impotence following aortic surgery. In Bernhard VM, Towne JB, eds. Complications in Vascular Surgery, 2nd ed. Philadelphia: WB Saunders, 1985, pp 311-324.)

thermore, once the diagnosis of organic impotence is established, the patient can be referred for a penile implant if appropriate correction of the specific problem is impossible.

History

Although many of the barriers that previously precluded frank discussion of erectile dysfunction have been dismantled, some patients are still reluctant to broach this problem with their physician. Since 70% to 80% of patients with aortoiliac arterial occlusive disease in some series have been impotent[15,16] and as many as 50% of diabetic patients under the age of 40 may be similarly disabled,[17] vascular surgeons must be prepared to initiate such discussions with their patients. This is especially important preoperatively, not only to permit modification of the operation to relieve impotence when possible, but also to document that the condition antedated the surgical procedure.

A careful and detailed history of the patient's

sexual dysfunction may suggest its etiology. *Organic impotence* is typically of gradual onset and results in complete inability to achieve erection. It is not partner specific, and masturbatory and morning erections are absent. The onset of the patient's symptoms cannot be related to any identifiable emotional stress and libido is typically retained. By contrast, *psychogenic impotence* may be rapid in onset, frequently less than 1 month, and may be intermittent in pattern. Partner specificity may be present, and erection can be achieved during masturbation. Morning erections occur and the onset of the patient's symptoms frequently can be related to an identifiable emotional stress. The presence of normal sexual drive may be quite variable.

In those patients with known organic impotence certain historical features help to differentiate those with a neurogenic vs. vasculogenic impotence. Patients suffering from *neurogenic* impotence are usually unable to achieve erections at all and may have decreased testicular sensation on palpation. Ejaculation with masturbation in such patients is generally absent. On the other hand, patients with *vasculogenic* impotence may be able to temporarily achieve an erection, but it is short-lived. Testicular pain on palpation is normal and masturbatory ejaculations are present. In patients with external iliac artery occlusion the ipsilateral internal iliac artery may be the major collateral blood supply to the lower extremity. Some of these patients may complain that although they are able to achieve a satisfactory erection during foreplay, when thrusting is initiated, the penis becomes flaccid and coitus becomes impossible. Presumably the increased demand for blood by the buttock and thigh muscles during active coitus shunts blood away from the genitalia, causing loss of erection.[16]

Nocturnal Penile Tumescence

This study is based on the observation that sexually potent men regularly have erections during the rapid eye movement (REM) phase of sleep.[18] The complete absence of tumescence during an adequate sleep study is strong evidence of organic impotence. Unfortunately, the failure of erection is often qualitative rather than complete and it has been difficult to standardize the quality of erections. Such studies are difficult to perform properly and are best carried out on an inpatient basis in specially equipped sleep laboratories.[19] Changes in penile circumference are monitored by means of mercury-filled strain gauges and/or video camera characterizations of the quality of the erection. The documentation of normal erections during REM sleep clearly establishes the psychogenic basis of the patient's erectile dysfunction and allows appropriate therapy.

Noninvasive Vascular Testing

Canning et al.[20] first emphasized that vascular insufficiency of the pelvic vessels, even in the presence of normal femoral pulses, could result in impotence. They attempted to identify such patients by palpating penile pulses and performing impedance plethysmography. Subsequently, other investigators assessed penile blood flow using mercury strain-gauge plethysmography, spectrographic or ultrasonic measurement of penile systolic pressure, and pulse

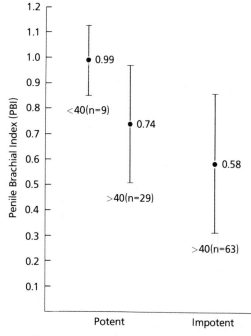

Fig. 12-4. Distribution of penile brachial index (mean ± SD) in patients by age and sexual potency. (Data from Kempczinski RF. Role of the vascular diagnostic laboratory in the evaluation of male impotence. Am J Surg 138:278, 1979.)

volume recordings.[21-24] When such studies are abnormal and the possibility of vasculogenic impotence is likely, more traditional noninvasive tests to exclude aortoiliac arterial occlusive disease should be performed. Kempczinski[24] studied 134 patients using the Doppler velocity meter to measure penile systolic pressure. This in turn was divided by brachial systolic pressure to obtain a penile brachial index (PBI). Pulse volume waveforms (PVW) of penile volume change with each cardiac cycle were also recorded. The influence of both sexual function and patient age on each of these parameters was then determined.

Age exerted a deleterious influence on all variables of penile blood flow independent of the status of sexual potency. Patients under the age of 40 had a mean PBI of 0.99 compared with a PBI of 0.74 for equally potent men over the age of 40. By contrast, impotent men over the age of 40 had a mean PBI of 0.58 (Fig. 12-4).

The PVW of patients under the age of 40 was of good to fair quality, and no poor quality waveforms were observed. With increasing age and sexual dysfunction, a greater percentage of patients had poor quality waveforms, but this difference was not statistically significant. The validity of these findings has been confirmed by numerous investigators, who have emphasized the importance of this type of testing in the evaluation of patients with erectile dysfunction.[25,26] However, the diagnosis of vasculogenic impotence cannot be established solely on the basis of such noninvasive measurements. Although mean PBIs differed significantly between the three groups, there was a great deal of overlap, and several patients were fully potent despite PBIs less than 0.6. Other researchers have similarly confirmed a lack of correlation between PBI and the degree of erectile dysfunction.[16] Although a low PBI is not sufficient to establish the diagnosis of vasculogenic impotence, the finding of a PBI greater than 0.8 confirms the adequacy of penile blood flow and suggests that vasculogenic impotence is extremely unlikely.

DePalma et al.[27] have placed greater emphasis on the diagnostic importance of the penile pulse volume waveform. Using a pneumoplethysmographic cuff containing a pressure transducer, they inflated the cuff to mean arterial pressure and recorded waveforms on a polygraph. A waveform amplitude greater than 6 mm and a systolic upstroke rate of 4 to 6 mm at a chart speed of 25 mm/sec were considered normal. Marked flattening of the waveforms with delayed upstroke greater than 6 mm and rounded waveforms were considered abnormal. Although they noted certain borderline categories in which diagnosis was equivocal, the technique was particularly helpful in cases in which the PBI was between 0.6 and 0.7.

Recently, Lue et al.[28] reported the use of duplex scanning in the evaluation of vasculogenic impotence. Using a high-resolution 10 MHz ultrasound probe, they were able to clearly visualize the cavernous arteries, dorsal veins, tunica albuginea, corpora cavernosa, and corpus spongiosum. The diameter of the arterial lumina, the thickness of the arterial walls, and the quality of their pulsations were assessed before and after papaverine injection. The pulsed Doppler was then used to study the blood flow through each of the penile arteries. Since this test can only be performed on the vessels distal to the pubis, further visualization of the pelvic vasculature with internal pudendal arteriography was required when ultrasonography suggested arterial disease.

Neurologic Testing

Since there are no direct measures of the neural pathways involved in erection, indirect measures must be employed. Fortunately, the autonomic pathways involved in micturition and erection are similar and *cystometrography* with measurement of bladder capacity and residual urine can be used as an indirect measure of penile innervation, assuming that involvement of the appropriate pelvic nerves is reflected by abnormalities in both areas. Using this technique, Ellenberg[17] confirmed neuropathy in 82% of impotent diabetic subjects.

The bulbocavernous reflex may be quantified by indirect measurement of pudendal nerve velocity *(sacral latency testing)*. Since this examination requires electrical stimulation of the penile skin with simultaneous electromyographic recording of the response in the bulbocavernous muscle, it must generally be performed with the patient under general anesthesia. The technique has been modified by using surface-mounted perineal electrodes, thus making measurement of somatosensory-evoked potentials (SEP) from the dorsal penile and posterior tibial nerves more comfortable. Values that are three standard deviations above the mean are considered abnormal.[27]

Intracavernous Papaverine Injection

This technique is useful in differentiating vasculogenic from psychogenic impotence.[12] However, it cannot distinguish psychogenic erectile dysfunction from neurogenic or hormonal impotence. It should be used only to supplement a careful history and physical examination, not to supplant it.

In patients with a penis of average size, 60 mg of papaverine, diluted with 2 to 5 ml of normal saline solution, is injected into the corpus cavernosum. A rubber band is wrapped tightly around the base of the penis before the injection to ensure that most of the drug remains in the corpus and it is left in place for 2 minutes after injection. The dose of papaverine may need to be adjusted in patients with an unusually large or small penis. In patients suspected of neurogenic impotence an initial test dose of 15 mg of papaverine should be used since they are prone to suffer priapism.

After the rubber band is removed, the patient is asked to stand to increase the venous pressure in the pelvis and to further reduce the entry of papaverine into the systemic circulation. If a full erection develops within 10 minutes and if it lasts for more than 30 minutes, the arterial, venous, and sinusoidal mechanisms can be assumed to be normal and vasculogenic impotence can be excluded. However, since a full erection may not develop in a nervous or anxious patient under the conditions of testing, a poor response does not infallibly confirm vasculogenic impotence.[12] When two or more injections fail to produce an adequate erection, an angiogram should be considered.

Angiography

The pelvic vasculature can be visualized using standard angiographic techniques with appropriate oblique projections. This should be the first procedure performed when large-vessel arterial occlusive disease or aortic aneurysm is suspected. Patency of the internal iliac artery on each side should be determined and the presence of significant lesions should be noted. Unfortunately, arteriographic findings correlate poorly with the patient's erectile function. In one study where these were compared, 23% of potent men undergoing aortic operation were noted to have bilateral iliac artery occlusions and an additional 36% had unilateral occlusion.[29] This is not surprising since routine angiograms rarely provide complete definition of the distal penile vasculature and cannot assess the adequacy of collateral blood flow around arterial occlusive lesions.

When no flow-reducing lesions are identified in the hypogastric arteries or their major branches, selective cannulation of the internal pudendal artery with the patient positioned in the appropriate degree of obliquity may be necessary. Since selective cannulation of this vessel may be difficult and the subsequent injection of dye may be painful, such studies are usually performed with the patient under epidural anesthesia.[30] Intra-arterial vasodilators, administered before the injection of contrast material, are important for improving visualization of the penile arteries (Fig. 12-5).

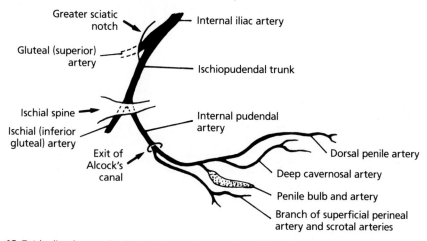

Fig. 12-5. Idealized normal subselective angiogram. Note filling of dorsal and deep penal arteries. The arteries of the corpus spongiosum do not visualize. (From DePalma RG, Emsellem HA, Edwards CM, Druy EM, Shultz SW, Miller HC, Bergsrud D. A screening sequence for vasculogenic impotence. J Vasc Surg 5:228, 1987.)

Corpus cavernosography, which can usually be performed with the patient under local anesthesia, may be used in the assessment of patients with erectile dysfunction, which is thought to be secondary to venous outflow problems. However, pulsed Doppler sonography should routinely be performed in such patients since only those with a normal sinusoidal system and arterial tree will have a good arterial response to papaverine.[12] If a patient does not achieve a full erection, the problem can be attributed to abnormal venous channels rather than to sinusoidal fibrosis. In addition, patients with congenital or acquired chordee may require cavernosography.[31]

PREVENTION

In order to ensure preservation of erectile function, surgical correction of aortoiliac occlusive disease must accomplish the following objectives: minimal disturbance of genital autonomic function, maintenance of adequate pelvic blood flow, and successful revascularization of the ischemic extremity. DePalma[32] has popularized a nerve-sparing approach to the infrarenal aorta that emphasizes approaching the abdominal aorta along its right lateral aspect, minimal division of longitudinal periaortic tissues to the left of the infrarenal aorta, avoidance of dissection at the base of the inferior mesenteric artery, and sparing of the nerve plexus that crosses the left common iliac artery (Fig. 12-6). Using such a nerve-sparing approach, several surgeons have achieved a notable reduction in postoperative impotence.[29,33-35]

Although the findings on preoperative angiograms correlate poorly with erectile function, preservation of adequate perfusion into at least one hypogastric artery appears to be a vital component of all operations that are successful in minimizing iatrogenic erectile dysfunction. When possible, direct antegrade perfusion of the internal iliac artery should be ensured. This may require thromboendarterectomy of the hypogastric artery orifice when appropriate. If

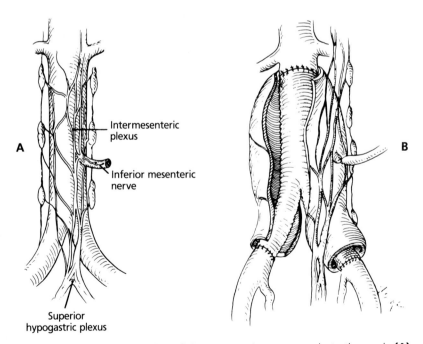

Fig. 12-6. Diagrammatic representation of the autonomic nerve supply to the penis **(A)** and suggested modification of the surgical approach to the aorta during resection of abdominal aortic aneurysms **(B)** to minimize damage to these structures. (From Weinstein MH, Machleder HI. Sexual function after aorto-iliac surgery. Ann Surg 181:787, 1975.)

both external iliac arteries are occluded or stenotic and a bypass into the common femoral arteries is anticipated, proximal aortic anastomosis should be performed in an end-to-side fashion since retrograde perfusion of the internal iliac artery would be impossible in such circumstances and significant reduction of pelvic blood flow would be likely. When proximal disease is so extensive that thromboendarterectomy is impractical and preoperative noninvasive testing has confirmed decreased penile perfusion, simple aortofemoral grafting may not always restore a pelvic collateral blood flow adequate to relieve vasculogenic impotence. Although preoperative recognition of such cases is not easy, when the probability seems likely, the surgeon should consider reimplanting the hypogastric artery into one limb of the aortofemoral graft or adding a jump graft into the distal hypogastric artery.[36]

In patients with unilateral iliac artery occlusive disease, the objectives of nerve sparing, extremity revascularization, and increased hypogastric artery perfusion may all be accomplished using femorofemoral bypass. Several investigators have confirmed the success of this procedure in improving penile blood flow and restoring erection.[25,37] Femorofemoral bypass is especially appropriate for young, sexually active men with unilateral disease since it avoids the necessity for any periaortic dissection.

When direct aortic reconstruction is necessary, it is important to avoid flushing atheromatous debris down the hypogastric artery.[29] Operative technique should be modified to adequately back-bleed the hypogastric arteries before completion of anastomoses. Unfortunately, emergent aortic surgery, such as the resection of a ruptured abdominal aortic aneurysm, rarely allows time for the careful anatomic dissection necessary to avoid nerve damage, and the incidence of iatrogenic impotence is accordingly higher.[38] Although rarely under the control of the vascular surgeon, emergent operations should be avoided whenever possible.

TREATMENT

Once organic impotence is confirmed, a precise etiologic diagnosis is essential before initiating appropriate therapy. If arteriograms confirm occlusion of the proximal pelvic arteries and the measured PBI is less than 0.6, bypass into a distal patent branch of the hypogastric artery on at least one side should be considered. If the PBI is less than 0.6 but no large-vessel occlusive lesions are identified, selective angiograms of the internal pudendal artery may document more distal occlusive lesions. If patent deep penile or dorsal penile arteries can be confirmed, consideration should be given to direct revascularization of the penis using the inferior epigastric artery and microvascular anastomosis into one of these vessels. Although the long-term durability of such procedures has not been documented, initial success has been reported in approximately 70% of such procedures.[39]

When neurogenic impotence is documented, patients may be managed by teaching them to perform self-injection of intracorporal papaverine or by implantation of a suitable penile prosthesis. In hypertensive patients who require ganglion-blocking drugs to control their disease and in whom impotence develops secondary to such medications, alternate forms of treatment should be found. If the hypertension is secondary to renal artery stenosis, renal revascularization should be considered.

RESULTS

In a collected series of 138 patients undergoing aortic reconstruction using standard vascular surgical techniques, Flanigan et al.[29] documented a 25% incidence of iatrogenic impotence. By minimizing periaortic dissection and emphasizing a nerve-sparing technique along with efforts to ensure perfusion of at least one hypogastric artery during the arterial reconstruction, they were able to eliminate this complication. Furthermore, retrograde ejaculation was reduced from 43% in the collected series to only 3% in the control group.

Since 80% of patients who present with aortoiliac arterial occlusive disease have significant erectile dysfunction, careful planning of the operative reconstruction to ensure hypogastric artery perfusion is essential if this symptom is to be relieved. Excluding patients with diabetes mellitus in whom neurogenic impotence is most likely, relief of preoperative erectile dysfunction can be anticipated in 30% of patients so afflicted.[15,29] Half of the patients who regained potency following revascularization were noted to have bilateral iliac artery occlusion on preoperative arteriogram.[29]

CONCLUSION

A multimodal diagnostic approach to the impotent patient is essential to ensure precise etiologic diagnosis and appropriate therapy. Furthermore, an understanding of the multiple factors involved in achieving a normal erection is essential if potency is to be preserved during the course of aortic surgery. Since nearly 25% of patients undergoing direct aortic reconstruction will suffer iatrogenic erectile dysfunction if appropriate technical modifications are not employed, the problem of iatrogenic impotence is not inconsequential. By appropriate nerve-sparing dissection of the infrarenal aorta and preservation of hypogastric perfusion, the postoperative development of erectile dysfunction can be virtually eliminated and improvement in preoperative impotence can be maximized. When postoperative impotence occurs despite every precaution, an attentive and objective approach can offer much comfort to the patient and his sexual partner. In only a small percentage of such cases will additional revascularization be necessary.

REFERENCES

1. Leriche R, Morel A. The syndrome of thrombotic obliteration of the aortic bifurcation. Ann Surg 127:193, 1948.
2. Harris JD, Jepson RP. Aorto-iliac stenosis: A comparison of two procedures. Aust NZ J Surg 34:211, 1965.
3. DePalma RG, Kedia K, Persky L. Vascular operations for preservation of sexual function. In Bergan JJ, Yao JST, eds. Surgery of the Aorta and Its Body Branches. Orlando, Fla.: Grune & Stratton, 1979.
4. Queral LA, Flinn WR, Bergan JJ, Yao JST. Sexual function and aortic surgery. In Bergan JJ, Yao JST, eds. Surgery of the Aorta and Its Body Branches. Orlando, Fla.: Grune & Stratton, 1979.
5. Weiss HD. The physiology of human penile erection. Ann Intern Med 76:793, 1972.
6. Kedia KR, Markland C, Fraley EE. Sexual function following high retroperitoneal lymphadenectomy. J Urol 114:237, 1975.
7. Krane RJ, Siroky MB. Neurophysiology of erection. Urol Clin N Am 8:91, 1981.
8. Willis EM, Ottesen B, Wagner G, Sundler F, Fahrenkrug J. Vasoactive intestinal polypeptide (VIP) as a possible neurotransmitter involved in penile erection. Acta Physiol Scand 113:545, 1981.
9. Adaikan PG, Kottegoda SR, Ratnam SS. Is vasoactive intestinal polypeptide the principal transmitter involved in human penile erection? J Urol 135:638, 1986.
10. Benson GS. Penile erection: In search of a neurotransmitter. World J Urol 1:209, 1983.
11. Conti G. L'erection due penis humain et ses bases morphologico vasculeries. Acta Anat (Basel) 14:17, 1952.
12. Lue TF, Tanagho EA. Physiology of erection and pharmacological management of impotence. J Urol 137:829, 1987.
13. Newman HF, Northrup JD, Devlin J. Mechanism of human penile erection. Invest Urol 1:350, 1964.
14. Michal V, Pospichal J. Phalloarteriography in the diagnosis of erectile impotence. World J Surg 2:239, 1978.
15. May AG, DeWeese JA, Rob CG. Changes in sexual function following operation on the abdominal aorta. Surgery 65:41, 1969.
16. Nath RL, Menzoian JO, Kaplan KH, McMillian TN, Siroky MB, Krane RJ. The multidisciplinary approach to vasculogenic impotence. Surgery 89:124, 1981.
17. Ellenberg M. Impotence in diabetes: The neurologic factor. Ann Intern Med 75:213, 1971.
18. Bohlen JG. Sleep erection monitoring in the evaluation of male erectile failure. Urol Clin N Am 8:119, 1981.
19. Karacan I, Salis PJ, Ware JC, Dervent B, Williams RL, Scott FB, Attia SL, Beutler LE. Nocturnal penile tumescence and diagnosis in diabetic impotence. Am J Psychiatry 135:191, 1978.
20. Canning JR, Bowers LM, Lloyd FA, Cottrell TLC. Genital vascular insufficiency and impotence. Surg Forum 14:298, 1963.
21. Abelson D. Diagnostic value of the penile pulse and blood pressure: A Doppler study of impotence in diabetics. J Urol 113:636, 1975.
22. Britt DB, Kemmerer WT, Robison JR. Penile blood flow determination by mercury strain gauge plethysmography. Invest Urol 8:673, 1971.
23. Gaskell P. The importance of penile blood pressure in cases of impotence. Can Med Assoc J 105:1047, 1971.
24. Kempczinski RF. Role of the vascular diagnostic laboratory in the evaluation of male impotence. Am J Surg 138:278, 1979.
25. Merchant RF Jr, DePalma RG. Effects of femorofemoral grafts on postoperative sexual function: Correlation with penile pulse volume recordings. Surgery 90:962, 1981.
26. Queral LA, Whitehouse WM, Flinn WR, Zarins CK, Bergan JJ, Yao JST. Pelvic hemodynamics after aorto-iliac reconstruction. Surgery 86:799, 1979.
27. DePalma RG, Emsellem HA, Edwards CM, Druy EM, Shultz SW, Miller HC, Bergsrud D. A screening sequence for vasculogenic impotence. J Vasc Surg 5:228, 1987.

28. Lue TF, Hricak H, Marick KW, Tanagho EA. Vasculogenic impotence evaluated by high-resolution ultrasonography and pulsed Doppler spectrum analysis. Radiology 155:777, 1985.

29. Flanigan DP, Schuler JJ, Keifer T, Schwartz JA, Lim LT. Elimination of iatrogenic impotence and improvement of sexual function after aorto-iliac revascularization. Arch Surg 117:544, 1982.

30. Ginestie JF, Romieu A. Radiologic Exploration of Impotence. The Hague: Martinus Nijhoff, 1978.

31. Fitzpatrick T. The corpus cavernosum intercommunicating venous drainage system. J Urol 113:494, 1975.

32. DePalma RG. Impotence in vascular disease: Relationship to vascular surgery. Br J Surg 69:514, 1982.

33. DePalma RG, Levine SB, Feldman S. Preservation of erectile function after aortoiliac reconstruction. Arch Surg 113:958, 1978.

34. Miles JR, Miles DG, Johnson G. Aortoiliac operations and sexual dysfunction. Arch Surg 117:1177, 1982.

35. Weinstein MH, Machleder HI. Sexual function after aorto-iliac surgery. Ann Surg 181:787, 1975.

36. Billet A, Dagher FJ, Queral LA. Surgical correction of vasculogenic impotence in a patient after bilateral renal transplantation. Surgery 91:108, 1982.

37. Schuler JJ, Gray B, Flanigan DP, Williams LR. Increased penile perfusion and reversal of vasculogenic impotence following femorofemoral bypass. Br J Surg 69:67, 1982.

38. Flanigan DP, Pratt DG, Goodreau JJ, Burnham SJ, Yao JST, Bergan JJ. Hemodynamic and angiographic guidelines in selection of patients for femoro-femoral bypass. Arch Surg 113:1257, 1978.

39. Michal V, Kramar R, Hejhal L. Revascularization procedure of the cavernous bodies. In Zorgomotti AW, Rossi G, eds. Vasculogenic Impotence: Proceedings of the First International Conference on Corpus Cavernosum Revascularization. Springfield, Ill.: Charles C Thomas, 1980.

13

Complications Following Juxtarenal and Upper Abdominal Aortic Branch Reconstructions

Ronald J. Stoney   **Chris Cunningham**   **Peter A. Schneider**

This chapter reviews complications occurring after juxtarenal and upper abdominal aortic operations. The usual lesions of these regions are described along with their commonly used primary surgical repairs. The vascular beds at risk during these operations include those of the kidneys, gastrointestinal tract, lower extremities, and spinal cord. The most devastating complications occur to these organs. Detection and management of operative complications are outlined. In addition, a review of the causes of these complications offers an opportunity to avoid their occurrence by using modifications of techniques during the primary operation. Both the prevention and treatment of complications of surgery in this challenging region of the abdominal aorta are addressed.

JUXTARENAL AORTIC DISEASES

Chronic juxtarenal aortic occlusion is the result of obstruction of the distal aorta or iliac arteries with retrograde thrombosis to the immediate subrenal aortic level. This may have been among the first lower abdominal aorta lesions to be managed with temporary suprarenal aortic control. When an infrarenal abdominal aortic aneurysm begins immediately below the renal artery level, there is no surgical neck and juxtarenal aortic management frequently is required. Aortic atherosclerosis involving the renal arteries selectively or in combination with infrarenal aortic disease also is managed as a juxtarenal aortic problem. The primary surgical objectives in the treatment of all these lesions are restoration of lower extremity flow, replace-

ment of the infrarenal aorta, and renal revascularization, or a combination of these. Temporary, obligatory renal ischemia is used to allow (1) removal of a juxtarenal intraluminal aortic thrombus, (2) attachment of a graft to the proximal nonaneurysmal subrenal aorta, or (3) a combined aortic and renal revascularization. The primary vascular beds at risk in these procedures are those of the limbs and kidneys. Colonic ischemia and pelvic ischemia are rare concerns, and their development depends on the status of the visceral arteries and the available collateral circulation.

UPPER ABDOMINAL AORTA AND BRANCH DISEASES

The upper abdominal aorta is susceptible to a varied group of lesions that affect the visceral circulation but they rarely cause simultaneous aortic luminal obstruction. Aortic atherosclerosis may affect the orifice of any or all of the major upper abdominal branches and predictably is located within the first 1 to 2 cm of the origin of the vessel. Aortic aneurysms also involve the upper abdominal aorta as an extension from either above or below. Infrequently these aneurysms have associated atherosclerotic obstruction of the aortic branches but not of the aorta itself. Coral reef atherosclerosis—a rare lesion so named because of its irregular polypoid, calcific, luminal appearance—does obstruct the suprarenal aortic lumen and the visceral branch orifices.

There are several nonatherosclerotic lesions that directly or indirectly impair flow through the upper abdominal aorta or the major aortic branches themselves. These include the middle aortic syndrome, which may be of congenital or inflammatory origin, fibrodysplastic lesions, and visceral artery compression by adjacent ligamentous or neural tissue.

PRIMARY OPERATIONS FOR JUXTARENAL AND UPPER ABDOMINAL AORTIC DISEASES

The operations commonly performed include prosthetic grafting, which is used to improve flow through the aortic branches or the aorta itself, and autogenous grafting (venous), which is routed in a retrograde manner to revascularize the renal arteries.

Thromboendarterectomy of the upper aortic branches through the aorta itself (transaortic visceral endarterectomy) is slowly being adopted by surgeons for treatment of atherosclerotic obstruction alone or in conjunction with an aortic reconstruction. Finally, extrinsic compression of the celiac axis, usually caused by the median arcuate ligament, can be managed by resection of the ligamentous constriction and transarterial dilation of the constricted celiac trunk.

The operative approach to the juxtarenal aorta usually is achieved through a transabdominal infracolic exposure or through the extraperitoneal route. Operations on the upper abdominal aorta may be accomplished using the transcrural route to the supraceliac aorta or using a thoracoabdominal or transabdominal route using left medial visceral rotation. Depending on the postoperative complication under consideration, the surgical route used for the primary operation may be an important factor in management of the problem.

COMPLICATIONS

Complications of all aortic operations can be grouped according to their time of appearance after surgery. *Perioperative* complications occur during or within 24 hours of operation. *Early* complications occur from 1 to 30 days after operation or during the hospitalization. *Late* complications appear remote from an operation, usually 1 or more years later.

Perioperative Complications
Bleeding

Bleeding may originate from vessels encountered during aortic exposure or from the vascular repair itself. When bleeding is undetected during or after the operation, hypovolemia with resulting shock occurs in the early postoperative period. Immediate reoperation and thorough exploration of the operative field allow detection of the bleeding site and simple ligation or suture. Intraoperative bleeding also may result from a coagulopathy associated with depletion or dilution of clotting factors, inadequate component replacement or prolonged hepatic ischemia associated with celiac axis, or supraceliac aortic clamping. Hypothermia may occur during the operation and adversely affect hemostasis. The use of cell mass, fresh frozen plasma, and platelets is an essential component for combating the bleeding state. Reversal of anticoagulants is guided by serial coagulation studies during the operation. Heating the operating room, using a warming blanket for the patient, and warm saline solution irrigation of the operative field are all efficacious. Fibrin glue made from cryoprecipitated plasma and thrombin can be used on oozing surfaces. This produces a thick, clear, jellylike coagulum, which over time or with the use of air drying and heat will become quite adherent and have a dramatic hemostatic effect.

Thrombosis

Thrombosis of any juxtarenal or visceral artery repair can now be detected in the operating room before wound closure. Arteriography has given way to intraoperative duplex scanning or handheld Doppler flow detection (Fig. 13-1). Sensitive ultrasound technology can detect abnormal flow or defects in the reconstruction itself. Defects can be visualized and appropriately repaired intraoperatively, preventing later occlusion and possible organ ischemia. Renal ischemia may be manifested postoperatively by anuria. Ischemic limb pain and paralysis or progressive acidosis and shock indicate failure of the repair and require immediate reexploration and revision.

The release of large emboli during aortic manipulation or clamping can cause serious

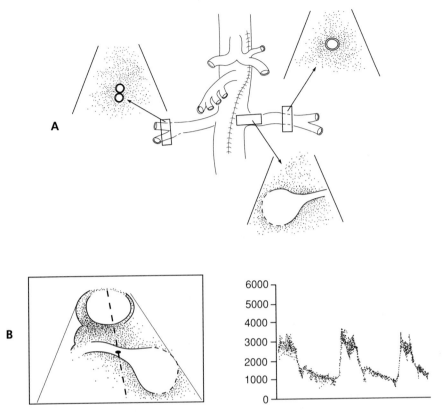

Fig. 13-1. Intraoperative duplex scanning. The combination of high-resolution real-time B-mode imaging and an integrated, pulsed Doppler is employed routinely to ensure the patency of reconstructed visceral and renal arteries. Technical defects can be readily identified and corrected. **A,** A 7.5 mm Hg transducer coupled with the appropriate acoustic gel is covered with a sterile drape to evaluate the reconstructed vessel. **B,** The B-mode image and Doppler waveform confirm the integrity of the reconstruction.

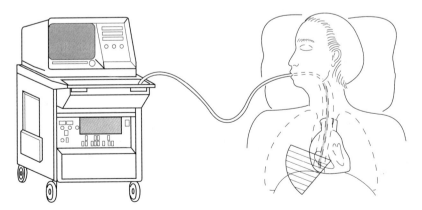

Fig. 13-2. Intraoperative cardiac imaging. Transesophageal two-dimensional echo (TEE) provides constant evaluation of the heart and is a sensitive indicator of wall motion abnormalities and myocardial ischemia. This may be particularly useful during supraceliac or suprarenal aortic cross-clamping in order to optimize the patient's hemodynamic status.

ischemia and present as sudden thrombosis of the reconstruction. Microembolic events resulting from dislodged friable atherosclerotic debris usually from within the aorta itself also may occur during the operation. Depending on the level of origin of embolic fragments, any aortic branch or the distal runoff iliac arteries may be affected. The end organ (gastrointestinal viscera, kidneys, spinal cord, or legs) may be threatened. Subclinical microembolic events probably occur during most aortic operations but go undetected unless they cause significant ischemia. However, ischemia from some microembolic fragments can be disastrous and even fatal. The viscera and lower extremities may survive noncritical ischemia but major or diffuse infarction of critical vascular beds can be lethal since it usually is nonreversible. Renal infarction may lead to an oliguric state, bowel infarction with perforation, vascular collapse, or sepsis, which are catastrophic consequences of microemboli.

Early Complications

Complications appearing within 30 days of operation are usually the result of arterial occlusion. The resulting ischemia may be caused by the embolization of atheromatous debris or clot in distal vascular beds, or by prolonged ischemia in organs at risk during the primary operation. Finally, distal thrombosis of the iliofemoral and femoropopliteal arterial tree beyond the reconstructive site may occur as a consequence of prolonged occlusion of the aorta and stasis in these diseased distal vascular beds. Depending on the time of complication occurrence and the resulting degree of ischemia, intervention may be optional or mandatory. Renal ischemia causing acute tubular necrosis may be supported with dialysis, particularly when the renal failure is nonoliguric in nature and renal perfusion is documented. Lower extremity ischemia may be nonthreatening and resolve, or may require intervention and distal thromboembolectomy or administration of lytic therapy to improve perfusion.

Impaired perfusion of the spinal cord after reconstructions of the upper abdominal aorta results from prolonged clamp ischemia of critical posterior intercostal vessels supplying the terminal cord, embolic occlusion of their ostia by aortic debris, or exclusion of these vessels following the reconstruction itself. There have been no definitive measures yet discovered to prevent these disastrous complications of paraparesis or paraplegia although intrathecal vasodilators, spinal cord drainage and pressure monitoring, reattachment of paired intercostal and lumbar arteries, and the use of somatosensory-evoked potentials have all been suggested as measures to avoid this problem. Once this complication has appeared, treatment is supportive. The patient may achieve independent ambulation with aggressive physical therapy after paraparesis but this rarely, if ever, occurs after profound paraplegia.

Certainly, cardiovascular and pulmonary complications are possible after any major aortic operation and for the most part they occur in the early postoperative period. Aggressive critical care monitoring has become routine following these operations, and prolonged ventilation often is required and may be lifesaving in patients with pulmonary insufficiency. Cardiac risk remains the leading cause of mortality after any aortic operation, but with the aggressive use of intraoperative hemodynamic monitoring and cardiac imaging, these complications now can be reduced to approximately 1% by an experienced anesthesiologist and a surgeon (Fig. 13-2). The use of vasodilators to protect the heart from increased afterload (caused by high aortic clamping), accurate hemodynamic assessment, and blood volume normalization are essential during surgery to minimize myocardial ischemic events. The use of a transesophageal two-dimensional echo allows the detection of segmental wall motion abnormalities that may be caused by myocardial ischemia. Reversal of these wall motion changes usually avoids postoperative myocardial events, whereas persistent intraoperative wall motion abnormalities are highly predictive of a postoperative myocardial infarction.

Infection is always a potential complication of prosthetic reconstructions of the juxtarenal and upper abdominal aortic branches. However, prosthetic graft infection is extremely rare in the early perioperative period and most septic problems that follow any aortic reconstruction appear 1 to 2 years afterward.

A wound infection is the most common septic consequence following aortic reconstruction and rarely involves the reconstruction itself. Management includes exploration of the involved wound, usually the groin, and thorough débridement of necrotic tissue. The wound can be loosely approximated and frequent packing of the superficial wound with Betadine-soaked gauze usually promotes secondary healing without subsequent involvement of the underlying graft.

Late Complications

Complications that appear late, more than 1 month and usually 1 or more years following reconstruction of the juxtarenal or upper abdominal aortic branches, are manifest by ischemia, bleeding, or infection (Table 13-1). They result from abnormal healing of the arterial or prosthetic repair or from the progression of arterial disease. Autogenous (endarterectomy) repairs are susceptible only to ischemia; prosthetic grafts may develop all three complications.

Ischemia

Ischemia following these aortic repairs usually involves the lower extremities and is the immediate result of graft limb or native iliofemoral artery occlusion. The onset, whether abrupt or gradual, may suggest the cause since sudden thrombosis of anastomotic false aneurysm, gradual occlusion of an anastomotic myointimal hyperplasia lesion, or progressive obstruction of the common femoral branches caused by atherosclerosis may all appear similar on examination or aortography.

Graft limb occlusion may result from compression or kinking at the inguinal ligament or redundancy at the graft bifurcation in the abdomen. Bilateral graft limb occlusion suggests either a proximal aortic anastomotic failure or obstruction in the proximal juxtarenal aorta above the graft resulting from an inadequate primary operation.

Ischemia of the kidneys or gastrointestinal tract usually is gradual and silent following aortic branch repair. The cause may be obstruction of the branch repaired by endarterectomy or prosthetic graft. Technical failure, anastomotic myointimal hyperplasia, and progressive disease are indistinguishable until they are observed directly.

Bleeding

Bleeding occurring late after prosthetic aortic reconstruction is rare. The site may be the retroperitoneum adjacent to the reconstruction and the usual cause is rupture of a false aneurysm, which may be infected. Gastrointestinal bleeding may originate in the upper or lower intestines, depending on the site of erosion or fistula formed between the intestine and an adjacent prosthetic graft. Massive hematuria may result from erosion of the ureter by an adjacent graft.

Table 13-1. Presentations of Late Complications of Surgery of the Upper Abdominal Aorta and Its Branches

Ischemia	Bleeding	Infection
Acute lower extremity ischemia	Hemodynamic instability	Wound infection/sinus tract
Lower extremity gangrene	False aneurysm	Fever—unknown etiology
Rest pain	Gastrointestinal bleeding	Gastrointestinal bleeding
Claudication	Intra-abdominal hemorrhage	False aneurysm
Acute intestinal ischemia	Hematuria	Septic emboli
Chronic visceral ischemia		Intra-abdominal abscess
Pancreatitis		Hydronephrosis
Renovascular hypertension		Pyuria
Azotemia		"Incidental" perigraft fluid

Infection

The most dreaded late complication of any prosthetic aortic reconstruction is infection. It can occur anytime but usually appears 1 to 2 years after implantation. It is apparent most often in the groin, where aortic prostheses frequently terminate. Progressive infection of any prosthesis may extend to the suture lines, where dehiscence with bleeding or false aneurysm results. A prosthetic repair confined to the abdomen usually involves the aorta or a major branch. Infection of such a retroperitoneal graft may be chronic and without clinical symptoms or signs. Septic distal emboli or fever of unknown origin should always suggest the possibility of a graft infection.

DETECTION AND MANAGEMENT OF COMPLICATIONS

The major challenge for the vascular surgeon confronted with a possible complication after an operation on the juxtarenal or upper abdominal aorta is to establish an accurate diagnosis. Whenever possible, the status of the operated aorta and its branches should be ascertained. If management of the complication is under the care of the surgeon who performed the original operation, he should review the original operative report and the hospital records. Whenever possible, the original hospital records and preoperative arterial studies should be examined so the treating surgeon is familiar with all details of the original operation as well as the current complication.

Aortography is mandatory for all late complications since many of these occur more than a year after surgery and the arterial anatomy is unknown. Retroperitoneal imaging is essential when infection, anastomotic aneurysm, or organ ischemia is likely. This may be achieved by computed tomography with contrast or magnetic resonance imaging. The perigraft region may contain air or fluid, and the contour of the reconstruction may be abnormal in course or alignment. Solid organ ischemia or infarction may be detected, thus preparing the surgeon to modify the operative plan accordingly.

The major complications that mandate emergent intervention are (1) critical ischemia of the extremities or any organ supplied by the reconstructed aorta and (2) continued hemorrhaging into the gastrointestinal tract from the reconstructed juxtarenal or upper aorta and its branches.

ISCHEMIA

Depending on the extent, degree, and duration of limb ischemia, the management may be elective or emergent based on the viability of the limb. It usually results from a graft limb occlusion. The aortogram confirms the diagnosis and guides the exposure of the distal graft anastomosis and native arteries, which are the important objectives in such an operation. Ischemia of any organ supplied by a prior aortic branch repair may be acute, causing infarction, or chronic, causing renal hypertension or intermittent impairment of the visceral circulation (abdominal angina).

Renal Revascularization

A new graft is used in late failures of aortorenal grafts or endarterectomy. The graft can originate from a replaced aortic graft or alternatively from the supraceliac aorta. In this location the graft limbs are routed behind the pancreas to join the distal renal artery near the renal hilus. Another site for graft origin that may avoid the previously operated pararenal area is the hepatic or splenic arteries. On the right the graft required to reach the renal hilus is short; on the left the splenic artery can be mobilized, transected distally without splenectomy, and positioned for anastomosis to the distal renal artery.

Revascularization by transaortic renal endarterectomy is not applicable if the juxtarenal or pararenal aorta was incorporated in the original reconstruction or if the renal artery continuity was interrupted by a previous graft.

Visceral Revascularization

The retrograde aortovisceral graft is the most common reconstruction to fail and is ideally managed by transaortic visceral endarterectomy. The old graft does not require removal and a durable visceral revascularization can be achieved in a previously undissected portion of the aorta. If bowel viability is questionable, immediate resection or a second look is planned.

The other visceral revascularization that can be used for any noninfective complication is antegrade aortovisceral bypass. The prosthetic graft originates from the supraceliac aorta and the limb(s) is attached to the transected distal celiac and superior mesenteric artery trunks beyond the orifice disease and the failed graft.

The intraoperative plan should provide adequate exposure of the failing reconstruction. The aortic component and the previously reconstructed artery are identified, as well as the termination of the reconstruction in the aortic branch itself. This may permit a determination of the cause of the reconstructive failure and suggest a more effective method of repeat repair, such as endarterectomy or a bypass graft extension or replacement. Since the functional recovery of the threatened organ may not be known at reoperation, aggressive repairs are advocated. Restoration of normal blood flow may result, allowing functional recovery not anticipated preoperatively. If viable, the revascularized kidney can be assessed later to determine its functional recovery. Intestinal viability at the time of reoperation may be incomplete or indeterminate. Nonviable segments always should be resected, whereas marginally viable segments may be retained and reevaluated at a second-look procedure in which a final decision may be more accurate.

BLEEDING

Bleeding related to a previous aortic reconstruction is the result of impaired prosthetic healing or host incorporation. A connection between a graft and the adjacent intestine (prosthetic enteric communication) may cause occult or exsanguinating gastrointestinal hemorrhage. Traditional treatment is used. A remote subcutaneous axillofemorofemoral prosthetic bypass is installed, followed by transabdominal graft removal as a second stage. The bowel is repaired and the aorta proximal to the graft resected or débrided to allow closure of the aortic stump. If the previous graft was anastomosed to the side of the aorta, local endarterectomy of the aortic anastomosis and direct or patch closure are indicated whenever distal aortic flow can be maintained.

Retroperitoneal bleeding late after any prosthetic upper aortic graft repair suggests an anastomotic false aneurysm disruption. This can be the result of occult perigraft infection and may be caused by suture failure or decreased tensile strength of the aortic wall itself. The surgical objective in these repairs is to establish the presence or absence of infection and excise the failed anastomosis and adjacent host aortic tissue. Interposition of a prosthetic graft segment is satisfactory unless infection is found, in which case autogenous repair or remote bypass is used. Occasionally, remote bypass of the upper abdominal aortic graft is not possible. In such instances following extensive soft tissue débridement, a new prosthetic graft is inserted. Long-term antibiotic therapy has resulted in prevention of further graft infection in a select number of these high-risk patients.

Infection complicating a prosthetic aortic graft repair may be associated with gastrointestinal bleeding secondary to graft erosion of the adjacent intestine but more commonly causes a perigraft space infection, often with a groin sinus. Since the majority of patients depend on the graft for limb viability, a substitute remote subcutaneous prosthetic bypass is mandatory, prior to graft removal, to avoid limb ischemia and amputation. Limb perfusion is ensured and chances for contamination by the infected aortic graft are greatly diminished. At the second stage transabdominal removal of the prosthesis and closure of the aortic stump are carried out. If the graft infection involves a prosthesis that is confined to the abdomen and supplies the visceral or renal branches, there are several direct methods of management: (1) the infected graft may be removed without a new graft replacement if there is adequate collateral flow to the vascular bed or organ in question, (2) the infected graft can be removed and replaced with an autogenous graft of native iliac artery or saphenous vein, and (3) the graft can be removed and endarterectomy used to restore flow in the diseased aortic branch that was grafted originally.

CONCLUSION

Complications of juxtarenal and upper abdominal aortic branch revascularization are rare but challenging. Perioperative complications usually are attributed to technical failures and commonly cause bleeding or ischemia due to thrombosis. Early complications (1 to 30 days after surgery) usually are related to ischemia. Late complications occurring 1 or more years after operation are caused by arterial healing abnormalities, anastomotic failures, prosthetic graft infection, or enteric erosion or fistula. Challenging problems in diagnosis and management are reviewed within the context of the type of primary operation that failed. Application of the principles discussed in this chapter should save nearly all the afflicted patients and provide successful treatment of their vascular problems caused by these complications.

14

Renal Revascularization: Errors in Patient Selection and Complications of Operation

James C. Stanley

Renal revascularization is undertaken for two principal reasons: to reduce hypertension and to improve renal function. It most commonly is performed in patients with renal arterial stenoses causing moderate or severe blood pressure elevations. The rate of beneficial responses in patients with severe hypertension ranges from 73% to 96% among different subgroups of properly selected patients.[1] Renal revascularization also may contribute to improved renal function and is of practical clinical importance.[2-4] Renovascular reconstructive procedures have become somewhat standardized, and individualized surgical therapy should be based on the patient's specific type and anatomic pattern of renal artery disease.[5] Because of the high incidence of bilateral disease and the known potential for progression of all forms of renal artery occlusive disease, performing routine nephrectomy in a patient with renal insufficiency clearly is undesirable in the management of renovascular hypertension.

Contemporary experience with renal revascularization justifies a surgical approach to the management of most patients with clinically important renal artery stenoses. Certainly the outcomes of operative therapy are the standard by which other therapeutic modalities must be judged. However, surgical results are often compromised by errors in patient selection and operative complications.[6-10] These latter issues are addressed in this chapter.

PATIENT SELECTION

The prevalence of renovascular hypertension among all patients with diastolic hypertension is less than 5%, although the frequency is higher among pediatric patients, women less than 50 years of age, and patients of both sexes with the onset of hypertension beyond the age of 50 years. Patients in these groups are unlikely to have essential hypertension; because of this fact, they are suspect for secondary hypertension. Clinical manifestations of renovascular hypertension are as varied as the heterogeneic group of diseases producing the stenoses and will result in many errors if used alone as the basis for pursuing diagnostic studies.[11] Nevertheless, patients with renovascular hypertension, when compared with essential hypertensive patients, are more likely to have (1) a negative family history of hypertension, (2) hypertension of shorter duration, (3) accelerated hypertension with grade III or IV retinopathy, and (4) abdominal or flank bruits. Undermining the value of these generalities is the fact that renovascular hypertension can affect both sexes at any age and its severity may range from mild to severe, with control with drug therapy usually possible if diligently pursued. Thus other data, in addition to clinical clues, are needed to establish a diagnosis of renovascular hypertension.

Procedures contributing to the diagnosis of renovascular hypertension may be divided into three categories: (1) functional studies related to diminished blood flow and urine production that are accompanied by reductions in renal mass or decreased clearances of various substances from the bloodstream; (2) tests documenting activation of the renin-angiotensin system with accompanying increased vasopressor activity; and (3) anatomic imaging of the renal artery.[8] No single test has served as a reliable marker to establish the diagnosis of renovascular hypertension. Indeed, the only infallible evidence of renovascular hypertension is the return of blood pressure to normal after a successful renal revascularization or nephrectomy; nevertheless, a thorough understanding of contemporary diagnostic and prognostic investigations for patients suspected of renovascular hypertension becomes critical in clinical practice.

Functional Studies
Hypertensive Urography

Rapid sequence excretory urography is supportive of renal ischemia in the presence of (1) unilateral delays in the appearance of contrast medium in the collecting system, (2) differences in renal length when the right kidney is 1.5 cm smaller than the left or the left is 2 cm smaller than the right, or (3) hyperconcentration of contrast medium in the collecting system on delayed films. In addition, ureteral notching caused by tortuous collateral vessels is an important, although inconsistent, finding of advanced renal artery occlusive disease.

Bilateral functionally important disease in approximately 15% of cases and the existence of segmental disease that does not interfere with the kidney's total excretory function limit the overall sensitivity of urography to 85% at best. The Cooperative Study on Renovascular Hypertension reported abnormal urograms in 78% of patients having renal artery stenoses greater than 50%.[12,13] This was in contrast to abnormal urograms in only 11% of this series' patients having essential hypertension. Most patients with renovascular hypertension in the study had unilateral atherosclerotic lesions, a condition most likely to place the entire affected renal mass at risk for ischemia. At the University of Michigan, Ann Arbor, a 72% fre-

Table 14-1. Hypertensive Urography in Renovascular Hypertension Cured by Surgery*

Condition	Abnormal urogram (%)	Normal urogram (%)
Pediatric disease	24	76
Adult fibrodysplastic disease	47	53
Arteriosclerotic disease	72	28

*Data from Stanley JC, Whitehouse WM Jr, Graham LM, Cronenwett JL, Zelenock GB, Lindenauer SM. Operative therapy of renovascular hypertension. Br J Surg 69:S63-S66, 1982.

quency rate of abnormal urograms among patients with arteriosclerotic disease was similar to that of the cooperative study.[14,15] However, abnormal urograms were evident in only 24% of pediatric and 47% of adult fibrodysplastic renovascular hypertensive patients in the Michigan experience (Table 14-1). Despite an occasional report documenting high specificity of urograms among renovascular hypertensive patients and an unusually low incidence of abnormal studies in essential hypertensive patients,[16] the use of rapid sequence excretory urography is unjustified for routine screening of patients suspected of renovascular hypertension.[17]

Split-Renal Function Tests

Individual kidney *p*-aminohippuric acid (PAH) and inulin clearance rates may be used to assess renal blood flow. However, because of the high incidence of abnormal tests in patients with nonrenovascular parenchymal disease, they have limited diagnostic applicability. The two studies used most often to evaluate renal ischemia are the Howard test, which documents greater sodium and creatinine concentrations and reduced volumes of urine from the ischemic kidney, and the Stamey test, which documents greater concentrations of PAH from the ischemic kidney after a urea-induced diuresis. The Vanderbilt group reported increased sensitivity of split-renal function studies with liberalization of the criteria for a positive test[18,19] (Table 14-2). Although application

Table 14-2. Split-Renal Function Studies in Essential Hypertension and Renovascular Hypertension Cured by Surgery*

Criteria†	Essential hypertension (% positive studies)	Renovasacular hypertension (% positive studies)
Classic	2	50
Half classic	2	72
Lateralizing	10	92

*Data from Dean RH, Rhamy RK. Split renal function studies in renovascular hypertension. In Stanley JC, Ernst CB, Fry WJ, eds. Renovascular Hypertension. Philadelphia: WB Saunders, 1984.
†Definition of criteria: (1) Classic—40% reduction in urine volume, 50% increase in creatinine concentration, 100% increase in PAH concentration; (2) Half Classic—25% reduction in urine volume, 25% increase in creatinine concentration, 50% increase in PAH concentration; (3) Lateralizing—consistent lateralization in each of three collection periods with decrease in urine volume and increase in creatinine and PAH concentrations.

of classic criteria resulted in very few positive studies in patients having essential hypertension, only half of those with renovascular hypertension exhibited positive studies. Use of less rigid diagnostic criteria resulted in greater test sensitivity but was accompanied by appreciable numbers of positive studies in patients without renovascular disease. Thus even though the sensitivity of split-renal function tests may be enhanced by liberalizing the definition of abnormal studies, unacceptably high false-positive rates limit their diagnostic use for renovascular hypertension.

Isotope Renography

Radionuclides provide another noninvasive means of assessing kidney function in suspected cases of renovascular hypertension.[20,21] Isotope renography allows direct imaging of the kidney and provides washout curves of various tracers, with iodine-131 orthoiodohippurate the most common. Such compounds are cleared in a manner reflecting both renal blood flow and excretory function, similar to that of PAH in split-renal function studies.

Unfortunately, false-positive radionuclide studies are common in patients with essential hypertension, with certain states of dehydration and instances of increased renal resistance causing flow abnormalities. Cooperative study data revealed 75% specificity and 76% sensitivity in patients suspected of renovascular hypertension[22] (Table 14-3). Renal perfusion–excretion ratios may enhance the usefulness of radionu-

Table 14-3. Isotope Renography in Essential Hypertension and Renovascular Disease*

Condition	Abnormal renogram (%)†
Essential hypertension	25
Renovascular disease, degree of stenosis	
<50%	44
50%-80%	69
>80%	77
100%	94

*Data from Franklin SS, Maxwell MH. Clinical work-up for renovascular hypertension. Urol Clin North Am 2:301-310, 1975.
†Renograms were abnormal in 76% of all renovascular cases having stenoses >50%.

clide screening for detecting renal ischemia. In more recent times technetium-99m DMSA and ^{99m}Tc DPTA renography has increased the accuracy of measuring differential excretory function. Angiotensin-converting enzyme inhibitors may decrease nuclide uptake in the ischemic kidney and increase the specificity of isotope renography in renovascular hypertension. Unfortunately, standards for use of this latter technology have not been forthcoming, and its widespread use has been limited.

Documentation of Activated Renin-Angiotensin System
Renin Assays

Renin is a proteolytic enzyme released from the juxtaglomerular apparatus of the kidney. In patients with renovascular hypertension this release is likely to occur as a consequence of baroreceptor response to decreased perfusion pressure. Increased sympathetic activity, low sodium level, and low intracellular calcium level also may contribute to renin release but are not considered the dominant causes of hyperreninemia in these patients. Renin acts on renin substrate, an α_2-globulin produced in the liver, to produce angiotensin I, a dectapeptide. This latter substance is converted to angiotensin II, an octapeptide, by converting enzyme. Angiotensin II is a potent vasopressor and is responsible for a vasoconstrictive element in renovascular hypertension. Angiotensin II also results in adrenal gland production of aldosterone, thus increasing sodium retention and contributing to a volume element in renovascular hypertension.

Documentation of excessive renin activity seems logical in establishing the presence of renin-mediated hypertension. Unfortunately, peripheral plasma renin activity has not been a reliable diagnostic finding in cases of suspected renovascular hypertension. In fact, approximately 15% of essential hypertensive patients have high circulating peripheral renins, and nearly 33% of proven renovascular hypertensive patients exhibit normal peripheral renin activity. Some of the latter patients might be identified as having abnormally high renin activity if their peripheral renin levels were indexed to urinary sodium levels. However, the latter procedure requires very careful assessments of sodium balance and withdrawal of certain drugs and has not been used much in clinical practice.

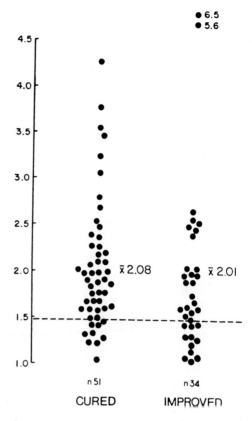

Fig. 14-1. Renal vein renin ratios in 85 patients with renovascular hypertension who responded to surgical intervention. Differences between cured and improved categories were not present. NOTE: 18% of cured and 32% of improved patients had ratios less than 1.48. (From Stanley JC, Gewertz BL, Fry WJ. Renal : systemic renin indices and renal vein renin ratios as prognostic indicators in remedial renovascular hypertension. J Surg Res 20:149-155, 1976.)

Renal Vein Renin Ratios

Comparing plasma renin activity from the effluent venous blood of one kidney to that of the other kidney has relevance in evaluating unilateral renal artery stenotic disease. Quantitation of renin activity in renal venous blood of essential hypertensive patients has revealed that each kidney contributes an average of 24% more renin to its effluent venous blood than it receives in the arterial blood supply.[23] Thus there is 48% more renin in the combined renal venous outflow than in the arterial inflow. A physiologically abnormal renal vein renin ratio

(RVRR) exists when this value becomes greater than 1.48. At this level circulating renin exceeds that which the liver can degrade in a manner to maintain a steady state. Compounding measurements of RVRR are errors incumbent to contemporary renin radioimmunoassays, which usually quantitate angiotensin I levels. Because of these assay errors, an RVRR approaching 2 may be necessary to confirm irrefutably the presence of excessive renin secretion.[24-26]

RVRRs are of limited use in diagnosing renovascular hypertension (Fig. 14-1). Two situations compromise the RVRR as an indicator of renovascular hypertension. First, in approximately 15% of patients there is advanced bilateral disease, causing abnormal elevation of renin production from both kidneys; however, the elevations may occur equally from each side. In these instances the RVRR may be 1, despite marked renin hypersecretion. Second, errors may occur in patients with an unstimulated renin-angiotensin system at the time of sampling. In these circumstances minimal variances in basal physiologic secretion during samplings may result in high ratios that for practical purposes are of no clinical relevance. This potential error may be lessened by stimulation of the renin-angiotensin system before blood sampling. This is usually accomplished by (1) reducing sodium intake to no more than 20 mEq/day for 3 days, (2) administering a natriuretic drug for 3 days, and (3) sampling venous blood from the patient when in the semiupright position. Simultaneous sampling also may lessen errors in these patients but has

proved too cumbersome for routine use. Agents inhibiting renal renin release such as β-adrenergic blockers should be discontinued before sampling blood for these assays. Some have suggested that administering angiotensin-converting enzyme inhibitors may increase the reliability of renin data as a diagnostic test.[27] Confirmation that renin data are more accurate when modified by the latter drugs has not been forthcoming.

Renal : Systemic Renin Indices

Renal:systemic renin indices (RSRI) document each kidney's individual contribution to total circulating renin[26]; thus the RSRI lessens the errors inherent to the RVRR. The RSRI is calculated by subtracting the value of systemic renin activity from that of the renal vein and dividing the remainder by the value of systemic renin activity. Unilateral hypersecretion occurs when the RSRI is greater than 0.48. Functionally important hyperreninemia also exists when the sum of the RSRI from both kidneys exceeds

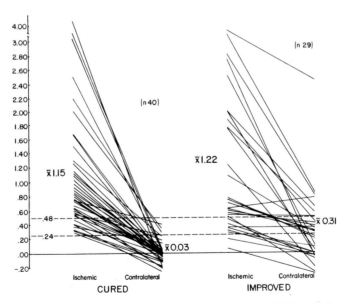

Fig. 14-2. Renal : systemic renin indices in 69 patients, comparing individual renal vein activity to systemic renin activity. Mean ischemic kidney hypersecretion in cured vs. improved groups (1.15 and 1.22, respectively) did not prove statistically different. Contralateral suppression of renin activity was obvious in cured group (0.03) and nonexistent in improved group (0.31). Differences in degree of suppression proved significant ($p < .01$). (From Stanley JC, Fry WJ. Surgical treatment of renovascular hypertension. Arch Surg 112:1291-1297, 1977. Copyright 1977 American Medical Association.)

0.48, even though either kidney's RSRI might be less than 0.48. In patients with unusually high levels of circulating renin, the upper limits of a normal RSRI may be less than 0.48.[23] Ischemic kidney renin hypersecretion (RSRI >0.48) with contralateral kidney renin suppression (RSRI approaching 0) allows determination of which patients who will be cured from those who will be improved after the operation[14,26,28] (Fig. 14-2). However, because of inconsistencies in patient preparation, variations in radioimmunoassay, and sampling errors, the diagnostic sensitivity of RSRI data is imperfect. Approximately 10% of known renovascular hypertensive patients do not exhibit abnormal ischemic kidney renin release, and 8% of patients who are cured fail to exhibit contralateral kidney renin suppression.[14] Although the RSRI represents an important refinement in the interpretation of renin activity, rigid application of this test to clinical decision-making is inappropriate.

Angiotensin-Converting Enzyme Inhibitors

In the past it was hoped that the presence of renovascular hypertension could be documented by inhibiting the converting enzyme with drugs and quantitating subsequent diminutions in blood pressure.[29] Unfortunately, the specificity of such diagnostic studies using converting enzyme inhibitors has proved unacceptable, primarily because these agents frequently decrease blood pressure in nonrenovascular hypertensive patients. This decrease occurs because converting enzyme is identical to kinase II, which is responsible for degradation of bradykinin. Thus administration of converting enzyme inhibitors results both in excess accumulations of vasodepressor bradykinin and in reductions in angiotensin II. The limited usefulness of these drugs as diagnostic agents does not lessen their value in treatment. However, an important complication of using converting enzyme inhibitors therapeutically is deterioration of renal function in patients with bilateral renal artery occlusive lesions or in those with a solitary kidney harboring a stenotic renal artery.[30] Whenever an abrupt decline in renal function occurs in patients administered converting enzyme inhibitors, renovascular hypertension should be suspected.

Renal Artery Imaging
Conventional Arteriography

Anatomic definition of diseased renal arteries is accomplished best by aortography and selective renal arteriography. The morphologic appearance of renal artery stenotic disease has prognostic implications, with considerable differences between arterial fibrodysplasia and spill-over aortic arteriosclerosis. More important are the diagnostic implications of certain anatomic arteriographic findings. Specifically, the presence of collateral vessels circumventing a stenosis is evidence of the hemodynamic importance of such a lesion (Fig. 14-3). Furthermore, existence of collaterals implies that the underlying stenosis is functionally important. Pressure gradients of approximately 10 mm Hg across a stenosis are necessary for collateral development, and this same degree of pressure change can cause excessive renin release from the kidney. Pharmacoangiographic manipulation of the renal circulation may facilitate visualization of collateral vessels and allow docu-

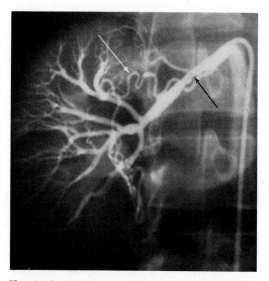

Fig. 14-3. Selective renal arteriogram revealing a benign-appearing stenosis (black arrow) associated with a large collateral vessel circumventing the lesion (white arrow) that documents the stenosis' hemodynamic significance.

mentation of otherwise equivocally important stenotic disease.[31] These latter studies can document functionally important stenoses if selective renal artery infusions of acetylcholine or epinephrine reverse blood flow in nonparenchymal branches originating beyond the stenosis.

Standard anteroposterior aortography may result in interpretive errors regarding the presence or absence of proximal renal artery disease. Oblique views often are required to demonstrate such lesions or distal segmental dysplastic disease. Renal artery origins are best demonstrated using the right posterior oblique projection, and studies without this view are incomplete.[32]

Digital Subtraction Arteriography

Computerized enhancement of radiographic images after intravenous administration of contrast agents initially was proposed as an accurate screening test for renal artery disease causing renovascular hypertension.[33,34] The sensitivity of these studies, approximately 80%, is limited. Unfortunately, ostial or segmental disease often is not evident because of the limited resolution of existing technology or the presence of overlying intestinal vessels. False-positive results occur in approximately 5% of studies. Because of these factors, intravenous digital subtraction studies are used less frequently in current times.

In contrast, intra-arterial digital subtraction angiography provides excellent definition of the main and proximal segmental renal vessels and often offers resolution of vascular detail comparable to that of conventional angiography. An important plus for intra-arterial digital subtraction arteriography is the smaller amounts of contrast agents administered, thus lessening the risk of contrast nephrotoxicity. The latter consideration is very important in the assessment of diabetic and azotemic patients.

Vascular Ultrasonography

Duplex scanning of the proximal renal arteries has been proposed as a reasonable means of recognizing stenotic disease.[35,36] Perhaps more important than confirming the presence of re-

nal artery occlusive disease is the exclusion of such disease in patients suspected of renovascular hypertension. At the present time the usefulness of this study as a diagnostic test has not been determined. The accuracy of deep abdominal ultrasonography of the aorta and its visceral branches often is technician dependent, yet the noninvasive aspects of this test offer great appeal for screening programs.

Assessments in Azotemic Patients

Patients in moderate or severe renal failure who are undergoing renal revascularization have much greater morbidity and mortality rates than those with normal or minimally compromised renal function.[37] Most patients with impaired renal function caused by diminished blood flow have severe stenotic lesions affecting their entire renal mass. Renal insufficiency and secondary hypertension as a complication of chronic total renal artery occlusion may occur in as many as 60% to 75% of patients.[4,38] Guidelines for assessing the potential value of renal revascularization in azotemic patients have not been defined fully.

Decreased kidney size is a known consequence of renal ischemia and deserves comment. This decrease may be a reflection of simple reductions in renal blood volume, reversible atrophy, or progressive cellular damage and fibrosis. Size alone is not a valid criterion by which to predict the response to surgical therapy. Indeed, small kidneys less than 9.5 cm in length may be revascularized successfully, resulting in improved renal function 50% of the time and a lessening of the hypertensive state 90% of the time.[4] The absolute minimal length of a retrievable ischemic kidney has not been defined but is approximately 7 cm in the average-sized adult. Kidneys smaller than this probably have incurred irreparable ischemic cortical injury. Intraoperative biopsy may reveal irreversible ischemic changes, including obliteration of all glomeruli, interstitial fibrosis, and loss of tubules. However, biopsies directed toward areas of ischemic injury may reveal mixed findings, including those of reversible atrophy. Because of such inconsistencies, biopsies alone are rarely the basis for choosing between nephrectomy and revascularization. Preoperative and intraoperative arteriography may predict accurately the potential for successful renal revascularization. Evidence of severe intraparenchymal arterial obstructions, extensive "pruning" of cortical vessels resulting from nephrosclerosis, or multiple infarctions often lends support to the performance of nephrectomy rather than revascularization.

General Sorting Strategy

Most contemporary diagnostic and prognostic studies in patients suspected of renovascular hypertension have limitations. Application of clinical and laboratory clues to patients with moderate or severe hypertension allows identification of candidates for arteriographic studies (Fig. 14-4). An algorithm is established that provides for the later use of renin assays as a means of identifying patients with important renal artery occlusive disease that otherwise appears equivocal on arteriographic studies. Although the specificity of many tests appears high, their sensitivity is not. Given the low prevalence of renovascular hypertension in the general population, most diagnostic studies have a very limited predictive value as screening tests. Interestingly, most large surgical series report beneficial outcomes after operative therapy that exceed 90%. Given the limited sensitivity of current diagnostic testing, this suggests that hypertensive patients with renovascular occlusive lesions are going unrecognized.

Another approach to establishing the diagnosis of renovascular hypertension is the use of a scoring system combining (1) one study related to renal excretion such as hypertensive urography, split-renal function tests, or isotopic renography, (2) another test related to anatomic studies such as conventional arteriography or digital subtraction arteriography, and (3) a physiologic test concerning angiotensin II generation such as peripheral renin activity related to urinary sodium or renal : systemic renin indices. Unfortunately, no scoring system using various combinations of studies assessing these different aspects of renal ischemia has been forthcoming.

COMPLICATIONS

Recurrent or persistent renovascular hypertension and kidney-threatening complications from earlier renal revascularizations usually necessitate reoperation. Patients subjected to such secondary operations usually present difficult

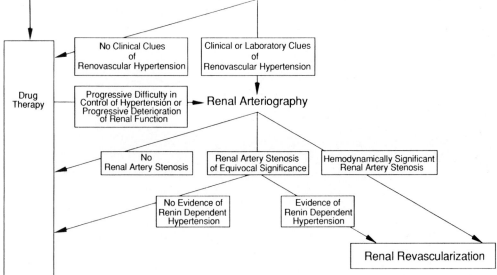

Fig. 14-4. Algorithm for management of renovascular hypertension.

management problems. The largest published experience on reoperative renovascular surgery is from the author's institution in which 72 secondary procedures for complications of prior renal artery reconstructive surgery were undertaken in 58 patients from 1961 to 1983.[10] Eventual benefits regarding hypertension were afforded 91% of these patients, and only one death occurred among the 72 patients. The 1.4% operative mortality rate in this series is more representative of contemporary practice than the 28% mortality rate accompanying reoperation in the cooperative study.[37]

Reoperative renal revascularizations often present formidable technical problems. However, this must not be viewed as a worse-case scenario to support nonsurgical management of renovascular hypertension but instead should be viewed in the overall context of contemporary surgical therapy of this disease. For instance, in a more recent Michigan experience the frequency of secondary operations was nearly half the previously reported rate of reoperation.[10] This is particularly noteworthy in that recently the extent of disease has been greater and technical details of the initial operation much more demanding than in earlier experiences.

Secondary renovascular procedures are complicated by two major factors. First, reoperation usually necessitates dissection in an operative field obscured by fibrous scar tissue. That this represents a commonly encountered feature of these secondary operations is an understatement. In such cases use of intraoperative Doppler ultrasonography to identify small arteries may be required to lessen the risk of vascular injury accompanying dissection. The second major complicating factor is that only a few millimeters of artery distal to the primary revascularization may be available as an entry point for the repeat revascularization. This situation is more likely to occur with reoperations for fibrodysplastic renovascular hypertension, the disease entity most often subject to secondary procedures.

Because the risks of reoperation are considerable, these procedures should be contemplated only when recurrent or persistent postreconstructive hypertension or in some cases deterioration in renal function has been documented as a consequence of an inadequate primary operative procedure.[7,10] Many complications requiring reoperation in the past occur rarely in contemporary practice. Nevertheless, the spectrum of complications with renal artery recon-

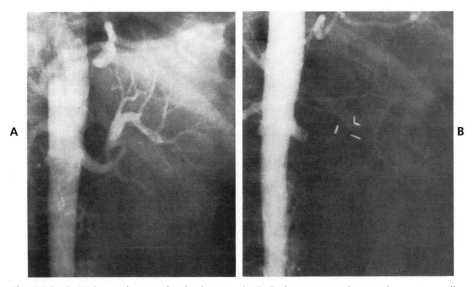

Fig. 14-5. A, Main renal artery dysplastic stenosis. **B,** Early postoperative arteriogram revealing ligated proximal renal artery and total occlusion of aortorenal bypass graft.

structions warrants the attention of all surgeons caring for patients with renovascular hypertension.

Acute Renal Arterial Graft Thrombosis and Stenosis

Early occlusion of aortorenal, iliorenal, hepatorenal, or splenorenal bypasses can occur with grafts of either autologous tissue or synthetic material (Fig. 14-5). The reported incidence of this complication is approximately 8% with vein grafts and slightly higher with synthetic prostheses. The current frequency of this event at our institution is less than 2%. Most graft thromboses occurring in the perioperative period are related to technical mishaps. Intimal flaps and dissections at the distal anastomosis

are the most common causes of these failures. Intimal thickening is present in most renovascular hypertensive patients as a consequence of turbulent flow beyond the stenotic lesions, and it predisposes the patient to these disruptions and dissections.

Distal graft–to–renal artery anastomotic stenoses are most often caused by faulty technique. Recognition of this type of narrowing necessitates early reintervention and refashioning of the anastomosis or performance of a patulous vein patch angioplasty at the anastomosis (Fig. 14-6). Delayed reoperation in these cases carries increased risks in that cicatricial formation associated with healing makes late dissection exceedingly difficult.

Creation of end-to-end ovoid distal anasto-

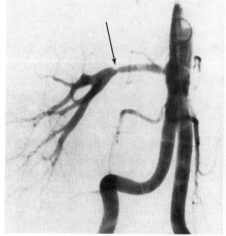

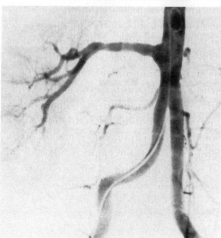

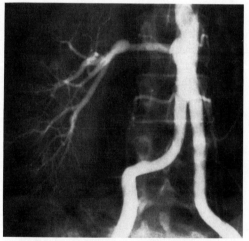

Fig. 14-6. A, Early postoperative arteriogram documenting distal anastomotic stricture (arrow) in a patient with fibrodysplastic renal artery disease who underwent aortorenal bypass with reversed autogenous saphenous vein. **B,** Arteriographic study 1 week after reoperation with vein patch angioplastic repair of anastomotic stricture. Note the generous character of the patch graft. **C,** Arteriographic study at 12 months documenting normal appearance of reconstruction. (From Stanley JC, Whitehouse WM Jr, Zelenock GB, et al. Reoperation for complications of renal artery reconstructive surgery undertaken for treatment of renovascular hypertension. J Vasc Surg 2:133-144, 1985).

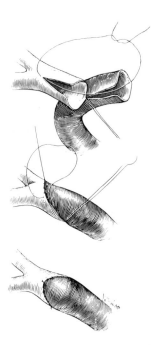

Fig. 14-7. Technique of end-to-end graft–to–renal artery anastomosis following spatulation of both conduits to facilitate creation of a generous ovoid anastomosis. (From Stanley JC, Graham LM. Renal artery fibroplasia and renovascular hypertension. In Rutherford RB, ed. Vascular Surgery, 2nd ed. Philadelphia: WB Saunders, 1984, pp 1145-1162).

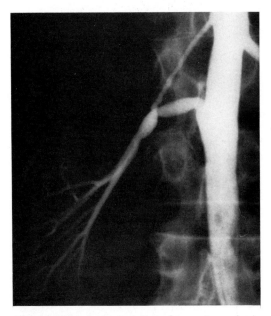

Fig. 14-8. Marked angulation of an aortorenal vein graft at distal end-to-side anastomosis.

moses by spatulation of both the graft and renal artery may lessen the frequency of early graft thromboses. These anastomoses are facilitated if the graft conduit is spatulated posteriorly and the renal artery anteriorly. Visualization of the renal vessel's interior with more precise placement of individual sutures is possible with this technique of end-to-end anastomosis (Fig. 14-7). Use of fine monofilament polypropylene suture is preferred. Excessive traction on this type suture should be avoided because it could cause "pursestring" constrictions of these anastomoses. End-to-side distal anastomoses are accompanied more commonly by kinking (Fig. 14-8) and are not favored in contemporary practice.

Severe aorta-to-graft angulation may compromise blood flow and represents an uncommon early complication of renal revascularization. Although excessive graft tension should be avoided, redundant graft lengths, especially with ptotic kidneys, may produce graft buckling and twisting (Fig. 14-9); thus particular attention should be directed toward the intraoperative positioning of grafts so that patency will not be compromised when patients assume an upright posture. Immediate correction of positioning abnormalities is preferable to reoperation. Certain aorta-graft anastomotic problems are lessened with the use of a "branch-patch" anastomosis. In this technique the saphenous vein used for bypass is removed with a branch inferiorly. Incision of this branch into the main trunk of the vein provides a generous anastomotic circumference (Fig. 14-10). This procedure facilitates a more perpendicular origin of the vein from the aorta and lessens the risk of acute proximal graft angulations.

Occasionally, conduits chosen for reconstructions are diminutive in size, and early thrombosis is more likely. Autogenous veins with diameters less than 4 mm and prosthetic materials with diameters less than 6 mm should not be used for main renal artery reconstructions. However, autologous veins of smaller diameters may be satisfactory for reconstruction of segmental vessels. Thromboses of arterial autografts, regardless of their size, are very uncommon.[39-41] Similarly, early splenorenal or hepatorenal bypass failures are unusual when preexistent celiac or splenic arterial narrowings

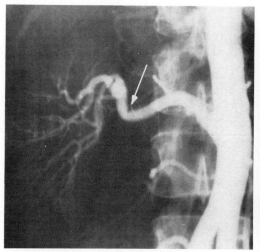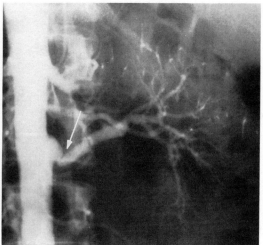

A   B

Fig. 14-9. A, Redundant saphenous vein–aortorenal graft resulting in sharp angulation distally (arrow). **B,** Proximal angulation of aortorenal vein graft (arrow) secondary to improper aortic anastomosis.

are not present.[42,43] Use of small-caliber prosthetic grafts for distal revascularizations has a high incidence of early occlusion.

Early thromboses of aortorenal grafts are sometimes quite obvious during the initial operative procedure. Doppler assessment of blood flow in arteries beyond the anastomosis or direct evaluation of the anastomoses by intraoperative duplex scanning in more subtle cases of occlusion or stenosis should afford more frequent recognition of correctable problems accompanying inadequate reconstructions.[44] More often occlusions become apparent during the immediate postoperative period, with persistent or early recurrence of diastolic hypertension. Hematuria may follow graft occlusion if the occlusion is associated with thromboembolization. However, this is not a universal finding. To the contrary, hematuria may accompany successful revascularizations as a result of insignificant operative renal parenchymal or collecting system trauma. Intravenous urograms or nuclide renograms and renal scans are of little value in determining graft patency in the early postoperative period. The latter studies may reveal relatively normal renal function and perfusion patterns in many patients with occluded grafts because of their extensive preexisting collateral circulation. Arte-

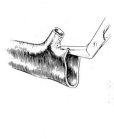
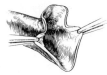
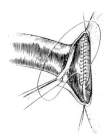

Fig. 14-10. Technique of end-to-side, graft-to-aorta anastomosis after creation of a common orifice between the branch lumen and central lumen of the saphenous vein. (From Stanley JC, Messina LM. Renal artery fibrodysplasia and renovascular hypertension. In Rutherford RB, ed. Vascular Surgery, 3rd ed. Philadelphia: WB Saunders, 1989, p 1258.)

riography is mandatory to diagnose early graft occlusion and should be undertaken without delay in instances of suspected early graft failure. Immediate anticoagulation and reoperation should be contemplated when this complication is recognized. Re-revascularization in situ is usually possible, although management of segmental vessel thromboses may require ex vivo repair.

Acute Postendarterectomy Arterial Thrombosis

Endarterectomy for renal or aortorenal arteriosclerotic occlusive disease is a durable means of renal revascularization in properly selected patients.[45,46] Arteriosclerosis at renal artery orifices is similar to that affecting other muscular vessels, and plaques extending for limited distances into this artery are common. Hazards of endarterectomy include arterial occlusions, which may be caused by excessive clot deposition on the exposed thrombogenic media or dissections of distal intimal flaps, and bleeding from an endarterectomy plane that is too deep. The incidence of postendarterectomy renal artery thrombosis is approximately 2%, and hemorrhage is rare.

Transaortic endarterectomy, either through the transected aorta during aortic reconstruction or through a "trap-door" aortotomy beginning lateral to the superior mesenteric artery on the left and extending anteriorly between both renal arteries, is the most common type of renal artery endarterectomy. Plaque extraction without visualization of the distal end-point of disease is often necessary during these procedures. Despite this limitation, a transaortic approach often is preferable to an axial arteriotomy limited to the renal vessels or to a transverse midrenal aortotomy extended onto the proximal renal arteries. The latter often requires patch-graft angioplasty of the renal arteries to prevent suture line stricture or vessel kinking. Although a direct approach to the renal artery facilitates completion of the distal endarterectomy, it entails a greater risk of renal ischemia and potential arterial narrowing with closure.

Operative arteriography may document dis-

tal intimal flaps or dissections, but it is not routinely used by those experienced in renal artery endarterectomy. Intraoperative duplex scanning may provide a better means of assessing the technical adequacy of renal artery endarterectomy.[44] Recognition of acute renal artery occlusion after endarterectomy warrants early reoperation. Re-revascularization using a conventional aortorenal bypass is most often undertaken in these secondary procedures unless a well-localized intimal flap is identified. In the latter circumstances an axial renal artery arteriotomy is performed; after the obstructing material is removed, the vessel is closed, usually with a vein patch.

Acute Arterial Thrombosis After Operative Dilation

Intraoperative dilation with advancement of rigid dilators through an open arteriotomy has proved useful, especially in the treatment of intraparenchymal stenoses caused by intimal fibroplasia. Complications of this technique have not been described in the literature but do occur. At the author's institution one insignificant dissection was identified among 28 patients undergoing either dilation alone or adjunctive dilation as part of a conventional bypass procedure.

Complications incumbent to arterial dilation are associated primarily with intimal flaps and occasional subintimal dissections. Small dilators may penetrate the intima and pass with relative ease into the vessel wall. To avoid these complications, dilators 2 mm in diameter or smaller should not be used. Similarly, excessively large dilators may be associated with intimal drag and may produce disruption of the inner vessel wall. Risks of vessel wall disruption may be lessened by using dilators not more than 1 mm larger than the normal renal vessel and by using lubricants such as a fine silicone solution to facilitate passage of the dilators. The presentation of thromboses after dilation is similar to that of acute occlusions after a bypass or endarterectomy. However, thromboses are more difficult to manage. These complications may require ex vivo reconstruction and frequently lead to partial or total nephrectomy.

Acute Occlusion After Renal Artery Resection and Aortic Reimplantation or Primary Reanastomosis

Resection of a stenotic renal artery and reimplantation of the vessel into the aorta or primary anastomosis of the artery's ends may be accompanied by anastomotic stricture and early occlusion (Fig. 14-11). A need for more extensive resection than indicated by arteriographic studies often contributes to this problem. Creation of generous ovoid anastomoses may be difficult under these circumstances because arterial ends may not be easily spatulated and approximated without excessive anastomotic tension. Occasionally, redundant vessels will allow successful completion of this form of renal revascularization, and in at least one report implantation was performed without any subsequent abnormalities noted arteriographically.[2] In the case of focal ostial stenoses in the pediatric-aged group, aortic reimplantation of the spatulated proximal renal artery may be preferable to more conventional bypass procedures because of complications associated with the latter.

Anastomotic strictures associated with reanastomosis or aortic reimplantation may be recognized intraoperatively or during the early postoperative period. Early intervention is necessary to prevent this complication from being compounded by late fibrosis around an already compromised anastomosis. Reoperation with conventional aortorenal bypass may be required in these patients. Percutaneous transluminal dilation during the early postoperative period should not be undertaken because of the risk of anastomotic disruption.

Perioperative Intraparenchymal Renal Arterial Thrombosis

An unusual but serious cause of renal revascularization failure is intraparenchymal thrombosis during an otherwise successful reconstruction (Fig. 14-12). A recognized cause of this complication is inadequate anticoagulation during the time of renal blood flow interrup-

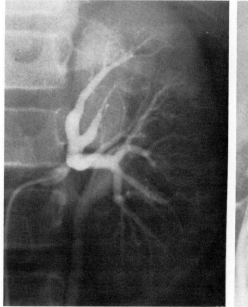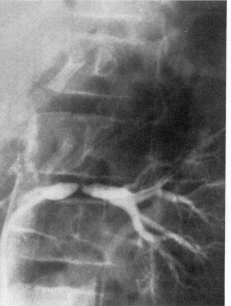

Fig. 14-11. A, Dysplastic stenosis at origin of primary segmental vessels. Poststenotic dilatation of superior polar vessels is evident. Obstructing lesion was resected and a primary end-to-end reanastomosis performed. **B,** Early postoperative arteriogram documenting high-grade anastomotic stricture with nonvisualization of superior pole vessels.

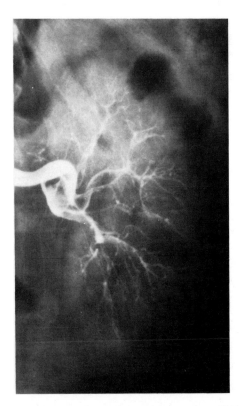

Fig. 14-12. Extensive intra-arterial thrombus within parenchymal vessels secondary to inadequate anti-coagulation therapy.

tion. Systemic anticoagulation with heparin is preferred to regional anticoagulation. The author recommends intravenous administration of 150 U/kg of sodium heparin. The local anticoagulant effect of regionally administered heparin frequently is lost with the abundant collateral circulation, causing an early washout of this drug from within the kidney. Early graft thromboses occur nearly twice as often after the use of regional anticoagulation compared with that after the use of systemic anticoagulation.[47]

Embolization of debris from proximal arteriosclerotic aortic or renal lesions during the operation and dislodged thrombi from surfaces of newly placed grafts may be responsible for other early intraparenchymal occlusions. Administration of antiplatelet agents during the immediate postoperative period may reduce the frequency of this complication, although

their efficacy remains undocumented. A less common cause of intraparenchymal thrombosis is trauma to vessels beyond the reconstruction. Use of miniature microvascular clamps or gentle traction slings rather than standard macrovascular clamps should lessen the likelihood of clamp-induced traumatic occlusions.

Renal infarction caused by intraparenchymal occlusions may be tolerated without undue consequences if limited to a small segment of the kidney. Unfortunately, most patients undergoing an operation for stenotic renal artery disease have abundant collateral vessels that prevent infarction and maintain the viability of parenchymal tissue distal to acute segmental occlusions. This ischemic tissue is often the source of continued renin release, resulting in persistent secondary hypertension. Nephrectomy or segmental kidney resections may be necessary if these patients are eventually to become normotensive. Fibrinolytic agents currently do not have an accepted role in the management of major perioperative thromboses affecting the kidney because of the serious hemorrhagic complications associated with their use.

Renal Failure After Renal Revascularization

Serious reductions in renal function are unusual after uncomplicated renal revascularizations. Complicated reconstructions accompanied by intraoperative hypotension and prior renal parenchymal disease are associated more often with this problem. The preexisting collateral circulation usually ensures adequate perfusion of the kidney during the time required to undertake a reconstruction. Clamping the main renal artery in this setting for 60 to 90 minutes rarely is associated with clinically significant renal dysfunction. However, if collateral vessels are interrupted during the operation or if significant systemic hypotension develops, renal perfusion may become marginal, with resultant glomerular and tubular injury.

Preoperatively, fluid balance should be assessed carefully in renovascular hypertensive patients. Many of these patients have contracted intravascular volumes as a result of long-term diuretic therapy. In addition to adequate preoperative and intraoperative hydration, administration of mannitol or a loop diuretic at the time of renal artery occlusion has been advocated. Such a maneuver appears to provide some protection against kidney injury if severe hypoperfusion occurs.

In contrast to in situ revascularizations, transient deterioration of renal function is common following ex vivo vascular repairs. This result has been attributed to the potentiation of ischemia with the disruption of collateral circulation in these cases. This transient deterioration is of little clinical importance with successful reconstructions.[48-50] However, early failures of ex vivo repairs after disruption of major collaterals may result in irreparable renal ischemia and loss of the kidney.

Acute Renal Venous Injury

Intraoperative tears of the renal vein requiring ligation represent an additional complication of renovascular surgery that leads to decreased renal function. This is particularly true if the right renal vein is interrupted or compromised significantly during the revascularization. Division of the left renal vein, because of its more numerous collaterals, may be of less importance, although doing so is not advised during renal artery reconstructive surgery. A nephrotic-like syndrome with proteinuria and hypertension, usually of brief duration, often accompanies acute renal vein occlusions. Although major segmental renal vein branches may be sacrificed with little effect during the course of reconstructing distal renal arteries, this practice should be discouraged unless absolutely necessary.

Late Aortorenal Graft Stenoses

Anastomotic strictures have become less common with improved vascular surgical techniques. In particular, creation of an ovoid end-to-end anastomosis with a circumference greater than that of the recipient artery has reduced the incidence of subsequent distal anastomotic strictures. During the early era of renovascular surgery distal anastomoses often were performed with no consideration for the inevitable anastomotic constriction accompanying the normal healing process. Use of interrupted sutures for pediatric reconstructions also has been important in lessening anastomotic narrowings and allows for unimpeded vessel growth in these young patients.[51,52]

Accumulation of dysplastic fibrous tissue around an anastomosis is another common cause of late graft stenosis (Figs. 14-13 and 14-14). Factors contributing to this complication are poorly understood. Turbulent flow with continual deposition of thrombus on a denuded graft or vessel surface may be important. The role of antiplatelet agents in lessening this complication is ill defined, although certain patients may benefit from this preventive therapy.

Three other specific operative events may lead to late graft stenoses. The first relates to graft trauma, especially application of clamps on autologous vein or artery conduits. The practice of completing an aortic anastomosis before the renal reanastomosis and then occluding the proximal graft while restoring aortic blood flow should be discouraged. The deleterious consequences of clamp placement on vein grafts has been well documented (Fig. 14-15). Similarly, overzealous use of dilators in treating stenoses or "sounding" segmental vessels beyond the site of anastomosis should be avoided. As is the case with external trauma, progression of fibrotic stenoses has been observed in arteries subjected to excessive intraluminal dilator trauma (Fig. 14-16). A second technical cause of late graft stenoses is related to a fibroproliferative process originating from a surrounding hematoma (Fig. 14-17). In addition to the constrictive effect as the hematoma becomes organized, a blood clot around vein grafts impedes neovascularization of these vessels; in such cases graft ischemia may occur and contribute to later narrowing. Meticulous hemostasis is mandatory to prevent this complication. This is particularly true if grafts are carried behind the vena cava where this complication seems to occur most often. The third operative event leading to late failures is graft malpositioning, resulting in sharp angulations. Progressive fibrous changes within the conduit, perhaps associated with turbulent flow, are apparent consequences of this complication.

Vein graft stenoses of varying degrees are relatively common postoperative findings.[53]

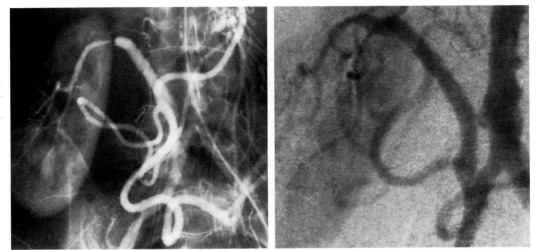

Fig. 14-13. A, Postoperative appearance at 124 months of iliorenal autogenous saphenous vein bypass to segmental renal artery demonstrating high-grade distal anastomotic stricture. A large collateral artery within the mesenteric circulation also is apparent. **B,** Digital subtraction arteriogram revealing satisfactory vein patch angioplasty of the distal stricture 1 week post-operatively.

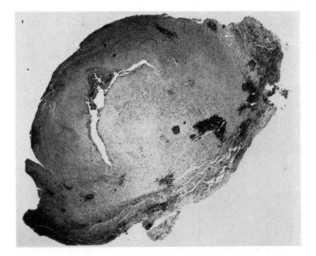

Fig. 14-14. Microscopic section of late vein graft stenosis revealing marked intimal fibroplasia causing near obliteration of lumen (hematoxylin-eosin stain, x16). (From Stanley JC, Ernst CB, Fry WJ. Fate of 100 aortorenal vein grafts: Characteristics of late graft expansion, aneurysmal dilatation, and stenosis. Surgery 74:931-944, 1973.)

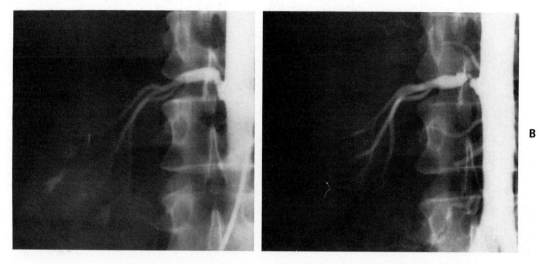

Fig. 14-15. A, Appearance of aortorenal graft immediately postoperatively. **B,** Late arteriographic evidence of proximal vein graft stenosis secondary to clamp trauma during implantation.

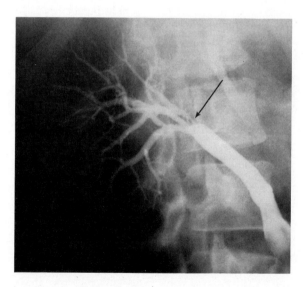

Fig. 14-16. Arteriographic appearance of segmental renal artery stenosis (arrow) secondary to trauma from operative passage of dilators.

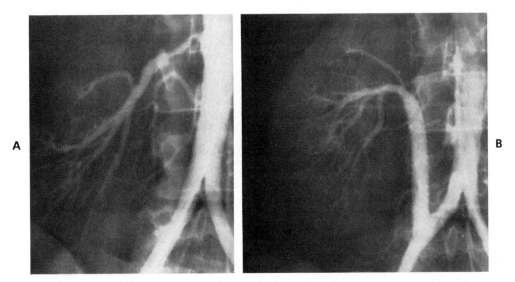

Fig. 14-17. A, Segmental stenosis of proximal aortorenal vein graft secondary to perigraft hematoma and fibrosis. **B,** Appearance after re-revascularization.

Late arteriographic studies have demonstrated development of clinically serious stenoses in 8% of aortorenal vein grafts.[47] Proximal vein graft stenoses are more common than distal stenoses. As might be anticipated, prosthetic grafts, in comparison to vein grafts, are more likely to become thrombosed long after implantation. Similarly, late occlusions after endarterectomy are unusual,[45,53] and late stenoses with arterial autografts are rare.[39,41,54]

Late graft strictures, regardless of the cause, usually are manifest by recurrent hypertension. Total occlusions are unusual because of the early clinical recognition of most of these stenotic lesions. Detailed assessment of recurrent hypertension in patients after earlier reconstructive procedures must include arteriographic studies to determine if graft failure is the cause. Approximately 20% of patients with arteriosclerotic stenoses and 15% of those with fibrodysplastic renal artery stenoses have or will develop bilateral lesions requiring revascularization of both kidneys. Thus development of hypertension after an initially successful operation may reflect progression of contralateral disease rather than graft failure.

Certain nonanastomotic graft stenoses caused by graft trauma, luminal thrombus accumulation, or degenerative changes adjacent to venous valves may be considered for treatment by percutaneous transluminal balloon dilation. Reoperations for this type complication range from simple local angioplastic procedures to replacement of the entire graft. Desmoplastic fibrous tissues surrounding the previously repaired renal arteries often make extensive dissection, including removal of the kidney for ex vivo repair, exceedingly difficult.

Late Aortorenal Graft Dilation

A number of reports have documented that 20% to 44% of saphenous vein grafts used during revascularization procedures undergo nonprogressive, uniform increases in graft diameter.[47,55] This change has been termed "expansion" and is viewed, perhaps erroneously, as a normal manifestation of vein graft arterialization. Distinct from these relatively insignificant changes are advanced aneurysmal changes in aortorenal vein grafts. This phenomenon has been documented in less than 6% of all cases[47] but occurs in nearly three times that number among pediatric-aged patients[52] (Figs. 14-18 and 14-19). Others have reported a lesser frequency of this complication.[55]

The cause of aneurysmal vein grafts remains

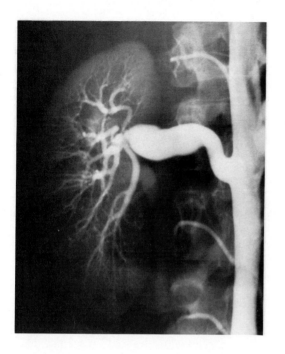

Fig. 14-18. Aneurysmal autogenous saphenous vein aortorenal graft in an adolescent. (From Ernst CB, Stanley JC, Marshall FF, et al. Autogenous saphenous vein aortorenal grafts. A ten-year experience. Arch Surg 105:855-864, 1972. Copyright 1972 American Medical Association.)

A

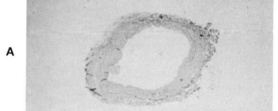

Fig. 14-19. Microscopic sections of saphenous vein segment removed at time of original operation **(A)** and aneurysmal aortorenal graft removed 18 months later **(B)** (same patient as in Fig. 14-18) (hematoxylin-eosin stain, x9). (From Ernst CB, Stanley JC, Marshall FF, et al. Autogenous saphenous vein aortorenal grafts. A ten-year experience. Arch Surg 105:855-864, 1972. Copyright 1972 American Medical Association.)

B

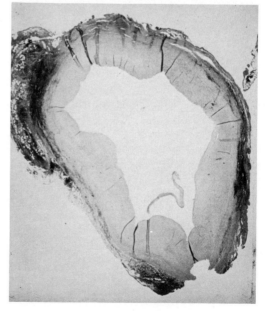

ill defined. The predisposition for dilation to affect pediatric patients may reflect peculiarities of their veins. Normal venous segments in the very young exhibit extensive adventitial networks of vasa vasorum with simple loops penetrating deep within the vessel wall. In adults attenuation of the adventitial plexuses occur, and the deep loops develop into complex superficial plexuses with interconnecting vessels. These differences in the intrinsic nutrient blood supply of veins may account for greater mural ischemia and injury to veins when they are transplanted in the younger patient. Although aneurysmal dilation has been reported to occur with transplanted autogenous arterial segments, the frequency of this event appears less than with veins.[39,55] This result would be anticipated if ischemia to the vessel wall were the major contributing factor to graft dilation. Muscular arteries derive their nourishment through vasa vasorum that originate at branchings; thus transplantation of an artery that has branches would be less disruptive to its nutrient blood supply than transplantation of a vein that obtains its vasa vasoral blood supply from an adjacent artery.

Injudicious procurement, preparation, and transplantation of autogenous vein grafts also have been considered potentially important in their later aneurysmal degeneration. Allowing veins to become desiccated after removal or extensive adventitial stripping before implantation will reduce their structural stability. Although early experimental evidence suggested benefits from intraoperative storage of excised veins in blood, no randomized clinical studies have been forthcoming about the effects of different storage media on the integrity of chronic implanted vein grafts.

Rupture of aneurysmal aortorenal vein grafts has not been reported. However, slowed flow along the dilated graft wall may result in microthrombus formation and distal embolization. It is because of the latter that aneurysmal dilation is considered serious. Although progressive dilation might be considered invariable once this complication develops, only 4 of 15 aneurysmal grafts encountered at the author's institution have continued to expand.

In a patient with advanced aneurysmal dilation it may be best to use either an arterial or synthetic graft to replace the deteriorated vein. As an alternative, plication of the aneurysmal vein graft has been advocated to reduce lateral wall pressures and further dilatation[9] (Fig. 14-20). Plication has appeared to limit progressive aneurysmal expansion, but the long-term durability of this procedure has not been estab-

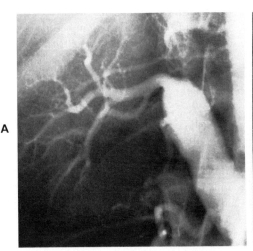
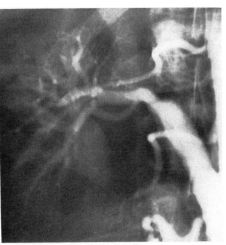

A

B

Fig. 14-20. A, Aneurysmal aortorenal autogenous saphenous vein bypass 16 months after implantation. **B,** Reduced vein graft diameter 18 months after plication of the dilated graft.

lished. Recently others have advocated surrounding vein grafts at the time of their implantation in children with Dacron mesh to prevent aneurysmal dilation.[56] The initial results of this technique also are encouraging, but longer follow-up will be necessary before it becomes accepted practice. Because of the unusually high incidence of vein graft dilation in childhood and adolescence, serious consideration always should be given to the initial use of autologous artery in these patients.

Late Aortorenal Prosthetic Graft Infection and Enteric Fistulization

Prosthetic grafts are proven reasonable conduits for many renal artery reconstructions.[57,58] A major disadvantage of prosthetic grafts relates to their being a foreign substance subject to infection. With the use of prophylactic antibiotics, late prosthetic aortorenal graft infections are uncommon but probably occur in 1% of cases. Another serious complication of artificial graft materials is their erosion into adjacent intestinal tract, usually the duodenum.[59-61] Removal of the prosthesis and revascularization of the kidney using autologous tissue in such instances are mandatory. Frequently re-revascularization is impossible, and nephrectomy is necessary. Manifestations of these two unusual complications include sepsis and, in the case of enteric erosions, intermittent gastrointestinal bleeding. Both have a clinical course identical to that encountered with similar complications involving aortic prosthetic grafts.

MORTALITY RATE

Operative deaths related to primary renal reconstructive surgery are uncommon. The overall mortality rate was 1.1% in a previous study from the author's institution.[14] No operative deaths in this series were associated with the more than 200 procedures performed in 159 patients having fibrodysplastic renal artery disease. This same series included an operative mortality rate of 2.9% among 105 patients treated for arteriosclerotic renovascular disease. Surgical mortality in this experience was in fact limited to a subgroup of 51 patients having clinically overt generalized arteriosclerotic cardiovascular disease. Among these patients pre-

existing cardiac disease represented a major operative risk factor. Caution is advised when considering renal reconstructive surgery in this subgroup without preoperative assessments of coronary artery disease and myocardial function. In patients with obvious myocardial ischemia, treatment of significant coronary artery disease usually should be undertaken before addressing treatment of the renal artery occlusive disease.

Currently, the overall operative mortality rate when treating renovascular hypertension at major centers has averaged 1.7% for all patients regardless of the type of disease.[1] This is in distinct contrast to the unacceptably high overall operative mortality rate of 5.9% and specific mortality rates of 3.4% and 9.3% among patients with fibrodysplastic and arteriosclerotic disease, respectively, as reported in the Cooperative Study on Renovascular Hypertension.[37] It is likely that diminution in mortality reflects contemporary advances in arterial reconstructive surgery. Alternatives to the operative treatment of renal artery stenotic disease in patients with secondary hypertension must be judged in light of the excellent long-term results and an up-to-date analysis of morbidity and mortality attributed to surgical interventions. In properly selected patients with renovascular hypertension the optimal therapy remains operative revascularization.

REFERENCES

1. Stanley JC, Ernst CB, Fry WJ. Surgical treatment of renovascular hypertension: Results in specific patient subgroups. In Stanley JC, Ernst CB, Fry WJ, eds. Renovascular Hypertension. Philadelphia: WB Saunders, 1984, pp 363-371.
2. Dean RH, Englund R, Dupont DW, Meacham PW, Plummer WD Jr, Pierce R, Ezell C. Retrieval of renal function by revascularization. Study of preoperative outcome predictors. Ann Surg 202:367-375, 1985.
3. Novick AC, Pohl MA, Schreiber M, Gifford RW Jr, Vidt DG. Revascularization for preservation of renal function in patients with atherosclerotic renovascular disease. J Urol 129:907-912, 1983.
4. Whitehouse WM Jr, Kazmers A, Zelenock GB, Erlandson EE, Cronenwett JL, Lindenauer SM, Stanley JC. Chronic total renal artery occlusions: Effects of treatment on secondary hypertension and renal function. Surgery 89:753-763, 1981.
5. Stanley JC, Messina LM, Wakefield TW, Zelenock GB. Renal artery reconstruction. In Bergan JJ, Yao

JST, eds. Techniques in Arterial Surgery. Orlando, Fla.: WB Saunders, 1990, pp 247-263.

6. Bergentz SE, Ericsson BF, Husberg B. Technique and complications in the surgical treatment of renovascular hypertension. Acta Chir Scand 145:143-148, 1979.

7. Ekestrom S, Liljeqvist L, Nordhus O, Tidgren B. Persisting hypertension after renal artery reconstruction. A follow-up study. Scand J Urol Nephrol 13:83-88, 1979.

8. Stanley JC, Graham LM, Whitehouse WM Jr. Limitations and errors of diagnostic and prognostic investigations in renovascular hypertension. In Bernhard VM, Towne JB, eds. Complications in Vascular Surgery, 2nd ed. New York: Grune & Stratton, 1985, pp 213-227.

9. Stanley JC, Whitehouse WM Jr, Graham LM. Complications of renal revascularization. In Bernhard VM, Towne JB, eds. Complications in Vascular Surgery, 1st ed. New York: Grune & Stratton, 1980, pp 189-218.

10. Stanley JC, Whitehouse WM Jr, Zelenock GB, Graham LM, Cronenwett JL, Lindenauer SM. Reoperation for complications of renal artery reconstructive surgery undertaken for treatment of renovascular hypertension. J Vasc Surg 2:133-144, 1985.

11. Simon N, Franklin SS, Bleifer KH, Maxwell MH. Clinical characteristics of renovascular hypertension. JAMA 220:1209-1218, 1972.

12. Bookstein JJ, Abrams HL, Buenger RE, Lecky J, Franklin SS, Reiss MD, Bleifer KH, Klatte EC, Varady PD, Maxwell MH. Radiologic aspects of renovascular hypertension. 2. The role of urography in unilateral renovascular disease. JAMA 220:1225-1230, 1972.

13. Bookstein JJ, Maxwell MH, Abrams HL, Buenger RE, Lecky J, Franklin SS. Cooperative study of radiologic aspects of renovascular hypertension. Bilateral renovascular disease. JAMA 237: 1706-1709, 1977.

14. Stanley JC, Fry WJ. Surgical treatment of renovascular hypertension. Arch Surg 112:1291-1297, 1977.

15. Stanley JC, Whitehouse WM Jr, Graham LM, Cronenwett JL, Zelenock GB, Lindenauer SM. Operative therapy of renovascular hypertension. Br J Surg 69:S63-S66, 1982.

16. Grim CE, Luft FC, Weinberger MH, Grim CM. Sensitivity and specificity of screening tests for renal vascular hypertension. Ann Intern Med 91:617-622, 1979.

17. Thornbury JR, Stanley JC, Fryback DG. Hypertensive urogram: A nondiscriminatory test for renovascular hypertension. Am J Roentgenol 138:43-49, 1982.

18. Dean RH, Foster JH. Criteria for the diagnosis of renovascular hypertension. Surgery 74:926-930, 1973.

19. Dean RH, Rhamy RK. Split renal function studies in renovascular hypertension. In Stanley JC, Ernst CB, Fry WJ, eds. Renovascular Hypertension. Philadelphia: WB Saunders, 1984, pp 135-145.

20. Giese J, Mogensen P, Munck O. Diagnostic value of renography for detection of unilateral renal or renovascular disease in hypertensive patients. Scand J Clin Lab Invest 37:307-310, 1975.

21. Machay A, Eadie AS, Cumming AMM, Graham AG, Adams FG, Norton PW. Assessment of total and divided renal plasma flow by ^{123}I-hippuran renography. Kidney Int 19:49-57, 1981.

22. Franklin SS, Maxwell MH. Clinical work-up for renovascular hypertension. Urol Clin North Am 2:301-310, 1975.

23. Sealy JE, Buhler FR, Laragh JH, Vaughan ED Jr. The physiology of renin secretion in essential hypertension. Estimation of renin secretion rate and renal plasma flow from peripheral and renal vein renin levels. Am J Med 55:391-401, 1973.

24. Marks LS, Maxwell MH, Varady PD, Lupu AN, Kaufman JJ. Renovascular hypertension: Does the renal vein renin ratio predict operative results? J Urol 115:365-368, 1976.

25. Marks LS, Maxwell MH. Renal vein renin: Value and limitations in the prediction of operative results. Urol Clin North Am 2:311-325, 1975.

26. Stanley JC, Gewertz BL, Fry WJ. Renal:systemic renin indices and renal vein renin ratios as prognostic indicators in remedial renovascular hypertension. J Surg Res 20:149-155, 1976.

27. Thibonnier M, Joseph A, Sassano P, Guyenne TT, Corvol P, Raynaud A, Seurot M, Gaux JC. Improved diagnosis of unilateral renal artery lesions after captopril administration. JAMA 251:55-60, 1984.

28. Vaughan ED, Buhler FR, Laragh JH, Sealey JE, Baer L, Bard RH. Renovascular hypertension: Renin measurements to indicate hypersecretion and contralateral suppression, estimate renal plasma flow, and score for curability. Am J Med 55:402-414, 1973.

29. Case DB, Wallace JM, Keim HJ, Weber MA, Drayer JIM, White RP, Sealey JE, Laragh JH. Estimating renin participation in hypertension: Superiority of converting enzyme inhibitor over saralasin. Am J Med 61:790-796, 1978.

30. Hricik DE, Browning PJ, Kopelman R, Goorno WE, Madias NE, Dzau VJ. Captopril-induced renal insufficiency in patients with bilateral renal-artery stenosis or renal-artery stenosis in a solitary kidney. N Engl J Med 308:373-376, 1983.

31. Bookstein JJ, Walter JF, Stanley JC, Fry WJ. Pharmacoangiographic manipulation of renal collateral blood flow. Circulation 54:328-334, 1976.

32. Gerlock AJ, Goncharenko V, Sloan OM. Right posterior oblique: The projection of choice in aortography of hypertensive patients. Radiology 127:45-48, 1978.

33. Havey RJ, Krumlovsky F, delGreco F, Martin HG. Screening for renovascular hypertension. Is renal digital-subtraction angiography the preferred noninvasive test? JAMA 254:388-393, 1985.

34. Hillman BJ. Digital imaging of the kidney. Radiol Clin North Am 22:341-364, 1984.

35. Kohler TR, Zierler RE, Martin RL, Nicholls SC, Bergelin RO, Kazmers A, Beach KW, Strandness DE Jr. Noninvasive diagnosis of renal artery stenosis by ultrasonic duplex scanning. J Vasc Surg 4:450-456, 1986.

36. Taylor DC, Kettler MD, Moneta GL, Kohler TR, Kazmers A, Beach KW, Strandness DE Jr. Duplex ultrasound in the diagnosis of renal artery stenosis: A prospective evaluation. J Vasc Surg 7:363-369, 1988.

37. Franklin SS, Young JD Jr, Maxwell MH, Foster JH, Palmer JM, Cerny J, Varady PD. Operative morbidity and mortality in renovascular disease. JAMA 231:1148-1153, 1975.

38. Lawson JD, Hollifield JH, Foster JH, Rhamy RK, Dean RH. Hypertension secondary to complete occlusion of the renal artery. Am Surg 44:642-649, 1978.

39. Lye CR, String ST, Wylie EJ, Stoney RJ. Aortorenal arterial autografts. Late observations. Arch Surg 110:1321-1326, 1975.

40. Novick AC, Stewart BH, Straffon RA. Autogenous arterial grafts in the treatment of renal artery stenosis. J Urol 118:919, 1977.

41. Stoney RJ, DeLuccia N, Ehrenfeld WK, Wylie EJ. Aortorenal arterial autografts: Long-term assessment. Arch Surg 116:1416-1427, 1981.

42. Chibaro EA, Libertino JA, Novick AC. Use of the hepatic circulation for renal revascularization. Ann Surg 199:406-411, 1984.

43. Khauli RB, Novick AC, Ziegelbaum M. Splenorenal bypass in the treatment of renal artery stenosis: Experience with sixty-nine cases. J Vasc Surg 2:547-551, 1985.

44. Okuhn SP, Reilly LM, Bennett JB III, Hughes L, Goldstone J, Ehrenfeld WK, Stoney RJ. Intraoperative assessment of renal and visceral artery reconstructions: The role of duplex scanning and spectral analysis. J Vasc Surg 5:137-147, 1987.

45. Stoney RJ. Transaortic renal endarterectomy. In Rutherford RB, ed. Vascular Surgery. Philadelphia: WB Saunders, 1977, pp 1001-1006.

46. Stoney RJ, Messina LM, Goldstone J, Reilly L. Renal endarterectomy through the transected aorta: A new technique for combined aortorenal atherosclerosis—A preliminary report. J Vasc Surg 9:224-233, 1989.

47. Stanley JC, Ernst CB, Fry WJ. Fate of 100 aortorenal vein grafts: Characteristics of late graft expansion, aneurysmal dilatation, and stenosis. Surgery 74:931-944, 1973.

48. Kent KC, Salvatierra O, Reilly LM, Ehrenfeld WK, Goldstone J, Stoney RJ. Evolving strategies for the repair of complex renovascular lesions. Ann Surg 206:272-278, 1987.

49. Novick AC, Straffon RA, Stewart BH. Surgical management of branch renal artery disease: In situ versus extracorporeal methods of repair. J Urol 123:311-316, 1979.

50. Sicard GA, Valentin LI, Freeman MB, Allen BT, Anderson CB. Renal autotransplantation: An alternative to standard renal revascularization procedures. Surgery 104:624-630, 1988.

51. Novick AC, Straffon RA, Stewart BH, Benjamin S. Surgical treatment of renovascular hypertension in the pediatric patient. J Urol 119:794-805, 1978.

52. Stanley JC, Fry WJ. Pediatric renal artery occlusive disease and renovascular hypertension: Etiology, diagnosis and operative treatment. Arch Surg 11B:669-676, 1981.

53. Ekelund J, Gerlock J Jr, Goncharenko V, Foster J. Angiographic findings following surgical treatment for renovascular hypertension. Radiology 126:345-349, 1978.

54. Kaufman JJ. Renovascular hypertension. The UCLA experience. J Urol 121:139-144, 1979.

55. Dean RH, Wilson JP, Burko H, Foster JH. Saphenous vein aortorenal bypass grafts: Serial arteriographic study. Ann Surg 130:469-478, 1974.

56. Berkowitz HD, O'Neill JA Jr. Renovascular hypertension in children. Surgical repair with special reference to the use of reinforced vein grafts. J Vasc Surg 9:46-55, 1989.

57. Kaufman JJ. Dacron grafts and splenorenal bypass in the surgical treatment of stenosing lesions of the renal artery. Urol Clin North Am 2:365-380, 1975.

58. Lagneau P, Michel JB, Charat JM. Use of polytetrafluoroethylene grafts for renal bypass. J Vasc Surg 5:738-742, 1987.

59. Campbell HC Jr, Ernst CB. Aortoenteric fistula following renal revascularization. Ann Surg 44:155-158, 1978.

60. Howard RJ, Leonard JJ, Howard BD. Renal artery–cholecystoduodenal fistula. A late complication of Dacron patch angioplasty for renal artery stenosis. Arch Surg 113:888-890, 1978.

61. Keeffe EB, Krippaehne WW, Rosch J, Melynk CS. Aorto-duodenal fistula: Complication of renal artery bypass graft. Gastroenterology 67:1240-1245, 1974.

15

Diagnosis and Management of Aortic Bifurcation Graft Limb Occlusions

Victor M. Bernhard   Earl D. Cottrell

Forty years have passed since the introduction of vascular grafts for the treatment of aneurysm and aortoiliac occlusive disease.[1] Although many advances in technique and prosthetic manufacture have had a remarkable impact on the durability of these aortoiliac replacements, thrombosis of one or occasionally both limbs of a graft continues to be the most common complication of aortoiliac bypass surgery. Occlusion occurs in 5% to 20% of patients within 5 years[2-8] and reaches 60% at 20 years.[5] It is tempting to incriminate the thrombogenicity of the graft surface; however, experience and study of graft materials suggest that this factor alone is a relatively minor issue. With the graft in the aortoiliac or aortofemoral position, those factors that reduce the rate of flow through these conduits have far greater implications as predictors of patency.

Although the affected limb frequently is at least marginally viable following acute graft occlusion, the degree of ischemia usually requires urgent, if not emergent, correction in the majority of patients. In the native vessels, where disease progression is generally gradual and chronic, collaterals develop to mitigate the severity of limb ischemia before total occlusion occurs. By contrast, when flow diminishes to its critical velocity in synthetic grafts, occlusion is generally abrupt and usually occurs before collateral recruitment reaches its full potential. Therefore the management of the patient presenting with thrombosis of an iliac or femoral limb of an aortic bifurcation graft requires a clear knowledge of the contributing factors so

that a rapid, direct approach can be implemented for the diagnosis and management of this form of extremity ischemia.

ETIOLOGY OF GRAFT LIMB FAILURE

The causes of both early and late graft failure can be logically divided into deficiency of inflow, problems inherent within the graft, hypercoagulability, and inadequacy of the outflow tract, the most common problem. The average reported interval from graft insertion to graft limb occlusion is 28 to 39 months.[9-12]

Problems of inflow are rare and generally result in total occlusion of the bifurcation graft. It is conceivable, however, that inflow could be impeded to a degree that would promote thrombosis only in the limb with the more severely reduced outflow while the other limb remains patent. All synthetic grafts are thrombogenic to varying degrees and even though slight differences in patency theoretically may be achievable with different materials, no major advantages in aortoiliac or aortofemoral graft patency have been demonstrated in any of the currently available prostheses.[13] The incidence of hypercoagulable states is not well known but may be as high as 9.5% in vascular surgery patients.[14] Nevertheless, the effect of a hypercoagulable state is less important in high-flow systems. Albeit rare, infection may play a role in graft limb thrombosis by creating anastomotic defects and enhancing local coagulability. In the vast majority of cases, the most important and most frequently encountered factor causing both early and late graft failure is an obstructed outflow tract. Reduced graft flow resulting from decreased cardiac output or hypovolemia may be a primary or contributing factor to graft limb thrombosis.

The 1% to 5% incidence of early (less than 30 days) graft failure is usually ascribed to technical problems such as twisting or kinking of the graft or poorly performed anastomoses (Fig. 15-1). Occasionally, however, no technical problem can be determined. Although these failures sometimes may be secondary to inadequate flushing before completion of the distal anastomosis, embolism from a proximal source, or an undiscovered hypercoagulable state, the most common cause in this circumstance is failure to establish good profunda femoris outflow in the presence of multilevel disease. The graft typically is sutured to a diseased common femoral artery with chronic occlusion of a superficial femoral artery and an overlooked stenosis of the profunda femoris. This cause of graft failure has led to an emphasis on the importance of performing some form of profunda-plasty as part of the original surgical procedure whenever compromised outflow exists.[15] Even in patients with localized profunda femoris disease and a patent superficial femoral artery, patency rates were improved when profunda femoris angioplasty was performed in association with the common femoral anastomosis.[2]

Gradual progression of disease in the outflow vessels accounts for more than 80% of subsequent occlusions. This is the result of progression of the atherosclerotic process or a steady buildup of neointimal fibrous hyperplasia at the distal anastomosis.[16] As outflow diminishes, a thickening layer of thrombus becomes adherent to the neointima of the graft, which further diminishes flow and contributes to graft thrombosis. Flow is eventually reduced below the critical level required to maintain patency in the synthetic conduit. In most patients with severely stenosed or occluded superficial femoral arteries, disease progression occurs at the orifice and the proximal segment of the profunda femoris artery. When the major outflow consists of a previously placed infrainguinal bypass, progression of disease and/or thrombosis in this distal conduit will result in

similar consequences. The progression of atherosclerosis is likely to be more rapid in those individuals who continue to be subjected to atherosclerotic risk factors such as smoking, hyperlipidemia, and diabetes.[17,18]

As previously noted, inflow is a rare cause of late aortic graft failure and accounts for no more than 5% of bifurcation graft limb failures.[9] This problem occurs most commonly

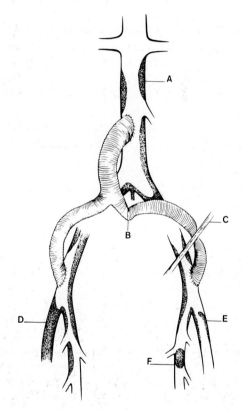

Fig. 15-1. Causes of thrombosis of aortofemoral grafts. *A,* Progression of atherosclerosis proximal to a low takeoff of the graft from the aorta. *B,* Kinking of graft limb caused by a low takeoff and wide angle required for limb to reach groins. *C,* Compression at inguinal ligament, which may be exaggerated by extreme crouch positions. *D,* Insufficient runoff due to superficial femoral artery occlusion and progressing stenosis of the profunda femoris. *E,* Dissection of intimal plaque in runoff vessel. *F,* Embolus. (From Bernhard VM. The failed arterial graft: Loss pulses and gangrene. In Condon RE, De Cosse JJ, eds. Surgical Care: A Physiological Approach to Clinical Management. Philadelphia: Lea & Febiger, 1980, pp 153-167.)

when the proximal anastomosis is placed in the distal abdominal aorta, an area with a propensity for atherosclerotic progression.[2,4] Additionally, placement of the graft low on the abdominal aorta requires a more obtuse angle for the limbs to reach the groins and therefore may predispose to obstruction caused by kinking.[10] It has been suggested that a proximal end-to-side anastomosis is more prone to thrombosis because of competitive flow; however, there are no data to support this contention. However, if the angle of takeoff of the aortic end-to-side anastomosis is too wide, overlying viscera may cause mechanical compression of the graft. Occasionally, a graft limb may be compressed by the inguinal ligament.

Other causes for aortofemoral thrombosis include emboli from the heart or proximal arteries that lodge distally and obstruct outflow. Interventional radiologic procedures may damage the outflow vessels adjacent to the femoral anastomosis and thereby induce graft failure. The placement of too large a graft or dilatation of the prosthesis may lead to stasis and thrombus formation. Aneurysm formation of the graft itself is rare but can lead to similar consequences.[19] The pseudointimal lining of the prosthesis can degenerate, fragment, and embolize distally to obstruct flow. Pseudoaneurysm formation caused by mechanical disruption or infection may be a source of embolism, thrombosis, or compression of the outflow vessels adjacent to the degenerating anastomosis.[20]

DIAGNOSIS

Most patients with acute thrombosis of a limb of a bifurcation graft will present with abrupt return of ischemic symptoms and absence of the femoral pulse, necessitating urgent evaluation. Indeed, 81% of patients in a recently reported series presented with severe limb ischemia and half of these required revascularization within 48 hours.[9] Occasionally, when the occlusion process is gradual and good collaterals are present, the patient may complain only of decreased exercise tolerance. Since some of these patients are severely debilitated with sedentary lifestyles, unilateral graft occlusion may go relatively unnoticed and become evident only by physical examination or noninvasive testing.

Thorough evaluation for coexisting disease states is essential since these may preempt or alter management. The absence of both femoral pulses indicates complete graft occlusion and suggests that the precipitating cause is either systemic or an inflow problem such as progressive disease above the graft or a large embolus. The patient's current cardiac status and rhythm may implicate significant reduction in cardiac outflow or an embolic source.

Reduced high-thigh Doppler pressures will confirm the diagnosis of acute thrombosis, although it is not usually necessary to obtain this study in most patients. The presence of Doppler flow in the pedal arteries suggests that limb perfusion is sufficient to permit the time delay required for appropriate pretreatment investigation. If limb viability is not immediately threatened, arteriography should be obtained before intervention in order to evaluate the proximal aortic anastomotic area, to rule out inflow problems, and to visualize the contralateral limb for outflow anastomotic stenosis, pseudoaneurysm, and emboli. If possible, the outflow tracts should be visualized to direct subsequent surgical angioplasty or bypass. Review of prior arteriograms may be helpful, especially if the current arteriogram does not demonstrate the status of the runoff bed because collateral flow is absent. However, when the profunda femoris and/or distal vessels are not visualized and the limb appears to be acutely nonviable, one should not conclude that the threatened leg cannot be salvaged. In most of these situations exploration of the affected limb will reveal a patent and acceptable distal profunda femoris or popliteal artery.

Evaluation with computed tomography (CT) can reveal pathologic findings that otherwise may not be suspected, such as proximal or distal pseudoaneurysms, severe graft dilatation or focal graft aneurysm, extrinsic compression of the graft, or perigraft fluid suggesting an infection. Finally, CT can also demonstrate proximal thrombus in the upper aorta or the aortic portion of the graft, a finding that may alter surgical management.

The patient who presents with absent Doppler flow and loss of motor function and sensation indicating profound limb ischemia requires urgent intervention to restore perfusion based on clinical and Doppler findings alone. The performance of arteriography can be omitted, unless time and logistics permit, in order to minimize the delay in restoring limb perfusion. The threat to the limb is more important than the information that can be attained with further diagnostic measures, and most unilateral occlusions can be managed through a groin incision with operative arteriography. Likewise, the patient with graft limb thrombosis in the perioperative period should be explored without angiography since it is rarely helpful.

MANAGEMENT OF THE PATIENT WITH AN OCCLUDED BIFURCATION LIMB

Since most patients presenting with thrombosis of an aortic bifurcation graft limb are elderly and have coexisting morbidities, their other medical problems must be evaluated and management optimized while diagnostic investigations are performed. Management strategies should be designed to reestablish limb perfusion without unnecessarily jeopardizing the health of the patient. This may dictate that nothing be done in the occasional patient who is at markedly increased risk from associated diseases, in whom the viability of the affected limb is not threatened, and who is relatively asymptomatic because of a sedentary lifestyle. However, generally revascularization is required to reestablish good leg circulation, and the severity of ischemia will dictate the urgency of revascularization.

As soon as acute occlusion has been identified by physical examination, heparin should be administered while other diagnostic procedures are performed. Heparin administration will prevent further propagation of the thrombus and help to maintain patency in low-flow vessels in the distal limb, which may be prone to thrombosis. Heparin should not be withheld for interventional studies since arteriography can be performed safely in the heparinized patient.

With the rare exception of an acute embolic event occluding one limb of the graft, simple operative or nonoperative clearing of the thrombus from the graft does not relieve the underlying cause of the problem. In the study by LeGrand et al.,[12] late patency of grafts that underwent either inflow graft replacement or thrombectomy without a complementary outflow procedure was nil. By contrast, those patients in whom both inflow and outflow procedures were performed had late patency rates of 77%.

Lytic Therapy

The role of local intra-arterial thrombolytic therapy for unilateral graft limb occlusions is not well established. Although there is little doubt that lysis can be achieved,[21] numerous factors limit its application to this problem. Often the severity of ischemia will not allow the delay of several hours required for lysis. In addition, lytic agents predispose the patient to bleeding complications, especially from arteriography puncture sites, even though the infusion is limited to the involved limb. Some investigators have documented transgraft hemorrhage even in old grafts[22,23] although this has been an infrequent problem. Cardiac emboli and chronic thrombus are much more resistant to lysis, making attempts at their clearance with lytic agents time consuming and frequently incomplete. Since mechanical thrombectomy is performed through the same incision in the groin required for outflow repair, the time delay and increased bleeding risk argue against routine application of preliminary lytic therapy. In the occasional poor-risk patient in whom the involved extremity is at least marginally viable and will tolerate a delay of several hours before circulation is restored, an attempt to clear the graft with lytic therapy can be planned in the hope that enough flow will be established and maintained with anticoagulation to improve the condition of leg. When the thrombus is lysed, distal visualization may demonstrate a lesion that can then undergo percutaneous endovascular ablation. Occasionally lytic therapy will allow better preoperative definition of the distal vasculature and thus permit the surgeon to approach the groin more methodically. However, surgical intervention will be required in most patients to restore adequate runoff regardless of the method used for elimination of thrombus from the proximal graft limb.

Operative Management

The most commonly performed surgical procedure for this problem is graft thrombectomy and profundaplasty. Adequate monitoring is required since these patients have a high incidence of coronary atherosclerosis and may be at greater risk than during the initial bifurcation graft surgery. Prophylactic antibiotic therapy is routinely administered. The abdomen, both groins, and the entire affected limb are prepared to permit access to the aorta, both iliac and femoral arteries, and the distal vasculature of the ischemic leg. Both the surgeon and the patient should be prepared for a more extensive procedure such as graft limb replacement, extra-anatomic bypass, extended profundaplasty,[24] or bypass to the popliteal or tibial vessels since this relatively limited groin procedure may not be sufficient to resolve both the inflow and outflow problems.

Initially, an incision is made through the previous scar in the groin of the affected limb and may be extended cephalad and caudad to facilitate exposure of the previous anastomosis and the proximal segment of the profunda femoris. The easiest approach may be to dissect down to the graft at the inguinal ligament and proceed along the graft to define the femoral artery anastomosis. Alternatively, the superficial femoral artery distal to the anastomosis can be exposed and the diseased artery traced toward the anastomosis. Dense perianastomotic scar makes this dissection tedious. Meticulous dissection is required in order to circumferentially expose the occluded graft and the common femoral, distal external iliac, and profunda femoris vessels. All branches of the common femoral and profunda femoris should be carefully preserved since these may be significant contributors to outflow. The profunda femoris is exposed distally to a point beyond obviously palpable atherosclerotic disease, which almost invariably requires division of the overlying lateral circumflex femoral vein (Fig. 15-2). The patient is heparinized with 100 U/kg of body weight and the external iliac artery and all branches of the femoral artery are occluded with elastic tapes or clamps. The previous suture line is disconnected and thrombus removed to expose the orifices of the profunda femoris and superficial femoral arteries. If preoperative angiography was not obtained or visualization of the profunda femoris and distal limb vasculature was inadequate, a single-injection angiogram may be obtained by direct injection of 20 to 25 ml of full-strength contrast into the profunda femoris. It is most important to visualize adequately the profunda femoris either preoperatively or during surgery to define the extent of disease in this vessel and determine whether it will provide sufficient runoff. If the profunda femoris appears inadequate because of extensive disease in the distal portion of the vessel, it may be necessary to expose the popliteal artery and repeat an angiogram to visualize the infrageniculate circulation for possible bypass.

Outflow Procedures

The importance of the profunda femoris to the long-term patency of aortobifemoral grafts cannot be overemphasized. This vessel supplies the large muscle bulk of the thigh, and in the presence of superficial femoral obstruction, its branches become the collaterals to the popliteal and tibial arteries to supply the leg and foot. When disease is present in the internal iliac system, the profunda femoris also supplies circulation to the gluteus and pelvis. Therefore, in the presence of superficial femoral artery occlusion, profunda femoris flow will be greater than the flow through the patent superficial femoral artery or through a femorodistal bypass.

When the profunda femoris has a focal stenosis only at its orifice, this can be relieved by limited endarterectomy and reattachment of the thrombectomized limb of the prosthesis as an extended tongue onto the proximal 1 to 2 cm of profunda femoris. If the disease is more extensive, an endarterectomy and patch angioplasty will be required. Autogenous vein or preferably an endarterectomized segment of the adjacent occluded superficial femoral artery are the patch materials of choice[25] (Fig. 15-3).

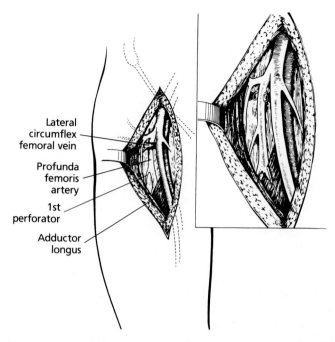

Fig. 15-2. Surgical exposure of the profunda femoris artery for profundaplasty requires transection of the large lateral circumflex femoral vein, which is anterior to the main portion of the profunda femoris. The distal portion of the profunda femoris at and beyond the level of the second perforator is exposed by incising the adductor longus muscle. (From Bernhard VM. The role of profundaplasty in revascularization of the lower extremities. Surg Clin North Am 59:681-692, 1979.)

Fig. 15-3. Endarterectomy and patch angioplasty for extensive obstructive disease in the proximal profunda femoris. Either vein or an endarterectomized segment of the adjacent occluded superficial femoral artery may be used for the patch material. (From Bernhard VM. Profundaplasty. In Rutherford RB, ed. Vascular Surgery, 3rd ed. Philadelphia: WB Saunders, 1989, pp 716-723.)

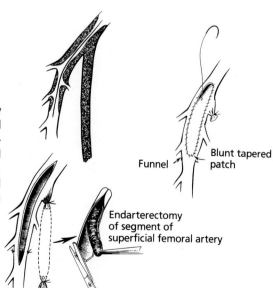

When neither of these autogenous sources is available, expanded polytetrafluoroethylene (PTFE) can be used. If scarring is extensive, bypass to the mid profunda femoris rather than an endarterectomy may be preferred. This portion of the profunda femoris beyond the obstruction and distal to the scar is readily exposed in healthy tissue through an approach lateral to the sartorius muscle.[26,27]

It has been suggested that adequacy of the profunda femoris as an outflow vessel may be demonstrated by the easy passage of a 4 mm probe to ensure its diameter[10] and passage of a deflated soft embolectomy catheter to a length of 20 to 25 cm.[9] When the profunda femoris is so diseased that it cannot be effectively repaired, the performance of a femoropopliteal or femorotibial bypass will be required to increase outflow and to ensure aortofemoral graft patency. Brewster et al.[9] found this to be the case in 32% of patients undergoing outflow reconstruction, whereas Bernhard, Ray, and Towne[10] and LeGrand et al.[12] noted that femoropopliteal or femorotibial bypass was necessary as an outflow procedure in only 5% of limbs. Both Bergan and Stoney,[9] in discussion of the report by Brewster et al., suggested that distal bypass was necessary infrequently and substantiated the prevailing opinion that profundaplasty is both possible and preferred in the vast majority of these patients. Nevertheless, there is some controversy regarding the importance of superficial femoral artery obstruction and the long-term patency of aortobifemoral grafts. Most investigators conclude that superficial femoral artery lesions have little influence on overall patency.[5,28,29] However, Harris[11,30] has argued to the contrary and performed femoropopliteal bypass in 57% of the occluded limbs in his series.

Inflow Procedures

There has been considerable disagreement regarding the best technique for reestablishing inflow after correction of outflow obstruction. Replacement of the entire graft or more commonly the occluded limb has been recommended in some reports[31-33] (Fig. 15-4). These are demanding procedures, with increased trauma produced by abdominal or retroperitoneal graft exposure and the potential for injury to adherent ureters, duodenum, and adjacent major veins.[32,34] Although the aortic graft limb can be approached transabdominally or retroperitoneally, the latter approach is technically easier and may be associated with fewer complica-

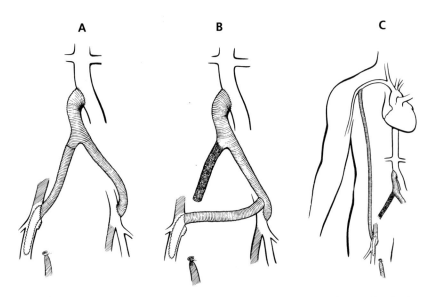

Fig. 15-4. Techniques for insertion of new grafts to restore inflow after profundaplasty. **A,** Resection of the entire graft or a single limb with in situ replacement. **B,** Femorofemoral bypass. **C,** Axillofemoral bypass. (From Bernhard VM, Ray LI, Towne JB. The reoperation of choice for aortofemoral graft occlusion. Surgery 82:867-874, 1977.)

tions. After the graft has been identified, its fibrous capsule is entered and the occluded limb traced back to its origin. The aortic portion of the graft can then be tangentially clamped to preserve flow to the contralateral limb and to prevent embolization of the thrombus, which may extend into the bifurcation. The graft is then divided a short distance distal to the bifurcation, thrombus is extracted from the proximal end, and a new graft is inserted.

Because of the potential difficulties and complications associated with direct graft replacement, extra-anatomic bypass is often advocated (Fig. 15-4). Axillofemoral grafts are almost never required and their use is less desirable because of the tendency of these long narrow grafts to occlude. Femorofemoral grafts have been extensively employed and generally have acceptable long-term patency rates.[35,36] The disadvantage of this approach is the need for scar dissection in the two previously operated groins.

The simplest and most widely used approach is direct mechanical thrombectomy of the occluded limb. Early critics of this technique cautioned that there would be a high incidence of rethrombosis because of residual neointima and thrombus that could not be reliably removed. Furthermore, cross-embolization to the contralateral limb was likely, and the graft wall might be damaged or a graft defect might be overlooked. These logical fears have not been substantiated and excellent results are obtainable with retrograde balloon catheter thrombectomy[10,12,24,37-40] (Fig. 15-5). Restored inflow is excellent and rarely is there any abnormality in the prosthesis itself. Furthermore, transgraft thrombectomy requires only one incision to correct both inflow and outflow. Although thrombectomy is more easily accomplished with occlusions of short duration, it can be applied as late as 6 months after graft limb thrombosis has occurred.

Retrograde graft limb thrombectomy is performed after outflow reconstruction has been accomplished. A No. 4 Fogarty catheter is inserted retrograde into the thrombosed graft limb and advanced through the clot into the patent aortic segment of the prosthesis. This maneuver is performed very gently to prevent pushing thrombus over the bifurcation. There is usually a cap on the thrombus that extends into the bifurcation, which can embolize. The balloon is fully inflated and withdrawn through the occluded graft to extract the thrombus. This maneuver is repeated with a No. 5 or No.

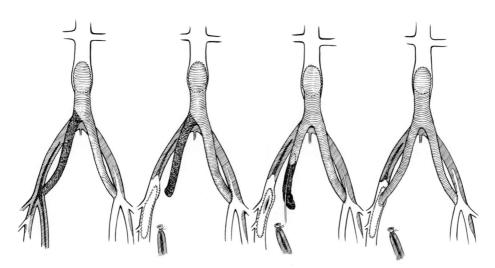

Fig. 15-5. Balloon catheter thrombectomy after restoration of outflow by profundaplasty. (From Bernhard VM, Ray LI, Towne JB. The reoperation of choice for aortofemoral graft occlusion. Surgery 82:867-874, 1977.)

6 Fogarty catheter until vigorous, unrestricted, pulsatile blood flow through the graft is achieved, indicating that the thrombotic obstruction has been relieved. When the bifurcation is approached during each passage of the catheter, an assistant should apply firm pressure to the contralateral groin to attempt to establish a static column of blood that will inhibit cross-embolization.

A dense neointimal thrombus lining, which can impede attempts at establishing good flow, develops in all grafts and is more prominent in patients with long-standing occlusions. This lining may significantly reduce the effectiveness of balloon catheter extraction of the obstructing thrombus. In order to facilitate effective disobliteration of the graft limb under these circumstances, Ernst and Daugherty[41] described the use of a loop endarterectomy device along with the Fogarty catheter to dislodge this persistently adherent fibrous material (Fig. 15-6). The deflated balloon catheter is first passed through the ring of the endarterectomy stripper and then upwards through the graft into its aortic portion. The balloon is then fully inflated and

withdrawn to the bifurcation, where it is wedged into the orifice of the involved limb to temporarily occlude it and prevent embolization to the opposite leg. The endarterectomy stripper, with a loop just small enough to pass through the prosthetic limb, is inserted into the graft limb over the catheter as a guide. It is passed up toward the balloon with a back and forth twisting motion. The balloon is then deflated slightly so that the balloon, loop endarterectomy device, and loosened thrombus can be withdrawn as a unit. This maneuver is repeated as necessary until the graft limb is fully cleared of obstructing material.

The effectiveness of thrombectomy can be confirmed with an intraoperative arteriogram by retrograde injection with 30 ml of full-strength contrast directly into the cleared graft limb while exposing the film.[9] More direct visualization of the lumen can be achieved with angioscopy[42] while the limb is occluded proximally with a balloon catheter. These monitoring techniques will direct further use of strippers and grabbers to remove residual debris that may be present.[43] Following these maneu-

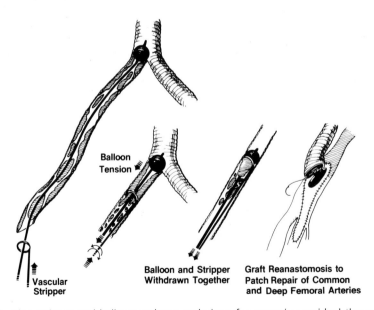

Balloon Tension

Vascular Stripper

Balloon and Stripper Withdrawn Together

Graft Reanastomosis to Patch Repair of Common and Deep Femoral Arteries

Fig. 15-6. Ring stripper and balloon catheter technique for removing residual thrombus and pseudointima from thrombosed graft limb. (From Bernhard VM. Late vascular graft thrombosis. In Bernhard VM, Towne JB, eds. Complications in Vascular Surgery, 2nd ed. Philadelphia: WB Saunders, 1985, pp 187-204.)

vers, when the graft limb has been effectively cleared of all obstructing material, the graft is resutured to the femoral artery.

A short segment of prosthetic material may be required to bridge the gap between the thrombectomized limb of the prosthesis and the repaired outflow tract. The runoff is generally repaired before graft thrombectomy since this avoids prolonged blood stasis in the prosthetic limb.[9,10] An occluded aortoiliac segment of a bifurcation graft may be handled in a similar manner as described for the aortofemoral occluded limb except for the proximal surgical exposure, which is obtained through a retroperitoneal incision. After thrombectomy, the graft should always be extended to the infrainguinal position to ensure satisfactory outflow through the common femoral artery and its branches.

Graft limb thrombectomy is successful in 90% to 95% of patients. However, for the infrequent case in which adequate thrombectomy is not possible, inflow can be effectively restored by direct replacement of the graft limb through a retroperitoneal incision or more commonly by femorofemoral bypass.

PREVENTION

Early graft thrombosis for the most part should be avoidable. Care should be taken to ensure that no kinks or redundancies exist. Grafts should be thoroughly flushed, and static blood within the graft for prolonged periods should be avoided. When the operative procedure appears to have been technically satisfactory or when there is intraoperative evidence of abnormal clotting, the coagulation system of the patient should be investigated. If a hypercoagulable state exists, therapy should be instituted as indicated by the nature of the defect.

The most important factor related to both long- and short-term patency, regardless of the type or positioning of the prosthesis, is the establishment and maintenance of adequate distal outflow. Early thrombosis is generally the result of failure to establish adequate outflow, whereas late failure is usually the result of anastomotic neointimal hyperplasia or progression of atherosclerosis. These causes of failure can be decreased by ensuring adequate profunda femoris flow, if necessary with profundaplasty

at the initial procedure. Cessation of smoking, control of hypertension and diabetes, dietary alteration, and pharmacologic control of hyperlipidemia when indicated should be aggressively pursued to inhibit the progression of atherosclerosis. Concomitant lumbar sympathectomy has not been demonstrated to enhance patency either acutely or chronically.[44,45]

All patients require close follow-up following aortofemoral or aortoiliac bypass grafting, which should include periodic noninvasive evaluation. Although a protocol that will reliably identify patients in danger of aortofemoral graft thrombosis has not been defined, we recommend routine clinical and laboratory evaluation at 6-month intervals for the first 2 years and yearly reexamination thereafter. Arteriography is liberally recommended for any recurrence of symptoms or clinical or laboratory findings suggesting outflow obstruction. Oblique filming of the femoral anastomoses should be requested in order to clearly demonstrate the profunda femoris orifice. If the superficial femoral artery is occluded and >50% profunda femoris stenosis is identified, prophylactic profundaplasty is recommended.

CONCLUSION

When dealing with the patient with a graft limb thrombosis, the surgeon should direct attention to the causes of failure and the knowledge of the techniques and the procedures available for reestablishing flow to help to diminish the risk of limb loss. Heparin should be given immediately upon diagnosis unless there is clear evidence of a contraindication such as heparin-induced platelet activation[46] or hemorrhagic diathesis. Preoperative imaging studies including angiography help in planning the most important part of the management of this complication, that is, the establishment of a better outflow tract, and in identifying proximal graft abnormalities and contralateral disease. However, adequate assessment can frequently be achieved by clinical examination and careful examination of the femoral anastomosis exposed through the groin incision. Outflow is generally addressed first and can usually be improved with various methods of profundaplasty. If the profunda femoris is occluded or diseased in its distal portion, bypass to the popliteal or tibial vessels is required. Inflow is usually obtained by retrograde thrombectomy, which may be facilitated by the use of a loop stripper. Adequacy of graft clearance can be assessed by operative arteriography or angioscopy. Thrombectomy is almost always possible, even in chronically occluded limbs, but if thrombectomy is not successful, inflow can be created with a femorofemoral bypass or direct graft limb replacement, preferably through a retroperitoneal incision.

Over 70% of thrombosed graft limbs are patent at 1 year after reoperation and 50% at 5 years. If failed grafts are subjected to additional reoperation, the continued patency can be 80% and 75% at 1 and 5 years, respectively. This translates into limb salvage rates of 70% vs. the dismal result that would be achieved if no revascularization was performed in these patients.

REFERENCES

1. Voorhees AB Jr, Jaretzki A, Blakemore AH. The use of tubes constructed from Vinyon "N" cloth in bridging arterial defects. Am Surg 135:332-336, 1951.
2. Malone JM, Moore WS. The natural history of bilateral aortofemoral bypass graft for ischemia of the lower extremities. Arch Surg 110:1300-1306, 1975.
3. Brewster DC, Darling RC. Optimal methods of aortoiliac reconstruction. Surgery 84:739-748, 1978.
4. Nevelsteen A, Suy R, Daenen W, Boel A, Stalpert G. Aortofemoral grafting: Factors influencing late results. Surgery 88:642-653, 1980.
5. Crawford ES, Bomberger RA, Glaeser DH, Saleh SA, Russell WL. Aortoiliac occlusive disease: Factors influencing survival and function following reconstructive operation over a twenty-five year period. Surgery 90:1055-1067, 1981.
6. Sonnenfeld T. Reconstructive vascular surgery for intermittent claudication. Acta Med Scand 212:145-149, 1982.
7. Rutherford RB, Jones DN, Martin MS, Kempczinski RF, Gordon RD. Serial hemodynamic assessment of aortobifemoral bypass. J Vasc Surg 4:428-435, 1986.
8. Piotrowski J, Pearce WH, Jones DN, Whitehill TA, Bell R, Rutherford RB. Aortobifemoral bypass: Operation of choice for unilateral iliac occlusion? J Vasc Surg 8:211-218, 1988.
9. Brewster DC, Meier GH III, Darling RC, Moncure AC, LaMuraglia GM, Abbott WM. Reoperation for aortofemoral graft occlusion: Optimal methods and long-term results. J Vasc Surg 5:363-374, 1987.
10. Bernhard VM, Ray LI, Towne JB. The reoperation of choice for aortofemoral graft occlusion. Surgery 82:867-874, 1977.
11. Harris PL. Aorto-iliac-femoral re-operative surgery: Supplementary surgery at secondary operations. Acta Chir Scand 538:51-55, 1987.
12. LeGrand DR, Vermilion BD, Hayes JP, Evans WE. Management of the occluded aortofemoral graft limb. Surgery 93:818-821, 1983.
13. Cintora I, Pearce DE, Cannon JA. A clinical survey of aortobifemoral bypass using two inherently different graft types. Ann Surg 208:625-630, 1988.
14. Donaldson MC, Weinberg DS, Belkin M, Whittemore A, Mannick JA. Screening for hypercoagulable states in vascular surgical practice: A preliminary study. J Vasc Surg 11:825-831, 1990.
15. Bernhard VM, Ray LI, Militello JP. The role of angioplasty of the profunda femoris artery in revascularization of the ischemic limb. Surg Gynecol Obstet 142:840-844, 1976.
16. LoGerfo FW, Quist WC, Nowak MD. Downstream anastomotic hyperplasia. Ann Surg 197:479-483, 1983.
17. Wray R, DePalma RG, Hubay CH. Late occlusion of aortofemoral bypass grafts: Influence of cigarette smoking. Surgery 70:969-973, 1971.
18. Myers KA, King RB, Scott DF, Johnson N, Morriss PJ. The effect of smoking on the late patency of arterial reconstruction in the legs. Br J Surg 65:267-271, 1978.
19. Nunn DB, Carter MM, Donahue MT, Hudgins PC. Postoperative dilatation of knitted Dacron aortic bifurcation grafts. J Vasc Surg 12:291-297, 1990.
20. Treiman GS, Weaver FA, Cossman DV, Foran RF, Cohen L, Levin PM, Treiman RL. Anastomotic false aneurysm of the abdominal aorta and iliac arteries. J Vasc Surg 8:268-273, 1988.
21. Van Breda A, Robinson G, Feldman L, Waltman AC, Brewster DC, Abbott WM, Athanasoulis CA. Local thrombolysis in the treatment of arterial graft occlusions. J Vasc Surg 1:103-112, 1984.
22. Perler B, Kinnison M, Halden W. Transgraft hemorrhage: A serious complication of low dose thrombolytic therapy. J Vasc Surg 3:936-938, 1986.
23. Rabe FE, Becker GJ, Richmond BD, Yune HY, Holden RW, Dilley RS, Klatte EC. Contrast extravasation through Dacron grafts: A sequela of low-dose streptokinase therapy. AJR 138:917-920, 1982.
24. Bernhard VM, Militello JM, Geringer AM. Repair of the profunda femoris artery. Am J Surg 127:676-679, 1974.
25. Malone JM, Goldstone J, Moore WS. Autogenous profundaplasty: The key to long-term patency in secondary repair of aortofemoral graft occlusion. Ann Surg 188:817-823, 1978.
26. Dardik H, Ibrahim M, Sussman BC, Israel M, Kahn M, Dardik I. Remote profunda femoral bypass for limb salvage. Surg Gynecol Obstet 151:625-629, 1980.
27. DePalma RG, Malgieri JJ, Rhodes RS, Clowes AW. Profunda femoris bypass for secondary revascularization. Surg Gynecol Obstet 151:387-390, 1980.
28. Martinez BD, Hertzer NR, Beven EG. Influence of distal arterial occlusive disease on prognosis following aortobifemoral bypass for intermittent claudication. Surgery 88:795-805, 1980.

29. Hill DA, McGrath MA, Lord RSA, Tracy GD. The effect of superficial femoral artery occlusion on the outcome of aorto-femoral bypass for intermittent claudication. Surgery 87:133-136, 1980.

30. Harris PL. Aorto-iliac-femoral re-operative surgery. Supplementary surgery at secondary operations. Acta Chir Scand 538:51-55, 1987.

31. Crawford ES, Manning LG, Kelly TF. "Redo" surgery after operations for aneurysm and occlusion of the abdominal aorta. Surgery 81:41-52, 1977.

32. Najafi H, Dye WS, Javid H, Hunter JA, Goldin MD, Serr C, Julian OC. Late thrombosis affecting one limb of aortic bifurcation graft. Arch Surg 110:409-412, 1975.

33. Szilagyi DE, Elliot JP Jr, Smith RF, Hageman JH, Sood RK. Secondary arterial repair: The management of late failures in arterial reconstructive surgery. Arch Surg 110:485-493, 1975.

34. Benhamou AC, Kieffer E, Tricot JF, Maraval M, Thoai ML, Natali J. "Redo" surgery for late aortofemoral graft occlusive failures. J Cardiovasc Surg 25:118-125, 1984.

35. Brouwer MHJ, Biemans RGM, Donders HPC. Long-term results of 44 cross-over bypasses. J Cardiovasc Surg 29:290-295, 1988.

36. Fahal AH, McDonald AM, Marston A. Femorofemoral bypass in unilateral occlusion. Br J Surg 76:22-25, 1989.

37. Lyons JH Jr, Weisman RE. Surgical management of late closure of aortofemoral reconstruction. N Engl J Med 278:1035-1037, 1968.

38. Cohn LH, Moore WS, Hall AD. Extra-abdominal management of late aortofemoral graft thrombosis. Surgery 67:775-779, 1970.

39. Harbrecht PJ, Ahmad W, Fry DE. Management of aortic bypass graft thrombosis: Utility of thrombectomy. Am J Surg 136:363-368, 1978.

40. Hyde GL, McCready RA, Schwartz RW, Mattingly SS, Ernst CB. Durability of thrombectomy of occluded aortofemoral graft limbs. Surgery 94:748-751, 1983.

41. Ernst CB, Daugherty ME. Removal of a thrombotic plug from an occluded limb of an aortofemoral graft. Arch Surg 113:301-302, 1978.

42. Towne JB, Bernhard VM. Techniques of intraoperative endoscopic evaluation of occluded aortofemoral grafts following thrombectomy. Surg Gynecol Obstet 148:87-89, 1979.

43. Ahn S. The use of grabbers, cutters, and shavers as an adjunct during endovascular surgery. In Moore WS, Ahn SS, eds. Endovascular Surgery. Philadelphia: WB Saunders, 1989, pp 514-517.

44. Satiani B, Liapi CD, Hayes JP, Kimmins S, Evans WE. Prospective randomized study of concomitant lumbar sympathectomy with aortoiliac reconstruction. Am J Surg 143:755-760, 1982.

45. Barnes RW, Baker NA, Shanik G, Maixner W, Hayes AC, Lin R, Clarke W. Value of concomitant sympathectomy in aorto-iliac reconstruction. Arch Surg 112:1325-1330, 1977.

46. Kappa JR, Fisher CA, Cottrell ED, Addonizio VP. Heparin-induced platelet activation in sixteen surgical patients: Diagnosis and management. J Vasc Surg 5:101-109, 1987.

16

Problems Related to Extra-anatomic Bypass Including Axillofemoral, Femorofemoral, Obturator, and Thoracofemoral Bypasses

James S.T. Yao   **William H. Pearce**   **Walter J. McCarthy III**

Extra-anatomic or extracavitary bypass is now an acceptable revascularization procedure. The procedure often is performed in patients who are poor surgical risks or as an alternate route to reconstitute flow to the lower extremity after removal of an infected aortic bypass graft. Extra-anatomic bypasses in use include axillofemoral, femorofemoral, obturator, and thoracofemoral grafts. Since these procedures often are performed in high-risk patients, additional complications can be devastating. This chapter reviews the diagnosis and management of complications commonly associated with these four procedures.

AXILLOFEMORAL BYPASS

The axillofemoral bypass graft was first introduced by Blaisdell and Hall[1] and Louw[2] in the early 1960s. Since then the procedure has become an alternate revascularization technique in patients with aortoiliac occlusion who are at risk for transabdominal aortic bypass grafting. The procedure is also an integral part of surgical technique in the management of an infected aortic graft.

Fortunately, complications after axillofemoral graft placement are rare. In a review of 916 axillofemoral grafts reported in the literature, Bunt and Moore[3] found a 1.6% incidence of complications (15 of 916). The reported complications include four emboli, two proximal pseudoaneurysms, and nine axillary/brachial artery thromboses. Only two of these 15 complications resulted in upper extremity amputation; none resulted in death.

Proximal Anastomotic Disruption

Disruption of the axillary anastomosis leading to acute bleeding or pseudoaneurysm formation is a serious complication. This complication often occurs during the early post-

This work is supported in part by the Alyce F. Salerno Foundation.

operative period and is always associated with exertion or extreme movement such as hyperextension of an arm or falling. Patients who have undergone an amputation are more susceptible, especially when transferring their weight on overhead bars. According to Daar and Finch,[4] when the upper extremity is fully abducted and there is maximal lateral flexion of the spine convex to the site of measurement, the graft pathway may increase in length from 4 to 12 cm. Unless the graft is placed in a more fixed position such as in the first part of the axillary artery, disruption of the graft or anastomosis pullout can occur. Unlike Dacron graft, the external ring–reinforced polytetrafluoroethylene (PTFE) graft is not stretchable. Consequently, the inelastic nature of the PTFE graft contributes to the possibility of rupture. This complication has been reported by several authors.[5,6] It is not only the anastomosis that can be disrupted: we also have observed disruption of the graft with the suture line of the anastomosis left intact. According to White et al.,[6] more than 40 such cases have been recorded, suggesting that this problem is not as rare as previously estimated.

Most would agree that the placement of the anastomosis is the key to avoiding anastomotic disruption. As stated clearly by Blaisdell and Hall[1] in their initial description and reemphasized recently,[7] the proximal anastomosis should be placed medially to the pectoralis minor tendon. This first part of the axillary artery has no branches, is less mobile, and should be the only site used for anastomosis. In addition, it must be stressed that division of the pectoralis minor muscle is not necessary and that such a maneuver to gain exposure only increases the risk of anastomotic complications. Compression of surrounding nerve structures can occur as a result of hematoma or pseudoaneurysm formation, causing transient or even permanent brachial plexus injury. Treatment of disruption includes the placement of a new interposed graft with reanastomosis of the axillofemoral graft to the new graft. A culture must be performed to ensure that infection does not play a role in the rupture.

Axillary Artery Thrombosis

Early or late thrombosis of the axillary artery is uncommon. Thrombosis may occur silently without symptoms. Johnson et al.[8] noted one asymptomatic axillary thrombosis in 56 grafts followed up for 5 years. Others also have reported this complication but the incidence is extremely low.[9,10] In the review by Bunt and Moore,[3] they found that two patients underwent amputation as a result of axillary artery thrombosis. Late severe ischemia following occlusion of axillofemoral bypass graft, though rare, is a serious complication[11] (Fig. 16-1). Once again, if the site for the anastomosis is appropriate, thrombosis seldom presents with upper extremity ischemia. The first part of the axillary artery is devoid of significant branches. All other areas proximal and distal to this segment of the artery have large collateral branches. If the anastomosis is placed in these segments and becomes thrombosed, perfusion of the arm could be jeopardized because of interruption of these collateral vessels. Thrombosis can occur in the body of the graft as a result of compression. The effect of body weight compression on

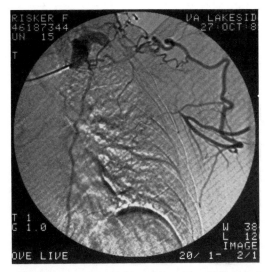

Fig. 16-1. Arteriogram in patient with axillofemoral graft. Note the occlusion of the axillary artery caused by acute thrombosis.

axillofemoral bypass patency has been reported by several investigators.[12,13] Using ankle pressure measurement, Jarowenko, Buchbinder, and Shah[13] found that no hemodynamic changes occurred after external body weight compression. With the increased use of external ring–reinforced PTFE grafts, compression by body weight is now seldom the cause of thrombosis.

Besides thrombosis of the graft at the site of axillary artery anastomosis, kinking or twisting of the body of the graft may cause stenosis leading to occlusion. Redundancy of the graft is the responsible factor for this complication. In elderly patients the combination of being in a sitting position and having mild kyphosis caused by degenerative changes of the spine may exaggerate the redundancy of the graft. As a result stenosis can occur in these patients. Treatment is simple: resection of the redundant graft followed by end-to-end anastomosis.

Graft Infection

Like axillary artery thrombosis, infection of the axillofemoral graft also is rare. In a review of 55 axillopopliteal bypass grafts, Ascer, Veith, and Gupta[14] found a 3.6% incidence of infection. Infection is often in the groin area, but midgraft infection has also been observed. Most of these infected grafts can be treated with local débridement, systemic antibiotic therapy, and local wound care. Because of the excellent incorporation of PTFE graft by surrounding tissue, removal of the entire graft is seldom needed. If necessary, the infected segment can be removed and replaced with an interposed short graft.

Distal Embolization

Distal embolization is an extremely rare complication. It often occurs when there is graft thrombosis. Embolization to the brachial artery can cause severe ischemia. This complication has been reported only sporadically by Bandyk, Thiele, and Radke,[15] who noted emboli to the extremity in one patient, and by Sheiner[16] in three patients. Fig. 16-1 illustrates brachial emboli in a patient in whom late thrombosis of the axillofemoral graft developed.

Perigraft Seroma

Perigraft seroma is an unusual complication and may develop in either Dacron or PTFE graft. Interestingly, it occurs only when the graft is placed in the subcutaneous position. Perigraft seroma, a nonpulsatile, painless mass overlying a graft, must be distinguished from pseudoaneurysm. The cause of perigraft seroma is unclear. Histologically, it is confined within a pseudocapsule consisting of a thin, fibrous membrane and fibroblasts. No inflammatory cells are present. The content is often serous, although gelatinous material has been reported.[17,18] Chronic perigraft seroma often becomes apparent about 4 to 8 weeks after graft implantation. Diagnosis can be made by duplex scan, infusion CT scan, or direct aspiration. Treatment is by excision with new graft replacement. Since perigraft seromas often are related to graft biofilm infections, special culture techniques are necessary for the diagnosis (see Chapter 17).

Structural Failure

Similar to an aortic Dacron graft, the axillofemoral graft also can suffer structural failure leading to gross dilatation of the graft or pseudoaneurysm formation of the body of the graft.[19,20] This complication most likely is related to the use of lightweight or knitted Dacron graft and is seldom encountered if PTFE graft is used. Of interest is the recent report of recurrent multiple aneurysms in an axillofemoral graft with coagulopathy.[21]

FEMOROFEMORAL GRAFT

When unilateral iliac artery occlusion is present, a femorofemoral graft is an acceptable alternative bypass procedure to aortofemoral reconstruction. In the young adult it is probably the procedure of choice when donor iliac arterial occlusive disease is minimal and avoidance of sexual dysfunction is thought to be important. Since the technique was introduced by Oudot and Beaconfield[22] and Freeman and Leeds[23] and popularized by Vetto,[24] the femorofemoral graft is now considered a permanent reconstructive procedure.

Early complications of femorofemoral grafting include hemorrhage, thrombosis, and local wound complication. Penile swelling or scrotal hematoma is another unpleasant complication; it occurs more frequently when one attempts to pass the graft retrofascially. Disruption of the venous plexus in the Retzius' space can cause marked swelling of the penis.

Kinking of the graft at the proximal or distal anastomotic site can occur if one is not careful about the alignment of the graft with the donor or the recipient artery. To avoid this complication the graft should be placed in the tunnel first. The arteriotomy is made based on the angle of the graft with the artery and whether the anastomosis is to be constructed in a C or S manner.

Late complications include the formation of anastomotic aneurysm, distal embolization, and the development of the steal phenomenon. With the increased use of PTFE grafts, it is now uncommon to encounter an anastomotic aneurysm in femorofemoral grafts. When thrombosis develops in a femorofemoral graft, distal embolization to the superficial femoral or popliteal artery has been reported.[25] Donor limb steal has been observed, especially when the graft is performed for intermittent claudication. The decrease of donor limb ankle pressure seen in our series[26] was caused by either unrecognized iliac disease or multilevel disease. For patients with intermittent claudication, ankle pressure of the donor limb must be evaluated by treadmill exercise. A decrease of ankle pressure after exercise of the donor limb increases the likelihood of steal phenomenon if a femorofemoral graft is performed. Other hemodynamic tests such as duplex scanning and intra-arterial pressure measurement of the femoral artery also may help to detect hemodynamically significant iliac artery disease.

As with all bypass grafts, infection of the femorofemoral graft can occur. Treatment requires graft removal with reconstitution of blood flow by another route.

OBTURATOR BYPASS

Obturator bypass often is performed in patients with an infected groin or dense scar tissue as a result of multiple groin dissections. The procedure first described by Shaw and Baue[27] is now an acceptable bypass procedure. Complications of the procedure include injury to the obturator artery, obturator nerve, or the genital urinary tract. The original description of the procedure called for passing the tunneling device from above after identification of the obturator foramen. Such a maneuver may be difficult and injury to the obturator nerve or artery during dissection is a real possibility. Injury to the obturator nerve can cause pain radiating from the groin to the medial aspects of the knee. Paresthesia and hyperesthesia also may occur. Motor dysfunction produces a wide-based gait that is the result of adductor muscle weakness. Electromyography or obturator nerve blocks are useful to establish the diagnosis.[28] Injury of the obturator artery may result in a retroperitoneal hematoma or excessive blood loss. The urologic complications that have been reported are perforation of the bladder and transection of the ipsilateral ureter.[16,28] We have observed bladder injury in one of 14 patients who underwent this procedure.[29] This patient had a history of pelvic surgery followed by radiation therapy and should not have been considered for this type of bypass. Fig. 16-2 shows the PTFE graft penetrating the bladder.

To simplify this procedure, we favor passing the tunneling device from below.[29,30] After an incision is made just below the adductor longus tendon in the midthigh, the tunnel is then created below the adductor longus and magnus muscles with the leg abducted and externally rotated. A large curved DeBakey clamp (14 inches long) then is passed upward from below and directed toward the obturator foramen. At this time the operator's hand is placed over the obturator foramen and the membrane is penetrated. The graft then is drawn from above into the thigh to be anastomosed to the popliteal artery.

One of the interesting complications of obturator bypass is interval gangrene of the thigh.[31] Unless there are sufficient collateral pathways connecting the popliteal and tibial trunks with the profunda femoris, proximal

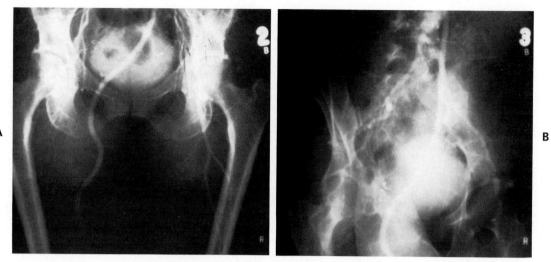

Fig. 16-2. Anteroposterior **(A)** and lateral **(B)** arteriograms in patient with PTFE graft penetrating the bladder after obturator bypass.

myonecrosis may occur because the obturator graft bypasses the profunda femoris artery at the groin. This complication can be avoided by including the profunda femoris artery in the reconstruction.

THORACOFEMORAL BYPASS

Extra-anatomic bypass from the descending thoracic aorta to the femoris was first introduced by Blaisdell, DeMattei, and Gauder[32] in 1961. Since then the procedure has been used by many surgeons for various indications. We use this type of bypass in patients for the following reasons: (1) conversion of existing or recently failed axillopopliteal or axillofemoral bypasses originally placed for septic abdominal aortic indications (infected aortic grafts or aortoduodenal fistulas), (2) avoidance of redissection of the retroperitoneum in patients after many other complex operations or infections, or (3) multiple failed aortofemoral bypasses. In each instance the infrarenal abdominal aorta is relatively inaccessible to reoperation.[33] The procedure is rather simple and the descending thoracic aorta is approached through thoracotomy. The graft is tunneled retroperitoneally to the left femoral artery and a femorofemoral bypass then is added to complete revasculariza-

tion. The technique has not been widely used, and therefore the incidence of complications is unknown. In our series there were two complications. Infection involving the thoracic aorta developed in one patient following conversion of the axillofemoral graft originally performed for aortoduodenal fistula. The other patient had a tear in the spleen during a tunneling maneuver, necessitating splenectomy. This patient later died of massive hemorrhage as a result of anastomotic disruption.

CONCLUSION

Extra-anatomic bypass grafts are useful and often provide an effective means to restore blood flow in special conditions. Although some of these grafts may be considered temporary, enough data have now been accumulated to demonstrate that femorofemoral grafts may be considered permanent reconstructions. Similarly, the frequent use of external ring–reinforced PTFE grafts may provide patients with a much better patency rate than previously reported. Extra-anatomic bypass represents an advance in techniques in vascular surgery. With the rather low incidence of complications, this procedure should remain a viable alternate surgical technique for revascularization.

REFERENCES

1. Blaisdell FW, Hall AD. Axillary-femoral artery bypass for lower extremity ischemia. Surgery 54:563-568, 1963.
2. Louw JH. Splenic to femoral and axillary to femoral bypass grafts in diffuse arteriosclerotic occlusive disease. Lancet 1:401-402, 1963.
3. Bunt TJ, Moore W. Optimal proximal anastomosis/tunnel for axillofemoral grafts. J Vasc Surg 3:673-676, 1986.
4. Darr AS, Finch DRA. Graft avulsion: An unreported complication of axillofemoral bypass grafts. Br J Surg 65:442-446, 1978.
5. Sullivan LP, Davidson PG, D'anna JA Jr, et al. Disruption of the proximal anastomosis of axillofemoral grafts: Two case reports. J Vasc Surg 10:190-192, 1989.
6. White GH, Donayre CE, Williams RA, et al. Exertional disruption of axillofemoral graft anastomosis—"The axillary pull-out syndrome." Arch Surg 125:625-627, 1990.
7. Blaisdell FW. Late axillary thrombosis in patients with occluded axillary-femoral bypass grafts. J Vasc Surg 2:925, 1985.
8. Johnson WC, LoGerfo FW, Vollman RW et al. Is axillobilateral femoral graft an effective substitute for aortobilateral iliac/femoral graft? An analysis of ten years' experience. Ann Surg 186:123-129, 1977.
9. Kempczinski R, Penn I. Upper extremity complication of axillofemoral grafts. Am J Surg 136:209-211, 1978.
10. Rashleigh-Belcher HJC, Newcombe JF. Axillary artery thrombosis: A complication of axillo-femoral bypass grafts. Surgery 101:373-375, 1987.
11. Farina C, Schultz RD, Feldhaus RJ. Late upper limb acute ischemia in a patient with an occluded axillofemoral bypass graft. J Cardiovasc Surg 31:178-181, 1990.
12. Cavallaro A, Sclacca V, Marzo LD, et al. The effect of body weight compression on axillo-femoral bypass patency. J Cardiovasc Surg 29:476-479, 1988.
13. Jarowenko MV, Buchbinder D, Shah DM. Effect of external pressure on axillo-femoral bypass grafts. Arch Surg 193:274-276, 1981.
14. Ascer E, Veith FJ, Gupta S. Axillopopliteal bypass grafting: Indications, late results, and determinants of long-term patency. J Vasc Surg 10:285-291, 1989.
15. Bandyk DF, Thiele BG, Radke HM. Upper extremity embolus secondary to axillofemoral bypass grafts. Arch Surg 118:673-676, 1983.
16. Sheiner NM. Peripheral vascular surgery: Alternate anatomical pathways and the use of allograft veins as arterial substitute. Curr Probl Surg 15:1-6, 1978.
17. Blumberg RM, Gelfand ML, Dale WA. Perigraft seromas complicating arterial grafts. J Cardiovasc Surg 24:372, 1983.
18. Borreor E, Doscher W. Chronic perigraft seromas in PTFE grafts. J Cardiovasc Surg 29:46-49, 1988.
19. Watanabe T, Kusabe A, Kuma H, et al. Failure of Dacron arterial prostheses caused by structural defects. J Cardiovasc Surg 24:95-100, 1983.
20. Orringer MB, Rutherford RB, Skinner DB. An unusual complication of axillofemoral artery bypass. Surgery 72:769-771, 1972.
21. Okadome SMK, Onohara T, Yamamura S, et al. Recurrent multiple aneurysms in an axillofemoral graft with coagulopathy. Acta Chir Scand 156:571-573, 1990.
22. Oudot J, Beaconfield P. Thrombosis of the aortic bifurcation treated by resection and homograft replacement. Arch Surg 66:365-374, 1953.
23. Freeman NE, Leeds FH. Operations of large arteries: Application of recent advances. Calif Med 77:229-233, 1952.
24. Vetto RM. The femoro-femoral shunt: An appraisal. Am J Surg 112:162, 1966.
25. Seeger JM, Kwab-Gatt CS, Lazarus HM, et al. Embolic and occlusive complications from thrombosed femorofemoral grafts. J Cardiovasc Surg 21:547-558, 1980.
26. Harris JP, Flinn WR, Rudo ND, et al. Assessment of donor limb hemodynamics in femorofemoral bypass for claudication. Surgery 90:764-773, 1981.
27. Shaw RS, Baue AE. Management of sepsis complicating arterial reconstructive procedures. Surgery 53:75-86, 1962.
28. Sheiner NM, Sigman H, Stilman A. An unusual complication of obturator foramen arterial bypass. J Cardiovasc Surg 10:324, 1969.
29. Pearce WH, Ricco JB, Yao JST. Modified technique of obturator bypass in failed or infected grafts. Ann Surg 197:344-347, 1983.
30. Pearce WH, McCarthy WJ, Flinn WR, et al. Obturator foramen bypass. In Bergan JJ, Yao JST, eds. Techniques in Arterial Surgery. Orlando, Fla.: WB Saunders, 1990, pp 367-371.
31. Rudich M, Gutierrez IZ, Gage AA. Obturator foramen bypass in the management of infected vascular prostheses. Am J Surg 137:657-660, 1979.
32. Blaisdell FW, DeMattei GA, Gauder PJ. Extraperitoneal thoracic aorta to femoral bypass graft as replacement for an infected aortic bifurcation prosthesis. Am J Surg 102:583-585, 1961.
33. McCarthy WJ, Rubin JR, Flinn WR, et al. Descending thoracic aorto-to-femoral artery bypass. Arch Surg 121:681-688, 1986.

17

Vascular Graft Infections: Epidemiology, Microbiology, Pathogenesis, and Prevention

Dennis F. Bandyk

Infection involving a vascular reconstruction is an infrequent but ominous complication. Despite refinements in arterial reconstructive surgery during the past two decades, including improved vascular prostheses and perioperative administration of antibiotics, infection has remained a nemesis for the vascular surgeon. When infection involves a biologic or prosthetic graft, the result can be a loss of organ function, amputation, or death. When a patient has a graft infection, the ultimate outcome depends on multiple factors but it is, in general, worse than the natural history of the vascular problem that led to graft implantation. Liekweg and Greenfield[1] cited an overall mortality rate of 34% and an amputation rate of 20% following treatment of aortic and peripheral prosthetic infections *despite* aggressive surgical and antibiotic therapy. Although most reports on graft infections have emphasized the surgical principles important in the prevention of early postoperative infection, vascular surgeons now realize that the risk of infection extends well beyond the perioperative period. Aortic graft infections, for example, typically present months to years after implantation as an anastomotic false aneurysm, groin sinus tract, or aortoenteric fistula.

The prevention of graft infection is an important axiom of vascular surgery that deserves emphasis, but achieving this goal may be unrealistic. Bacteria come into contact with the vascular reconstruction at many stages during the operative procedure, the period of wound healing, and as bacteremias anytime following operation. Prevention also requires an understanding of the pathobiology of graft infections, which has improved steadily during the last decade. Recent studies have provided strong evidence that bacteria present in diseased artery walls at the time of graft implantation may be an important source of the bacteria that can colonize vascular prostheses and produce late-appearing graft infections.[2,3] Although surgeons have been made aware of the importance of *Staphylococcus aureus* as a pathogen, contemporary reviews of the problem of graft infection now also emphasize the role of coagulase-negative staphylococci (CNS), particularly in the pathogenesis of late graft infections.[4,5] Infections caused by CNS, such as *Staphylococcus epidermidis*, differ from classic graft sepsis unless there is involvement with the gastrointestinal tract. Bacterial colonization is confined to prosthetic surfaces; systemic signs of infection are absent; and the number and virulence of the infecting organism are low.

This chapter reviews the epidemiology, bacteriology, and pathobiology of vascular graft infections. Pathogenetic mechanisms, both known and hypothesized, are discussed since clinical manifestations and selection of treatment options depend on the anatomic characteristics of the infectious process and pathogen(s) involved. Similarly, if graft infections are to be prevented, the route and mechanisms by which bacteria colonize vascular grafts and the role of a foreign body as a potentiator of infection must be understood.

EPIDEMIOLOGY

The reported incidence of prosthetic graft infections ranges from 0.7% to 3.5%, a level significantly higher than the infection rate (less than 1%) of autologous vein grafts[4,6-12] (Table 17-1). The type of graft material, method of graft fabrication, implant site, use of antibiotic prophylaxis, immune status and nutritional state of the patient, presence of remote infection, and pathogenicity of contaminating organisms are all factors that influence the risk of graft infection. Reports from institutions with extended follow-up of more than 1500 aortic graft implantations indicate a minimal incidence of 1%, including both early- and late-appearing infections.[7-9] By comparison, the reported incidence of infection involving prosthetic lower extremity grafts and extra-anatomic bypass grafts is higher (2% to 5%); vascular grafts implanted in the neck or upper extremity (grafts placed for hemodialysis excluded) rarely become infected.[4,10-12] The actual incidence of prosthetic graft infection may be higher than the level reported in these retrospective observational studies because of the rarity of the

complication, the variable time interval (days to years) between the primary procedure and the recognition of graft sepsis, and the mobility of the patient population. A patient with a graft implanted at one hospital that subsequently becomes infected may be managed elsewhere and not included in the complication statistics of the original institution or the surgeon.

Infection can follow any vascular reconstructive procedure but it occurs more frequently when prosthetic material is used and the grafting procedure extends into the groin. The propensity of graft infection in groin wounds is not unexpected considering the microflora in this region of the body, the frequency of poor hygiene in obese patients, and the colonization of lymphatic channels draining infected lesions of the feet. It is important to emphasize that any arterial reconstruction, with or without a prosthetic graft, can become infected if colonized by a sufficient concentration of a pathogen. In a canine model of femoral artery reconstruction, Fry and Lindenauer[13] demonstrated high infection rates (in excess of 80%) of simple arteriotomy closure, vein patch angioplasty, or prosthetic patch closure following a 10^4 to 10^5 inoculum of *S. aureus* applied topically to the vascular repair before wound closure. In clean and clean-contaminated surgical wounds, autogenous tissues, such as saphenous vein and endarterectomized arterial segments, are far less likely to become involved with sepsis compared with vascular prostheses. As a result antibiotic prophylaxis is mandatory whenever prosthetic grafts are implanted. Goldstone and Moore[4] noted a decrease in graft infection from 4.1% to 1.5% after routine institution of antibiotic prophylaxis. If the early (less than 4 months) graft infection rate of an individual surgeon or institution exceeds 1.5%, review of surgical technique, operating room environment, and antibiotic prophylaxis regime is indicated since this level is higher than the expected incidence of wound infection following clean surgical cases.[14]

Vascular surgeons can expect to see more graft infections in their practice as the number of implant and reoperative procedures increases and the life expectancy of patients with

Table 17-1. Incidence of Vascular Graft Infections

Study	Graft type	Location	Incidence (%)
Hoffert et al.[6] (1965)	Prosthetic	Aortoiliac/femoral	2.2
		Femoropopliteal	12
Szilagyi et al.[7] (1972)	Prosthetic	Aortoiliac	0.7
		Aortofemoral	1.6
		Femoropopliteal	3
	Vein	Femoropopliteal	0.4
Goldstone and Moore[4] (1974)	Prosthetic	Aortofemoral	1.5
		Axillofemoral	3.1
Lorentzen et al.[8] (1985)	Prosthetic	Aortoiliac	0
		Aortofemoral	3
		Femoropopliteal	3.5
O'Hara et al.[9] (1986)	Prosthetic	Aortoiliac	0.4
		Aortofemoral	1.3
Durham et al.[10] (1986)	Prosthetic	Femoropopliteal	2.8
Edwards et al.[11] (1987)	Prosthetic	Femoropopliteal	2.9
Johnson et al.[12] (1988)	Vein	Femoropopliteal	0
	Prosthetic	Femoropopliteal	5.7

vascular disease is prolonged. Improvements in prosthetic materials, formal training in vascular surgery, and routine antimicrobial prophylaxis have reduced the incidence of early postoperative infections.[15-17] Lindenauer et al.[18] noted a relative change in both the timing and pathogens of graft infection with perioperative antibiotic administration. More infections were caused by gram-negative bacteria and the time till appearance of clinical signs increased from an average of 1.5 months to 11 months. At present the majority of aortic graft infections are recognized beyond 1 year after graft implantation. The mean time interval from primary procedure to onset of clinical manifestations has been reported in the range of 25 to 41 months with no difference in the symptom-free interval of patients with perigraft infections and those with paraprosthetic-enteric erosion or fistula.[9] In a 10-year review of aortofemoral graft infection, Bandyk et al.[5] found that 27 of 30 infections presented more than 4 months after operation; in 18 (66%) of these cases, *S. epidermidis* was documented as the infecting organism. A more recent study of the etiologic

factors involved in the formation of anastomotic femoral pseudoaneurysms documented occult infection as a contributing factor in 27 of 45 patients (60%) who underwent correction of this complication 10 to 173 months (mean, 95 months) after graft placement or revision.[19] *S. epidermidis* was the most common bacterial isolate being recovered from 18 of the explanted grafts. These observations confirm that the risk of prosthetic graft infection persists for many years after implantation. The attitude of vascular surgeons regarding surveillance of bypass grafts for hemodynamic failure should be extended to the early detection of graft-healing complications associated with infection, such as perigraft inflammation and anastomotic false aneurysm.

When infection involves prosthetic material, it is persistent and in most instances requires graft removal. Infection involving aortic grafts has the highest reported mortality (40% to 75%) because of hemorrhage from anastomotic dehiscence and graft-enteric fistula, sepsis, and complications resulting from multiple operative procedures.[1,5,8,9] By contrast, infection involving lower limb grafts has an associated mortality rate of less than 10%.[10] Early recognition of graft infection and meticulous surgical technique can reduce mortality and limb loss. Reports from institutions with extensive experience in the management of graft infections indicate that eradication of the infectious process and long-term survival can be anticipated in the majority of patients. Use of staged procedures or preliminary extra-anatomic bypass or endovascular procedure, optimization of cardiopulmonary function, and nutritional support coupled with aggressive artery wall débridement and prolonged antibiotic administration have reduced both the operative mortality and late limb loss associated with treating vascular graft infections.[8,20-22] The nemesis of infection in vascular surgery can be reduced as surgeons achieve an understanding of the factors responsible for graft colonization and knowledge of the microorganisms likely to be implicated and as they become convinced that cure is possible with aggressive therapy.

MICROBIOLOGY

Although any organism can infect a vascular graft, *S. aureus* is reported to be the prevalent pathogen in most series (Table 17-2). The landmark reports of Szilagyi et al.[7] in 1972 and Liekweg and Greenfield[1] in 1977 emphasized the importance of *S. aureus* as a pathogen, accounting for 33% and 50% of graft sepsis, re-

spectively. Gram-negative bacteria, including *Escherichia coli, Klebsiella, Enterobacter, Pseudomonas,* and *Proteus,* were cultured from approximately 40% of infected grafts, and mixed gram-positive and gram-negative infections occurred in 10% to 15% of cases. During the past two decades, the microbiology of graft infections has changed. Infections caused by CNS and gram-negative bacteria have increased in frequency and now account for more than two thirds of infections involving prosthetic grafts. Also of note, reviews on the microbiology of graft infections now cite a 5% to 20% incidence of sterile cultures.[4,5,9,11] The inability to identify a pathogen is most commonly associated with late-onset infections and the result of prosthesis colonization by CNS, which are harbored and survive within a biofilm on the biomaterial surfaces. The perigraft inflammation produced by a bacterial biofilm infection has been erroneously attributed to an immune-mediated foreign body reaction. Standard culture techniques, such as swabs of graft surfaces or perigraft exudate imprinted on agar media, result in a significant sampling error because of low numbers of bacteria within the surface biofilm and the absence of perigraft invasion. Culture of graft material in broth media with mechanical disruption of the bacterial-laden surface biofilm has been shown to enhance the recovery of CNS associated with late-appearing graft infections.[23] When managing a patient with clinical signs of graft infection, the surgeon should not insist on a positive preoperative culture to establish the appropriate diagnosis. Likewise, negative cultures do not exclude the diagnosis of graft infection.

Early (within 4 months) graft infections typically have as their origin a wound infection and develop most commonly in the inguinal region. *S. aureus* is usually the pathogen initially isolated. With hospitalization, local wound care, and antibiotic administration, nosocomial colonization with gram-negative bacteria (*Proteus, Pseudomonas, Serratia,* and *Enterobacter*) can occur. *Pseudomonas* species have been associated with virulent infections involving both prosthetic and autologous vein grafts. Using a canine model to study the differential responses of *Pseudomonas* and *S. epidermidis* infections on

Table 17-2. Organisms Recovered From Prosthetic Graft Infections*

Organism	No.	%
S. aureus	162	44
S. epidermidis	60	16
E. coli	48	13
Streptococcus sp.	34	9
Klebsiella/Enterobacter	20	5
Pseudomonas	18	5
Proteus	16	4
Bacteroides	4	1
Corynebacterium	2	<1
Other gram negative sp.	9	2

*Cumulative data from references 1, 6, 13-19.

vein and prosthetic grafts, Geary et al.[24] report-ed a high incidence of anastomotic disruption (5 of 10 grafts) and vein wall necrosis (two of five grafts) within 10 days of direct inoculation of *Pseudomonas aeruginosa* (10^8 colony-forming units) onto the grafts. By contrast, no prosthetic or vein graft inoculated with *S. epidermidis* developed graft or anastomotic disruption. The virulence of *Pseudomonas* species is associated with their ability to produce destructive pro-teases (elastase, alkaline protease) that break down elastin, collagen, fibronectin, and fibrin, thereby leading to compromised structural in-tegrity of artery and vein graft walls. Coagulase-positive staphylococci also can produce lysins, which are hemolytic and produce both cell necrosis and the killing of mobilized leuko-cytes. The invasion of perigraft tissues, in-cluding adjacent native artery, in established infections caused by *S. aureus* or gram-nega-tive organisms accounts for the negligible mi-crobiologic sampling error with routine culture techniques. The pathogen(s) responsible can be readily identified by Gram's stain and cul-ture of wound drainage, perigraft exudate, or tissue. Unexplained sepsis, prolonged ileus, or abdominal distention and tenderness may be the only clinical signs of an early aortic graft infection.

The microbiology of late-appearing graft in-fections depends on clinical presentation. The most common manifestations are an inflamma-tory process (e.g., sinus tract, perigraft exudate or cavity) involving the groin incision of an aortofemoral or prosthetic femorodistal graft, or an anastomotic false aneurysm. One third of patients with late aortic graft infections present with gastrointestinal bleeding caused by ero-sion of the prosthesis into the upper or lower gastrointestinal tract.[25] The most common or-ganisms responsible for late graft infections are CNS, including *S. epidermidis*, *Staphylococcus hominis*, and *Staphylococcus warneri*. We also have observed a similar infectious process in an aortic graft infected by *Candida* organisms. Un-like *S. aureus* and gram-negative bacteria, CNS sequester and grow primarily within a biofilm adherent to prosthetic surfaces; they do not produce toxins or products capable of tissue autolysis and in the presence of normal host

defenses, do not invade perigraft tissues. Colo-nization of aortic prostheses with enteric or-ganisms *(E. coli, Klebsiella)* occurs rapidly after erosion into the bowel. Sepsis with positive blood cultures can develop and if an adjacent graft-artery anastomosis becomes infected, fis-tula formation or aortic rupture will eventually occur. Microbiologic confirmation of graft in-fections caused by CNS requires the use of sensitive culture techniques (broth media, me-chanical disruption of surface biofilms). Cul-ture of excised graft material in broth media will isolate microorganisms from more than 80% of late-appearing graft infections despite the find-ings of only white blood cells on Gram's stain of perigraft exudate and a sterile swab culture.[3,23]

PATHOGENESIS

Any mechanism that exposes a vascular re-construction to bacterial contamination can result in infection. These mechanisms include local routes of contamination via the operative wound during implantation and in the postop-erative period of wound healing or via a hematogenous route from transient bacter-emias. Malone et al.[26] demonstrated in experi-mental animals that a single intravenous infu-sion of *S. aureus* resulted in positive graft cul-tures in 100% of animals up to 1 month after graft implantation. A pseudointima developed with time and the susceptibility of grafts to infection from bacteremic sources decreased to a 75% incidence and a 30% incidence at 4 months and 1 year, respectively. Grafts with a complete pseudointima lining were resistant to infection from bacteremia. Despite these con-vincing experimental data, the clinical evidence of bacterial seeding of an implanted graft is primarily anecdotal.

Bacterial contamination at the time of graft implantation remains the most important pathogenetic mechanism for graft sepsis. Al-though it is difficult to establish with certainty the origin of organisms in individual patients, potential sources include (in order of impor-tance) the skin, contaminated lymphatics, or-ganisms harbored in diseased arteries, breaks in surgical technique during the operation, and improperly sterilized grafts or instrument packs. Performance of a concomitant surgical procedure (e.g., incidental appendectomy, cholecystectomy, colon resection) at the time of graft implantation also will increase the risk of colonization by the patient's enteric flora. Despite bactericidal and mechanical preparation of the skin for operation, significant numbers of organisms will remain on the skin surface and within the dermal layer. Contact of prosthetic graft with the skin or its cut edge risks colonization by the skin flora at that site. We have demonstrated that the majority of vascular surgery patients admitted to the hospital for bypass grafting are colonized with multiple strains of mucin- or slime-producing CNS.[27] Exposure to the hospital environment, including perioperative antibiotic administration, increased the incidence of methicillin-resistant *S. epidermidis* strains from 15% on admission to 50% following operation. This selection process can decrease the effectiveness of routine antibiotic prophylaxis regimens in patients with prolonged hospitalization before operation and in those requiring reoperation.

Infected lymph nodes and lymphatic channels are other important sources of potential pathogens.[28] Femoral anastomoses are particularly vulnerable to this route of contamination, especially when infection, ulceration, or gangrene is present distally in the extremity. The lymphatics can transport bacteria directly to the operative wound and vascular graft when transected during operative dissection or to the systemic circulation via lymphatovenous communications, producing a hematogenous route for graft contamination. Disrupted lymph channels can continue to bathe the surgical wound and graft after operation until wound healing occurs. Careful isolation, ligation, and transection of inguinal lymphatics can minimize both bacterial colonization via this route and the development of a lymphocele in the surgical wound after operation.

The majority of early graft infections, particularly those involving lower extremity bypasses, are associated with wound healing complications (hematoma, lymphocele, skin edge and subcutaneous fat necroses, wound dehiscence). Risk factors identified as contributing to the development of wound and subsequent graft infections include chronic steroid therapy, ipsilateral limb ulcer, subcutaneous placement of the graft, bypass to a pedal artery, and, in the case of autologous vein grafting, use of the in situ bypass technique.[29,30] Patients with advanced limb ischemia often have concomitant systemic disorders, such as diabetes mellitus, poor nutrition, and nosocomial infections, which further predispose to poor wound healing. When a prosthetic vascular graft becomes exposed to the ambient environment as a result of a wound complication, the graft should be considered infected and excision may be necessary. Ouriel et al.[31] found that the fate of exposed saphenous vein grafts was highly dependent on the bacterial flora of the infectious process. Vein graft disruption was frequent in patients with gram-negative infections. The development of local skin necrosis or ischemia, wound infection, lymph fistula, and lymphocele can be minimized with preoperative control of infection in the ischemic limb coupled with meticulous attention to operative technique and wound closure. These measures are vital in subcutaneous prosthetic or autologous vein (in situ saphenous vein method) graft procedures because infection of overlying skin can result in morbid sequelae of graft exposure, hemorrhage, limb loss, or death.

Late-appearing graft infections are the result of colonization of the prosthesis by CNS, most commonly *S. epidermidis*. Bacterial contact with the graft most likely occurs at the time of implantation or in the perioperative period. Cultures of skin, adipose tissue, diseased artery wall, mural thrombus of arterial aneurysms, and lymph nodes from patients undergoing prosthetic graft placement have demonstrated a significant incidence of colonization by CNS. Macbeth et al.[2] reported that positive cultures were obtained from 43% of arterial walls explanted during clean, elective vascular reconstructive procedures. *S. epidermidis* was the isolate recovered in 71% of positive cultures. Ernst et al.[32] documented that the incidence of aortic graft infection in patients undergoing abdominal aortic aneurysm repair increased from 2% to 10% when culture of aneurysm contents was positive. Coagulase-negative bacteria from these various sources can attach and become sequestered on prosthetic surfaces, surviving within an adherent biofilm. The bacterial-laden biofilm is composed of coalescing microcolonies enclosed in an extracellular nutrient glycocalyx that is produced by the organisms. Bacterial biofilm infections are not unique to vascular prostheses. A variety of biomaterials and devices routinely implanted in humans have been reported to be involved with a surface biofilm caused by CNS, including hip and knee prostheses,[33] prosthetic heart valves,[34] cerebrospinal fluid shunts,[35] and indwelling venous catheters.

The infection of a vascular prosthesis by a bacterial biofilm is a complex process involving colonization of the biomaterial and activation of host defenses by both the microorganisms and their products of metabolism and the foreign body. Chronic inflammation surrounds the graft and extends into the surrounding tissue. Important components of this process include a bacterial-laden biofilm on prosthetic surfaces, abnormal perigraft tissues with a sterile exudate, and a pathologic interaction of the colonized graft with adjacent artery at anastomotic sites (Fig. 17-1). Fulfillment of these anatomic and microbiologic criteria, in combination with the absence of systemic signs of infection, is necessary to establish the diagnosis of vascular prosthesis infection caused by bacterial biofilms. Chronic activation of host defenses produces autolysis of the tissue surrounding the

graft, accounting for the absence of graft incorporation and perigraft cavity formation. Because of host defenses and the virulence of the organisms, the CNS do not invade the perigraft tissue and their low numbers in the perigraft exudate make recovery by standard microbiologic culture techniques unlikely. Chronic perigraft inflammation can result in pathologic conditions involving anastomotic sites (false aneurysm formation), interaction with adjacent bowel (graft-enteric fistula or erosion), and overlying subcutaneous tissue and skin (graft–cutaneous sinus tract). In canine models of aortic graft infection, *S. epidermidis* has been demonstrated to be capable of producing a graft infection with the anatomic (perigraft inflammation and anastomotic disruption) and microbiologic characteristics (sterile perigraft exudate, bacterial-laden biofilm) of late-appearing graft infections in humans.[36,37] At present the preoperative diagnosis of graft infection caused by bacterial biofilm must be based on clinical presentation and the anatomy of the infectious process. A characteristic of patients with bacterial biofilm graft infections is a history of multiple reoperations for hematoma, graft thrombosis, or false aneurysm.

Adhesion of bacteria to the surface of a prosthetic implant is a necessary inceptive stage in the pathogenesis of clinical infection. Factors

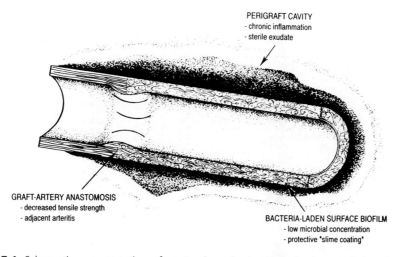

PERIGRAFT CAVITY
- chronic inflammation
- sterile exudate

GRAFT-ARTERY ANASTOMOSIS
- decreased tensile strength
- adjacent arteritis

BACTERIA-LADEN SURFACE BIOFILM
- low microbial concentration
- protective "slime coating"

Fig. 17-1. Schematic representation of anatomic and microbiologic characteristics of vascular prosthesis infections caused by bacterial-laden biofilm.

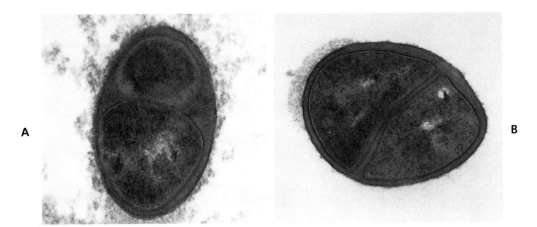

Fig. 17-2. Scanning electron micrographs of mucin-producing **(A)** and nonmucin-producing **(B)** *S. epidermidis* bacteria, demonstrating differences in morphology and thickness of capsule caused by production of extracellular glycoproteins (mucin).

contributing to bacterial adherence include the bacterial species, production of exopolysaccharide, physical-chemical character of the biomaterial, duration of microbial exposure, and the use of antibiotic prophylaxis. *S. aureus* has been demonstrated to have a greater adherence to suture material (as high as 100 times greater in number) than *E. coli*.[38] Likewise, strains of CNS that produce large amounts of polysaccharide extracellular material, or mucin, have been demonstrated in vitro to adhere in greater numbers to both polytetrafluoroethylene (PTFE) and Dacron vascular grafts compared with nonmucin-producing strains[39] (Fig. 17-2). In addition to promoting bacterial adherence, mucin production protects the organisms against antibodies, antibiotics, and phagocytes. Mucin-producing *S. epidermidis* is the primary pathogen recovered from late-onset graft infections and mucin production also is involved with *S. aureus* and *P. aeruginosa* infections.

Graft fabrication also can affect quantitative bacterial adherence. Bacterial strains have been shown to have greater affinity (10 to 100 times) for Dacron compared with PTFE.[39] The observed decrease in adherence of mucin- and non-mucin-producing *S. epidermidis* strains to preclotted and albumin-coated knitted Dacron grafts compared with unclotted Dacron grafts indicates porosity, and coating the graft with serum and tissue proteins also alters bacterial cell–biomaterial interactions.[40] Recently Tojo, Goldman, and Pier[41] isolated a capsular polysaccharide from a mucin-producing *S. epidermidis* strain that appears to mediate bacterial adherence. Antibody to this adhesin inhibited adherence of adhesin-producing strains to Silastic catheter tubing. The ability to identify specific cell surface glycoproteins responsible for initial bacterial adherence is an important step in our understanding of the mechanisms involved in the colonization of biomaterials. It is important to emphasize that the vascular prosthesis is not an innocent bystander in the infectious process: it augments the inflammatory response and provides an environment conducive to bacterial survival and proliferation. The acidic and relatively ischemic environment surrounding vascular prostheses induced by a foreign body reaction provides nutritional sources for the bacteria and inhibits penetration of phagocytes and lysosomal enzymes that normally would be bactericidal.

Infections involving prosthetic grafts can be classified into three groups based on anatomic signs, mode of onset, and pathogen(s) involved (Table 17-3). Failure to recognize the protean signs of a perigraft infection within the abdomen risks development of an aortoenteric fistula or anastomotic false aneurysm and the poten-

Table 17-3. Classification of Vascular Graft Infection

	Time interval after implantation	Pathogens
Perigraft infection	<4 mo	S. aureus
		Streptococcus sp.
		E. coli
		Klebsiella
		Pseudomonas
	>4 mo	S. epidermidis
Graft-enteric erosion	>4 mo	E. coli
		Enterococcus
		Bacteroides
Graft-enteric fistula	<4 mo	E. coli
		S. aureus
	>4 mo	E. coli
		Klebsiella
		S. epidermidis

tial for exsanguination. The virulence of infecting organisms and the extent of graft-artery involvement are critical factors that influence clinical manifestations of graft sepsis. When bacterial colonization is confined to prosthetic surfaces, systemic signs of infection are absent and the number and virulence of organisms are low. As such, this type of graft infection may be safely managed by treatment methods other than total graft excision, such as partial graft excision with muscle flap coverage or in situ replacement. By contrast, failure to diagnose early or late graft infections with gastrointestinal involvement and delays in operative management of these infections are associated with decreased patient survival.

PREVENTION

Measures to prevent vascular graft infections must begin before operation and continue at operation and into the postoperative period. Every possible effort should be made to restore nutritional and immune deficiencies before operation. Hypovolemia, anemia, hypoxemia, uremia, and intercurrent infection are known to impair wound healing and thereby promote infection. Infected or necrotic lesions on the toes and the feet should be aggressively treated before operation, including débridement or amputation if necessary. Appropriate cultures should be taken and specific antibiotic therapy prescribed in order to sterilize tissues adjacent to the site of graft implantation. The operation should begin with preparation of the skin, particularly in the groins. Patients should bathe with an antibacterial soap (hexachlorophene, iodophor, chlorhexidine gluconate) for several days before bypass grafting is performed.

At operation, contamination of the graft by the patient's flora, the surgical team, and the operating room environment must be minimized and if possible eliminated. Although laminar air flow systems have been advocated for the reduction of prosthetic device infection, careful studies have not proved their benefit. Of course, surgeons or assistants with active infections should not participate in prosthetic arterial reconstructions. Preparation of skin at the planned incision sites and patient draping are important components of the operation. Shaving the skin should be done just before the operation; the skin should be prepared by mechanical cleansing and disinfected with agents such as povidone-iodine, 1% iodine in 70% ethyl alcohol, hexachlorophene, or chlorhexidine gluconate. Despite skin preparation bacteria harbored in hair follicles and sweat glands can repopulate the operative field. Plastic surgical drapes and abdominal wound protectors are useful adjuncts to prevent vascular prostheses from contacting the skin. Surgical sponges saturated in antibiotic solution (50,000 units bacitracin and 1 gm kanamycin/1 L of normal saline solution) can be used to line the incisions and protect tissues from retractor trauma. Use of plastic bags to enclose and protect the small bowel and thereby improve surgical exposure has been implicated in increasing the potential for graft infection. Ernst et al.[32] noted a high incidence of positive cultures when they submitted for culture the transudate fluid that accumulated in the bag during abdominal aortic operations. In addition, atheromatous and thrombotic materials should be removed before closure of the retroperitoneum. Aortic prostheses should be covered carefully by retroperitoneal tissue or if necessary the omentum to prevent contact between the prosthesis and duodenum or small intestine. No drains should be placed adjacent to prosthetic grafts.

In operations on the femoral artery and in lower limb arterial bypass procedures, awareness of major risk factors associated with wound complications is vital. Autogenous reconstruction should be used whenever possible. Careful tissue handling, hemostasis, lymphatic tissue ligation or excision, and wound closure, including avoidance of creating ischemic skin flaps, should be practiced. If a continuous incision is used for exposure of the saphenous vein for in situ bypass grafting, preoperative mapping with duplex ultrasonography can minimize inadvertent creation of skin flaps. Groin incisions should be closed in multiple layers using interrupted absorbable (polyglycolic acid) sutures to ensure that no dead space remains. Skin edge approximation using staples or continuous 4-0 or 5-0 polyglycolic acid sutures is preferred to transcutaneous sutures and gives an excellent cosmetic result. Following operation a dry surgical dressing should be used to cover the incisions until no further wound drainage is identified on daily dressing changes. If wound drainage is persistent, coverage of the suture line with antibiotic ointment should be added to the dry dressing regimen. Noninfectious complications arising from groin incisions such as seroma or lymph fistula should be managed using meticulous aseptic technique on the hospitalized patient.

Antibiotics are an important adjunct in the armamentarium of vascular surgeons for the prevention of infection. Newer drugs exhibit bactericidal activity over a broad range of microorganisms and are less toxic. Proper dosage and administration of antibiotics minimize the development of toxic side effects and the consequences of bacterial resistance. Ideally, an antibiotic administered for prophylaxis during vascular graft implantation should be bactericidal for potential pathogens, achieve therapeutic serum and tissue concentrations at the operative site, and maintain these levels for the duration of the procedure. Based on the microbiology of graft infections, which was discussed previously, antibiotic therapy should be directed at *Staphylococcus* species, both coagulase-positive and coagulase-negative, *E. coli*, and *Streptococcus* species. These four organisms are responsible for more than 80% of all prosthetic graft infections.

First- and second-generation cephalosporins remain the agents of choice for antibiotic prophylaxis during arterial reconstruction procedures. Of note, the clinical studies often quoted to support prophylactic use of antibiotics in arterial reconstructive surgery have documented a decrease in the occurrence of wound infections and an absence of infections involving the implanted graft material. Kaiser, Clayson, and Mulherin,[15] in a prospective randomized study, compared cefazolin (1 gm before operation and four doses after operation) and placebo. Although the incidence of wound infection was less in the patients administered cefazolin (0.9%) compared with those given placebo (6.8%), the number of graft infections in the two patient groups was not significantly different despite the absence of graft infection in patients administered antibiotics. Pitt et al.,[16] in a prospective randomized, blind study, also demonstrated decreased groin and incisional infections among patients undergoing vascular procedures who received prophylactic antibiotics by either topical, systemic, or combined administration of cephradine. No patient in this study developed an infection involving the vascular graft during a follow-up period ranging from 10 to 35 months. The findings of these studies have been extrapolated to support routine use of antibiotic prophylaxis in vascular surgery based on the hypothesis that a reduction of wound infections correlates with decreased incidence of graft infections. Recommendations for prophylactic antibiotic administration are listed in Table 17-4.

There are many unanswered questions regarding antibiotic prophylaxis in vascular surgery. The most efficacious duration of antibiotic administration after graft insertion is not known. Clinical studies to date have not followed patients for sufficient duration to determine whether 1 to 3 days of antibiotic administration is adequate prophylaxis to prevent graft colonization by *S. epidermidis* and other pathogenic CNS strains. We continue postoperative administration of antibiotics for 5 to 7 days in patients undergoing lower extremity bypass grafting when a distal ulceration or gangrene is present. Patients hospitalized for prolonged periods before operation or those undergoing early reoperation for a failed primary reconstruction may harbor different flora than patients admitted for elective procedures. Although we have documented the emergence of antibiotic-resistant strains of *S. epidermidis* in patients undergoing prosthetic grafting procedures, the *S. epidermidis* isolates recovered by skin culture after operation remained susceptible to cefazolin, the antibiotic used as prophylaxis.

The development of a vascular prosthesis that is resistant to infection has considerable appeal. Techniques have been developed to bind antibiotics directly to graft surfaces.[42-44] These approaches have been shown both in vitro and in experimental animal models to inhibit the growth of organisms on graft surfaces and increase an implanted graft's resistance to infection of bacteremic origin and by direct inocula-

tion of the graft. It is not known whether bacteria coming in contact with the graft are actually killed or suppressed by the antibacterial activity. Further study is required to determine whether binding antibiotics to graft surfaces can reliably prevent CNS from becoming sequestered within the surface biofilm of an implanted prosthesis, thereby decreasing the significant problem of late graft infections.

Table 17-4. Prophylaxis for Prosthetic Vascular Graft Implantation

Standard regimen	Cefazolin 1 gm 1hr before, then 1 gm every hr for three doses
Penicillin allergy	Vancomycin 1 gm IV slowly over 1 hr, plus gentamicin 1.5 mg/kg IV 1 hr before procedure, then every 8-12 hr for three additional doses

REFERENCES

1. Liekweg WG Jr, Greenfield LF. Vascular prosthetic infection: Collected experience and results of treatment. Surgery 81:335-342, 1977.
2. Macbeth GA, Rubin JR, McIntyre KE, et al. The relevance of arterial wall microbiology to the treatment of prosthetic graft infections: Graft infection vs arterial infection. J Vasc Surg 1:750-756, 1984.
3. Durham JR, Malone JM, Bernhard VM. The impact of multiple operations on the importance of arterial wall cultures. J Vasc Surg 5:160-169, 1987.
4. Goldstone J, Moore WS. Infection in vascular prosthesis. Am J Surg 128:225-233, 1974.
5. Bandyk DF, Berni GA, Thiele BL, et al. Aortofemoral graft infection due to *Staphylococcus epidermidis*. Arch Surg 119:481-486, 1984.
6. Hoffert PW, Gensler S, Haimovici H. Infection complicating arterial surgery. Personal experience with 12 cases and review of the literature. Arch Surg 90:427-435, 1965.
7. Szilagyi DE, Smith DF, Elliott JP, et al. Infection in arterial reconstruction with synthetic grafts. Ann Surg 176:321-333, 1972.
8. Lorentzen JE, Nielsen OM, Arendrup H, et al. Vascular graft infection: An analysis of sixty-two graft infections in 2,411 consecutively implanted synthetic vascular grafts. J Vasc Surg 98:81-86, 1985.
9. O'Hara PJ, Hertzer NR, Beven EG, et al. Surgical management of infected abdominal aortic grafts: Review of a 25-year experience. J Vasc Surg 3:725-731, 1986.
10. Durham JR, Rubin JR, Malone JM. Management of infected infrainguinal bypass grafts. In Bergan JJ, Yao JST, eds. Reoperative Arterial Surgery. Philadelphia: WB Saunders, 1986, pp 359-373.
11. Edwards WH, Martin RS, Jenkins JM, et al. Primary graft infections. J Vasc Surg 6:235-239, 1987.
12. Johnson JA, Cogbill TH, Strutt PJ, et al. Wound complications after infrainguinal bypass: Classification, predisposing factors and management. Arch Surg 123:859-862, 1988.
13. Fry WJ, Lindenauer SM. Infection complicating the use of plastic arterial implants. Arch Surg 94:600-609, 1967.
14. Cruse PJE. Incidence of wound infection on the surgical services. Surg Clin North Am 55:1269-1275, 1973.

15. Kaiser AB, Clayson KR, Mulherin JL. Antibiotic prophylaxis in vascular surgery. Ann Surg 188:283-289, 1978.

16. Pitt HA, Postier RG, MacGowan WA, et al. Prophylactic antibiotics in vascular surgery: Topical, systemic, or both. Ann Surg 192:356-364, 1980.

17. Hasselgren PO, Ivarsson L, Risberg B, et al. Effects of prophylactic antibiotics in vascular surgery: A prospective randomized, double-blind study. Ann Surg 200:86-92, 1984.

18. Lindenauer SM, Fry WJ, Schaub G, et al. The use of antibiotics in the prevention of vascular graft infection. Surgery 62:487-492, 1967.

19. Seabrook GR, Schmitt DD, Bandyk DF, et al. Anastomotic femoral pseudoaneurysm: An investigation of occult infection as an etiologic factor. J Vasc Surg 11:629-634, 1990.

20. Turnipseed WD, Berkoff HA, Detmer DE, et al. Arterial graft infections: Delayed versus immediate vascular reconstruction. Arch Surg 118:410-414, 1983.

21. Edwards MJ, Richardson JD, Klamer TS. Management of aortic prosthetic infections. Am J Surg 155:327-330, 1988.

22. Schmitt DD, Seabrook GR, Bandyk DF, et al. Graft excision and extra-anatomic reconstruction: The treatment of choice for the septic aortic prosthesis. J Cardiovasc Surg 31:327-330, 1990.

23. Bergamini TM, Bandyk DF, Govostis D, et al. Identification of *Staphylococcus epidermidis* vascular graft infections: A comparison of culture techniques. J Vasc Surg 9:665-670, 1989.

24. Geary KJ, Tomkiewicz ZM, Harrison HN, et al. Differential effects of a gram-negative and a gram-positive infection on autogenous and prosthetic grafts. J Vasc Surg 11:339-347, 1990.

25. Bandyk DF. Aortic graft infection. Semin Vasc Surg 3:122-132, 1990.

26. Malone JB, Moore WS, Campagna G, et al. Bacteremic infectability of vascular grafts: The influence of pseudointimal integrity and duration of graft function. Surgery 78:211-216, 1975.

27. Levy MF, Schmitt DD, Edmiston DE, et al. Sequential analysis of staphylococcal colonization by body surface cultures on patients undergoing vascular surgery. J Clin Microbiol 28:664-669, 1990.

28. Rubin JR, Goldstone J, Malone JM. The role of the lymphatic system in acute prosthetic graft infections. J Vasc Surg 2:92-98, 1985.

29. Johnson JA, Cogbill TH, Strutt PJ, et al. Wound complications after infrainguinal bypass. Arch Surg 123:859-862, 1988.

30. Wengrovitz M, Atnip RG, Gifford RRM, et al. Wound complications of autogenous subcutaneous infrainguinal arterial bypass surgery: Predisposing factors and management. J Vasc Surg 11:156-163, 1990.

31. Ouriel K, Geary KJ, Green RM, et al. Fate of the exposed saphenous vein graft. Am J Surg 160:148-150, 1990.

32. Ernst CB, Campbell HC, Daugherty MS, et al. Incidence and significance of intraoperative bacterial cultures during abdominal aortic aneurysmectomy. Ann Surg 185:626-635, 1977.

33. Gristina AG, Costerton JW, McGanity PL. Bacteria-laden biofilms: A hazard to orthopedic prostheses. Infect Surg 3:655-662, 1984.

34. Slaughter L, Morris JE, Starr A. Prosthetic valvular endocarditis: A 12 year review. Circulation 47:1319-1325, 1973.

35. Schoenbaum SC, Gardner P, Shillito J. Infection of cerebrospinal fluid shunts: Epidemiology, clinical manifestation, and therapy. J Infect Dis 131:543-551, 1975.

36. Bergamini TM, Bandyk DF, Govostis D, et al. Infection of vascular prostheses caused by bacterial biofilms. J Vasc Surg 7:21-30, 1988.

37. Martin LF, Harris JM, Fehr DM, et al. Vascular prosthetic infection with *Staphylococcus epidermidis:* Experimental study of pathogenesis and therapy. J Vasc Surg 9:464-471, 1989.

38. Chih-Chang C, William DF. Effects of physical configuration and chemical structure of suture materials on bacterial adhesion. Am J Surg 147:197-204, 1984.

39. Schmitt DD, Bandyk DF, Pequet AJ, et al. Mucin production by *Staphylococcus epidermidis:* A virulence factor promoting adherence to vascular grafts. Arch Surg 121:89-95, 1986.

40. Siverhus DJ, Schmitt DD, Edmiston CE, et al. Adherence of mucin and nonmucin producing staphylococci to preclotted and albumin-coated velour knitted vascular grafts. Surgery 107:613-619, 1990.

41. Tojo M, Goldman DA, Pier GB. Isolation and characterization of a capsular polysaccharide adhesion from *Staphylococcus epidermidis.* J Infect Dis 157:713-722, 1988.

42. Moore WS, Chavapil M, Sieffert G, et al. Development of an infection-resistant vascular prosthesis. Arch Surg 116:1403-1407, 1981.

43. White JV, Benvenisty AI, Reemtsma K, et al. Simple methods for direct antibiotic protection of synthetic vascular grafts. J Vasc Surg 1:372-380, 1984.

44. Shenk JS, Ney AL, Tsukayama DT, et al. Tobramycin-adhesive in preventing and treating PTFE vascular graft infections. J Surg Res 47:487-492, 1989.

18

Management of Vascular Graft Infections

Joseph J. Piotrowski   **Victor M. Bernhard**

Vascular graft infection represents one of the most challenging clinical problems in vascular surgery. Seemingly opposing goals of therapy are (1) maintaining adequate distal tissue perfusion while (2) treating sepsis involving a prosthesis originally placed for inadequate perfusion. This requires a thoughtful common sense approach and considerable technical expertise. All vascular surgeons encounter this complication, but because of its relative infrequency, reported series are generally small and usually span two or more decades during which graft materials, antibiotics, and anesthetic management have undergone dramatic changes. The recent statement by H. Brownell Wheeler to the New England Society for Vascular Surgery[1] on common sense in carotid surgery is equally appropriate for the management of vascular infections:

There is a tendency to use composite average data to make highly individual decisions. There is a tendency to denigrate clinical judgement. . . . There is, and can be, no replacement for a wise and compassionate surgeon when a patient faces a difficult decision about surgery.

Appropriate management of a vascular graft infection depends on a well–thought-out plan. This requires thorough investigation of the extent of the infection (see Ch. 17). Preoperative arteriography is needed to determine the presence and location of suitable inflow and outflow arteries in order to plan the most efficacious method of revascularization. This study may also identify sources of autogenous graft material by demonstrating an occluded iliac or superficial femoral artery. These otherwise useless segments can be readily converted by eversion endarterectomy into conduits for in situ placement as an alternative to prosthetic extra-anatomic bypass, which might be cumbersome or not feasible. In general, if autogenous graft material or extra-anatomic routes are available, graft excision, aggressive débridement, and direct or remote revascularization is the most prudent management strategy. Alternate approaches such as local antibiotic and antiseptic irrigation and in situ prosthetic grafting may be appropriate for limited indications. Additional important supportive measures include hyperalimentation and precise antibiotic therapy.

The following case history illustrates the complexity of this problem. A 65-year-old man with a right femoral–to–distal popliteal in situ vein bypass performed 2 years previously underwent cardiac angioplasty. He presented with acute hemorrhage from the right groin 7 days later associated with an indurated, erythematous, pulsatile mass and a 1 cm opening in the overlying skin. The bleeding had stopped and a duplex scan revealed a large pseudoaneurysm at the proximal anastomosis of the bypass. Arteriography revealed a widely patent bypass with good iliac inflow and runoff as well as an occluded superficial femoral artery. The left saphenous vein had been harvested previously for coronary revascularization and no suitable arm veins were present. The skin defect was closed over the hematoma and isolated from the field with an impermeable dressing. An incision was then made in the right flank to obtain proximal control of the external iliac artery. The occluded superficial femoral artery was excised through clean tissue planes and converted into a 20 cm conduit by eversion endarterectomy, and the harvest wound was closed and covered with an impermeable dressing. The groin was then explored and the infected pseudoaneurysm and adjacent segments of the common femoral, proximal in situ graft, and proximal profunda femoris were resected back to normal-appearing vessels. Aggressive local débridement of the infected periarterial tissues was performed. Small portions of the remaining and normal-appearing arterial wall were sent to the laboratory for culture and sensitivity. The endarterectomized superficial femoral artery was used to bridge the defect between the common femoral artery, the distal vein graft, and the distal profunda femoris. After completion arteriography (Fig. 18-1), the wound was closed over suction drains. *Pseudomonas* was detected in cultures of the arterial wall and the patient was treated with specific antibiotics intravenously for 6 weeks followed by oral antibiotics for an additional 3 months. Recov-

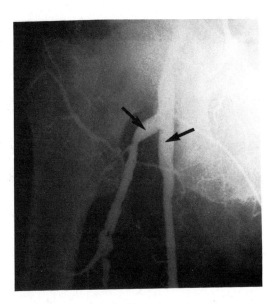

Fig. 18-1. Repair of vein graft infection with excision of the proximal graft, wound débridement, and restoration of vascular continuity. An endarterectomized segment of occluded superficial femoral artery (left arrow) was placed in situ between the common femoral artery, distal graft, and profunda femoris (right arrow).

ery was uneventful and at 6-months' follow-up he was well with a normally perfused limb. This case illustrates the need for careful preoperative assessment and planning, aggressive débridement, arterial reconstruction, and appropriate supportive care.

DEFINITIONS AND GUIDELINES

There are numerous reports of methods for the management of vascular infections; however, they are invariably retrospective, usually describe small series of patients, and span one or more decades. There have been no prospective randomized trials comparing different treatment options. Terminology is often imprecise and inconsistently employed. For instance, the meaning of the term "in situ" may indicate removing a synthetic graft and replacing it with a new one in the same bed or leaving the old graft in place and treating it with topical agents. Therefore we have established several guidelines in order to compile and evaluate information derived from our own experience and a review of the literature.

Only original studies descriptive enough to identify the type of graft material, location of the infection (aortic or infrainguinal), presence or absence of enteric fistulas, treatment performed, and outcome have been used for statistical comparison. Review articles have been included only to evaluate added cases from the authors' own experience. Several excellent articles could not be used in the summary tables because of the inability to separate treatment outcomes for aortic graft infections (AGIs) vs. aortoenteric fistulas (AEFs),[2,3] for aortic vs. peripheral grafts,[4] or prosthetic extra-anatomic bypass (EAB) vs. autogenous reconstruction.[2] With minor exceptions, primarily from the more recent literature, long-term outcome is difficult to determine since information regarding character and duration of follow-up frequently was not recorded.

All studies were examined to identify the intent of the *initial* treatment plan as the basis for determining eventual outcome. For example, if a determined attempt to treat with local therapy failed and was subsequently followed by graft excision, the patient's outcome was recorded as failure of the former therapy. This contrasts with reports of others.[5,6]

AGIs included tube grafts, aortobi-iliac, aortobifemoral, and aortoiliofemoral synthetic prostheses. AEFs were analyzed separately and only those secondary to a previous synthetic bypass were included. Peripheral graft infections included iliofemoral, femorofemoral, axillofemoral, femoropopliteal, and femorodistal bypasses with synthetic material and femoral or profunda patch angioplasty if synthetic patch material was used. Autogenous peripheral arterial repair infection is discussed separately.

"Excision" implies complete graft removal without revascularization. "Local care" includes any combination of aggressive wound care treatments including débridement, antibiotic or antiseptic irrigation, and suture or patching of a disrupted anastomosis if the prosthesis was left in place. "In situ" indicates complete or nearly complete graft removal and insertion of prosthetic material in the same location. "Excision and EAB" refers to complete graft removal and prosthetic EAB either sequentially at one operation or as a staged-remote procedure. Finally, "excision and autogenous reconstruction" implies complete or partial graft removal and use of autogenous material for revascularization either in situ or in an extra-anatomic location.

MANAGEMENT OF AUTOGENOUS GRAFT INFECTIONS

There are relatively few publications regarding autogenous bypass graft infections, probably because of the relative infrequency of this complication compared with the incidence of prosthetic infections.[7] Furthermore, these infections are usually the result of early postoperative wound complications rather than being primary infections of the graft itself and therefore are more likely to respond to local measures.[8,9] Finally, autogenous graft infections are almost invariably associated with infrainguinal bypass procedures for which autogenous reconstruction is more feasible.

The extent of infection, presence and degree of direct involvement of the graft wall, and presence of associated pseudoaneurysm can usually be detected at the time of débridement and excision of overlying necrotic skin. Angiography and/or noninvasive testing is required for late-appearing infection to identify inflow or outflow stenoses. In the presence of pseudoaneurysm or acute hemorrhage, immediate excision and débridement are required. Débridement must be aggressive enough to ensure complete excision of obviously infected arterial wall and the adjacent involved segment of vein graft. A biopsy of a portion of the retained vessel wall at the edge of the débrided area should be obtained with clean instruments and cultured in trypticase soy broth as well as on agar plates to detect residual infection directly invading the vessel wall.[10] If the arterial wall culture is positive, long-term specific antibiotic therapy is indicated to reduce the incidence of secondary arterial rupture.[11]

Revascularization should be delayed if the limb is clinically viable, Doppler pedal arterial flow is present, and collateral circulation that was previously sufficient for limb viability has not been sacrificed. If immediate revascularization is required, autogenous repair is preferred. This may be limited to vein patch angioplasty of the common and profunda femoris arteries or may require insertion of a segment of an autogenous vein to maintain continuity of the previous venous bypass. This is feasible if all grossly infected tissue can be excised and the repair covered with healthy tissue, preferably a muscle pedicle. The alternative is to perform autogenous bypass through clean tissue planes via an extra-anatomic route. When autogenous tissue is not available, a prosthesis can be used. However, this will require an available alternate route through uncontaminated tissue, effective sealing of the infected wound from the other incisions, repreparing and draping of the patient, and the use of fresh instruments in order to avoid contamination of the new prosthesis.

In patients with an intact graft, split-thickness skin or preferably rotational muscle flaps should be used to cover the exposed vessels as soon as local wound care has decreased the local bacterial flora. Extrapolating from the burn literature, Mixter et al.[12] suggest a level of bacteria less than 10^5/gm as the criterion for determining the successful healing of a rotated muscle flap. The rectus femoris muscle is advocated for groin coverage; it has a consistent proximal blood supply from the profunda femoris artery, whereas the sartorius muscle is more segmentally supplied. The rectus abdominis muscle is also available. The gastrocnemius and soleus muscles can be used for distal wounds.

MANAGEMENT OF PROSTHETIC AORTIC GRAFT INFECTIONS

The incidence of AGI in the absence of AEF varies between 0.5% and 2%. This complication occurred in 1.4% of 1662 implanted Dacron grafts at the Henry Ford Hospital.[7]

Determination of the extent of infection in this location by CT scan is important since autogenous reconstruction is generally less feasible in this situation and treatment options vary widely depending on whether the proximal body of the graft is involved or whether the process is limited to the distal portion of one graft limb. The use of magnetic resonance imaging (MRI) has also been helpful, and in a recent report MRI defined the extent of infection in 14 of 16 cases based on demonstration of perigraft fluid collections.[13] As this technology improves, MRI may become the method of choice for preoperative planning. Fine needle aspiration of perigraft fluid collections may be useful for tailoring antibiotic coverage.[14] A culture-negative specimen may represent chronic coagulase-negative staphylococci (CNS) infections rather than healing problems or graft vs. host reaction.[15] Therefore the inability to culture organisms, especially in a perigraft fluid collection that persists more than 3 months after bypass, should not dissuade one from using aggressive therapy.

Angiography should be performed to define runoff and also to locate sources of autogenous material. Occluded or severely diseased native vessels such as aorta and iliac arteries can be converted into vascular conduits by endarterectomy if the bypass was placed for occlusive disease. However, most of the completely autogenous reconstruction options are possible only if the infection is limited to the groin or iliac vessels. Frequently, none of these options is feasible and the primary therapeutic decision involves excision alone, excision and EAB, or excision and in situ prosthetic grafting.

Local Treatment

Local treatment is an attractive option since it avoids subjecting an ill patient to a severe hemodynamic insult as well as the technical problems of graft excision and EAB. Application of this management regimen is usually limited to infections confined to the distal limb of an aortobifemoral graft. A review of all reported cases in which local treatment was employed indicates that 83% were limited to the groin (Table 18-1).

This method of therapy consists of operative exploration of the infected graft limb to define the limits of the local septic process followed by aggressive débridement of necrotic and infected perigraft tissues and irrigation with antiseptic- or antibiotic-containing solutions.[16,23,24,26] The wound is left open in most cases to provide access for frequent antibiotic- or antiseptic-soaked dressing changes and daily local débridement by the surgeon. Alternatively, if the initial débridement appears to have eradicated all necrotic and infected tissue, the wound may be closed over suction drains with continuous antibiotic irrigation. Direct coverage of the exposed graft with a well-vascularized muscle flap may be performed immediately or delayed until the septic process has receded. Specific antibiotic therapy based on the results of wound culture should be given intravenously for at least 2 weeks or until the infectious process appears to have resolved. Although the need for prolonged oral antibiotic therapy thereafter has not been clearly defined, continued specific antibiotic treatment for at least 3 months is appropriate in order to eliminate bacteria that may be trapped in the interstices of the graft material.

An often cited series by Carter, Cohen, and Whelan[16] in 1963 included four cases of AGI, all confined to the groin. Local care, consisting of continuous antibiotic irrigation via polyethylene catheters, was administered with successful results in each case. However, these infections appeared long after the original aortic bypass was performed and manifested as a consequence of secondary thrombectomy or revision limited to the groin area that subsequently became infected.

There are only six reported cases of infection involving the full extent of the prosthesis in which local care was employed exclusively. Of these, three were not primary graft infections but involved grafts contaminated later by a primary gastrointestinal process (one ruptured appendix, two small bowel perforations).[25,26]

Table 18-1. Local Treatment for Aortic Graft Infection (Graft Not Removed)

Author	No. of patients	Healed	Diec	Amputation	Follow-up (yr)	Comments
Schramel and Creech[6] (1959)	1	0	0	1	NS	Groin
Carter et al.[16] (1963)	4	4	0	0	1	Groin; remote original operation
Shaw and Baue[17] (1963)	2	0	0	0	NS	Subsequent excision
Conn et al.[18] (1970)	3	2	1	0	NS	One groin healed; one abdominal healed
Szilagyi et al.[7] (1972)	1	1	0	0	NS	CNS by history
Becker and Blundell[19] (1976)	5	0	3	2	NS	Groin
Liekweg and Greenfield[20] (1977)	4	3	0	1	1	Groin mostly
Yashar et al.[21] (1978)	1	1	0	0	NS	Groin
Connolly et al.[22] (1981)	1	0	1	0	NA	Groin originally; subsequent AEF led to death
Kwaan and Connolly[23] (1981)	5	5	0	0	1	Groin
Almgren and Eriksson[24] (1981)	3	3	0	0	3	Shaft also
Renvall and Havia[25] (1981)	2	2	0	0	3	Not primary AGIs; acute appendicitis; bowel perforation
Hinton and Bryant[26] (1981)	1	1	0	0	NS	Died SBO 6 mo; groin
Knight et al.[27] (1983)	1	1	0	0	2	Perforated bowel; not primary AGI; shaft
Lorentzen et al.[28] (1985)	18	7	9	2	1.2	Groin mostly
Mixter et al.[12] (1989)	11	10	1	0	3	Groin; muscle flap closure
TOTAL	63	40 (63%)	15 (24%)	6 (10%)		83% groin infections only

NS, not stated; NA, not applicable; CNS, coagulase-negative staphylococci; AEF, aortoenteric fistula; AGI, aortic graft infection; SBO, small bowel obstruction.

Therefore, based on only three cases of primary AGI successfully treated with local care by Almgren and Eriksson[24] in 1981, it is difficult to recommend this approach with any certainty for cases in which the entire graft is involved.

Local care has been associated with an acceptable healing rate (63%), a low amputation rate, and an operative mortality of 24% in the published anecdotal experiences (Table 18-1).

Local care is contraindicated when healing fails to progress, suggesting extension of infection; when an anastomosis is or becomes involved based on anastomotic bleeding or false aneurysm formation; when the graft limb is thrombosed; or when signs of ongoing sepsis persist. Even when healing appears complete, continued routine surveillance for recurrent infection is required. Although guidelines for follow-up evaluation have not been defined, our current routine is to perform CT scans covering the full extent of the aortic graft at 4- to 6-month intervals for at least 2 to 3 years in addition to frequent clinical examination.

Excision Without Immediate Revascularization

When the entire aortoiliac or aortofemoral prosthesis is involved, excision with or without revascularization remains the mainstay of therapy. Excision alone is a particularly attractive option when the graft is occluded and collaterals are sufficient to permit limb survival. If the graft was initially inserted with an end-to-side aortic anastomosis for occlusive disease, aortic endarterectomy or patch closure in the area of proximal anastomosis may be feasible.[2,4,5] The intent of this procedure is to retain flow through the previously undisturbed native circulation and its collaterals. However, the potential for anastomotic rupture must be considered if the arterial wall is invaded with bacteria.[11]

In general, excision has been associated with both high mortality (49%) and amputation rates (28%) (Table 18-2). The morbidity rates in this category are probably falsely elevated since these patients would have been reassigned to the excision and remote EAB, autogenous, or in situ reconstruction categories by most investigators if they had survived excision with viable extremities. Many of these patients may have

Table 18-2. Graft Excision Without Immediate Revascularization for Aortic Graft Infection

Author	No. of patients	Healed	Died	Amputation	Follow-up (yr)	Comments
Schramel and Creech[6] (1959)	1	0	1	1	NA	
Van de Water and Gaal[29] (1965)	1	0	0	NS	1	
Cohn and Angell[30] (1968)	1	0	1	0	NA	
Najafi et al.[31] (1969)	4	3	1	1	NS	All groin infections
Conn et al.[18] (1970)	4	0	2	1	NS	
Becker and Blundell et al.[19] (1976)	4	0	2	2	NS	
Szilagyi et al.[7] (1972)	9	0	6	3	NS	Aortic stump blow-out in 2
Jamieson et al.[32] (1975)	3	0	1	1	NS	Continued chronic drainage in 1
Liekweg and Greenfield[20] (1977)	3	0	3	0	NA	
Fulenwider et al.[33] (1983)	6	6	0	NS	3	
Lorentzen et al.[28] (1985)	3	0	0	3	1.2	
Thomas and Baird[34] (1986)	1	0	1	0	NA	
O'Hara et al.[35] (1986)	13	1	12	0	1	Stump rupture
Reilly et al.[36] (1987)	15	5	3	7	NS	2 AEFs included
TOTAL	68	16 (24%)	33 (49%)	19 (28%)		

NA, not applicable; NS, not stated; AEF, aortoenteric fistula.

been too ill for more extensive procedures. However, Bennion et al.[37] reported five patients who survived initial graft excision with intact extremities, which were apparently adequately perfused immediately after graft removal. Delayed revascularization was performed 2 months later using EAB, with recovery in all. Unfortunately, most authors are not as specific regarding the interval from excision to reconstruction and therefore it is not possible to evaluate fully excision alone as a treatment option.

Excision alone is an option to be considered if the preoperative status suggests that collateral circulation will be adequate to maintain limb viability after graft removal, usually in patients with established graft occlusion and viable limbs, and these collaterals are not destroyed in the process of graft excision. However, current methods for determining limb viability immediately after aortic graft excision may not be entirely reliable and the presence of pedal arterial flow on Doppler examination coupled with physical findings and clinical judgment may not be sufficient to determine that EAB can be delayed. Furthermore, colon ischemia may occur concomitant with limb necrosis if perfusion is inadequate because of loss of retrograde flow through pelvic collaterals.[38] An immediate sequential approach is almost always necessary when the original operative procedure was resection of an abdominal aortic aneurysm since the presence of adequate collateral flow is unlikely.

Excision and EAB

EAB for an infected prosthetic bifurcated graft was first reported in 1961 by Blaisdell, DeMattei, and Gauder,[39] who used a thoracic aorta–to–femoral artery route. Subsequently Blaisdell and Hall[40] modified this procedure to the more common axillofemoral bypass.

Excision and EAB is the most common treatment for AGI (Fig. 18-2). The 18% mortality rate and 21% amputation rate may be considered acceptable for this extremely difficult patient management group (Table 18-3). The primary causes of death in most series were uncontrollable sepsis and aortic stump rupture. In the series reported by Reilly et al.,[2] 54 pa-

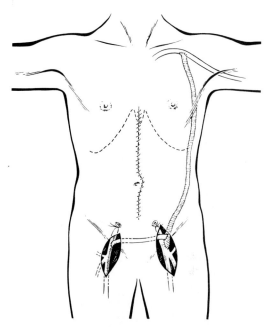

Fig. 18-2. Axillobifemoral bypass can be performed in the standard fashion when the aortic prosthesis is confined entirely to the abdomen. When graft excision is carried out first, the abdominal incision is closed and sealed with plastic drapes before the EAB is carried out to prevent contamination. (From Bernhard VM. Aortoenteric fistulas. In Bergan JJ, Yao JST, eds. Operative Techniques in Vascular Surgery. Orlando, Fla.: WB Saunders, 1980, pp 193-202.)

tients underwent excision and EAB. There were six perioperative deaths (myocardial infarction in three, and exsanguination, persistent infection, and multisystem failure in one each). However, two additional patients died of recurrent sepsis, and therefore of the eight deaths, 50% were caused by sepsis. This excellent series is not included in Table 18-3 since 72% were autogenous EAB reconstructions and results were not separately analyzed. The two largest series in Table 18-3 are those of Lorentzen et al.[28] and O'Hara et al.[35] Both report a significant incidence of recurrent sepsis involving the EAB itself: 13% and 25%, respectively.

Because of concern for both the duration of the procedure and the possibility of contamination of the EAB, the question of the sequence of bypass and excision and delay between the

Table 18-3. Graft Excision and Extra-anatomic Bypass for Aortic Graft Infection

Author	No. of patients	Healed	Died	Amputation	Follow-up (yr)	Comments
Shaw and Baue[17] (1963)	1	1	0	0	NS	Obturator bypass
Veith et al.[41] (1964)	1	1	0	0	1	
Fry and Lindenauer[42] (1966)	1	0	1	0	NA	Groin only
Najafi et al.[31] (1969)	1	1	0	0	NS	CNS by history
Dietrich et al.[43] (1970)	3	3	0	0	NS	
Conn et al.[18] (1970)	1	0	0	1	NS	
Szilagyi et al.[7] (1972)	3	1	2	0	NS	
Jamieson et al.[32] (1975)	5	3	2	0	NS	In the 2 patients who subsequently died, partial excision of one graft limb was attempted
Spanos et al.[44] (1976)	2	2	0	0	3	
Liekweg and Greenfield[20] (1977)	3	1	2	1	NS	Amputation led to 1 death
Yashar et al.[21] (1978)	4	2	1	2	NS	Amputation led to 1 death
Fulenwider et al.[33] (1983)	8	4	0	4	3	2 delayed in situ grafts were late due to repeated axillofemoral thrombosis
Bennion et al.[37] (1983)	5	5	0	0	2.2	All remote groin infections and delayed EAB
Trout et al.[45] (1984)	3	1	2	0	4	13 days, 3rd stump rupture
Lorentzen et al.[28] (1985)	20	13	2	3	1.2	2 patients chronically infected but doing well
Yeager et al.[46] (1985)	3	1	1	1	1	Infected axillofemoral bypass
O'Hara et al.[35] (1986)	32	20	4	8	1	8 patients with recurrent infection in EABs
Thomas and Baird[34] (1986)	1	0	1	0	NA	
TOTAL	97	59 (61%)	18 (18%)	20 (21%)		

NS, not stated; NA, not applicable; CNS, coagulase-negative staphylococci; EAB, extra-anatomic bypass.

former and the latter have received attention.[35,36,45,46] The larger series[35,36] have shown no significant differences in the incidence of EAB infection or operative mortality with either an initial bypass followed by either immediate or remote graft excision or the sequence of graft excision followed immediately by EAB. Whether the staged EAB and remote excision approach is less stressful, with a lower morbidity and mortality, is unclear since an inherent bias colors all retrospective analyses. There were no differences in survival between these groups reported by O'Hara et al.,[35] and these results were similar to those of Reilly et al.,[36] who registered a 24% mortality in the immediate-sequential vs. 26% in the staged-remote group. Similar problems plague retrospective analysis of amputation rates. O'Hara et al.[35] reported an amputation rate of 41% in the immediate-sequential EAB group and only a 7% amputation rate in the staged-remote EAB group; similar findings were noted by Reilly et al.[36] Therefore it may be advantageous to establish EAB before graft excision to reduce the amputation rate.

The technique employed for EAB depends on the location of the septic process with regard to the groins. If the process is limited to the intra-abdominal retroperitoneum and the groins are not involved, axillofemoral bypass can be carried out in the standard fashion (Fig. 18-2). This is the usual situation when dealing with aortic tube or aortoiliac bifurcation grafts. When the graft extends to one or both of the femoral arteries, it is important to rule out occult extension of the infection to the groin areas by CT scan and indium-111 white cell scanning in addition to clinical examination. If these studies are negative, the patient is hemodynamically stable, and there is little or no doubt that the diagnosis of graft infection is correct, it is appropriate to proceed with axillofemoral bypass first. At the time of femoral exposure, the portions of the prior graft in the groin should be grossly evaluated for infection, and segments of graft and arterial wall at the old anastomosis should be excised for culture.[10] After femoral anastomoses are completed, the distal limbs of the old graft are ligated and tucked well up behind the inguinal ligaments, and healthy tissue is reapproximated around the femoral artery. This may help to seal off the new graft and femoral anastomoses from contamination when the distal limbs of the old graft are subsequently drawn up into the septic area at the time of abdominal exploration and graft removal.

When abdominal AGI extends to the groin, the technique of EAB must be designed to avoid contamination of the new extra-anatomic prostheses. Considerable ingenuity is often required to permit satisfactory limb revascularization without graft contamination. This may

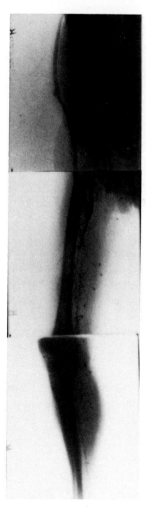

Fig. 18-3. Composite Dacron and arm vein axillo-profunda bypass inserted before excision of diffusely infected aortofemoral and femoropopliteal Dacron prostheses.

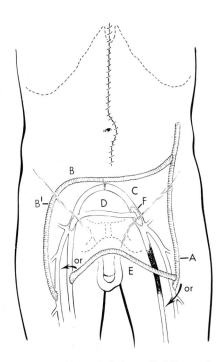

Fig. 18-4. Variations of the axillobifemoral technique to avoid contamination from the groin wounds from an infected aortofemoral graft. *A,* Lateral placement of the axillofemoral limb just medial and deep to the anterior superior iliac spine with anastomosis to the midprofunda or distal femoropopliteal segment. *B,* High takeoff of the femorofemoral limb tunneled between the distal end of the abdominal incision and the pubis but sufficiently proximal to the old femoral incisions to remain in fresh uncontaminated tissue. *B¹,* The descending limb is placed laterally. *C,* Iliac arteries may be anastomosed to each other to provide transpelvic crossover. *D,* Autogenous saphenous vein femorofemoral bypass through contaminated groin wounds. This graft is not inserted until the wounds for the lateral axillofemoral graft have been closed. *E,* Femorofemoral graft tunneled through clean tissue medial and distal to the groin wounds and crossing over to the opposite thigh below the pubic prominence. *F,* Vein patch closure of common femoral defect after excision of an aortofemoral graft limb. (From Bernhard VM. Aortoenteric fistulas. In Bergan JJ, Yao JST, eds. Operative Techniques in Vascular Surgery. Orlando, Fla.: WB Saunders, 1980, pp 193-202.)

require lateral bypass to the distal profunda femoris or popliteal artery (Fig. 18-3) combined with autogenous in situ repair within the infected groin fields. The various strategies applied under these circumstances are depicted in Fig. 18-4.

The obturator foramen may be the optimal route for EAB when graft sepsis is clearly limited to the distal few centimeters of one aortofemoral graft limb and satisfactory runoff can be achieved through the popliteal artery. After the infected area is carefully sealed off, the proximal portion of the graft is exposed through a transperitoneal or retroperitoneal approach to determine that it is well incorporated, indicating that there is no evidence of infection at this level. It is transected and the proximal end is sutured to a new prosthesis, which is tunneled through the obturator membrane and deep to the adductor longus muscle to the point of anastomosis to the popliteal artery.[17,38a]

Excision and EAB remains the best available treatment option for the majority of cases of AGI when the septic process is not limited to one limb of the graft.

Excision and Autologous Reconstruction

Although not possible in the majority of cases, good results have been reported with this treatment option (Table 18-4).[46-48] In 1979, an extension of an earlier series, Ehrenfeld et al.[47] reported on 24 patients (15 of whom had AGIs) treated by excision and autogenous reconstruction with a 20% mortality rate and 13% amputation rate. The operative techniques employed in this series included native vessel endarterectomy, arterial autograft replacement or bypass in situ, and vein patch angioplasty. In some instances, autogenous repair was combined with an EAB prosthesis or composite graft.

Good early results were also obtained by Seeger et al.,[48] who performed eversion endarterectomy on the excised aorta and used saphenous vein to create a new bifurcation, which was placed in situ to achieve total autogenous repair (Table 18-4). However, half of these patients (5 of 10) had a coagulase-negative staphylococcal graft infection, which may be less aggressive in the presence of native tissue repair. Furthermore, 67% of these patients required

Table 18-4. Graft Excision and Autologous Reconstruction for Aortic Graft Infection

Author	No. of patients	Healed	Died	Amputation	Follow-up (yr)	Comments
Ehrenfeld et al.[47] (1979)	15	10	3	2	1.4	Arterial autografts predominant
Seeger et al.[48] (1983)	10	8	1	1	0.2	5 CNS by description; 6 needed subsequent revisions
Yeager et al.[46] (1985)	3	1	2	0	3	
TOTAL	28	19 (68%)	6 (21%)	3 (11%)		

CNS, coagulase-negative staphylococci.

subsequent procedures for recurrent distal ischemia resulting from graft-related problems.

Overall recorded results for autologous repair in a total of 28 patients collected from the literature was healing in 68%, death in 21%, and amputation in 11% (Table 18-4).

Excision and In Situ Replacement

In situ prosthetic graft replacement for AGIs has been infrequently recommended except for a recent report by Bergamini et al.[49] (Table 18-5). In their experience with 15 cases of late (greater than 4 months) coagulase-negative staphylococcus (CNS) infection, 12 were confined to one limb of an aortobifemoral graft. Remarkable success was achieved with in situ placement of a new prosthesis. However, rigid criteria were used for patient selection and patients were excluded if they presented early (less than 4 months after graft insertion), had systemic signs of sepsis, or had residual bacterial tissue invasion as determined by gram-positive stain or culture. All patients presented with a normal white count and were afebrile. The primary clinical finding indicating infection in these patients was the demonstration of failure of graft incorporation in the groin. In many of these cases, CNS was cultured in trypticase soy broth only after ultrasound treatment of the excised graft. This suggests that some of the previously reported cases of perigraft seroma[15] may indeed represent CNS infection. Treatment consisted of excision of the involved segment of graft, extensive débridement of perigraft tissues and adjacent artery, and in situ replacement with a new prosthetic graft limb of polytetrafluoroethylene (PTFE). The skin was closed primarily. Parenteral antibiotics followed by oral antibiotics were administered for 6 to 12 weeks.

Late follow-up with a mean of 18 months (range, 5.5 to 34 months) documented continued success with this very select group of patients. When the specific conditions described by Bergamini et al. are not present, the application of this therapeutic regimen is questionable since there are very few successful cases to support in situ prosthetic treatment of AGIs when obvious and extensive sepsis involves the proximal graft.[9,23,33-35]

Table 18-5. Graft Excision and In Situ Replacement for Aortic Graft Infection

Author	No. of patients	Healed	Died	Amputation	Follow-up (yr)	Comments
Blaisdell et al.[39] (1961)	1	0	1	0	NA	
Shaw and Baue[17] (1963)	1	0	1	0	NA	
Veith et al.[41] (1964)	1	0	0	0	NA	Required subsequent removal
Szilagyi et al.[7] (1972)	3	3	0	0	NS	All groin infections
Thomas and Baird[34] (1986)	1	1	0	0	1.5	
Bergamini et al.[49] (1991)	12	12	0	0	1.5	CNS only; all groin
TOTAL	19	16 (84%)	2 (11%)	0		

NA, not applicable; NS, not stated; CNS, coagulase-negative staphylococci.

AORTOENTERIC FISTULAS

The management of aortoenteric fistula (AEF) presents a unique challenge since treatment decisions such as staged-remote vs. immediate-sequential bypass depend on the presence and severity of active gastrointestinal bleeding in addition to the degree of sepsis. Overall results are generally poorer than with AGIs in all categories (Tables 18-6 through 18-9). For the purposes of this review, secondary AEFs are discussed separately from AGIs. In addition, it is important to distinguish treatment of primary AEF, usually caused by aneurysm erosion into the gastrointestinal tract, from graft-enteric fistula. Two excellent reports[50,51] have documented the safety of in situ graft placement for *primary* AEF.

Local Treatment

Local surgical treatment has been reported for AEF by several authors (Table 18-6) and is appealing since additional hemodynamic stress from surgery is minimized in these patients, who are frequently in shock, and distal perfusion is not interrupted. Unfortunately this approach is generally associated with a high mortality because of sepsis and recurrence of the fistula.

Kleinman, Towne, and Bernhard[38] reported the results of various treatment options in 20 patients with secondary AEFs in 1979. None of the patients in whom the aortic prosthesis was left in place survived; death was caused by recurrent AEF. Champion et al.,[62] in a large series of AEFs, also reported that death occurred in all five patients who received local repair. The one notable exception is a report in the British literature by Thomas and Baird[34] in 1986. In a series of seven patients, four had closure of the duodenum, direct suture repair of the aortic defect, and omental interposition. With good follow-up, three patients have had no further difficulty. One patient with recurrence of the AEF at 3 months was successfully re-repaired and was well for 3 years thereafter. However, the overall reported AEF-related mortality with this approach is 72%. Only 8 of 43 patients treated in this fashion have survived. Therefore, despite good results from one small series, this approach is not recommended.

Table 18-6. Local Aortic and Bowel Repair for Aortoenteric Fistula (Graft Not Removed)*

Author	No. of patients	Healed	Died	Amputation	Follow-up (yr)	Comments
MGH#45282/45522[52] (1959)	2	1	1	0	NS	
Cordell[52] (1960)	1	0	1	0	NA	
DeWeese[52] (1962)	2	0	2	0	NA	
Humphries et al.[52] (1963)	5	0	5	0	NA	
Garrett et al.[53] (1963)	1	0	0	0	2	Recurrent AEF at 19 mo
Ferris et al.[54] (1965)	1	0	0	0	NA	Recurrent AEF at 3 mo
Van de Water and Gaal[29] (1965)	1	1	0	0	NS	
Tobias and Daicoff[55] (1973)	1	1	0	0	4	
Elliott et al.[56] (1974)	4	1	3	0	NS	
Brenner et al.[57] (1974)	1	1	0	0	NS	
Yashar et al.[21] (1978)	1	0	1	0	NA	Dacron patch
Dean et al.[58] (1978)	1	0	1	0	NA	
Busuttil et al.[59] (1979)	1	0	1	0	NA	
Kleinman et al.[38] (1979)	2	0	2	0	NA	2 deaths from recurrent AEF at 1 mo and 2 mo
Buchbinder et al.[60] (1980)	2	0	2	0	NA	
O'Mara et al.[61] (1981)	3	0	2	0	NS	1 recurrent AEF at 1 yr
Champion et al.[62] (1982)	5	0	5	0	NS	
Flye and Thompson[63] (1983)	2	0	2	0	NA	
O'Hara et al.[35] (1986)	3	0	3	0	NA	
Thomas and Baird[34] (1986)	4	3	0	0	3	1 recurrent AEF at 3 mo
TOTAL	43	8 (19%)	31 (72%)	0		

NS, not stated; NA, not applicable; AEF, aortoenteric fistula.
*No homografts.

Excision

In an extensive series of late failures after reconstruction for occlusive disease, Crawford et al.[64] described two cases of secondary AEF treated by graft excision alone. Although both patients survived, unilateral amputation was required in one patient as a result of ischemia. Subsequently reported results by others using this technique have been poor, and the overall collected mortality is 79% (Table 18-7). The low amputation rate reflects the low number of survivors and in many reports was not documented. By contrast with AGIs, more AEFs occur after prosthetic replacement for aneurysmal disease. Since collateral flow would be expected to be poor in these patients, this may be a factor contributing to the high mortality rate.

Although the numbers are small and the reported experience is merely a collection of anecdotes, the generally poor results suggest that closure of the enteric defect and graft excision alone should not be recommended.

Excision and EAB

The first case of graft AEF managed by graft excision and EAB was reported by Blaisdell, DeMattei, and Gauder[39] in 1961. Sporadic reports followed during the 1960s. The publication of a relatively large experience by Kleinman, Towne, and Bernhard[38] in 1979 and subsequent reports by others have documented the utility of this technique (Table 18-8).

Kleinman, Towne, and Bernhard[38] reported seven patients who underwent graft excision, closure of the bowel defect, and placement of a knitted Dacron axillobifemoral bypass graft. Two patients had intraoperative hypotension: renal failure developed in one and the other patient suffered a myocardial infarction; both subsequently died. Five patients (71.5%) survived. Buchbinder et al.[60] had similar results (64% survival) in a group of 14 patients treated in this fashion.

The largest reported series using this method is that by O'Hara et al.[35] and covers a 25-year experience at the Cleveland Clinic. In their experience with 84 AGIs, 33 patients were treated for AEFs. Nine were managed by a variety of techniques in which prosthetic material was not

Table 18-7. Graft Excision Without Limb Revascularization for Aortoenteric Fistula

Author	No. of patients	Healed	Died	Amputation	Follow-up (yr)	Comments
Crawford et al.[64] (1960)	2	1	0	1	NS	
Garrett et al.[53] (1963)	1	1	0	0	4	
Cohn and Angell[30] (1968)	1	0	1	0	NA	
Elliott et al.[56] (1974)	2	0	2	0	NA	Both deaths from stump rupture
Dean et al.[58] (1978)	1	0	1	0	NA	
Busuttil et al.[59] (1979)	2	0	2	0	NA	
Kleinman et al.[38] (1979)	4	1	3	0	1	Stump rupture at 7 mo
O'Mara et al.[61] (1981)	1	0	1	0	NA	
Champion et al.[62] (1982)	4	0	4	0	NA	
Flye and Thompson[63] (1983)	1	0	1	0	NA	Recurrent AEF
TOTAL	19	3 (16%)	15 (79%)	1 (5%)		

NS, not stated; NA, not applicable; AEF, aortoenteric fistula.

Table 18-8. Graft Excision and Extra-anatomic Bypass for Aortoenteric Fistula

Author	No. of patients	Healed	Died	Amputation	Follow-up (yr)	Comments
Conn et al.[18] (1970)	1	0	1	0	NA	
Elliott et al.[56] (1974)	2	2	0	0	NS	
Spanos et al.[44] (1976)	4	2	2	0	3	
Yashar et al.[21] (1978)	1	0	1	0	0.5	Late death from EAB infection
Dean et al.[58] (1978)	1	1	0	0	1	
Kleinman et al.[38] (1979)	7	4	2	0	1.5	1 late death from recurrent AEF
Buchbinder et al.[60] (1980)	14	9	5	0	NS	2 deaths from recurrent AEF or stump rupture
O'Mara et al.[61] (1981)	8	2	6	0	3	1 late death from stump rupture at 4 mo
Connolly et al.[22] (1981)	4	2	2	0	1	
Champion et al.[62] (1982)	6	3	3	1	NS	
Fulenwider et al.[33] (1983)	7	1	3	3	3	
Flye and Thompson[63] (1983)	10	3	7	0	NS	
Trout et al.[45] (1984)	4	3	2	0	1.1	1 death from ruptured thoracic aneurysm at 10 days
Yeager et al.[46] (1985)	8	4	3	1	2	
O'Hara et al.[35] (1986)	22	10	12	NS	1	4 late deaths in first year
Aarnio and Hannukainen[65] (1989)	3	2	1	0	1	
TOTAL	102	48 (47%)	43 (47%)	5 (5%)		

NA, not applicable; NS, not stated; EAB, extra-anatomic bypass; AEF, aortoenteric fistula.

Table 18-9. Graft Excision and In Situ Revascularization for Aortoenteric Fistula

Author	No. of patients	Healed	Died	Amputation	Follow-up (yr)	Comments
Sharf[52] (1959)	1	0	1	0	NA	Nylon graft
Thistlewaite et al.[67] (1960)	1	0	1	0	NA	Died during surgery
Blaisdell et al.[39] (1961)	1	0	1	0	NA	
Hershey[52] (1962)	1	0	1	0	NA	
Sproul[68] (1962)	1	1	0	0	NS	
Humphries et al.[52] (1963)	4	0	4	0	NA	
Garrett et al.[53] (1963)	2	1	1	0	4	
Ferris et al.[54] (1965)	1	1	0	0	NS	
Rosato et al.[69] (1967)	1	1	0	0	0.5	Died at 6 mo of MI; no autopsy
Cohn and Angell[30] (1968)	2	1	1	0	NS	
Conn et al.[18] (1970)	1	0	1	0	NA	
Pinkerton[70] (1973)	1	1	0	0	0.5	
Elliott et al.[56] (1974)	5	2	2	0	NS	In 1 patient, graft was subsequently excised and EAB performed
Yashar et al.[21] (1978)	1	0	1	0	NA	
Dean et al.[58] (1978)	3	2	1	0	1	Recurrent AEF at 2 yr; led to death
Busuttil et al.[59] (1979)	1	0	1	0	2	
Kleinman et al.[38] (1979)	2	0	2	0		Deaths from recurrent fistula at 1 mo and 7 mo
O'Mara et al.[61] (1981)	3	0	3	0	NA	1 died at 15 mo from recurrent AEF
Champion et al.[62] (1982)	3	1	1	0	NS	One chronically infected but doing well
Flye and Thompson[63] (1983)	3	1	2	0	NS	
O'Hara et al.[35] (1986)	6	0	6	0	NA	
Thomas and Baird[34] (1986)	1	1	0	0	5	
Walker et al.[66] (1987)	23	16	7	0	5	2 aortic ruptures at 1 mo, 3 mo
TOTAL	68	29 (43%)	37 (54%)	0		

NA, not applicable; NS, not stated; MI, myocardial infarction; EAB, extra-anatomic bypass; AEF, aortoenteric fistula.

entirely removed. Eight died and one was lost to follow-up. Two patients had excision alone. Twenty-two patients were treated by graft excision, duodenal repair, and EAB. Eight (36%) died within 30 days and another four (18%) within the first year. The major causes of death were not specified by treatment type but the overall cause of mortality for AEF was sepsis in 48%, ruptured aortic stump in 32%, and myocardial infarction in 16%. Aortic stump ruptures occurred at a mean 94 days following surgical repair, emphasizing the need to adequately débride the aortic stump before closure.

Overall mortality with excision and EAB in the collected series in Table 18-8 is 47%, which compares favorably to either local surgical treatment (72% mortality) or excision alone (79% mortality). The amputation rate of 5% is remarkably low in comparison to that of the other techniques. These data and the fact that these prostheses are infected by a wide variety of enteric as well as other organisms suggest that this technique is the most reliable method of management.

Excision and In Situ Revascularization

Although the grossly contaminated graft with extensive perigraft infection caused by AEF should be treated with excision and EAB, controversy exists regarding the optimal treatment when contamination is minimal. New graft replacement in situ has been recommended under these conditions and requires graft excision, aggressive débridement of locally infected tissues and of the aorta back to what grossly appears to be healthy, noninfected arterial wall, and repair of the enteric defect. Aortic continuity is then restored by in situ placement of a new prosthesis, and a tongue of greater omentum is placed between the graft and the overlying bowel. Collected results with this method (Table 18-9) are not noticeably different than excision and EAB (Table 18-8). However, the largest reported series of in situ replacement under these circumstances had somewhat better results.[66] Walker et al.[66] employed this treatment in 23 *consecutive* patients with a 30% mortality, mainly from sepsis or recurrent hemorrhage.

Except for this report, all other investigators

with more than 15 patients advocate excision and EAB[38,60,62] based on discouraging results with in situ grafts and local care. Nevertheless, in situ grafting may be a valuable option in selected cases and is deserving of further study. Furthermore, the use of long-term antibiotic coverage in cases where positive arterial wall cultures indicate residual bacterial invasion beyond the point of débridement may improve results regardless of technique used.[11]

In situ grafting and excision with EAB are not equivalent alternatives for the management of AEFs. Clinical judgment regarding the degree of local contamination and the adequacy of distal runoff to support an EAB provide the best clues for selecting optimal management in the individual case.

AORTIC STUMP AND ANASTOMOTIC RUPTURE

Rupture of a closed aortic stump or of a repaired arterial anastomotic site has frequently occurred after excision of an infected graft for either AGI or AEF.[35,38,56] This problem appears to be the result of inadequate débridement of the vessel back to healthy noninfected arterial wall.[11] The thoroughness of arterial wall débridement should be monitored by the gross appearance of the vessel and by culture of a specimen of the residual wall after what appears to be satisfactory excision (Fig. 18-5). If this culture is negative, antibiotic therapy may be discontinued when the acute septic process is clinically resolved, which usually occurs within 2 weeks. However, if the arterial wall culture is positive, specific antibiotic therapy should be administered intravenously for 4 to 6 weeks and continued orally for 6 months. Closure of the aortic stump is depicted in Fig. 18-6. If adequate aortic stump débridement is limited by proximity to the renal arteries, then either hepatorenal bypass on the right side with saphenous vein and/or splenorenal bypass on the left side can be performed to permit more proximal arterial excision[71] (Fig. 18-7).

Retrospective analysis of the experience from our institution revealed that aortic stump or reanastomosis disruption did not occur if these criteria were applied.[11] Data are insufficient at this time to define a more precise dura-

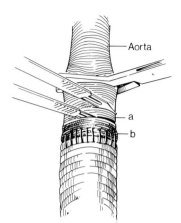

Aorta

a

b

Fig. 18-5. Aortic stump débridement. The anastomosis to the infected graft is resected back to healthy tissue *(b)*. A biopsy specimen is obtained for culture of the remaining aortic stump *(a)*. (From Bernhard VM, Parent FN. Treatment of aortic graft infection. In Ernst CB, Stanley JC, eds. Current Therapy in Vascular Surgery, 2nd ed. Philadelphia: BC Decker, 1991, pp 435-440.)

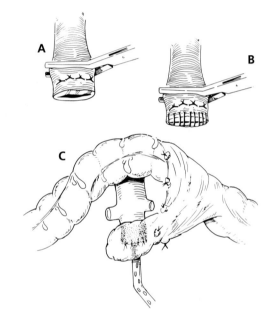

Fig. 18-6. A and **B**, Closure of aortic stump in two layers and omental coverage **(C)** after adequate débridement. A suction drain is placed below the stump in the former prosthetic bed **(C)**. (From Bernhard VM, Parent FN. Treatment of aortic graft infection. In Ernst CB, Stanley JC, eds. Current Therapy in Vascular Surgery, 2nd ed. Philadelphia: BC Decker, 1991, pp 435-440.)

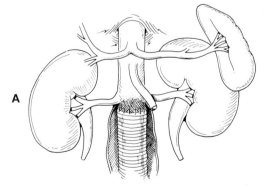
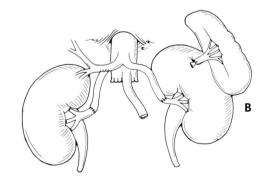

Fig. 18-7. When aortic wall sepsis extends up to or proximal to the renal orifices **(A),** hepatorenal and splenorenal autogenous bypass can be employed to preserve renal function **(B).**

tion of long-term antibiotic therapy when stump cultures are positive.

INFRAINGUINAL GRAFT INFECTIONS

The mortality rates reported for prosthetic graft infections in this location are much lower than for AGIs. However, amputation rates are higher (Tables 18-10 and 18-11). The primary decision involved in the management of a peripheral graft infection is whether primary amputation or an aggressive attempt to maintain perfusion for limb salvage is indicated.[9] Clinical judgment must be individualized, taking into consideration the associated medical conditions, the patency of the bypass graft, and the extent of proximal and distal native vessel disease.

Local Treatment

In 1972, Szilagyi et al.[7] developed a classification of wound infections related to bypass grafts in a review of 3347 "arterioplastic" operations. Grade I infections (1.7%) involved the dermis, Grade II infections (2%) extended to the subcutaneous region, and Grade III infections (1.5%) involved the graft itself. All Grade I and II infections healed promptly with local care. Grade III infections were more problematic.

In 1959, Schramel and Creech[6] treated two peripheral graft infections with local care. In one patient, in whom a crimped nylon femoropopliteal bypass was performed, an infection in the popliteal region developed that failed to heal with local care and a sartorius muscle flap. Although the patient survived, graft excision was necessary to control sepsis, and amputation at the hip was required. By contrast, a popliteal abscess developed in a second patient, who was successfully treated with continuous antibiotic irrigation. Many authors have reported their experiences with local care of prosthetic infections, with a collected mortality of 8% and amputation rate of 10% (Table 18-10). Although this is better than reported results from excision alone (Table 18-11), these groups are not comparable. In patients receiving local care, infections were usually caused by early wound breakdown, anastomoses were generally not in-

volved, the graft was functioning, and the limb was viable. By contrast, patients in whom excision alone was performed had thrombosed grafts and/or nonviable extremities. It is difficult to determine the contribution of infection as an independent variable relating to outcome in some reports since graft patency was not consistently documented. Patients with occluded grafts and infections have a worse outcome than those with infections in patent grafts.

Smith, Lowry, and Perdue[73] treated nine patients with prosthetic infrainguinal infections with aggressive local wound care including the topical application of betadine and achieved healing in eight. All grafts were patent at the time of initial treatment. Kwaan and Connolly[23] treated five groin infections (three axillofemoral, two femorofemoral) with local povidone-iodine irrigation, resulting in successful healing in all cases. All grafts were patent on initial presentation. Lorentzen et al.,[28] however, reported one death and two amputations in five patients treated, but no mention was made of graft patency at the time of presentation. Mixter et al.[12] achieved excellent results in eight patients treated with rotational muscle flaps in the groin. All of these grafts were patent at the time of treatment. Calligaro et al.[75] treated eight patients with *patent* grafts with povidone-iodine or antibiotic-soaked dressings and was successful in six patients; however, one died of sepsis and another had a nonhealing wound at 5 weeks.

Local care is the initial treatment of choice for peripheral graft infections when the graft is patent and there is no associated anastomotic dehiscence or bleeding.

Excision

Excision has been associated with a higher amputation rate (59%) (Table 18-11) than local care; however, this difference is probably the result of the bias of case selection. Szilagyi et al.[7] treated 12 iliofemoral and femoropopliteal synthetic bypass grafts with excision, which resulted in five amputations but no mortality. It is unclear what percentage of these were occluded at the time of presentation. Samson et al.[76] excised the occluded, infected prosthesis in 19 patients, leaving a small stump of graft so that the under-

Table 18-10. Local Treatment for Infrainguinal Graft Infection

Author	No. of patients	Healed	Died	Amputation	Follow-up (yr)	Comments
Schramel and Creech[6] (1959)	3	2	0	1	7 mo	No culture information
Shaw and Baue[17] (1963)	1	1	0		NS	
Hoffert et al.[72] (1965)	4	2	0	1	NS	2 failures; 1 *E. coli*; no culture information for 1
Smith et al.[73] (1967)	9	8	0	0	1.5	No problems
Conn et al[18] (1970)	3	1	2	1	NA	1 late death following amputation
Szilagyi et al.[7] (1972)	1	1	0	0	NS	No culture information
Yashar et al.[21] (1978)	1	1	0	0	NS	No anastomosis involvement
Popovsky and Singer[74] (1980)	3	3	0	0	3	2 axillofemoral, 1 femoral patch; all groin
Kwaan and Connolly[23] (1981)	5	5	0	0	1	3 axillofemoral, 2 femorofemoral
Almgren and Eriksson[24] (1981)	1	1	0	0	3	
Lorentzen et al.[28] (1985)	5	2	1	2	1.2	
Mixter et al.[12] (1989)	8	7	0	0	3	Muscle flap
Calligaro et al.[75] (1990)	8	6	1	0	1	
TOTAL	52	40 (77%)	4 (8%)	5 (10%)		

NS, not stated; NA, not applicable.

Table 18-11. Graft Excision Without Revascularization for Infrainguinal Graft Infection

Author	No. of patients	Healed	Died	Amputation	Follow-up (yr)	Comments
Schramel and Creech[6] (1959)	1	1	NS	NS	NS	
Carter et al.[16] (1963)	1	1	NS	NS	1	
Hoffert et al.[72] (1965)	6	1	1	5	NS	
Conn et al.[18] (1970)	4	1	NS	3	NS	
Szilagyi et al.[7] (1972)	12	7	NS	5	NS	
Yashar et al.[21] (1978)	2	NS	NS	2	NA	
Yeager et al.[46] (1985)	5	2	2	2	NS	
Lorentzen et al.[28] (1985)	10	1	2	7	NS	
Kikta et al.[77] (1987)	32	2	7	26	NS	
Samson et al.[76] (1988)	19	9	2	5	NS	Partial graft excision
Samson et al.[76] (1988)	4	3	0	1	NS	Total graft excision
TOTAL	96	28 (29%)	14 (15%)	56 (59%)		

NS, not stated; NA, not applicable.

lying native artery could provide collateral flow. Healing with an intact limb was achieved in nine (Table 18-5). Kikta et al.[77] treated 32 patients with primary prosthetic graft infections with excision. In 11 cases "reconstructive procedures to maintain axial blood flow" were performed but these consisted exclusively of vein patch angioplasty. Although not stated by the authors, these were presumably at the common femoral bifurcation and patch repair was apparently employed to maintain flow through the profunda femoris artery. Since 87% of the original bypasses were for "limb salvage," limb perfusion was lost when the infected graft was removed. Therefore it is not surprising that they reported a 79% amputation rate and a 22% mortality rate. If a patient presents with a nonviable extremity and an infected occluded bypass graft, amputation and either partial[43] or preferably total graft excision are indicated. If a patient presents with an ischemic but viable extremity and an occluded infected graft, it is unrealistic to assume that anything short of complete graft removal will be successful.

Excision and Revascularization

The majority of infrainguinal bypasses are performed using autogenous material to begin with and therefore those patients in whom infection develops in a prosthetic bypass frequently have no other source of autogenous material. This may explain the relative paucity of data regarding autogenous reconstruction under these circumstances. Exclusive of sporadic case reports, the only series of autogenous revascularization after prosthetic peripheral graft removal is that by Yeager et al.[46] and encompasses only five patients treated in this manner. Four survivors healed and a single patient died from sepsis. This patient had subtotal graft excision as opposed to the survivors whose grafts were completely removed. Autogenous reconstruction after prosthetic graft removal should be performed when possible.

When autogenous material is unavailable, revascularization with a prosthesis, usually PTFE, may be feasible if a satisfactory runoff vessel can be identified in the distal uninfected area and there is an alternate bypass route available through healthy tissue.

Calligaro et al.[75] treated six patients with occluded infected grafts by excision and prosthetic EAB, presumably through clean tissue planes with resultant healing in five and one amputation. However, one of the patients who had healed, presented with anastomotic disruption 2 years later.

CONCLUSION

Inherent methodologic problems in all collective reviews of vascular graft infection including this one *do not* allow for strict comparisons of results by various treatment methods. Although this review is helpful in providing clues for appropriate therapy, sound clinical judgment is needed to manage these difficult problems. The following general principles can be derived from previously recorded experiences.

Aortic Graft Infections (AGIs)

1. Aortic prosthetic infections limited to the distal limb in the groin without anastomotic involvement are frequently amenable to local care.

2. Aortic prosthetic infections in already occluded grafts or in cases in which collateral flow can be expected to be adequate for distal perfusion can be treated with excision alone.

3. Most aortic prosthetic infections should be treated by *total* graft excision and EAB.

4. Except for localized and minimal CNS infections, in situ prosthetic replacement is not advisable.

Aortoenteric Fistulas

1. In the presence of gross contamination, excision of all graft material and EAB is recommended.

2. In selected cases with minimal contamination, graft excision, débridement of all infected and nonviable tissue, and in situ regrafting may be indicated.

Peripheral Graft Infections

1. In the absence of anastomotic involvement, pseudoaneurysm, or a thrombosed graft, an initial trial of local care is warranted.

2. Pseudoaneurysm, hemorrhage, or a thrombosed graft requires prompt graft removal and revascularization when feasible or amputation.

No set of recommendations can improve on a well–thought-out plan and appropriate preoperative preparation. Determining the extent of infection with preoperative angiography and imaging studies, identifying sources of autogenous material, planning extra-anatomic routes, aggressive perigraft tissue débridement, adequate resection of infected arterial wall, and appropriate supportive measures are all components of a successful outcome.

REFERENCES

1. Wheeler HB. Presidential address: Common sense and carotid endarterectomy. J Vasc Surg 11:735-744, 1990.
2. Reilly LM, Altman H, Lusby RJ, Kersh RA, Ehrenfeld WK, Stoney RJ. Late results following surgical management of vascular graft infection. J Vasc Surg 1:36-44, 1984.
3. Turnipseed WD, Berkoff HA, Detmer DE, Acker CW, Belzer FO. Arterial graft infections: Delayed vs. immediate vascular reconstruction. Arch Surg 118: 410-414, 1983.
4. Goldstone J, Moore WS. Infection in vascular prosthesis: Clinical manifestations and surgical management. Am J Surg 128:225-233, 1974.
5. Bunt TJ. Synthetic vascular graft infections. I. Graft infections. Surgery 93:733-746, 1983.
6. Schramel RJ, Creech O. Effects of infection and exposure on synthetic arterial prosthesis. Arch Surg 78: 1028, 1959.
7. Szilagyi DE, Smith RR, Elliott JP, Vrandecic MP. Infection in arterial reconstruction with synthetic grafts. Am Surg 176:321-333, 1972.
8. Wengrovitz M, Atnip RG, Gifford RRM, Neumeyer MM, Heitjan DR, Thiele BL. Wound complications of autogenous subcutaneous infrainguinal arterial bypass surgery: Predisposing factors and management. J Vasc Surg 11:156-163, 1990.
9. Rubin JR, Folsom D. The management of lower extremity graft infections. Semin Vasc Surg 3:114-121, 1990.
10. Durham JR, Malone JM, Bernhard VM. The impact of multiple operations and the importance of arterial wall cultures. J Vasc Surg 5:160-169, 1987.
11. Malone JM, Lalka SG, McIntyre KE, Bernhard VM, Pabst TS. The necessity for long term antibiotic therapy with positive arterial wall cultures. J Vasc Surg 8:262-267, 1988.
12. Mixter RC, Turnipseed WD, Smith DJ, Acker CW, Rao VK, Dibbal DG. Rotational muscle flaps: A new technique for covering infected vascular grafts. J Vasc Surg 9:472-478, 1989.

13. Olofson PA, Auffermann W, Higgins CB, Robakie GN, Tavores N, Stoney RJ. Diagnosis of prosthetic aortic graft infection by magnetic resonance imaging. J Vasc Surg 8:99-105, 1988.

14. Cunat JS, Haaga JR, Rhodes R, Bekemy J, El Yousef S. Perigraft fluid aspiration for recognition of infected graft. AJR 139:251-253, 1982.

15. Blumenberg RM, Gelfand ML, Dale WA. Complicating arterial grafts. Surgery 97:194-203, 1985.

16. Carter SC, Cohen A, Whelan TJ. Clinical experience with management of the infected Dacron graft. Am Surg 58:249-255, 1963.

17. Shaw RS, Baue AE. Management of sepsis complicating arterial reconstructive surgery. Surgery 53:75-86, 1963.

18. Conn JH, Hardy JD, Chavez CM, Fain WR. Infected arterial grafts: Experience in 22 cases with emphasis on unusual bacteria and technics. Ann Surg 171: 704-714, 1970.

19. Becker RM, Blundell PE. Infected aortic bifurcation grafts: Experience with fourteen patients. Surgery 80:544-549, 1976.

20. Liekweg WG, Greenfield LJ. Vascular prosthetic infections: Collected experience and results of treatment. Surgery 81:335-342, 1977.

21. Yashar JJ, Weyman AK, Burnard RJ, Yashar J. Survival and limb salvage in patients with infected arterial prostheses. Am J Surg 135:499-504, 1978.

22. Connolly JE, Kwaan JHM, McCort PM, Bromwell DA, Levore ER. Aortoenteric fistula. Am Surg 194: 402-412, 1981.

23. Kwaan JHM, Connolly JE. Successful management of prosthetic graft infection with continuous povidone-iodine irrigation. Arch Surg 116:716-720, 1981.

24. Almgren B, Eriksson I. Local antibiotic irrigation in the treatment of arterial graft infections. Acta Chir Scand 147:33-61, 1981.

25. Renvall S, Havia T. Prevention of arterial prosthetic graft infection by lavage and peritoneal dialysis in diffuse peritonitis: A report of two cases. Br J Surg 68:615-616, 1981.

26. Hinton PJ, Bryant LR. Preservation of an infected arterial graft with combination systemic-topical antibiotic therapy. Am Surg 47:511-514, 1981.

27. Knight CD, Farnell MB, Hollier LH. Treatment of aortic graft infection with povidone-iodine irrigation. Mayo Clin Proc 58:472-476, 1983.

28. Lorentzen JE, Neilson OM, Arendrup H, Kimose HH, Bille S, Anderson J, Jensen CH, Jacobsen R, Roder OC. Vascular graft infection: An analysis of sixty-two graft infections in 2411 consecutively implanted synthetic vascular grafts. Surgery 98:81-86, 1985.

29. Van de Water JM, Gaal PG. Management of patients with infected vascular prostheses. Am Surg 31:651-658, 1965.

30. Cohn R, Angell WW. Late complications from plastic replacement of aortic abdominal aneurysms. Arch Surg 97:696-698, 1968.

31. Najafi H, Javid H, Dye WS, Hunter JA, Julian OC. Management of infected arterial implants. Surgery 65:539-547, 1969.

32. Jamieson GG, DeWeese JA, Rob CG. Infected arterial grafts. Ann Surg 181:850-852, 1975.

33. Fulenwider JT, Smith RB, Johnson RW, Johnson RC, Salam AA, Perdue CD. Reoperative abdominal arterial surgery: A ten-year experience. Surgery 93:20-27, 1983.

34. Thomas WEG, Baird RN. Secondary aortoenteric fistulae: Towards a more conservative approach. Br J Surg 73:875-878, 1986.

35. O'Hara PJ, Hertzer NR, Beven EG, Krawjevski CP. Surgical management of infected abdominal aortic grafts: Review of a 25-year experience. J Vasc Surg 3:725-731, 1986.

36. Reilly LM, Stoney RJ, Goldstone J, Ehrenfeld WK. Improved management of aortic graft infection: The influence of operative sequence and staging. J Vasc Surg 5:421-431, 1987.

37. Bennion RS, Hiatt JR, Williams RA, Wilson SE. Surgical management of unilateral groin infection after aortofemoral bypass. Surg Gynecol Obstet 156:724-728, 1983.

38. Kleinman LH, Towne JB, Bernhard VM. A diagnostic and therapeutic approach to aortoenteric fistulas: Clinical experience with treating patients. Surgery 86:868-880, 1979.

38a. Rutherford RB, Baue AE. Extra-anatomic bypass. In Rutherford RB, ed. Vascular Surgery, 3rd ed. Philadelphia: WB Saunders, 1989, pp 711-713.

39. Blaisdell RW, DeMattei GA, Gauder PJ. Extraperitoneal thoracic aorta to femoral bypass graft as replacement for an infected aortic bifurcation prosthesis. Am J Surg 102:583-585, 1961.

40. Blaisdell RW, Hall AD. Axillary femoral artery bypass for lower extremity ischemia. Surgery 54:563-568, 1963.

41. Veith FJ, Hartsuch JM, Crane C. Management of aortoiliac reconstruction complicated by sepsis and hemorrhage. N Engl J Med 270:1389-1391, 1964.

42. Fry WJ, Lindenauer SM. Infection complicating the use of plastic arterial implants. Arch Surg 94:600-609, 1966.

43. Dietrich EB, Noon GP, Liddicoat JE, DeBakey ME. Treatment of infected aortofemoral arterial prosthesis. Surgery 68:1044-1052, 1970.

44. Spanos PK, Gilsdorf RB, Sako Y, Najarian JS. The management of infected abdominal aortic grafts and graft enteric fistulas. Am J Surg 183:397-400, 1976.

45. Trout HH, Kozloff L, Giordano JM. Priority of revascularization in patients with graft enteric fistulas, infected arteries or infected arterial prostheses. Am Surg 199:669-683, 1984.

46. Yeager RA, McConnell DB, Sasohi TM, Vetto RM. Aortic and peripheral prosthetic graft infections: Differential management and causes of mortality. Am J Surg 150:36-43, 1985.

47. Ehrenfeld WK, Wilbur BG, Olcott CN, Stoney RJ. Autogenous tissue reconstruction in the management of infected prosthetic grafts. Surgery 85:82-92, 1979.

48. Seeger JM, Wheeler JR, Gregory RT, Snyder SO, Gayle RG. Autogenous graft replacement of infected prosthetic graft in the femoral position. Surgery 93:39-45, 1983.

49. Bergamini TM, Bandyk DF, Schmitt DD, Seabrook GR, Kinney EV, Towne JB. In situ replacement of vascular prosthesis infected by bacterial biofilms. J Vasc Surg (accepted for publication).

50. Daugherty M, Shearer GR, Ernst CB. Primary aortoduodenal fistula: Extraanatomic vascular reconstruction not required for successful management. Surgery 86:399-401, 1979.

51. Sweeney MS, Godacy JR. Primary aortoduodenal fistula: Manifestation, diagnosis and treatment. Surgery 96:492-497, 1984.

52. Humphries AW, Young JR, DeWolfe VG, Lefevre FA. Complications of abdominal aortic surgery. Arch Surg 86:43-50, 1963.

53. Garrett HE, Beall AC, Jordon GL, DeBakey ME. Surgical considerations of massive gastrointestinal tract hemorrhage caused by aortoabdominal fistula. Am J Surg 105:6-12, 1963.

54. Ferris EJ, Koltay MRS, Koltay OP, Sciammas FD. Abdominal aortic and iliac graft fistulae. Am J Roentgenol 94:416-420, 1965.

55. Tobias JA, Daicoff GR. Aortogastric and aortoiliac fistulas repaired by direct suture. Arch Surg 107:909-911, 1973.

56. Elliott JP, Smith RF, Szilagyi DE. Anastomotic and paraprosthetic enteric fistulas. Arch Surg 108:479-490, 1974.

57. Brenner WI, Richman H, Reed GE. Roof patch repair of an aortoduodenal fistula resulting from suture line failure in an aortic prosthesis. Am J Surg 127:762-764, 1974.

58. Dean RH, Allen TR, Foster JH, Maltinly S, Clayson KR, Edwards WH. Aortoduodenal fistula: An uncommon but correctable cause of upper gastrointestinal bleeding. Am Surg 44:37-43, 1978.

59. Busuttil RW, Rees W, Baser JD, Wilim SE. Pathogenesis of aortoduodenal fistula: Experimental and clinical correlates. Surgery 85:1-13, 1979.

60. Buchbinder D, Leather R, Shah D, Karmody A. Pathologic intervention between prosthetic aortic grafts and the gastrointestinal tract. Am J Surg 140:192-198, 1980.

61. O'Mara CS, Williams GM, Ernst CB. Secondary aortoenteric fistula. Am J Surg 142:203-209, 1981.

62. Champion MC, Sullivan SN, Coles JC, Goldbach M, Watson WC. Aortoenteric fistula. Am Surg 195:314-317, 1982.

63. Flye MW, Thompson WM. Aortic graft-enteric and paraprosthetic-enteric fistulas. Am J Surg 146:183-187, 1983.

64. Crawford ES, DeBakey ME, Morris GC, Garrett E. Evaluation of late failures after reconstructive operations for occlusive lesions of the aorta and iliac, femoral and popliteal arteries. Surgery 47:79-104, 1960.

65. Aarnio P, Hannukainen J. Aortic graft enteric fistula. Ann Chir Gynecol 78:329-331, 1989.

66. Walker WE, Cooley DA, Duncan JM, Hollman GL, Ott DA, Reul GH. The management of aortoduodenal fistula by in situ replacement of the infected abdominal aortic graft. Am Surg 205:727-732, 1987.

67. Thistlewaite JR, Hughes RK, Smyth NP, Cornwell EE. Spontaneous arteriovenous fistula between the abdominal aorta and vena cava. Arch Surg 81:61-64, 1960.

68. Sproul G. Rupture of an infected aortic graft with jejunum: Resection and survival. JAMA 182:1118-1120, 1962.

69. Rosato FE, Barker E, Roberts B. Aorto-intestinal fistula. J Thorac Cardiovasc Surg 53:511-514, 1967.

70. Pinkerton JA. Aortoduodenal fistula. JAMA 225:1196-1199, 1973.

71. Moncure AC, Brewster DC, Darling RC, Atnip RG, Newton WD, Abbott WM. Use of the splenic and hepatic arteries for renal revascularization. J Vasc Surg 3:196-203, 1986.

72. Hoffert PW, Gensler S, Haimovici H. Infection complicating arterial grafts. Arch Surg 90:427-435, 1965.

73. Smith RB, Lowry K, Perdue GD. Management of the infected arterial prosthesis in the lower extremity. Am Surg 33:711-714, 1967.

74. Popovsky J, Singer S. Infected prosthetic grafts. Arch Surg 115:203-205, 1980.

75. Calligaro KD, Veith RJ, Gupta SK, Ascer E, Dietzek AM, Franco CA, Wengerter KR. A modified method for management of prosthetic graft infections involving an anastomosis to the common femoral artery. J Vasc Surg 11:485-492, 1990.

76. Samson RH, Veith RJ, Janko GS, Gupta SK, Scher LA. A modified classification and approach to the management of infections involving peripheral arterial prosthetic graft. J Vasc Surg 8:147-153, 1988.

77. Kikta MJ, Goodson SR, Bishara RA, Meyer JP, Schuler JJ, Flanigan DP. Mortality and limb loss with infected infrainguinal bypass grafts. J Vasc Surg 5:566-571, 1987.

VIII Infrainguinal Reconstructive Grafts

19

Detection and Management of Failing Autogenous Grafts

Thomas M. Bergamini   **Jonathan B. Towne**

A significant decline in primary patency of autogenous grafts invariably occurs over time because of the development of fibrointimal hyperplasia of the vein conduit or anastomotic sites and the progression of atherosclerotic disease of the native arteries. The incidence of lesions that threaten the long-term patency of both in situ and reversed saphenous vein bypasses ranges from 20% to 26%.[1-3] Anatomic and hemodynamic alterations that require revision will develop in approximately 5% of vein bypasses per year; the majority of these will occur within the first 2 years after bypass.[4] The failure to detect and correct lesions that threaten bypass patency before graft thrombosis significantly decreases long-term patency of the autogenous graft. The long-term patency for revisions of autogenous grafts after thrombosis is dismal. The 3-year patency rate of revision of thrombosed in situ and reversed saphenous vein grafts ranges from 22% to 47% in recent reports.[1,5,6]

By contrast, the results of revisions on hemodynamically failing but patent conduits are excellent: secondary patency rates are equivalent to those for bypasses that never undergo revision.[1] Secondary procedures on patent grafts normalize the hemodynamics at the revision site and are associated with a low incidence of restenosis; long-term patency rates range from 80% to 93%.[1,7-9] The excellent durability of secondary procedures on the patent but hemodynamically abnormal bypass coupled with the dismal results of revision of the thrombosed bypass underscores the significant impact of monitoring graft hemodynamics with a surveillance protocol and elective bypass revision. This chapter discusses the definition and detection of autogenous graft failure by intraoperative and postoperative surveillance and details the surgical principles and results of management of the failing autogenous graft.

ETIOLOGY OF AUTOGENOUS GRAFT FAILURE

The etiology of autogenous graft failure differs according to the time of occurrence. Perioperatively (up to 30 days), autogenous graft failure most commonly is caused by technical errors, an inadequate inflow or outflow artery, or an inadequate vein. From 30 days to 2 years postoperatively, stenosis of the vein conduit or the anastomotic sites caused by fibrointimal hyperplasia is the most common cause of graft failure. Autogenous graft failure occurring more than 2 years postoperatively is likely a result of atherosclerotic disease progression of the inflow or outflow artery. Lesions associated with a diameter-reducing stenosis of the graft or native artery, regardless of the cause, can be identified reliably by abnormal graft hemodynamics. Occasionally autogenous graft thrombosis occurs despite normal hemodynamics because of thromboembolism, anastomotic pseudoaneurysm formation, aneurysmal degeneration of the conduit, infection, or a hypercoagulable state.

Perioperative

Perioperative failure of the autogenous graft is related to technical errors and the quality of the arterial and venous systems used for bypass. Technical errors in constructing the proximal and distal anastomoses and preparing the conduit can occur. Dissecting and clamping the inflow and outflow arteries can raise intimal flaps, which can create luminal stenoses and/or thromboses. Errors in performing the proximal and distal anastomoses can result in suture line bleeding, pseudoaneurysm formation, or suture line stricture. Likewise, proximal occlusive disease in the aortoiliac segment can cause graft failure. Technical imperfections of the vein conduit include luminal thrombus, platelet aggregates, graft torsion, kinking of the graft, graft entrapment, inadequate ligation of venous branches, and vein injury from dissection or valve ablation.

The quality of the vein and artery used for the bypass is important for success of the autogenous graft. A poor-quality vein (i.e., one with sclerotic segments, varicosities, or a small diameter) can predispose to technical errors in handling the venous conduit and result in graft thrombosis. Sclerotic vein segments can have a thrombogenic flow surface and also can result in significant luminal stenosis, both of which

can result in graft failure. Veins less than 2 mm in diameter are inadequate for long bypasses with both the in situ and reverse techniques. Inadequate arterial outflow caused by florid tibial and pedal occlusive disease can cause high outflow resistance resulting in low graft flow and subsequent graft failure.

Postoperative

Beyond the perioperative period, the two main disease processes that result in autogenous graft failure are fibrointimal hyperplasia of the vein conduit or anastomotic sites and the progression of atherosclerotic disease of the inflow or outflow vessel. From 1 to 24 months postoperatively, fibrointimal hyperplasia is the most common cause of vein graft stenosis: the incidence is 5%/year. Approximately one half of the lesions causing hemodynamic failure are located in the vein conduit itself. The remaining sites involve the proximal or distal anastomosis or the adjacent inflow or outflow artery. Lesions such as anastomotic stenoses, valve leaflet fibrosis, and focal or extensive fibrotic stenoses of the vein result in significant diameter-reducing stenosis with time. Beyond 2 years the incidence of significant graft stenoses decreases to 1% to 3%/year. During this time interval atherosclerotic disease progression is the most common cause of late graft failure. Atherosclerosis can progress in the native arterial inflow and outflow vessels, resulting in significant diameter-reducing stenosis and decrease in blood flow. Atherosclerosis also can develop in the vein bypass itself, resulting in aneurysmal dilatation or stenoses. The progression of fibrointimal hyperplasia and atherosclerotic disease results in stenosis of the vein graft and native arteries, which yields hemodynamic abnormalities that can be detected and corrected during postoperative surveillance.

GRAFT SURVEILLANCE PROTOCOL

The ideal autogenous graft surveillance protocol should be noninvasive, associated with minimal complications, and highly accurate and reliable in identifying graft lesions that threaten patency. Based on the time course of occurrence of graft failure, surveillance of the autogenous graft should be most frequent during the perioperative period and the first 2 years postoperatively. The graft surveillance techniques should be applicable intraoperatively, immediately postoperatively, and throughout the postoperative follow-up period. The results should be reproducible and correlate with one another on serial examinations. Follow-up of autogenous grafts based on the recurrence of symptoms of limb ischemia is inadequate in identifying grafts at risk for thrombosis. In studies of the in situ saphenous vein bypass, Bandyk and associates[7,10] have documented that only one third of patients had recurrence of symptoms despite noninvasive vascular laboratory studies indicating hemodynamic graft failure. In a study of reverse vein grafts, Minh-Chau et al.[2] documented that only 29% of limbs with low graft flow velocities (less than 45 cm/sec) had recurrence of symptoms. Thus for both in situ and reversed autogenous grafts the reliance on the recurrence of symptoms alone would mean that up to two thirds of the patients with autogenous grafts at risk for thrombosis would be missed. Hemodynamic assessment with use of noninvasive vascular laboratory testing is essential for the postoperative surveillance protocol (see box).

Surveillance protocols of autogenous grafts include hemodynamic monitoring of the arterial systolic pressure of the limb and the blood flow velocities of the venous conduit and native arteries. Ankle systolic pressure measurements correlate with the clinical symptoms of limb

ischemia and are predictive of healing of ulcers or amputation sites, but they are unable to localize the obstructive lesion to the inflow conduit or outflow. Also, because of the high incidence of diabetic patients requiring lower limb bypass, the presence of incompressible calf vessels makes measurement of ankle pressures impossible. Blood flow velocity analysis with the use of the duplex scanner can evaluate the venous conduit, anastomotic sites, and adjacent arteries for hemodynamic abnormalities of flow. Unlike limb pressures the duplex scan can reliably identify the location and anatomy of the lesions by ultrasound and quantitate the severity of flow disturbance and stenosis. Systolic pressure measurement and blood flow velocity analysis are complementary tests that can aid in the prediction of recurrence of symptoms or graft thromboses; both should be used during postoperative surveillance of the autogenous graft.[10,11]

Hemodynamic surveillance should be used intraoperatively, perioperatively, and during the postoperative follow-up period for both in situ and reversed autogenous grafts.[1,2,7,10] Intraoperative hemodynamic assessment of the in situ saphenous vein bypass can be performed with high-frequency (20 MHz), pulsed Doppler spectral analysis. The sterilized probe contains a small ultrasonic transducer with a pulsed Doppler sample volume of approximately 0.2 mm[3] that can be coupled to the vessel wall with the use of saline solution. Placement of the sample volume midstream in the lumen of the autogenous graft permits analysis of the velocity waveform and calculation of the peak systolic and diastolic velocities. The examination begins with the location of patent arteriovenous fistulas (AVFs). With the Doppler probe placed on the proximal graft, the distal graft is occluded with finger pressure. Persistence of forward flow anywhere along the conduit indicates AVF between the point of the Doppler and the point of finger occlusion. The Doppler probe then is passed down the length of the graft and the persistence of diastolic forward flow proximal to the AVF is noted. Once past the fistula the diastolic forward flow diminishes. When the fistulas are ligated, there should be

---

CLINICAL AND HEMODYNAMIC CRITERIA OF THE FAILING AUTOGENOUS GRAFT

Recurrence of symptoms of limb ischemia
Low peak systolic graft flow velocity (<45 cm/sec)
Decrease of flow velocity >30 cm/sec
Ankle/brachial index >0.15 on serial examinations

no diastolic forward flow with distal finger pressure occlusion. The high-frequency probe then is used to analyze the proximal and distal anastomoses, the inflow and outflow arteries, and the flow along the entire graft conduit, especially at the valve incision sites. Anatomic and technical defects are identified and quantitated according to the extent of spectral broadening and increase of peak systolic frequency. Mild-to-moderate flow disturbances are associated with spectral broadening during systole and peak systolic frequency less than 16 kHz. Severe flow disturbances are associated with spectral broadening during systole and diastole and peak systolic frequency greater than 16 kHz. With the in situ technique, partial valve lysis is associated with severe flow disturbances just distal to the valve site. Sclerotic vein segments, graft torsion, platelet aggregates, and anastomotic stenosis often are associated with severe flow disturbances at the site and just distal to the abnormal graft segment. The location, length, and severity of stenosis can be identified precisely with intraoperative spectral analysis.

Postoperative graft surveillance should be performed before hospital discharge using limb blood pressure measurement and duplex scanning. Systolic pressure measurements are ob-

tained by measuring the ankle/brachial index (ABI). Duplex scanning of the proximal and distal anastomoses, inflow and outflow arteries, and the entire autogenous conduit can be performed. Velocity waveform analysis can be performed by placing the sample volume in the center of the vessel lumen at the desired Doppler beam angle. Calculation of the graft flow velocities at designated sites with normal arterial flow patterns, where the vessel diameter does not vary, is necessary for reliable and reproducible results from one examination to the next. Flow velocity should be measured with the patient in the supine position, the limbs slightly externally rotated, and the knee bent and at rest.

Vein graft lesions detected in this time period include AVFs, residual intact valve leaflets, and graft or anastomotic stenosis. AVFs are recognized by high diastolic flows proximally located, increased flow turbulence at the site, and decreased or absent diastolic flow distal to the site of the fistula. Stenotic lesions of the graft conduit or anastomotic site are identified by increases in spectral broadening and peak systolic and diastolic velocities at, or just distal to, the site (Table 19-1). In addition to identifying hemodynamically significant lesions predisposing to early graft failure, early duplex scan-

Table 19-1. Duplex Scan Classification of Severity of Stenosis

Classification	Velocity waveform analysis
<20% DR	No increase in peak systolic velocity compared with adjacent proximal segment; spectral broadening during systole
20% to 50% DR	>30% increase in peak systolic velocity compared with adjacent proximal segment; spectral broadening during systole and diastole
50% to 75% DR	>100% increase in peak systolic velocity (Vp >125 cm/sec) compared with adjacent proximal segment; end-diastolic velocity <100 cm/sec; spectral broadening during systole and diastole
>75% DR	>100% increase in peak systolic velocity (Vp >125 cm/sec) compared with adjacent proximal segment; end-diastolic velocity >100 cm/sec; spectral broadening during systole and diastole

DR, diameter reduction; Vp, velocity peak.

ning provides a baseline on which to base subsequent graft surveillance studies. Serial evaluations with postoperative hemodynamic surveillance should be performed at 6 weeks postoperatively, every 3 months for the first 2 years, and every 6 months thereafter. Each examination should include limb pressure measurements and determination of peak systolic flow velocities at the mid and distal graft, and the results should be compared with prior studies. Autogenous grafts that exhibit abnormal hemodynamics (low graft flow velocity, >50% graft stenoses, significant decrease of peak systolic frequency on serial examinations, greater than 30 cm/sec, or ABI greater than 0.15) should be evaluated by complete duplex scanning of the entire graft and arteriography.

The failure to identify and revise a graft with a hemodynamically significant lesion before thrombosis is associated with poor patency. Long-term patency rates are improved markedly for autogenous grafts revised while patent compared with long-term patency rates for revision of thrombosed bypass conduits. The secondary patency rates for bypasses patent at

the time of revision are equivalent to those for bypasses that never undergo revision. Revision of the thrombosed reversed or in situ saphenous vein bypass uniformly results in poor long-term patency. In a study of 109 autogenous grafts, Whittemore et al.[12] reported that revision of the patent but failing autogenous graft yielded an 85% 5-year patency rate compared with a 37% 5-year patency rate for revision of the thrombosed bypass. In a study of 95 bypasses that underwent revision, Bergamini et al.[1] found a significant decline in the secondary patency for bypasses thrombosed at the time of revision (47%) compared with that for bypasses patent at the time of revision (93%) (Fig. 19-1). Compulsive bypass surveillance can identify the failing autogenous graft and permit elective revision, a practice that has significant impact on long-term patency.

The superior long-term patency rates of both in situ and reversed autogenous grafts also were related directly to improved surgical technique and the experience of the vascular surgeon.[1,13,14] Increasing surgical experience was associated with a significant decrease in the

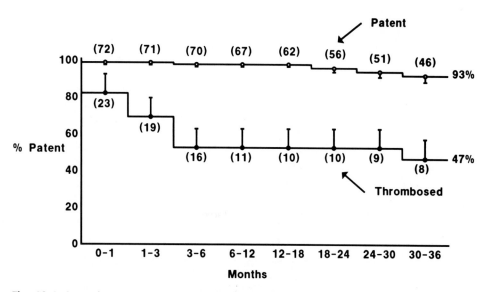

Fig. 19-1. Secondary patency of in situ saphenous vein bypasses that were patent at time of revision (open circles) was significantly higher ($p < .0000005$) compared with that of bypasses that were thrombosed at time of revision (closed circles).

number of technical errors encountered with vein preparation[1] (Table 19-2). Increasing surgical experience also was associated with a significant improvement in the secondary patency rate (92%) compared with the secondary patency rate of the first half of the series (80%) at 3 years (Fig. 19-2). Taylor, Edwards, and Porter[14] also have attributed the recent improvement in long-term patency of reversed autogenous grafts to improvements in surgical technique and increasing surgical experience. Long-term patency rates of the in situ and reversed autogenous grafts are improved with careful operative technique, meticulous postoperative graft surveillance, and increasing surgical experience.

EFFECT OF SITE OF DISTAL ANASTOMOSIS

In contrast to the patency for in situ saphenous vein bypass, the long-term patency for the reversed vein graft was significantly decreased for infrapopliteal bypasses, long bypasses performed with vein less than 3 mm in diameter, and reversed vein grafts in diabetic patients. Taylor, Edwards, and Porter[14] reported a significant decline in primary patency for autogenous reversed grafts to the infrapopliteal arteries (69%) compared with that for below-knee popliteal arteries (80%). The secondary patency for infrapopliteal arteries (77%) also was decreased compared with that for below-knee popliteal artery grafts (86%). Rutherford et al.[15] also showed a decrease in the cumulative patency rate at 3 years for reversed vein grafts (63%) compared with that for in situ (88%) vein bypasses to the tibial outflow artery.

Table 19-2. Incidence of Technical Errors With In Situ Saphenous Vein Bypass: First Half of Series vs. Latter Half*

Technical error	1981-1985	1986-1990
Valvulotome injury	20	9
Anastomotic stenosis	5	0
Bypass torsion	4	0
Residual valve leaflet	4	0
TOTAL[†]	33 (18%)	9 (5%)

*In the first half of the series (1981-1985) there were 179 cases; in the second half (1986-1990) there were 182 cases.
†Total number of technical errors for the first half compared with the second half is significantly different: $p = .0001$ (χ^2-analysis).

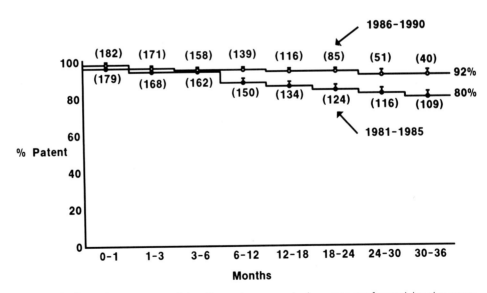

Fig. 19-2. Secondary patency of in situ saphenous vein bypasses performed by the more experienced surgeon from 1986 to 1990 (open circles) was significantly higher ($p < .02$) compared with that of bypasses in the earlier years from 1981 to 1985 (closed circles).

EFFECT OF VEIN GRAFT DIAMETER AND DIABETES MELLITUS

The long-term patency of reversed autogenous grafts with vein diameters less than 3 mm is decreased significantly compared with that for reversed autogenous grafts with greater vein diameters.[16] The in situ autogenous graft is not affected by vein size.[1,13]

Long-term patency and limb salvage are adversely affected by the presence of diabetes in patients with reversed autogenous grafts.[9,14,17] On the other hand, in situ autogenous graft long-term patency and limb salvage are not significantly different for the diabetic patient compared with those for the nondiabetic patient.[1]

OPERATIVE MANAGEMENT OF THE PATENT BUT FAILING AUTOGENOUS GRAFT

The goals of intraoperative modification or postoperative revision of the patent but failing autogenous graft should be correction of the anatomic abnormality, restoration of normal hemodynamics of the autogenous graft, and maintenance of long-term bypass patency. The principles and techniques of treatment of a graft stenosis are the same for the in situ and reversed saphenous vein grafts. Graft revisions require a clear understanding of the cause, location, and extent of the lesion.[7] Secondary procedures require meticulous dissection and technical precision. Regional or general anesthesia is preferred over local anesthesia to perform the revision with minimal patient discomfort. The use of scalpel dissection is essential to expose the autogenous graft without vein injury. After dissection of the abnormal segment of the autogenous graft, intraoperative spectral analysis can be performed to confirm the precise location and extent of the lesion. After exposure and control of bleeding points, the patients are heparinized systemically. Secondary procedures on the distal graft, distal anastomotic site, or native outflow artery are enhanced by the use of a pneumatic tourniquet as a substitute for vascular clamps for proximal and distal control in the scarred tissue planes.[18] The limb is exsanguinated by leg elevation and the use of an elastic wrap before inflation of the tourniquet (40 to 50 mm Hg above brachial systolic pressure). The secondary procedure then can be performed without the necessity to dissect the proximal and distal conduits circumferentially for control and without the need to work around the vascular clamps. Just before completion of the revision, the tourniquet should be deflated to confirm the presence of back-bleeding from the distal conduit. Intraoperative spectral analysis and arteriography are performed routinely to document the restoration of normal graft hemodynamics and anatomic configuration.

Modification of the Failing Autogenous Graft During the Primary Procedure

During the performance of the primary in situ or reversed autogenous graft, intraoperative modification of the venous conduit is performed to correct technical errors or a poor-quality vein. The key to successful treatment is recognition and correction of the lesion before graft thrombosis occurs. The intraoperative occurrence of the low-flow state can be caused by problems with the inflow artery, vein conduit, anastomotic site, or outflow artery. Significant stenosis of the inflow artery can be identified by intraoperative measurement of the systolic pressure by insertion of an 18- to 20-gauge needle in the common femoral artery connected to the arterial line monitor. A significant gradient (greater than 20 mm Hg) at rest or after injection of 20 mg papaverine between the inflow artery pressure and the brachial systolic pressure confirms the presence of a poor inflow artery. Improved inflow can be achieved by a proximal aortic bypass, extra-anatomic bypass, or intraoperative balloon angioplasty if a short segmental lesion is present.

The low-flow state caused by lesions of the vein conduit or anastomotic sites can be detected by complete survey of the graft from the proximal to the distal anastomosis with high-frequency spectral analysis. Technical errors or poor-quality vein segments are associated uniformly with increased peak systolic frequency and spectral broadening. Anastomotic stenoses are caused by technical errors, such as missing the endothelium, incorporation of adventitial tissue in the intraluminal flow surface, poorly placed stitches resulting in suture line stricture or bleeding, and intimal flaps or raised plaques.

The distal anastomotic stricture usually involves the toe of the end-to-side anastomosis. This is best corrected by reconstructing the entire anastomosis. Endarterectomy of the native artery to correct intimal flaps or atherosclerotic plaques sometimes is necessary. With the in situ technique, proximal anastomotic strictures can be a result of partial lysis of the first valve. This is corrected by the insertion of the valvulotome and repeat valve incision. With the reversed vein graft, meticulous technique is mandatory in anastomosing the larger end of the reversed vein to the smaller outflow artery.

Intraoperative modification of the venous conduit for both in situ and reversed autogenous grafts is performed to correct a poor-quality vein or technical error. Sclerotic veins have been treated by vein patching of the sclerotic segment or resection of sclerotic segment and replacement with a translocated vein segment from another source. If the endothelium of the sclerotic segment is abnormal and an adequate diameter and quality alternate vein source are available, resection and replacement of the sclerotic vein segment is preferred. Varicosities of the vein are treated with plication of the wall or a partial resection and vein patch angioplasty. Small-diameter vein segment or previously used segments of vein in the leg should be replaced with an alternate source of vein. The translocated vein segments used for interposition replacement should be of good quality with a thin-wall vein, greater than 2 mm in diameter, and a glistening endothelial flow surface. Intraoperative modification caused by technical failure of the in situ bypass is most commonly performed for retained valve leaflets or AVFs. The retained valve leaflet can be incised simply by reinserting the valvulotome through a side branch or directly into the vein conduit via an 18-gauge needle puncture hole. Sclerotic valves prompt valve excision under direct vision through a longitudinal venotomy. The venotomy is closed primarily if it is technically achievable without creating luminal stenosis or if it is possible with a vein patch. AVFs are treated simply by ligation. Injured segments of vein during dissection are repaired simply with lateral venorrhaphy, vein patch angioplasty, resection and primary anastomo-

sis, or resection and interposition grafting. The key to treatment of this technical problem is to resect all abnormal endothelium and injured vein wall and then reconstruct the bypass graft without creating luminal stenosis. Vein conduit torsion is best treated by transecting the conduit, untwisting the conduit, and performing a primary reanastomosis. Minor kinks or twists of less than 90 degrees in the bypass are treated with vein patch angioplasty across the twisted segment. Graft entrapment is detected by the presence of normal graft velocities with the knee flexed, but the development of a low-flow state with absence of diastolic flow with the knee extended is seen in patients who spend significant amounts of time in wheelchairs. Treatment of this complication includes a myotomy of the tendons and muscles in which the vein bypass is entrapped. The formation of platelet aggregates along the endothelial flow surface caused by heparin-induced platelet aggregation should be treated with reversal of the heparin, low-molecular-weight dextran drip, removal of the platelet aggregates by means of longitudinal venotomy, and subsequent primary or vein patch closure of the venotomy. Intraoperative thrombosis of the vein graft without the presence of a poor inflow artery, technical errors, or poor-quality vein should prompt a search for evidence of a hypercoagulable state (antithrombin III deficiency, heparin-induced platelet aggregation, abnormal plasminogen) or a poor outflow artery. Conduits with a poor outflow artery have a low-flow state and an absence of diastolic forward flow caused by high outflow resistance.[19] The best management is a translocated vein sequential graft or jump graft from the vein bypass to an alternate outflow artery, if available, to increase the outflow and decrease the resistance. Following the secondary graft procedures, intraoperative pulsed Doppler spectral analysis and arteriography should be repeated to make sure that there is normalization of the bypassed hemodynamic and anatomic abnormalities.

Secondary Procedures for Revision of the Failing Autogenous Graft

During postoperative surveillance, operative management of the failing but patent autogenous graft depends on the anatomy and location of the lesion. Stenoses of the graft conduit are secondary to fibrointimal hyperplasia at the anastomotic sites, valve sites, or areas of intraoperative vein injury. The areas of graft stenosis can vary from focal to extensive, affecting a long segment of the graft conduit (Fig. 19-3). Focal stenosis in the in situ saphenous vein bypass occurs at fibrotic valve sites. The formation of lesions caused by fibrointimal hyperplasia usually is associated with technical errors or injury in preparing the venous conduit for bypass. If focal stenosis develops in the vein conduit, sufficient length usually is present to permit resection of the lesion and primary end-to-end anastomosis to restore bypass patency. The amount of redundant graft is less for reversed autogenous grafts, making resection and primary reanastomosis an infrequent option.[7] If there is inadequate vein length or the stenosis is immediately adjacent to an anastomotic site, the focal stenosis is treated by a longitudinal venotomy across the length of the stenosis and vein patch angioplasty reconstruction. Stenoses of the proximal and distal anastomoses are treated with a vein patch angioplasty extending distally onto the native artery. A third treatment option for focal graft stenosis is percutaneous transluminal angioplasty (PTA). PTA is especially suitable for treatment of focal stenosis in

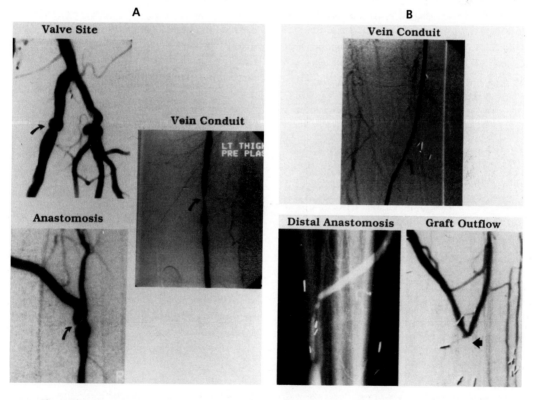

Fig. 19-3. A, Focal stenotic lesions of the failing autogenous graft detected during postoperative surveillance were caused by fibrointimal hyperplasia. Valve site stenosis was treated by excision and end-to-end reanastomosis. Vein conduit stenosis was treated with percutaneous balloon angioplasty. Anastomotic stenosis was treated by vein patch angioplasty. **B,** Extensive stenotic lesions of the failing autogenous graft detected during postoperative surveillance. Segmental stenotic lesions of the vein conduit and distal anastomosis caused by fibrointimal hyperplasia were treated with resection and interposition translocated vein graft. Extensive disease of the outflow artery caused by progression of atherosclerotic disease was treated with sequential/jump grafting to a more distal outflow artery site.

high-risk patients or in the native arteries proximal or distal to the graft.

More extensive lesions include long sclerotic vein segments, multiple stenotic lesions, and fibrointimal hyperplasia or atherosclerosis involving a long segment of the distal anastomosis or outflow artery. Long or multiple stenotic lesions of the vein conduit are treated by vein patch angioplasty or resection and interposition of a translocated vein segment if an alternate quality vein of similar diameter is available. Long stenotic lesions of the distal anastomosis are treated with vein patch angioplasty across the stenotic segment. Extensive lesions of the distal vein conduit and outflow artery are treated with a jump graft (extension of the graft to the same outflow artery) or a sequential graft (translocated vein segment to a different outflow artery) using translocated vein (greater saphenous, lesser saphenous, cephalic). The technical success of secondary procedures is evaluated by intraoperative spectral analysis and angiography to ensure achievement of normal graft hemodynamics and anatomic reconstruction.

PERIOPERATIVE RESULTS OF MANAGEMENT OF THE PATENT BUT FAILING AUTOGENOUS GRAFT

The early patency (30 days) of the autogenous graft is excellent if intraoperative normal hemodynamics and arteriography are achieved with the revascularization procedure.[20] In a study of in situ saphenous vein bypasses, the 30-day patency for the 83 bypasses in the series with normal intraoperative hemodynamics was 100%. Initially, 77 of the 83 in situ saphenous vein grafts had normal intraoperative hemodynamics, with a peak systolic velocity of greater than 40 cm/sec and biphasic (hyperemic flow) waveform. Six (7%) of the bypasses had low peak systolic blood flow velocity (less than 40 cm/sec) and an absence of hyperemic flow, a predictor of early failure of the in situ bypass.[21] Correction of the underlying causes (AVF, intact valve leaflet, poor-quality vein segment) resulted in early bypass patency with normal hemodynamics after modification in these six bypasses. The short-term patency was dependent on intraoperative identification and correction of the lesions causing flow abnormalities.[20] The determination of normal intraoperative hemodynamics of the autogenous graft is a highly accurate predictor of early patency following lower extremity revascularization. The primary and secondary patencies for both in situ and reversed autogenous grafts are decreased when intraoperative modification of the vein conduit is required to complete the lower extremity arterial reconstruction.[1,14]

FACTORS THAT AFFECT LONG-TERM PATENCY RATE OF AUTOGENOUS GRAFTS

The use of a postoperative surveillance protocol of in situ and reversed autogenous grafts allows the study of the pathophysiology of autogenous graft failure and also the analysis of factors that adversely affect long-term patency. The determinant factors that significantly affect long-term patency for both the in situ and reversed saphenous vein grafts are modification of the venous conduit at the initial operation to correct a poor-quality vein with patch angioplasty or vein interposition, technical error caused by injury to the vein during valve ablation, failure to revise the bypass before thrombosis during the surveillance period, and experience of the vascular surgeon in performing the autogenous graft. The long-term patency of autogenous grafts is decreased significantly when the ipsilateral saphenous vein is not adequate and requires some modification. In a recent large series of reversed saphenous vein grafts, Taylor, Edwards, and Porter[14] found that the ipsilateral greater saphenous vein was inadequate in 45% of the cases. The ipsilateral saphenous vein was inadequate because the vein was removed previously, the available vein was too short, the available vein was too small, or the vein contained sclerotic segments. Techniques practiced in performing the reversed vein graft in patients with inadequate ipsilateral saphenous vein were to use a more distal inflow artery, perform a venovenous anastomosis after removal of the abnormal segment, or use another source of vein—contralateral greater saphenous vein, cephalic vein, or lesser saphenous vein. The primary patency of the reversed vein grafts that had inadequate ipsilateral saphenous veins was 68%, a significant decrease compared with the 80% primary patency of those grafts that had adequate ipsilateral saphenous veins. The secondary patency of the grafts with inadequate veins requiring a modification technique was 77%, which also was decreased compared with the 84% patency of the reversed vein grafts with nonmodified conduits. Similarly, in a recent large series of in situ saphenous vein bypasses,[1] the primary and secondary patency rates also were decreased significantly for those bypassed veins undergoing modification at the time of bypass. Modification of the in situ saphenous vein conduit was performed in 23% of the total cases: 10% for an inadequate vein and 13% for technical problems with the vein. Modification of an inadequate vein was performed to correct sclerotic segments, previously used vein segments, small-diameter vein, or varicosities. Modification of an adequate vein necessitated by technical failure was performed for vein injury, anastomotic stenoses, retained valves, bypass torsion, platelet aggregates, or low-flow states caused by inadequate inflow or outflow arteries. The necessity to modify the vein conduit because of a technical failure or inadequate vein

was associated with a significant increase in the incidence of late appearing bypass stenosis and revision. The bypass stenoses were most commonly caused by the occurrence and progression of fibrointimal hyperplasia resulting from the injurious effects of the bypass modification (Fig. 19-4). The primary (50%) and secondary (72%) patencies of the in situ saphenous vein bypasses that required modification were decreased significantly compared with the primary (70%) and secondary (84%) patency rates of bypasses that did not undergo modification at the time of the bypass procedure. This increase in incidence of graft stenoses, bypass revision, and decline in primary and secondary patencies was believed to be caused by the occurrence of fibrointimal hyperplasia associated with the injurious effects of the bypass modification. The long-term patency of these conduits is dependent on a meticulous postoperative surveillance protocol identifying correctable lesions before thrombosis, permitting elective revision of patent conduits. Reversed and in situ autogenous grafts that have modified conduits mandate close postoperative surveillance to identify the development of lesions that threaten graft patency.

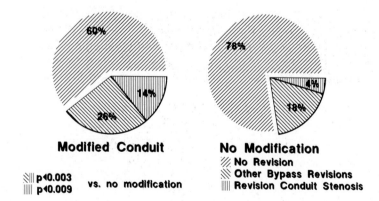

Modified Conduit   **No Modification**

⫷ No Revision
⫸ Other Bypass Revisions
|||| Revision Conduit Stenosis

⫸ p⊲0.003
|||| p⊲0.009   vs. no modification

Fig. 19-4. Modification to correct an inadequate vein or technical failure during the in situ saphenous vein bypass procedure was associated with a significant increase in the number of bypasses in which graft stenoses developed and that required revision during the postoperative surveillance period. Late-appearing stenoses occurred in 12 of 86 modified conduits (14%) compared with only 12 of 269 in situ bypasses (4.5%) not undergoing modification at the time of initial modification. During the postoperative surveillance period revision of the bypasses with modified conduits (34 of 86; 40%) was significantly more frequent compared with revision of bypasses with no modification of conduits (60 of 269; 22%).

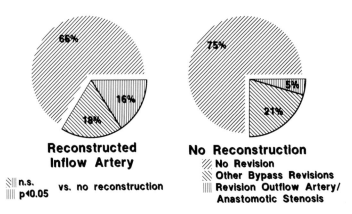

Fig. 19-5. In situ saphenous vein bypass revisions performed to correct anastomotic or outflow artery stenosis was significantly more frequent for grafts with reconstructed inflow arteries (7 of 44; 16%) compared with bypasses originating from nonreconstructed inflow arteries (14 of 310; 4.5%). Revision for graft stenosis was not significantly different for bypasses with reconstruction of inflow arteries (15 of 44; 34%) and those without (78 of 310; 25%).

For in situ saphenous vein bypasses, severe atherosclerotic disease of the common femoral artery was associated with a decline in primary patency but did not significantly alter secondary patency.[1] Severe disease of the common femoral artery necessitated endarterectomy, replacement with an interposition prosthetic or vein graft, or closure with a patch angioplasty in order to perform the proximal anastomosis. Bypasses originating from a reconstructed inflow artery had a significant increase in the number of revisions performed to correct anastomotic or outflow artery stenosis compared to bypasses with no reconstruction of the inflow artery (Fig. 19-5). With postoperative surveillance and elective revision, the secondary patency was not decreased significantly for the bypasses originating from a reconstructed inflow artery.

Long-term patency of the failing autogenous graft can be maintained if revision is performed before graft thrombosis occurs. Several studies have demonstrated that secondary procedures to revise the failing autogenous graft can be performed safely and are associated with an excellent long-term patency.[7,12] The results of the secondary procedure to revise the failing autogenous graft were dependent on the technical ability to correct the underlying cause. At-

tempts to treat focal short-segment stenoses of the autogenous vein conduit by total excision of the short segment of diseased vein and primary end-to-end reanastomosis were highly successful, with no occurrence of late restenosis or bypass failure.[7] The treatment of graft stenosis with vein patch angioplasty also resulted in excellent long-term patency (greater than 80%)[7,12] but was associated with an increased incidence of late restenosis at the revision site itself. In a recent study Bandyk et al.[7] demonstrated that 8 of 31 stenotic lesions (24%) treated by vein patch angioplasty resulted in restenosis; most occurred more than 3 months after the secondary procedure. PTA of focal vein graft stenosis also was associated with early bypass patency[8]; however, recurrent stenosis did occur in at least one half of the cases.[6,7,22,23] Because of the high incidence of recurrent graft stenosis, PTA should be used primarily for high-risk patients with a failing autogenous graft caused by focal lesion or for the management of atherosclerotic lesions in the native arteries. Restenosis of a vein patch angioplasty or PTA site was best treated by resection of the diseased, stenotic segment of vein and replacement with a translocated interposition vein graft.

Secondary procedures used to treat extensive lesions of the graft, distal anastomosis, or outflow artery also result in maintenance of long-term patency. In a recent study by Bandyk et al.,[7] recurrent stenosis and graft failure occurred less frequently after resection and interposition grafting compared with a sequential or jump graft procedure. Only 1 of 17 of the interposition grafts had a recurrent stenosis or graft failure. However, 11 of 21 sequential or jump grafting procedures were associated with recurrent stenosis or autogenous graft failure. The difference in patency was partially explained by the fact that the interposition grafts were placed for fibrointimal hyperplasia of the graft that was resectable and reconstructible, but the sequential or jump grafts were placed primarily for progression of atherosclerotic disease of the outflow artery. The bypass of the failing graft caused by progression of atherosclerotic disease of the outflow arteries with sequential or jump grafting was the least durable procedure: 5 of 21 grafts eventually failed.

Graft revision uniformly resulted in the restoration of normal hemodynamics of the autogenous graft. The ABIs and the peak systolic velocities returned to comparable levels that were present for the graft before the occurrence of the graft stenosis. The ABI was usually in the range of 0.6 before the secondary procedure and increased to greater than 0.9 following revision in 85% of the lower extremities. The peak systolic velocity was less than 45 cm/sec in 84% of the autogenous grafts in this series and uniformly increased to a level comparable to the initial postoperative studies.[5,7]

Secondary procedures for revision of the patent but failing autogenous graft were associated with a 5-year patency greater than 85% in many series.[1,7,12] The success of graft revision was dependent on excision of the lesion, use of autogenous tissue for reconstruction, confirmation of achievement of normal hemodynamics of the vein conduit after revision, and continued postoperative surveillance.

CONCLUSION

Long-term patency of the autogenous vein graft hinges on the detection and correction of the failing bypass before thrombosis. The development of fibrointimal hyperplasia of the graft or progression of atherosclerosis of the native arteries can result in diameter-reducing stenoses that threaten bypass patency. The necessity for intraoperative reconstruction of the inflow artery and for modification of the vein conduit during the bypass procedure because of a technical error or poor-quality vein significantly increases the risk of late-appearing stenoses and the need for bypass revision. The long-term patency of the autogenous vein grafts that develop hemodynamically significant lesions (low graft flow velocity, >75% stenosis) that threaten bypass patency is dependent on the identification and correction of the lesions before thrombosis. The secondary patency rates for the revision of a *patent* but hemodynamically failing autogenous graft have been equal to those of bypasses that do not undergo revision.[1,7] The secondary patency of revision of the *thrombosed* autogenous graft has been uniformly poor.[1,5] The success of graft revision is dependent on excision of the lesion, use of autogenous tissue for reconstruction, restoration of normal hemodynamics, and continued postoperative surveillance. Secondary procedures to correct the failing autogenous graft result in excellent long-term patency—greater than 85% at 5 years.[7,12] Secondary procedures should restore normal graft and hemodynamics with the excision of the pathoanatomic lesion and the use of normal autogenous tissue for reconstruction.

REFERENCES

1. Bergamini TM, Towne JB, Bandyk DF, et al. Experience with in situ saphenous vein bypasses from 1981-1989: Determinant factors of long-term patency. J Vasc Surg (in press).
2. Minh-Chau L, Friedman EI, Figg-Hoblyn L, et al. Decreased graft flow is a reliable predictor of impending failure of reversed vein grafts. J Vasc Technol 12:133, 1988.
3. Sladen JG, Gilmour JL. Vein graft stenosis. Am J Surg 141:549, 1981.
4. Bandyk DF, Kaebnick HW, Stewart GW, et al. Durability of the in situ vein arterial bypass: A comparison of primary and secondary patency. J Vasc Surg 5:256, 1987.
5. Belkin M, Donaldson MC, Whittemore AD, et al. Observations on the use of thrombolytic agents for thrombotic occlusion of infrainguinal vein grafts. J Vasc Surg 11:289, 1990.

6. Cohen JR, Mannick JA, Couch NP, et al. Recognition and management of impending vein-graft failure. Arch Surg 121:758, 1986.

7. Bandyk DF, Bergamini TM, Towne JB, et al. Durability of vein graft revision: A comparison of secondary procedures. J Vasc Surg (in press).

8. Berkowitz HD, Hobbs CL, Roberts B, et al. Value of routine vascular laboratory studies to identify vein graft stenosis. Surgery 90:971, 1981.

9. Veith FJ, Weiser RK, Gupta SK, et al. Diagnosis and management of failing lower extremity arterial reconstructions prior to graft occlusion. J Cardiovasc Surg 25:381, 1984.

10. Bandyk DF, Schmitt DD, Seabrook GR, et al. Monitoring patency of in situ saphenous vein bypasses: The impact of a surveillance protocol and elective revision. J Vasc Surg 9:286, 1989.

11. Green RM, McNamara J, Ouriel K, et al. Comparison of infrainguinal graft surveillance techniques. J Vasc Surg 11:207, 1990.

12. Whittemore AD, Clowes AW, Couch NP, et al. Secondary femoropopliteal reconstruction. Ann Surg 193:35, 1981.

13. Leather RP, Shah DM, Chang BB, et al. Resurrection of the in situ saphenous vein bypass: 1000 cases later. Ann Surg 208:435, 1988.

14. Taylor LM, Edwards JM, Porter JM. Present status of reversed vein bypass grafting: Five-year results of a modern series. J Vasc Surg 11:193, 1990.

15. Rutherford RB, Jones DN, Bergentz S-E, et al. Factors affecting the patency of infrainguinal bypass. J Vasc Surg 8:236, 1988.

16. Wengerter KR, Veith FJ, Gupta SK, et al. Influence of vein size (diameter) on infrapopliteal reversed vein graft patency. J Vasc Surg 11:525, 1990.

17. Cutler BS, Thompson JE, Kleinsasser LJ, et al. Autologous saphenous vein femoro-popliteal bypass: Analysis of 298 cases. Surgery 79:325, 1976.

18. Bernhard VM, Boren CH, Towne JB. Pneumatic tourniquet as a substitute for vascular clamps in distal bypass surgery. Surgery 87:709, 1980.

19. Bandyk DF. Postoperative surveillance of infrainguinal bypass. Surg Clin North Am 70:71, 1990.

20. Schmitt DD, Seabrook GR, Bandyk DF, et al. Early patency of in situ saphenous vein bypasses as determined by intraoperative velocity waveform analysis. Ann Vasc Surg 4:270, 1990.

21. Bandyk DF, Kaebnick HW, Bergamini TM, et al. Hemodynamics of in situ saphenous vein arterial bypass. Arch Surg 123:477, 1988.

22. Greenspan B, Pillari G, Schulman ML, et al. Percutaneous transluminal angioplasty of stenotic deep vein arterial bypass grafts. Arch Surg 120:492, 1985.

23. Sheridan J, Thompson J, Gazzard S, et al. The role of transluminal angioplasty in the management of femoro-distal graft stenosis. Br J Radiol Suppl 62:S64, 1989.

20

Early and Late Infrainguinal Autogenous Vein Graft Thrombosis

Anthony D. Whittemore   **Magruder C. Donaldson**   **John A. Mannick**

Since routine arterial reconstruction became feasible in 1948, increasingly complex arterial reconstructions have continued to provide effective palliation for intermittent claudication and significant salvage of threatened limbs.[1-8] Despite numerous technical improvements, however, 20% to 25% of autogenous reconstructions still fail during the first 5 years following surgery.[9-12] This persistent failure rate is in part the result of the steadily advancing age of our patient population and the necessity to perform reconstructions to increasingly distal locations in more severely diseased limbs. For the vascular surgeon confronted with an increasing number of patients having a diminished supply of autogenous tissue, the management of thrombosed vein grafts represents a considerable challenge.

Nearly 10 years ago, the examination of retrospective data retrieved from our registry at the Peter Bent Brigham Hospital revealed a series of 109 failed reversed femoropopliteal vein grafts; further investigation allowed us to determine the probable cause of failure in the majority of these cases based on angiographic evidence or direct observation during secondary surgery.[11] These grafts were equally divided between above-knee and below-knee reconstructions, but none were carried to the distal tibioperoneal system. Although we were unable to identify a probable cause for failure in nearly one third of these individuals, the most likely causes in the remaining 78 are indicated in Table 20-1. It had long been recognized that early failures result from technical errors at the time of the initial reconstruction and those occurring later most often result from the inevitable progression of distal atherosclerotic disease.[9,10] In 1973, Szilagyi et al.[10] emphasized the critical nature of intrinsic alterations within the vein graft in the pathogenesis of graft thrombosis. Our previous experience confirmed this finding and demonstrated that vein graft stenosis tended to occur after the first 6 postoperative months but within 2 years of the initial surgery.[11] These localized stenotic lesions were often found at the site of a fibrotic valve or within the narrowest portion of the reversed vein graft just distal to the proximal anastomosis. Late failures that occurred more than 2 years postoperatively were most often attributed to the progression of distal atherosclerotic disease with subsequent increase in outflow resistance.

Of the initial 109 graft failures, limb viability was clearly jeopardized in 72 and prompted subsequent secondary reconstruction. The

Table 20-1. Causes of Thrombosis in 109 Reversed Vein Grafts*

Mechanism	No. of patients (%)
Vein graft stenosis	27 (25%)
Technical errors	20 (18%)
Progression of disease	15 (14%)
Miscellaneous	16 (14%)
Indeterminate	31 (28%)

*Modified from Whittemore AD, Clowes AW, Couch NP, et al. Secondary femoropopliteal reconstruction. Ann Surg 193:35-42, 1981.

overall 5-year limb salvage rate for the entire group approximated 50%, although individual 5-year cumulative patency rates associated with most methods of secondary reconstruction were more limited (35%). It became apparent from a subgroup of grafts that were failing from localized stenotic lesions that repair with simple patch angioplasty before graft thrombosis yielded an 86% 5-year patency rate. In dramatic contrast, the same patch angioplasty preceded by catheter thrombectomy required for removal of thrombus resulted in a markedly reduced 19% 5-year patency rate. During the past decade several groups have reported similar results, which underscores the importance of identifying a failing graft before actual thrombosis occurs.[13-18] These studies have prompted the adoption of graft surveillance protocols for monitoring autogenous grafts at frequent intervals. For a variety of reasons, however, a significant residual number of failing grafts escape detection before thrombosis, and patients continue to arrive in the emergency room with acutely threatened limbs.[19-21] At present, there is little debate regarding the worth of aggressive reoperative management for such failed reconstructions but much debate with regard to the optimal method. Several general principles applicable to secondary intervention have nevertheless emerged during the past decade.

In our earlier series, virtually all early failures occurring within 30 days of surgery were directly attributable to either technical errors occurring at the time of surgery or poor patient selection (i.e., patients with inadequate distal outflow).[11] The advent of routine completion arteriography performed in the operating room following reconstruction has reduced but not eliminated the incidence of technical failures (Fig. 20-1). Of our most recent series of 411 in situ vein grafts, 27 (7%) failed within 30 days of surgery (Table 20-2), a rate similar to prior reports employing routine completion arteriography. Thus, although the total number of early failures may not have changed appreciably, the etiology certainly has.[3,22] Failure could be ascribed to a documented technical difficulty in only six (22%) of the patients, a vast improvement over our earlier experience.

Table 20-2. Causes of Early Vein Graft Failure in 27 (7%) of 411 In Situ Vein Grafts

Mechanism	No. of patients (%)
Hypercoagulopathy	9 (33%)
Inadequate runoff	7 (26%)
Technical error	6 (22%)
Systemic hypotension	5 (19%)
TOTAL	27 (100%)

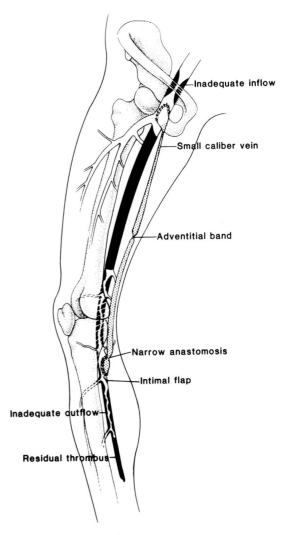

Fig. 20-1. Schematic illustration of technical errors responsible for early infrainguinal graft failure yet potentially detectable with intraoperative completion angiography.

These technical errors consisted of a perianastomotic intimal flap, a graft kink, one instance of suture line hemorrhage, a retained valve cusp, and graft injury with the valvulotome in two patients with small-caliber grafts. Four of these six failures occurred during the first 2 years of our in situ experience, and all are potentially avoidable.

An additional seven patients, 26% of all early failures, had grafts that were associated with severely limited runoff, and five might not be considered appropriate candidates for reconstruction today because they presented early in our experience with in situ grafts when limits of the technique were being defined. Systemic hypotension associated with myocardial infarction and/or a low cardiac output developed in an additional five patients (19%). Although prevention of postoperative hypotension is axiomatic, an irreducible number of early graft failures associated with this mechanism will undoubtedly persist.

As technical failures become less common and patient selection more realistic, a variety of less frequently encountered problems that contribute to early postoperative failure, including hypercoagulopathy,[23] hyperviscosity syndromes,[24] and distal spasm,[25] are now being addressed. The most common cause of early vein graft failure in our most recent series appeared to be associated with a relatively hypercoagulable state. Although the identification and management of a number of hemorrhagic diatheses have improved dramatically, a comparable understanding of acute thrombotic disorders remains embryonic.[23] Primary or congenital hypercoagulable disorders include deficiencies of antithrombin III,[26-28] protein C,[29] and protein S,[30] as well as a variety of fibrinolytic disorders and dysfibrinogenemia.[31] A significant number of less well-defined secondary hypercoagulable states may impact negatively on early graft patency and include abnormalities of platelet function[32] associated with myeloproliferative disorders, hyperlipidemias, diabetes, and heavy tobacco use, as well as heparin-induced thrombocytopenia[33-35] and lupuslike anticoagulant.[36,37]

Hyperviscosity syndromes such as the polycythemia and those associated with the induction of acute phase reactants by many surgical

Table 20-3. Hypercoagulable States in 272 General Vascular Surgery Patients

Mechanism	No. of abnormalities
Antithrombin III deficiency	3
Protein C deficiency	11
Protein S deficiency	4
Plasminogen abnormality	1
Lupuslike anticoagulant	18
Heparin-induced platelet activation	5
TOTAL	42*

*There were 42 abnormalities in 37 patients (13.6%).

procedures may also play an important role in early graft failure.[24] In an attempt to identify specific deficiencies to improve systemic anticoagulation in patients with primary coagulopathy, we embarked on a screening effort for all patients admitted for vascular surgical intervention.[38] Hypercoagulable states were initially identified in 15 of 158 patients (9.5%), and of these, 137 underwent reconstruction, 56 of which were infrainguinal bypass grafts. Five patients sustained graft thrombosis within 30 days (10%), three of whom had documented abnormal coagulation results. Thus early graft thrombosis occurred in 27% of patients with abnormal preoperative test results, a rate significantly higher than that of those patients with normal tests (2%).

We have recently updated our experience with 272 patients screened for hypercoagulopathy. Thirty-seven patients (14%) demonstrated detectable disorders (Table 20-3) that were associated with a significantly higher incidence of postoperative thrombotic events ($p < .0001$). Ninety-two individuals underwent infrainguinal bypass procedures, and graft occlusion developed in seven (8%) within 30 days. Thrombotic disorders were detected preoperatively in four of these seven patients ($p < .05$).

Of the 27 early failures in our in situ experience, nine (33%) were associated with hypercoagulopathy. Heparin-induced platelet aggregation was present in two patients, one of which also had protein S deficiency; a third patient exhibited the presence of a lupuslike anticoagulant; and a fourth demonstrated antithrombin III deficiency. Two patients were considered hypercoagulable on the basis of associated malignancy and systemic collagen-vascular disease; perianastomotic platelet plugs formed in three others and patency was subsequently sustained following simple thrombectomy with chronic platelet antiaggregation therapy.

It thus appears that hypercoagulable disorders exist in approximately 10% of the general vascular surgical population and are associated with a significantly higher incidence of early postoperative graft thrombosis and other postoperative thrombotic complications than that observed in patients without such deficits. Lupuslike anticoagulant and heparin-induced platelet aggregation appear to be the two most significant disorders of clinical impact and justify appropriate preoperative hematologic studies. Recurrent thrombosis warrants a more thorough search for some of the less frequently encountered coagulation disorders.

Arterial spasm, although not a common problem, may be associated with catheter thrombectomy or manipulation of the distal outflow bed in an occasional patient (Fig. 20-2) and may sometimes be responsible for thrombosed grafts for which no identifiable cause can be found.[25] In a series of 212 infragenicular vein grafts, Walsh et al.[39] found that 16 (7.5%) required thrombectomy within 30 days of surgery. The majority of these were in situ grafts. Four grafts failed for technical reasons including twist, intimal tear, suture line failure, and external compression. No cause for failure was apparent in the remaining 12 grafts, 10 of which underwent intragraft drug infusion with heparin and nitroglycerine following repeat thrombectomy. Eight of these infused grafts remained patent for a mean of 1.5 years; most of the grafts were treated with chronic anticoagulation. Walsh et al. believed that both anticoagulant infusion and vasolytic therapy contributed significantly to the sustained patency of 80% of the thrombosed vein grafts in their study.

Prevention of these early 30-day failures requires routine completion angiography to detect and repair technical errors, proper patient selection (i.e., excluding individuals with hopelessly restricted outflow), meticulous avoidance of hypotension, and identification and specific therapy for hypercoagulopathy or marked distal spasm. Since technical errors may occasionally escape detection with intraoperative arteriography, routine duplex scanning may prove beneficial in identifying potentially thrombogenic lesions.

More commonly, vein grafts fail during the 6- to 18-month postoperative interval, during which fibrous intimal hyperplasia develops. The resulting stenotic lesions have been the apparent cause for vein graft thrombosis in some 25% of all failures.[11] This process can

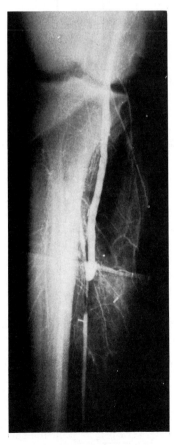

Fig. 20-2. Example of marked arterial spasm occurring just beyond the distal anastomosis of an in situ vein graft.

result in highly localized lesions amenable to patch angioplasty following thrombectomy (Fig. 20-3) or might involve a longer segment of vein graft more diffusely and necessitate an interposition graft. In our earlier experience and as subsequently documented by others, the 5-year patency rate associated with secondary reconstructions for this process was limited to 20% to 40%.[11-16] These secondary reconstructions consisted of patch angioplasty for localized lesions and extension vein grafts for more diffuse processes following initial catheter thrombectomy (Fig. 20-4). The use of saphenous vein, arm vein, or a portion of the original thrombectomized vein graft all yielded approximately the same 35% 5-year patency rate. Although these methods resulted in the salvage of 50% of affected limbs and justified continued aggressive intervention for failed grafts, it became readily apparent that if suitable autogenous vein graft was available, an entirely new vein graft would provide more durable results.[19-21] Because of the prevalence of coronary bypass and prior reconstructions in this patient population, however, autogenous tissue in the form of an undisturbed contralateral saphenous vein is not reliably available. Autogenous reconstruction then requires a diligent search for appropriate tissue such as lesser saphenous vein, residual portions of greater saphenous vein, and arm vein.[7,21]

In view of the excellent results achieved with secondary intervention for failing grafts before thrombosis contrasted with the poor results following graft thrombosis, we hypothesized that initial catheter thrombectomy required for thrombosed grafts might be responsible for triggering subsequent smooth muscle cell proliferation as demonstrated both in the laboratory[40] and clinically.[41-43] With the advent of thrombolytic agents, we had hoped that results from secondary intervention in occluded grafts might be improved with initial thrombolysis, thereby avoiding the potential injurious complications associated with balloon catheter thrombectomy.[44-46] An initial experience with 44 failed grafts, 25% of which were autogenous vein, demonstrated the superiority of urokinase

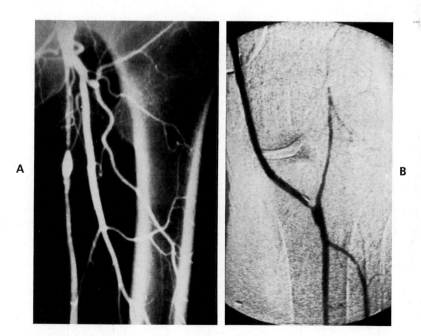

Fig. 20-3. Localized stenotic lesions occurring in the midportion of a vein graft **(A)** and at the distal popliteal anastomosis **(B),** both of which are amenable to simple patch angioplasty.

over streptokinase in providing more rapid dissolution of thrombus with fewer bleeding complications.[47] Although an initial success rate of 77% was achieved in this group, the long-term durability of this modality remains undetermined. Several theoretical advantages remain attractive. In addition to obviating the mechanical trauma inherent in the use of balloon embolectomy catheters, initial thrombolysis in the angiography suite allows more precise visualization of the causative lesion than is ordinarily possible in the operating room. Although angioscopy may ultimately prove equally precise, its use is not without considerable endothelial trauma. Thrombolytic therapy may also provide more complete dissolution of all thrombus within the graft in contrast to

catheter thrombectomy, which often leaves significant residual thrombus attached to the vein graft wall.[48] Finally, the administration of thrombolytic agents may result in more complete resolution of thrombus within the runoff bed beyond the reach of embolectomy catheters.

We have recently administered thrombolytic therapy to 35 patients with occluded vein grafts.[49] Initial thrombolysis was successfully achieved in 63%, and the majority underwent subsequent procedures designed to correct the responsible graft lesion. These secondary interventions included percutaneous transluminal angioplasty of short-segment localized stenoses, surgical vein patch angioplasty, and the implementation of vein interposition or extension grafts. Unfortunately, the 3-year vein graft patency rate remained limited to 23%, which is no improvement whatsoever over that achieved with initial balloon catheter thrombectomy in our earlier study.

The most effective and durable management therefore for an occluded vein graft beyond the initial 30-day postoperative period is its replacement with an entirely new graft.[7,13,21] In the absence of an intact contralateral saphenous vein, however, a diligent search for autogenous tissue may not yield a vein of adequate length or caliber and may justify the continued use of thrombolytic therapy in order to establish a more distal origin for a secondary bypass, from either the original vein graft or the superficial or deep femoral artery. Thrombolytic therapy may also be appropriate in individuals with extensive distal arterial thrombosis evident on initial arteriography and in those patients with a known hypercoagulopathy disorder whose graft thrombosis may not be associated with a specific causative lesion. Finally, for patients with a limited life expectancy, a temporizing nonsurgical approach with thrombolytic agents may provide a more expeditious solution to a limb-threatening situation.

Progression of atherosclerotic disease in the distal runoff bed results in an increasing number of graft thromboses, which most often requires an entirely new graft in accordance with the principles outlined above. In the absence of adequate vein, however, patch angio-

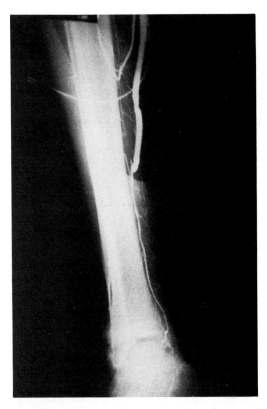

Fig. 20-4. Following initial catheter thrombectomy, this diffusely stenotic distal vein graft required an extension graft, in this case using cephalic vein, from the proximal original vein graft beyond the progressive atherosclerosis in the distal tibial artery.

plasty of the distal anastomosis or the use of a new extension graft to a more distal site may be appropriate alternatives.[7,50] Risk factors associated with the progression of atherosclerosis are well known and increased attention to smoking cessation, adequate control of hypertension, and reduction of lipid levels may yet translate into improved vein graft durability.

REFERENCES

1. Kunlin JL. Le traitement de l'artérite oblitérante par la greffe veineuse. Arch Mal Coeur 42:371, 1949.
2. Linton RR, Darling RC. Autogenous saphenous vein bypass grafts in femoropopliteal obliterative arterial disease. Surgery 51:62-72, 1962.
3. Maini BS, Mannick JA. Effect of arterial reconstruction on limb salvage: A ten-year appraisal. Arch Surg 113:1297, 1978.
4. Fogle MA, Whittemore AD, Couch NP, et al. A comparison of in situ and reversed saphenous vein grafts for infrainguinal reconstruction. J Vasc Surg 5:46-52, 1987.
5. Bandyk DF, Kaebnick HW, Stewart GW, et al. Durability of the in situ saphenous vein arterial bypass: A comparison of primary and secondary patency. J Vasc Surg 5:256-268, 1987.
6. Taylor LM Jr, Edwards JM, Porter JM. Present status of reversed vein bypass grafting: Five-year results of a modern series. J Vasc Surg 11:193-206, 1990.
7. Kent KC, Whittemore AD, Mannick JA. Short-term and mid-term results of an all-autogenous tissue policy for infrainguinal reconstruction. J Vasc Surg 9:107-114, 1989.
8. Pomposelli FB, Jepsen SJ, Gibbons GW, et al. The efficacy of the dorsalis pedis bypass for limb salvage in diabetic patients. J Vasc Surg 11:745-752, 1990.
9. Szilagyi DE, Elliot JP, Smith RF, et al. Secondary arterial repair: The management of late failures in reconstructive arterial surgery. Arch Surg 110:485-493, 1975.
10. Szilagyi DE, Elliot JP, Hageman JM, et al. Biological fate of autogenous vein implants as arterial substitutes. Ann Surg 178:232-246, 1973.
11. Whittemore AD, Clowes AW, Couch NP, et al. Secondary femoropopliteal reconstruction. Ann Surg 193:35-42, 1981.
12. O'Mara CS, Flinn WR, Johnson ND, et al. Recognition and surgical management of patent but hemodynamically failed arterial grafts. Ann Surg 193:467-476, 1981.
13. Brewster DC, LaSalle AJ, Robison JG, et al. Femoral-popliteal graft failures: Clinical consequences and success of secondary reconstructions. Arch Surg 118:1043-1047, 1983.
14. Veith FJ, Weiser RK, Gupta SK, et al. Diagnosis and management of failing lower extremity arterial reconstructions prior to graft occlusion. J Cardiovasc Surg 25:381-384, 1984.

15. Wolfe JHN, Thomas ML, Jamieson CW, et al. Early diagnosis of femorodistal graft stenoses. Br J Surg 74:268-270, 1987.
16. Cohen JR, Mannick JA, Couch NP, et al. Recognition and management of impending vein-graft failure: Importance for long-term patency. Arch Surg 121:758-759, 1986.
17. Berkowitz HD, Greenstein SM. Improved patency in reversed femoro-infrapopliteal autogenous vein grafts by early detection and treatment of the failing graft. J Vasc Surg 5:755-761, 1987.
18. Bandyk DF, Schmitt DD, Seabrook GR, et al. Monitoring functional patency of in situ saphenous vein bypasses: The impact of a surveillance protocol and elective revision. J Vasc Surg 9:286-296, 1989.
19. Green RM, Ouriel, K, Ricotta JJ, et al. Revision of failed infrainguinal bypass graft: Principles of management. Surgery 100:646-653, 1986.
20. Bartlett ST, Olinde AJ, Flinn WR, et al. The reoperative potential of infrainguinal bypass: Long-term limb and patient survival. J Vasc Surg 5:170-179, 1987.
21. Edwards JE, Taylor LM Jr, Porter JM. Treatment of failed lower extremity bypass grafts with new autogenous vein bypass grafting. J Vasc Surg 11:136-145, 1990.
22. Stept LL, Flinn WR, McCarthy WJ III, et al. Technical defects as a cause of early graft failure after femorodistal bypass. Arch Surg 122:599-603, 1987.
23. Schafer AI. The hypercoagulable states. Ann Intern Med 120:814-828, 1985.
24. Schwartz JA, Keagy BA, Johnson G. Effect of acute phase reaction on blood viscosity after infrainguinal arterial bypass. Am J Surg 152:158-164, 1986.
25. Samson RH, Gupta SK, Scher LA, et al. Arterial spasm complicating distal vascular bypass procedures. Arch Surg 117:973-975, 1982.
26. Karl R, Garlick I, Zarins C, et al. Surgical implications of antithrombin III deficiency. Surgery 89:429-433, 1981.
27. Towne JB, Bernhard VM, Hussey CV, et al. Antithrombin III deficiency: A cause of unexplained thrombosis in vascular surgery. Surgery 89:735-742, 1981.
28. Flinn WR, McDaniel MD, Yao JST, et al. Antithrombin III deficiency as a reflection of dynamic protein metabolism in patients undergoing vascular reconstruction. J Vasc Surg 1:888-895, 1984.
29. Tollefson DFJ, Friedman KD, Marlar RA, et al. Protein C deficiency: A cause of unusual or unexplained thrombosis. Arch Surg 123:881-884, 1988.
30. Comp PC, Esmon CT. Recurrent venous thromboembolism in patients with a partial deficiency of protein S. N Engl J Med 331:1525-1528, 1984.
31. Towne JB, Bandyk DF, Hussey CV, et al. Abnormal plasminogen: A genetically determined cause of hypercoagulability. J Vasc Surg 1:896-902, 1984.
32. McDaniel MD, Pearce WH, Yao JST, et al. Sequential changes in coagulation and platelet function following femorotibial bypass. J Vasc Surg 1:262-268, 1984.

33. Kappa JR, Fisher CA, Berkowitz HD, et al. Heparin-induced platelet activation in sixteen surgical patients: Diagnosis and management. J Vasc Surg 5:101-109, 1987.

34. Makhoul RG, Greenberg CS, McCann RL. Heparin-associated thrombocytopenia and thrombosis: A serious clinical problem and potential solution. J Vasc Surg 4:522-528, 1986.

35. Laster J, Cikrit D, Walker N, et al. The heparin-induced thrombocytopenia syndrome: An update. Surgery 102:763-770, 1987.

36. Ahn SS, Kalunian K, Rosove M, et al. Postoperative thrombotic complications in patients with the lupus anticoagulant: Increased risk after vascular procedures. J Vasc Surg 7:749-756, 1988.

37. Greenfield LJ. Lupus-like anticoagulants and thrombosis. J Vasc Surg 7:818-819, 1988.

38. Donaldson MC, Weinberg DS, Belkin M, et al. Screening for hypercoagulable states in vascular surgical practice: A preliminary study. J Vasc Surg 11:825-831, 1990.

39. Walsh DB, Swolak RM, McDaniel MD, et al. Intragraft drug infusion as an adjunct to balloon catheter thrombectomy for salvage of thrombosed infragenicular vein grafts: A preliminary report. J Vasc Surg 11:753-760, 1990.

40. Clowes AW, Karnovsky MJ. Suppression by heparin of smooth muscle cell proliferation in injured arteries. Nature 265:625-626, 1977.

41. Foster JH, Carter JW, Graham CP, et al. Arterial injuries secondary to the use of the Fogarty catheter. Ann Surg 171:971-978, 1980.

42. Dobrin PB. Mechanisms and prevention of arterial injuries caused by balloon embolectomy. Surgery 106:457-466, 1989.

43. Bowles CR, Olcott C IV, Pakter RL, et al. Diffuse arterial narrowing as a result of intimal proliferation: A delayed complication of embolectomy with the Fogarty balloon catheter. J Vasc Surg 7:487-494, 1988.

44. van Breda A, Robison JC, Feldman L, et al. Local thrombolysis in the treatment of arterial graft occlusions. J Vasc Surg 1:103-112, 1984.

45. McNamara TO, Fischer JR. Thrombolysis of peripheral arterial and graft occlusions: Improved results using high-dose urokinase. AJR 144:769-775, 1985.

46. Graor RA, Risius B, Young JR, et al. Peripheral artery and bypass graft thrombolysis with recombinant human tissue-type plasminogen activator. J Vasc Surg 3:115-124, 1986.

47. Koltun WA, Gardiner GA Jr, Harrington DP, et al. Thrombolysis in the treatment of peripheral arterial vascular occlusions. Arch Surg 122:901-905, 1987.

48. White GH, White RA, Kopchok GE, et al. Angioscopic thromboembolectomy: Preliminary observations with a recent technique. J Vasc Surg 7:318-325, 1988.

49. Belkin M, Donaldson MC, Whittemore AD, et al. Observations on the use of thrombolytic agents for thrombotic occlusion of infrainguinal vein grafts. J Vasc Surg 11:289-296, 1990.

50. Taylor LM Jr, Edwards JM, Brant B, et al. Autogenous reversed vein bypass for lower extremity ischemia in patients with absent or inadequate greater saphenous vein. Am J Surg 153:505-510, 1987.

21

The Management of Failed Infrainguinal Arterial Reconstructions

Frank J. Veith   Sushil K. Gupta   Steven P. Rivers
Kurt R. Wengerter   Ross T. Lyon   Thomas F. Panetta

Infrainguinal arterial reconstructions for lower extremity ischemia include axillofemoral and femorofemoral procedures and bypasses to the popliteal and infrapopliteal arteries. All of these operations have an intrinsic tendency to fail or become ineffective as time elapses. The proportion of such operations failing increases with time and is greater for reconstructions terminating more distally in the arterial tree. Because a number of patients undergoing these operations will suffer circulatory deterioration in their lifetime and because this deterioration is often associated with disabling or limb-threatening manifestations, appropriate management of this condition has become an important aspect of vascular surgery and one to which the competent vascular surgeon must be committed to serve his patients' interests well. This chapter discusses the general principles and strategies of this management with a specific focus on the aspects of reoperative vascular surgery that differ from a primary approach to lower extremity ischemia.

INDICATIONS

In general, arterial reconstructions should rarely be performed for intermittent claudica-tion.[1] One reason arterial reconstruction is not indicated is the relatively high inevitable failure rate of these operations and the fact that failure may be associated with ischemia more severe than that which prompted the original opera-tion. This and the increased difficulty and complication rate associated with most second-ary operations, particularly if arteries must be redissected, seem to justify a conservative ap-proach toward *primary* operations for intermit-tent claudication. This attitude, however, is by no means universal, and present practice ac-cepts "truly disabling" claudication as an indi-cation for primary arterial reconstruction to at least the popliteal level. In contrast, almost all vascular surgeons would tend to avoid second-ary arterial operations for intermittent claudi-cation. Thus gangrene, a nonhealing ischemic ulcer, or severe rest pain are the indications for most *secondary* arterial reconstructions, espe-cially those below the inguinal ligament. Inter-estingly, occasional patients with these classic limb-threatening manifestations and poor non-invasive indices can be effectively managed by conservative measures for protracted periods,[2] and such treatment, if possible, is particularly appropriate in patients who are faced with the need for a difficult distal reoperation. Thus, ex-cept for the special circumstances occurring with a "failing graft," unquestionable imme-diate limb salvage should be the indication for secondary arterial reconstruction.

Supported by The Manning Foundation, The Anna S. Brown Trust, the Renate & Allan B. Hunter Fund, and the New York Institute for Vascular Studies.

ETIOLOGY
Early Reoperations (Within 30 Days)

The need to reintervene soon after a primary arterial reconstruction can arise for several reasons.[3] First, the original operation can thrombose or fail in the early postoperative period, that is, within 30 days. Generally this is caused by a technical flaw in the operation or by the poor choice of inflow or outflow sites. In addition, thrombosis may occur for no apparent reason, presumably as a result of the inherent thrombogenicity of the graft in a low-flow setting. Usually this occurs only with polytetrafluoroethylene (PTFE) and other prosthetic grafts, but it can occur with a vein graft also. A transient fall in cardiac output, hypotension, or increased coagulability can contribute to such unexplained thrombosis. Also, a patent bypass graft can fail to provide hemodynamic improvement sufficient to relieve the patient's symptoms. This in turn can be the result of performing the wrong operation (e.g., the performance of an aortofemoral bypass in a patient whose femoral artery pressure was normal and who actually needed a femoropopliteal bypass). Alternatively, such hemodynamic failure could also occur in the presence of multisegment disease and extensive foot gangrene or infection. In this setting uninterrupted arterial circulation to the foot may be required and a primary or secondary sequential bypass may be indicated.[1,4,5]

Late Reoperations (After 30 Days)

Bypass graft thrombosis can occur at any time in the postoperative period. After the first postoperative month it is usually caused by the development of a flow-reducing lesion within the bypass graft or in its inflow or outflow tract. Intimal hyperplasia is a prominent cause of failure and graft thrombosis and can occur with all kinds of grafts at all levels in the arterial tree. The etiology of this process is poorly understood, and fortunately it does not affect most arterial reconstructions. When intimal hyperplasia does occur, it usually produces infrainguinal graft failure between 2 and 18 months after operation.[3,6,7] It can involve any portion of a vein graft in a focal or diffuse manner or anastomoses of either vein or prosthetic grafts. Because the lumen of the distal artery is smaller, this site is most vulnerable to flow reduction by this process. After 18 months postoperatively progression of the atherosclerotic disease process involving the inflow or outflow tract of the arterial reconstruction becomes the predominant cause of failure and graft thrombosis. After 3 to 4 years postoperatively a variety of other degenerative lesions can also afflict autogenous vein grafts and umbilical vein grafts, leading to wall changes and aneurysm formation with thrombosis or embolization.[6,8,9] These lesions are rare in autogenous vein grafts but extremely common in umbilical vein grafts.

FAILING GRAFT CONCEPT

Anastomotic intimal hyperplasia, progression of atherosclerotic disease of inflow and outflow vessels, and lesions within the vein graft itself can produce signs and symptoms of hemodynamic deterioration without producing concomitant thrombosis of the bypass graft.[10-13] We refer to this as a "failing graft" because graft thrombosis will almost certainly occur if the lesion is not corrected.[10] The importance of the failing graft concept lies in the fact that many difficult lower extremity revascularizations can be salvaged for protracted periods by relatively simple interventions if the lesion responsible for the circulatory deterioration and diminished graft blood flow can be detected and treated before graft thrombosis occurs.

We have now been able to detect more than 275 failing grafts and to correct the lesion before graft thrombosis has occurred.[10,35] The majority of these grafts were vein grafts, but approximately one third were PTFE or Dacron grafts. Invariably the corrective procedure is simpler than the secondary operation that would be required if the bypass went on to thrombose. Many lesions responsible for the failing state could be remedied by percutaneous transluminal angioplasty (PTA), although some require a vein patch angioplasty, a short bypass of a graft lesion, or a proximal or distal graft extension.[10,14] Some transluminal angioplasties of these lesions have failed and required a second reintervention; others have remained effective, some for more than 5 years. If the failing graft is a vein bypass, detection of the failing state permits accurate localization and definition of the responsible lesion by arteriography and allows salvage of any undiseased vein. On the other hand, if the graft is permitted to thrombose, the responsible lesion may be difficult to identify, the vein may be difficult or impossible to clear of thrombus, and the patient's best graft, the ipsilateral greater saphenous vein, may not be salvageable, rendering any secondary operation more difficult to perform, with poorer short- and long-term results. Most importantly, the results of reinterventions for failing grafts, both in terms of continued cumulative patency and limb salvage rates, have been far superior to the results of reinterventions for grafts that have thrombosed and failed.[7,10,12,14]

The marked improvement in graft patency of revised failing grafts as opposed to the patency of reoperated thrombosed grafts mandates frequent clinical postoperative graft surveillance in patients with infrainguinal bypass grafts. Ideally, noninvasive laboratory tests should be performed with similar frequency. If noninvasive test results demonstrate a deterioration, the pulse examination changes, or recurrence of the patient's symptoms occurs, urgent arteriography is necessary to detect and correct the cause of the failing graft.

MANAGEMENT STRATEGIES FOR PATIENTS WITH PRESUMED INFRAINGUINAL GRAFT FAILURE

Patients with circulatory deterioration after an infrainguinal arterial reconstruction present with recurrent symptoms, a decrease in pulses in the involved limb, signs of ischemia on physical examination, or a decrease in noninvasive vascular laboratory values. These manifestations may occur at any time postoperatively and are presumptive evidence that the arterial reconstruction has thrombosed. However, these symptoms could also occur in the absence of

graft thrombosis when there is a lesion proximal or distal to the bypass graft, that is, with a failing graft.

Presumed Early Failure (Within 30 Days)

If the primary operation was performed for limb salvage indications, early graft failure or thrombosis will always be associated with recurrent limb ischemia, often more severe than preoperative levels. If the original preoperative arteriogram was satisfactory, repeat arteriography is not performed. The patient is given intravenous heparin and returned to the operating room as expeditiously as possible. Since vein grafts can be injured by ischemia associated with intraluminal clot, which is difficult to remove, prompt reoperation is necessary for a patient with failed autogenous vein grafts. Signs of impending tissue necrosis such as calf muscle tenderness or neurologic changes require immediate attempts at revascularization. In patients with prosthetic grafts without signs of impending tissue loss, reoperation should be undertaken within 12 hours.

Vein Grafts

The distal incision of the arterial reconstruction is reopened and the graft thrombosis is confirmed by palpation. Control of the artery proximal and distal to the distal anastomosis is obtained, and a full anticoagulating dose of intravenous heparin (7500 IU) is given. A linear incision is made in the hood of the graft (Fig. 21-1) to visualize the interior of the distal anastomosis. Balloon catheters are gently passed retrograde in the graft to remove clot (Fig. 21-2). If necessary, clot is removed from the proximal and distal adjacent artery, and any visualized anastomotic defect is repaired. Valves in the vein graft may prevent retrograde passage of the catheter, or it may be impossible to restore adequate, normal prograde arterial flow through the graft. In either event the proximal incision is opened and the same procedures are performed at the proximal anastomosis. When flow is restored, the graft is closed with fine running monofilament suture. An intraoperative arteriogram is performed to visualize the

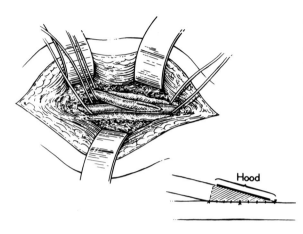

Fig. 21-1. Operative exposure of the distal anastomosis. The incision in the hood of the graft is made to within 1 mm of the distal end of the graft. This provides optimal exposure of the distal anastomosis and facilitates thrombectomy. (From Collier P, Ascer E, Veith FJ, et al. Acute thrombosis of arterial grafts. In Bergan JJ, Yao JST, eds. Vascular Surgical Emergencies. New York: Grune & Stratton, 1987.)

graft and the outflow tract. Adequacy of the reconstruction and the inflow tract is demonstrated by direct arterial pressure measurements at the distal end of the graft. A gradient over 20 mm Hg between the distal end of the graft and the brachial or radial artery indicates unacceptable inflow. Any gradient in excess of 25 mm Hg should be localized to the inflow tract or the graft by appropriate needle placement. If there is a gradient in the vein graft, it should be eliminated by revision. If this is impossible, the graft should be replaced with a prosthetic (PTFE) graft. Unexplained gradients are often caused by recanalized, thrombophlebitic segments of vein. Unless replaced, recurrent failure will result. If an inflow gradient is present, a suitable inflow bypass (aortofemoral, femorofemoral, or axillofemoral) should be constructed, or in some cases an intraoperative or postoperative balloon angioplasty of the aortoiliac segment should be performed.

Progression of disease in the outflow tract as the presumed cause of graft failure is best treated by a graft extension to a more distal, less diseased segment of the same or another outflow artery (Fig. 21-3). If no defect is detected by arteriography or pressure measurements,

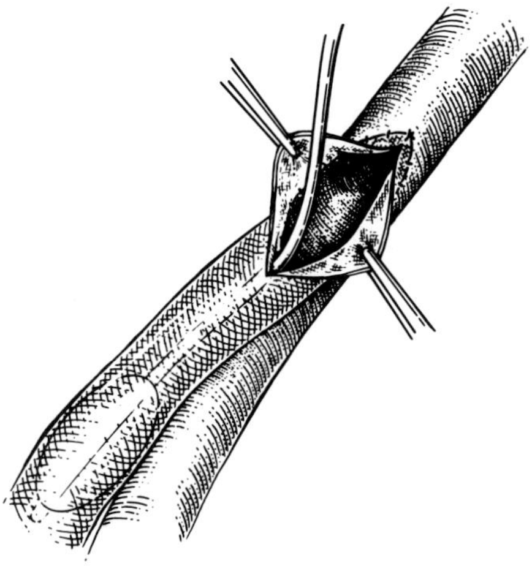

Fig. 21-2. Thrombectomy alone is performed through the distal graft incision when no cause for graft failure is identified. Clot is removed from the graft and if needed from the artery both proximally and distally. (From Collier P, Ascer E, Veith FJ, et al. Acute thrombosis of arterial grafts. In Bergan JJ, Yao JST, eds. Vascular Surgical Emergencies. New York: Grune & Stratton, 1987.)

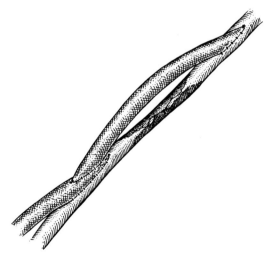

Fig. 21-3. If disease in the outflow tract is detected, a graft extension is performed. (From Ascer E, Collier P, Gupta SK, Veith FJ. Reoperation for PTFE bypass failure: The importance of distal outflow site and operative technique in determining outcome. J Vasc Surg 5:298-310, 1987.)

the procedure is terminated. Despite evidence to the contrary,[15] an occasional vein graft will undergo early failure for no apparent reason and will remain patent indefinitely after simple thrombectomy. Perhaps the unexplained thrombosis was caused by undetected decreased cardiac output with hypotension and decreased arterial flow. As our ability to perform distal bypasses to disadvantaged outflow tracts has increased,[1,16,17] we have had some patients whose distal grafts failed early for no apparent reason other than high outflow resistance. In some of these instances thrombectomy and extension of the graft to another outflow vessel as a sequential graft have resulted in long-term graft patency and limb salvage.[18]

PTFE and Other Prosthetic Grafts

Early thrombosis of PTFE grafts is managed in essentially the same fashion as already

described for early failure of vein grafts.[3,14] With prosthetic grafts, however, graft defects are not a cause of failure, although occasionally a PTFE graft will be compressed, kinked, or twisted because of poor tunneling technique and malposition around or through some of the tendinous structures in the region of the knee. In addition, graft thrombosis resulting from no apparent cause is more common with PTFE grafts than vein grafts and occurred in 38 of our 61 early failures in a series of 822 infrainguinal PTFE grafts.[19] Simple thrombectomy of the graft by the techniques already described resulted in patency rates in excess of 50% after 3 years when no defect was found and the distal anastomosis was above the knee joint.[3,14] The secondary operative treatment in the remaining 23 cases was designed to correct the cause of early failure. In one case treatment consisted of a patch angioplasty for outflow stenosis (Fig. 21-4), and in 22 cases a graft extension for inflow or outflow disease was performed.[19]

Presumed Late Failure (After 30 Days)

All patients with presumed late graft failure should undergo a standard transfemoral or translumbar arteriogram with visualization of all arteries from the renal arteries to the forefoot.[1] If a failing graft is found, it is urgently treated by reintervention as already discussed. If a failed or thrombosed graft is present, the patient is not subjected to reinterventional treatment unless the limb is unequivocally threatened. Surprisingly, in some cases even though the original operation was performed for limb salvage with critical ischemia,[20] the limb may not be in the critical limb ischemia category when the original arterial reconstruction occludes.[3] Ten percent to 25% of patients will be able to tolerate occlusion of a limb salvage bypass and function effectively indefinitely. This percentage seems to rise as the interval between the primary operation and its failure increases. Presumably this phenomenon occurs because the original limb-threatening lesion has healed as a result of the bypass and does not recur with the renewed ischemia. Alternatively, in some cases collateral vessels are more efficient after graft failure than before the operation for reasons that remain obscure.

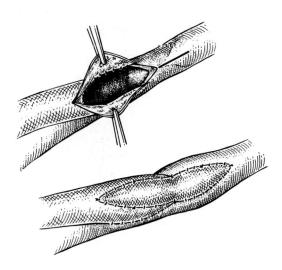

Fig. 21-4. Stenosis just distal to the anastomosis can be caused by an unrecognized atherosclerotic lesion. This can be corrected by extending the graft incision distally across its apex and down the recipient artery until its lumen is no longer narrowed. A patch of PTFE or vein is then placed across the stenosis to widen the lumen. Similar treatment is appropriate for intimal hyperplasia, which can cause late graft occlusion. (From Ascer E, Collier P, Gupta SK, Veith FJ. Reoperation for PTFE bypass failure: The importance of distal outflow site and operative technique in determining outcome. J Vasc Surg 5:298-310, 1987.)

When graft thrombosis is associated with renewed critical ischemia and an imminently endangered lower extremity, aggressive reintervention is indicated in order to achieve optimal limb salvage results.[1] Management strategies differ depending on the type of graft and its location.

Axillofemoral and Femorofemoral Grafts

When failure of one of these graft occurs, the inflow tract of the graft should be examined angiographically. With axillofemoral grafts it is possible to perform an aortic arch arteriogram by the translumbar route.[21] A similar examination should be performed to evaluate the inflow or donor iliac system in failed femorofemoral grafts. If significant inflow disease is found, it may be corrected by PTA, or a new bypass from an alternate site must be constructed. For example, if inflow iliac disease causes failure of a femorofemoral graft, it can be corrected by PTA or an aortobifemoral bypass, or an aortic limb can be brought to the thrombectomized femorofemoral graft.

The same arteriogram should be used to evaluate the outflow bed for evidence of progression of occlusive outflow disease and to define patent distal segments that can be used for jump or sequential grafts. For example, in a patient with progression of occlusive disease in a deep femoral artery that provides outflow for an axillofemoral or femorofemoral bypass, the popliteal artery should be evaluated angiographically, and thrombectomy of the graft should be followed by a profundaplasty or graft extension to the undiseased deep femoral or popliteal artery.

At operation, the graft is opened over the hood of the distal anastomosis so the interior of the distal anastomosis can be inspected. With axillofemoral grafts this access is facilitated if the original femorofemoral limb is placed over the distal end of the axillary limb. In this way a single opening in the graft permits thrombectomy of all prosthetic grafts, thrombectomy of arteries in one groin, and diagnosis and correction of anastomotic problems at one distal anastomosis. Although occasionally successful, the practice of blind balloon catheter thrombectomy of any distal anastomosis via an opening in the graft remote from the anastomosis is to be condemned. Since the chance of damaging the anastomosis, intimal injury, or plaque disruption in the adjacent artery is too great with remote blind balloon catheter thrombectomy, the anastomosis and its adjacent arteries must be dissected free and controlled despite the fact that this procedure may be difficult because of scarring.

If distal anastomotic intimal hyperplasia is detected as the cause of graft failure, graft extension or patch angioplasty of the hyperplastic lesion is preferred (Fig. 21-4). Patch angioplasty is performed by incising across the lesion. Since the superficial femoral artery is usually occluded, the arteriotomy is usually placed across the origin of the deep femoral artery.

If no cause of failure is found on preoperative arteriography or intraoperative inspection, an intraoperative arteriogram is performed. If no defects or partially obstructing lesions are found, as is often the case with failed axillofemoral grafts, the reoperative procedure is terminated and good results can be expected. Reoperations for failed extra-anatomic bypasses have substantially increased late patency rates,[22] with a 3-year *additional* patency rate, calculated from the time of reoperation, of 75%.[14]

If multiple failures occur, an alternative approach is to perform a totally new bypass using different inflow and outflow arteries. In this regard the ascending or descending thoracic aorta, retroperitoneally approached aorta, or iliac arteries are useful options to provide inflow. The distal portions of the deep femoral artery and the laterally approached popliteal artery are good options to provide outflow.

GENERALITIES APPLYING TO REOPERATIONS OR SECONDARY OPERATIONS AFTER LATE FAILURE OF FEMOROPOPLITEAL OR INFRAPOPLITEAL BYPASSES

If graft thrombosis is confirmed by arteriography, reintervention is only undertaken if the limb is in immediate jeopardy. If this is the case, complete contrast arteriography must precede any secondary operation to provide some information, albeit perhaps incomplete, as to why the graft failed and to define possible therapeutic options by imaging remaining patent distal arterial segments and by demonstrating the quality of undissected proximal arteries, which may be used for bypass origin such as the mid or distal portions of the deep femoral artery.[23,24]

Bilateral contrast venography should also precede reoperation to define the length and quality of the remaining superficial veins.[25] This can be helpful in patients with failed vein grafts by revealing unused accessory greater saphenous veins, short saphenous veins, and occasionally an unused main saphenous trunk. Duplex ultrasonography can be useful in predicting the length and diameter of usable upper or lower extremity venous segments. In addition, venography is indicated preoperatively in patients who have had a prosthetic bypass. Often in such cases the greater saphenous vein has been damaged at the first operation or was damaged by scarring in the perioperative period.

The standard surgical approaches to arteries in patients who have undergone previous failed bypasses are often rendered more difficult or even impossible because of surgical scarring and/or infection. For that reason a variety of unusual approaches to the infrainguinal arteries through virginal tissue planes have been developed.[23] These approaches avoid scarred standard access routes and can be essential if a previous operation was complicated by infection. These unusual approaches include direct access routes to the second and third portions of the deep femoral artery medial or lateral to the sartorius muscle.[23,24] These routes obviate the need to use a scarred or infected groin to trace the deep femoral artery down from its origin. They also permit the distal portions of the artery to be used to provide inflow for a distal shorter vein graft. We have now used these direct distal approaches to the deep femoral artery in more than 70 secondary cases.

Lateral access to the above-knee or below-knee popliteal artery is possible.[26] This approach is particularly appropriate in the presence of medial incision sepsis and permits the popliteal artery to be used for bypass inflow or outflow even in the presence of groin and medial thigh infection.[26] In addition, all three leg arteries can be approached medially or laterally and adequate exposure can be obtained to perform an anastomosis. The lateral approach, which involves fibula resection, allows access to all parts of the tibial and peroneal arteries.[26-28]

Recently we devised a method for adequately exposing the lower third of the peroneal artery from a medial approach. This technique involves division of the long flexor muscles and tendons to the toes and foot and is particularly suited if an in situ bypass to the distal third of the peroneal artery is to be performed.

Finally, we have developed surgical approaches to the terminal branches of the posterior tibial artery and the dorsalis pedis artery.[23,29] These branches include the medial and lateral plantar branches of the posterior tibial artery and the lateral tarsal and deep metatarsal arch branches of the dorsalis pedis artery, all of which can be used for secondary bypass operations.[16] The deep metatarsal arch is accessed via a dorsal incision, with removal of portions of the shaft of the second and perhaps third metatarsal bones.

Another principle that is particularly useful for secondary procedures is the short vein graft or distal origin bypass concept. Every bypass to the popliteal or infrapopliteal vessels need not originate from the common femoral artery.[1,30] Grafts to these distal arteries may originate from the superficial femoral, popliteal, or even tibial arteries without compromising late patency results, provided no serious inflow disease is present.[16,30]

Such short vein grafts are particularly useful in secondary bypass operations since they allow the surgeon to avoid previously scarred or infected areas, facilitate the use of the limited remaining superficial veins as bypass conduits, and are more durable than prosthetic grafts.[31] Moreover, it has recently been shown that short vein grafts probably have better patency rates than long vein grafts, particularly when they are used as bypasses to disadvantaged outflow tracts.[16,17]

Two types of secondary arterial reconstructions are available to the vascular surgeon who is planning reintervention for a failed infrainguinal bypass. The first is termed a "reoperation" and employs some form of graft thrombectomy and revision or graft extension in an effort to save all or as much of the original graft as possible. The other type of secondary operation involves placement of a totally new secondary bypass graft, preferably, but not necessarily, using previously undissected patent arteries for the origin and insertion of the bypass. The choice of secondary bypass depends on a number of variables, including the type of primary bypass (PTFE or autogenous vein), the nature and location of the lesion responsible for the failure of the primary operation, the surgeon's training and experience, the residual arterial and superficial venous anatomy, and most important the location of the primary bypass. Because of the importance of primary bypass location, the management of different kinds of failed primary operations that require reintervention will be considered separately.

Failed Femoropopliteal or Infrapopliteal Autogenous Vein Grafts

In this setting thrombectomy of the occluded vein graft is not attempted unless the graft is only partially thrombosed or the thrombosis has been present for less than 36 hours. Occasionally a vein graft can be salvaged in these circumstances; otherwise a totally new bypass is performed. If a patent isolated popliteal artery segment is present, a bypass to that segment is attempted. An effort to perform a bypass with a vein graft from the ipsilateral extremity is made using a remnant of the greater saphenous or the lesser saphenous vein. Use of the distal deep femoral or superficial femoral artery for inflow requires a shorter segment of vein, enabling autogenous reconstruction when vein availability is limited. If no ipsilateral lower extremity vein of adequate length is available, a PTFE graft offers good prospects of remaining patent and providing long-term salvage, particularly if inserted above the knee.[31] In this location it would be appropriate to use a PTFE graft in preference to vein from the opposite leg or upper extremities.

If foot necrosis or infection is extensive, a sequential femoral-to-popliteal-to-tibial bypass should be performed with a short vein jump graft if possible. It is important to establish pulsatile flow to the most proximal patent infrapopliteal artery that courses without significant obstruction to its terminal end. For these procedures autogenous vein from any extremity is used even if it is only 2 to 3 mm in diameter when distended.[16,32]

PTFE grafts should only be used for bypasses to infrapopliteal arteries if no autogenous vein is available. However, a secondary arterial reconstruction with a prosthetic graft has some chance of remaining patent for several years and a moderate chance of saving the involved limb.[31] Recent research suggests that late patency rates for prosthetic grafts can be improved by postoperative anticoagulation therapy.[33]

Failed Above-Knee Femoropopliteal PTFE Bypass

When failure of such a bypass results in a threatened limb, it is our present belief that a reoperation with an attempt at graft salvage is justified and indicated.[3,14] If the preoperative arteriogram indicates an inflow problem, PTA or a proximal graft extension is performed. The distal end of the graft is redissected along with its adjacent arteries (Fig. 21-1), and after administration of 7500 IU of heparin, a vertical incision is made in the distal hood of the graft to permit balloon catheter thrombectomy of the graft and of the popliteal artery proximally and distally (Figs. 21-1 and 21-2). Great care is exercised to use minimal balloon inflation when passing the catheter in arteries to avoid intimal injury. A proximal incision is made only if adequate flow cannot be restored in the graft. If a distal lesion is detected on inspection of the anastomosis or preoperative arteriography, it is treated. An incision across the lesion and patch angioplasty are performed for intimal hyperplasia (Fig. 21-4), and a graft extension to a distal patent artery with a PTFE or vein graft (Fig. 21-3) is performed for distal disease progression. Although this approach requires a difficult redissection of the distal anastomosis (which may be more technically demanding than performing a totally new bypass), it is justified by the 3-year patency results and by the fact that it preserves the maximal amount of undissected patent distal arterial tree should further problems develop.[14] On the other hand, if excessive scarring or infection is present or if the surgeon's preference dictates, a new bypass to patent unused arterial segments may be the best operation in this setting.

Failed Below-Knee Femoropopliteal or Infrapopliteal PTFE Bypass

When failure of such a procedure results in the need for a secondary arterial reconstruction, the best treatment is an entirely new secondary bypass, preferably employing an autogenous vein graft using some of the strategies already discussed to minimize graft length and permit use of previously unused segments of arteries or segments approached through virginal tissue planes. The primary reason for departing from our previous strategy[3] of performing a reoperation with attempted graft salvage is the poorer additional patency that can be obtained with reoperations on these below-knee grafts as compared with the better results (over 40% 2-year patency) achieved when a totally new secondary bypass is employed.[14] A second reason for not using the reoperation strategy is the high infection rate (6%) with such procedures compared with the infection rate for a new secondary bypass of less than 1%.[14]

Failure of Secondary Arterial Reconstructions

Although some vascular surgeons are reluctant to undertake multiple attempts at arterial reconstruction to salvage a threatened limb in the belief that the risks of infection and knee loss outweigh the potential benefits, we and others disagree. The results show that many patients can benefit from multiple limb salvage operations and that the benefits outweigh the risks and disadvantages if the principles and strategies already advocated are employed.*

CONCLUSION

Secondary interventions play an important role in achieving the ultimate goal of limb salvage after primary infrainguinal interventions

fail. If the described strategies and principles for secondary arterial reconstructions below the inguinal ligament are employed, good results in terms of patency of the reoperated primary reconstruction or the secondary reconstruction can be obtained with significantly improved limb salvage at a low cost in operative morbidity and mortality. These results mandate that vascular surgeons maintain an aggressive attitude toward the use of these secondary operations when a primary procedure fails to achieve or maintain its intended goal and a patient is faced with imminent limb loss because of distal ischemia.

REFERENCES

1. Veith FJ, Gupta SK, Samson RH, et al. Progress in limb salvage by reconstructive arterial surgery combined with new or improved adjunctive procedures. Ann Surg 194:386-401, 1981.
2. Rivers SP, Veith FJ, Ascer E, Gupta SK. Successful conservative therapy of severe limb-threatening ischemia: The value of nonsympathectomy. Surgery 99:759-762, 1986.
3. Veith FJ, Gupta SK, Daly V. Management of early and late thrombosis of expanded polytetrafluoroethylene (PTFE) femoro-popliteal bypass grafts: Favorable prognosis with appropriate reoperation. Surgery 87:581-587, 1980.
4. Veith FJ, Gupta SK, Daly V. Femoro-popliteal bypass to the isolated popliteal segment: Is polytetrafluoroethylene graft acceptable? Surgery 89:296-303, 1981.
5. Flinn WR, Flanigan DP, Verta MJ, et al. Sequential femoral-tibial bypass for severe limb ischemia. Surgery 88:357-365, 1980.
6. Szilagyi DE, Smith RF, Elliott JP, et al. The biologic fate of autogenous vein implants as arterial substitutes: Clinical, angiographic and histopathologic observations in femoro-popliteal operations for atherosclerosis. Ann Surg 178:232-244, 1973.
7. Whittemore AD, Clowes AW, Couch NP, et al. Secondary femoro-popliteal reconstruction. Ann Surg 193:35-42, 1981.
8. Karkow WS, Cranley JJ, Cranley RD, et al. Extended study of aneurysm formation in umbilical grafts. J Vasc Surg 4:486-492, 1986.
9. Hasson JE, Newton WD, Waltman AC, et al. Mural degeneration in the glutaraldehyde-tanned umbilical vein graft: Incidence and implications. J Vasc Surg 4:243-250, 1986.
10. Veith FJ, Weiser RK, Gupta SK, et al. Diagnosis and management of failing lower extremity arterial reconstructions. J Cardiovasc Surg 25:381-384, 1984.

*References 1, 3, 7, 14, 34, 35.

11. O'Mara CS, Flinn WR, Johnson ND, et al. Recognition and surgical management of patent but hemodynamically failed arterial grafts. Ann Surg 193:467-476, 1981.

12. Smith CR, Green RM, DeWeese JA. Pseudoocclusion of femoro-popliteal bypass grafts. Circulation 68(Suppl II): 88-93, 1983.

13. Berkowitz HD, Hobbs CL, Roberts B, et al. Value of routine vascular laboratory studies to identify vein graft stenosis. Surgery 90:971-979, 1981.

14. Ascer E, Collier P, Gupta SK, Veith FJ. Reoperation for PTFE bypass failure: The importance of distal outflow site and operative technique in determining outcome. J Vasc Surg 5:298-310, 1987.

15. Craver JM, Ottinger LW, Darling C, et al. Hemorrhage and thrombosis as early complications of femoro-popliteal bypass grafts: Causes, treatment, and prognostic implications. Surgery 74:839-838, 1973.

16. Veith FJ, Ascer E, Gupta SK, et al. Tibio-tibial vein bypass grafts: A new operation for limb salvage. J Vasc Surg 2:552-557, 1985.

17. Ascer E, Veith FJ, Gupta SK, et al. Short vein grafts: A superior option for arterial reconstruction to poor or compromised outflow tracts. J Vasc Surg 7:370-378, 1988.

18. Ascer E, Veith FJ, Morin L, et al. Components of outflow resistance and their correlation with graft patency in lower extremity arterial reconstructions. J Vasc Surg 1:817-828, 1984.

19. Collier P, Ascer E, Veith FJ, et al. Acute thrombosis of arterial grafts. In Bergan JJ, Yao JST, eds. Vascular Surgical Emergencies. New York: Grune & Stratton, 1987, pp 517-528.

20. Working Party of the International Vascular Symposium. The definition of critical ischaemia of a limb. Br J Surg 69(Suppl):S2, 1982.

21. Calligaro KD, Ascer E, Veith FJ, et al. Unsuspected inflow disease in candidates for axillo-femoral bypass operations: A prospective study. J Vasc Surg 11:832-837, 1990.

22. Ascer E, Veith FJ, Gupta SK, et al. Comparison of axillo-unifemoral and axillobifemoral bypass operations. Surgery 97:169-177, 1985.

23. Veith FJ, Gupta SK, Ascer E, et al. Alternative approaches to the deep femoral, the popliteal and infrapopliteal arteries in the leg and foot. In Bergan JJ, Yao JST, eds. Techniques in Arterial Surgery. Philadelphia: WB Saunders, 1990, pp 145-156.

24. Nunez A, Veith FJ, Collier P, et al. Direct approach to the distal portions of the deep femoral artery for limb salvage bypasses. J Vasc Surg 8:576-581, 1988.

25. Veith FJ, Moss CM, Sprayregen S, et al. Preoperative saphenous venography in arterial reconstructive surgery of the lower extremity. Surgery 85:253-259, 1979.

26. Veith FJ, Ascer E, Gupta SK, et al. Lateral approach to the popliteal artery. J Vasc Surg 6:119-123, 1987.

27. Veith FJ, Gupta SK. Femoral-distal artery bypasses. In Bergan JJ, Yao JST, eds. Operative Techniques in Vascular Surgery. New York: Grune & Stratton, 1980, pp 141-150.

28. Dardik H, Dardik I, Veith FJ. Exposure of the tibial-peroneal arteries by a single lateral approach. Surgery 75:372-382, 1974.

29. Ascer E, Veith FJ, Gupta SK. Bypasses to plantar arteries and other tibial branches: An extended approach to limb salvage. J Vasc Surg 8:434-441, 1988.

30. Veith FJ, Gupta SK, Samson RH, et al. Superficial femoral and popliteal arteries as inflow sites for distal bypasses. Surgery 90:980-990, 1981.

31. Veith FJ, Gupta SK, Ascer E, et al. Six-year prospective multicenter randomized comparison of autologous saphenous vein and expanded polytetrafluoroethylene grafts in infrainguinal arterial reconstructions. J Vasc Surg 3:104-114, 1986.

32. Wengerter KR, Veith FJ, Gupta SK, et al. Influence of vein size (diameter) on infrapopliteal reversed vein graft patency. J Vasc Surg 11:525-531, 1990.

33. Flinn WR, Rohrer MJ, Yao JST, et al. Improved long-term patency of infragenicular polytetrafluoroethylene grafts. J Vasc Surg 7:685-690, 1988.

34. Bartlett ST, Olinde AJ, Flinn WR, et al. The reoperative potential of infrainguinal bypass: Long-term limb and patient survival. J Vasc Surg 5:170-179, 1987.

35. Veith FJ, Gupta SK, Wengerter KR, et al. Changing arteriosclerotic disease patterns and management strategies in lower limb-threatening ischemia. Ann Surg 212:402-414, 1990.

22

Wound Complications Following Vascular Reconstruction

Kenneth E. McIntyre, Jr.

Of the many complications associated with vascular reconstruction, none is more worrisome to the vascular surgeon than the development of a wound complication. The spectrum of wound problems may vary from a minor healing problem to one of complete wound breakdown, graft exposure, and even limb loss or death. When a wound does not heal primarily, disruption of the protective covering of an underlying vascular reconstruction may occur. Breakdown of the integument may lead to infection, which may compromise a bypass, even if the conduit used for bypass is autogenous. Healing of wounds has always been a vital interest of surgeons and is especially important for the vascular surgeon. There are many factors contributing to wound healing that, when altered, may lead to necrosis and healing failures. The goal of this chapter is to examine the incidence of wound complications in the vascular surgery patient, review the etiologic factors responsible, and discuss methods of prevention and treatment.

CLASSIFICATION OF WOUNDS

The classic description and definition of a wound complication following a vascular surgical procedure were proposed by Szilagyi et al.[1] in 1972. They surveyed all of their arterial reconstructive operations over a 20-year period from 1952 to 1971. The authors described the infectious processes under three headings, according to the depth of involvement: grade I infections involve only the dermis; grade II in-

fections extend from the dermis into the subcutaneous region but do not involve the arterial implant; grade III infections involve not only the wound overlying the vascular implant, but also the vascular implant itself. This wound classification became important to the clinician because treatment of grade I and grade II infections is not difficult. However, with grade III infections, management strategy becomes more complicated, and risk to both life and limb is significant.

A more recent classification of wound complications following infrainguinal arterial bypass was proposed by Johnson et al.[2] in 1988. Their classification system included four categories: class 1 is wound erythema or seroma formation without separation of the incision; class 2 is ischemic necrosis of the suture line without apparent infection; class 3 is ischemic necrosis and wound breakdown with overt infection; class 4 is an open, infected wound with exposed graft material. The classification proposed by Johnson et al. is more thorough because it recognizes a group of wound complications that are not infected (classes 1 and 2) and yet have the potential to develop into more serious problems (class 3 or 4).

INCIDENCE

There are two important scenarios in which failure of an incision to heal becomes clinically important: following vascular reconstructive operations and following saphenous vein excisions for aortocoronary bypass procedures.

Johnson et al.[2] describe a 33% incidence of wound complications following infrainguinal bypass. They studied 135 patients who underwent infrainguinal bypass procedures during a 3-year period to determine the incidence of wound complications after such procedures. Sixty-seven percent healed without incident. Class 1 (15%) and class 2 (13%) infections were more common than class 3 (3%) or class 4 (2%) infections, and more severe problems occurred following bypasses with polytetrafluoroethylene (PTFE) conduits than with autogenous vein grafts.

Schwartz, Harrington, and Schanzer[3] reviewed their experiences with wound complications in 93 patients who had undergone 98 in situ bypass operations. Wound problems developed in 31 cases (31.6%). In addition, Wengrovitz et al.[4] recognized 28 wound complications (17%) among 163 subcutaneous autogenous bypass grafts. They classified wound complications according to a modified Szilagyi system for grading the severity of wound infections following prosthetic arterial reconstruction.[1] Wound complications occurred in 28 patients and were classified as grade I in 10 (36%), grade II in six (21%), and grade III in 12 (43%).

The vascular surgeon often is asked to treat patients who have undergone aortocoronary bypass grafting and have developed wound problems with the sites used to harvest the saphenous vein. Utley et al.[5] found significant impairment of wound healing in saphenous vein harvest incisions in 254 of 1047 patients (24.3%) who underwent aortocoronary bypass grafting. In their study wound healing impairment included an entire spectrum of wound problems: inflammation, separation, cellulitis, lymphangitis, drainage, necrosis, and abscess formation. Using identical criteria to define impaired wound healing, they were able to identify only 8 (0.8%) of the same patients with impaired sternal wound healing. Similarly, Angelini et al.[6] documented an infection rate of the saphenous vein excision wound in 4.5% of 113 patients undergoing aortocoronary bypass grafting. Other authors have recognized wound problems following saphenous vein excision but believe them to be uncommon.[7-10] How-

ever, when wound healing impairment occurs, the problem tends to be serious.[7,8]

Healing impairment of wounds in vascular reconstructive operations and saphenous vein harvest wounds for aortocoronary bypass grafting is not an uncommon problem. Depending on the severity of the wound complication, the vascular surgeon may be faced with a nuisance or a serious threat to the vascular reconstruction, limb, or even life of the patient. Wound healing impairment is a multifactorial problem and many factors have been identified that directly affect the ability of an incisional wound to heal. In the following section, factors that influence successful healing are identified.

ETIOLOGIC FACTORS
Surgical Technique

Although the method of performing an operation often is based on dogma, basic surgical principles should be followed to achieve the best results in terms of primary wound healing. The method of wound closure is one area in which much controversy exists.

Angelini et al.[6] performed a prospective, randomized study using four different methods of leg wound skin closure after excision of the greater saphenous vein in 113 patients who underwent aortocoronary bypass grafting. The four methods of skin closure used were (1) continuous nylon vertical mattress suture, (2) continuous subcuticular absorbable suture, (3) metal skin staples, and (4) adhesive sutureless skin closure (Op-Site). Wounds were examined by independent observers at 5, 10, and 45 days after operation. The authors noted an established wound infection rate of 4.5% overall, but no infections were noted in the wounds closed with a continuous subcuticular absorbable suture. They concluded that the continuous subcuticular absorbable suture was more effective than either metal staples or nylon vertical mattress sutures. In addition, the continuous subcuticular suture was superior to nylon vertical mattress sutures and skin staples in terms of final cosmetic result and equally effective as Op-Site sutureless skin closure.

Wengrovitz et al.[4] found a lower incidence of wound complications when interrupted incisions, rather than a continuous incision, were used for vein harvest. In their series 163 subcutaneous autogenous bypass grafts were analyzed and wound complications developed in 28 (17%). All wound complications were classified according to a modification of Szilagyi's grading system for infection after prosthetic arterial reconstruction.[1] Wound complications developed in 23 of 83 patients (27.7%) who had continuous incisions for vein harvest. Wound infections developed in 5 of 52 patients (9.6%) with separate incisions for vein harvest. This difference proved statistically significant (*p* >.05). Schwartz, Harrington, and Schanzer[3] examined wound complications following in situ bypass in 93 patients. Some wound complications developed in 33%. They noted wound complications in 23 of 54 patients (42.5%) who underwent in situ bypass with a continuous leg incision over the saphenous vein. However, there were wound complications in only 8 of 39 patients (20.5%) in whom interrupted incisions were used. This difference was statistically significant (*p* <.05). Furthermore, staple closure of the skin was found to be an independent predictor of wound complications by logistic regression analysis.

By contrast, DeLaria et al.[8] reported a different experience with saphenous vein harvest incisions in patients undergoing coronary bypass. Wound complications that required additional care following saphenous venectomy developed in only 1% of 2545 patients. All incisions used for vein harvest were continuous.

As part of the surgical decision-making process, one must decide on the type of conduit to be used if a bypass procedure is to be performed. Autogenous saphenous vein is considered the most appropriate graft for distal bypass because of its prolonged patency when compared with prosthetic conduits. An additional benefit may be that if a wound complication develops, the potential for the development of graft infection may be reduced if a venous conduit has been used for the bypass. Johnson et al.[2] used reversed autogenous vein grafts in 79 of 135 patients (58.5%) who underwent infrainguinal bypass. During the same time period, they performed 53 (39%) infrainguinal

bypasses using PTFE and 3 (2%) composite bypasses. Wound complications occurred in 39 of 113 femoropopliteal bypasses (35%) and 5 of 20 femorotibial bypass grafts (25%). In 23 of 53 PTFE bypass grafts (43%), wound complications developed, whereas wound complications occurred in only 21 of 79 patients (27%) with vein grafts, a statistically significant difference (*p* <.05). They used the four-category grading system described previously. The incidence of wound breakdown in combined classes 2 through 4 was 26% for PTFE grafts and 13% for vein grafts. In addition, six of seven infected wounds (86%) (classes 3 and 4) and all three graft infections occurred only in patients with PTFE grafts.

Lorentzen et al.[11] examined infections that occurred in 62 of 2411 consecutively implanted synthetic vascular grafts (2.6%) over a 4-year period. The incidence of infection was not influenced by the type of graft material used. However, local wound complications, including superficial infection, skin necrosis, hematoma, and lymphocele, were predisposing factors in 30 patients (48.4%) with graft infections. In addition, graft infections occurred only in those patients who had undergone groin incisions as part of their arterial reconstructive operation. Although the authors incriminate "surgical technique" as the common denominator, specific causes of wound breakdown and methods of prevention were not identified.

The success of healing of saphenous vein harvest incisions often is dependent on surgical technique. Utley et al.[5] and DeLaria et al.[8] stressed the importance of making a vertical incision through the skin and subcutaneous tissue directly over the greater saphenous vein to avoid the creation of skin flaps. Creation of a large skin flap may lead to ischemia of the undermined skin even if the patient has no objective evidence of vascular occlusive disease. Creation of skin flaps is a more common problem in the thigh because the saphenous vein is in a deeper location, thereby making it more difficult to locate and thus predisposing the patient to a wide and skin-devascularizing dissection. In addition, lack of meticulous hemostasis may be a greater problem after creation of a large skin flap because of the potential dead space that has been created.

Planning the appropriate incision to harvest the saphenous vein is extremely important. Saphenous vein mapping with real-time duplex ultrasound may be an appropriate preoperative maneuver to reduce the incidence of poorly placed venectomy incisions. Ruoff et al.[12] used this technique to evaluate 102 greater saphenous veins before in situ infrainguinal revascularization, not only to determine their suitability as conduits, but also to precisely map their location and thus ensure the location of a proper skin incision.

In summary, different types of surgical techniques have been used to facilitate saphenous vein harvesting for either coronary or peripheral vascular bypass operations. A continuous incision as opposed to smaller interrupted incisions for vein excision seems to carry a higher risk of wound complications. Moreover, a direct vertical incision through the dermis and subcutaneous tissue directly over the saphenous vein will reduce the chance of creating large skin flaps. Hemostasis must be meticulous and often it is preferable (in the coronary bypass situation) to leave the vein harvest incision open until the heparin used for cardiopulmonary bypass has been reversed with protamine sulfate. Mapping of the saphenous vein with duplex scanning before a proposed operation will facilitate proper location of the incision directly over the vein and will identify veins that are unsuitable so that unnecessary dissection can be avoided. The vein harvest incision should be closed in layers with absorbable sutures. Finally, the skin is best closed with a continuous subcuticular suture of absorbable material.

Diabetes

Diabetes often has been implicated as a risk factor for the development of wound infection after surgery. Unfortunately, there is very little objective evidence to support this concept. In fact, when examined as an independent risk factor for wound infection, diabetes seldom is incriminated. In the study of Johnson et al.[2] of 135 patients who underwent infrainguinal bypass during a 3-year period, 31% had diabetes

mellitus. However, the presence of diabetes mellitus did not influence wound healing or the incidence of wound infection. In addition, Schwartz, Harrington, and Schanzer,[3] in a survey of wound complications following in situ bypass, noted that 64% of their 93 patients had diabetes mellitus and demonstrated that diabetes was not an independent predictor of wound complications. DeLaria et al.[8] did not identify an increased frequency of diabetes mellitus or other chronic diseases associated with poor wound healing as predisposing factors in patients with wound complications.

By contrast, Wengrovitz et al.[4] found a significant association between wound morbidity and the presence of diabetes mellitus, regardless of insulin status. In addition, Utley et al.[5] found a significant correlation between impaired wound healing after saphenous vein excision for coronary bypass and diabetes mellitus. Edwards et al.[13] noted that diabetes was present in one third of their patients with graft infections. In addition, wound complications developed in one third of their patients following vascular reconstruction. Although it would appear that the incidence of diabetes affected the development of graft infection, it is not clear whether diabetes also affected the rate of wound infection.[13] Cruse and Foord[14] examined the rate of infection for clean surgical incisions in a population of patients both with and without diabetes mellitus. They found a tenfold increase in the rate of infection for clean surgical incisions in diabetic patients. Verta et al.[15] also found an increase in wound failure following minor amputations in diabetic patients.

Goodson and Hunt[16] demonstrated the value of insulin therapy in the early stage of wound healing. The early stage of wound healing involves an inflammatory response dependent on leukocyte chemotaxis and phagocytosis. It is well known that in animal models with experimental diabetes and in diabetic patients whose glucose is not well controlled, there is a defect in this inflammatory response that may lead to poor wound healing. Although the addition of insulin will improve blood glucose levels, leukocyte chemotaxis may improve but will remain mildly impaired.[17]

In summary, diabetic patients whose blood sugar is poorly controlled may have defects in leukocyte chemotaxis and phagocytosis that reduce their ability to heal wounds and fight infection. These defects are improved but not alleviated with careful control of blood glucose. Unfortunately, studies that have documented an increased rate of wound complications among diabetic patients have not stratified their patients in terms of quality of blood glucose control. If long-term and perioperative control of blood glucose is present in diabetic patients undergoing elective operations, the likelihood that diabetes mellitus, as an independent variable, will influence wound complication rate may be significantly reduced or eliminated.

Groin Incisions

Several studies have indicated that wounds involving the groin crease have a higher incidence of complications. In large part this may be caused by the proximity of the groin to the perineum. This intertriginous zone is moist, the skin is often unhealthy, and poor hygiene contributes to an increase in bacterial skin flora in this area. Moreover, the groin may never "see the light of day" when covered by the large panniculus in obese patients. Excellent preoperative hygiene may lower the risk of a wound complication developing after a groin incision. Preoperative showering with an antiseptic soap was shown to decrease the wound infection rate from 2.3% to 1.3% by Cruse and Foord.[14] In addition, they documented a lower wound infection rate (2% vs. 1.2%) when povidone-iodine was used as the surgical scrub rather than hexachlorophene-ethanol. Specifically, in vascular surgery patients, Kaiser et al.[18] noted a wound infection rate of 10.3% with a preoperative surgical scrub of hexachlorophene-ethanol vs. a 2.8% rate when povidone-iodine was used. Clearly, crossing the groin with an incision during a vascular operation creates an additional risk of wound complication to the patient's hospital course. However, the cause for the increased risk of wound complication may require a more complex explanation than the fact that an incision was made in a potentially contaminated area.

Role of Lymphatics and Open Ulcers

The lymphatic system may play a role in the development of wound complications following vascular surgical reconstructions. First, many lymphatics are interrupted during the course of mobilization of the femoral arteries in the groin. Although many of the lymphatics are divided, few are actually ligated and yet groin seromas or lymphoceles are relatively uncommon. However, seroma formation, when it does occur, may predispose the patient to necrosis and skin separation and inhibit incorporation of tissue into prosthetic grafts, making them more susceptible to infection.

The contained seroma itself may be nothing more than a nuisance following a vascular reconstruction, and reoperation seldom is indicated. Extremity elevation, which lowers venous pressure and lymphatic flow, usually will help to solve the problem. Seromas must be aspirated under sterile conditions to establish beyond question that the fluid is not infected. If there is seepage of fluid through the skin incision, this area must be covered with dry, sterile dressings to avoid subsequent contamination. In addition, leg elevation will reduce drainage through the wound.

The lymphatic system serves as an effluent channel for egress of bacteria from foot ulcers. Rubin, Malone, and Goldstone[19] evaluated the role of the lymphatic system in prosthetic graft infections. In a greyhound model, they were able to document the contribution of lymphatics contaminated with bacteria to the development of positive blood and graft cultures. Careful isolation, transection, and ligation of the inguinal lymphatics during the groin dissection would appear to minimize this risk.

Although the risk of wound complications was increased by contaminated lymphatics in Rubin, Malone, and Goldstone's animal model, other authors have evaluated the effect of open, contaminated ulcers on the rates of wound complication after arterial reconstruction. Johnson et al.[2] found no difference in the rate of wound complications based on the presence of an open foot ulcer. However, Wengrovitz et al.[4] identified an ipsilateral ulcer as a factor that predicted a cumulatively increasing risk of wound complications. Edwards et al.[13] found that 33% of those patients with graft infections had distal limb wound infections that complicated their vascular reconstruction. Moreover, 5 of 24 patients (20.8%) had an open ulcer or gangrene at the time of the initial reconstruction. Liekweg and Greenfield[20] noted that an open foot ulcer was present in 20 of 60 reported cases of prosthetic vascular graft infections. Moreover, similar bacteria were cultured from both foot wounds and from the prosthetic graft. Lorentzen et al.[11] also found preoperative infection in a foot ulcer or toe gangrene to be a predisposing factor for graft infection. Twenty-two of 62 patients (35.5%) who developed infections had an infected ulcer or toe gangrene at the time of the initial vascular operation.

From these reported experiences, one can conclude that the following management techniques should be used to reduce the lymphatic contribution to groin wound complications: (1) peripheral septic foci should be drained, cultured, and treated with appropriate antibiotics before limb revascularization; (2) careful groin dissection should minimize transection of lymphatics; and (3) meticulous ligation of divided lymphatic trunks must be accomplished.

Preoperative Transcutaneous Arteriography

Although not commonly implicated as a cause of wound morbidity following vascular reconstruction, preoperative arteriography performed by a transfemoral percutaneous technique may be a factor. Landreneau and Raju[21] examined the relationship between the arteriography site and the incidence of subsequent groin infection in 1173 patients. Wound complications included hematoma in 26, seroma in four, abscess in seven, and aneurysm in two, for a total of 39 (3.3%). One hundred fifty-eight (13.5%) underwent arteriography by the transaxillary route. However, all other procedures were performed through a percutaneous transfemoral approach. There was a significant increase in the incidence of postoperative groin wound complications in those patients who underwent transfemoral, as compared with transaxillary, arteriograms. Moreover, 81% of wound complications occurred in the same groin site as the preoperative arteriographic

skin puncture site. Timing of the operation following arteriography also was found to be important. The incidence of wound complications was lower if surgery was carried out within 24 hours after arteriography or if there was a delay of greater than 7 days between arteriography and surgery. Although the authors have documented the effect of preoperative arteriography on the incidence of groin wound complications following arterial reconstruction, the mechanisms have not been investigated. Furthermore, there have been no other studies to either support or contradict this finding.

Arteriographic puncture sites in the area of a proposed incision may be a contributing factor to wound complications because of hematoma formation, bacterial contamination, or interruption of lymphatics. Finally, it is imperative to carefully inspect an arteriographic puncture site in the area of a proposed incision before performing a vascular bypass.

Postarterial Reconstruction Extremity Edema

Although leg edema is not uncommon after infrainguinal arterial reconstructive operations, the edema may create an environment in which tissue healing becomes compromised. This edema is seen most commonly in the calf, foot, and ankle. Therefore skin incisions in these areas may be compromised if significant edema ensues. There are two theories put forth to explain postbypass extremity edema. First, there is increased fluid production from the altered capillary hemodynamics occurring as a consequence of lower extremity ischemia. Second, obstruction to fluid outflow as a result of lymphatic obliteration occurs during the course of arterial dissection. Schubart and Porter[22] conclude that significant limb edema does not occur unless capillary hemodynamics and lymphatic transport are deranged simultaneously. Although little can be done about microcirculatory hemodynamics, there are several ways to avoid extensive lymphatic disruption.

Vaughn, Slavotinek, and Jepson[23] compared lymphatic trunks in healthy persons with those of patients who had undergone femoropopliteal bypass. They identified an average of 9.5 patent lymphatic trunks in the healthy subjects compared with an average of 1.7 patent trunks following femoropopliteal bypass. In addition, the most common sites for lymphatic disruption were the medial thigh and knee. Both Porter, Lindell, and Lakin[24] and Stillman et al.[25] found that meticulous surgical technique with preservation of inguinal and popliteal lymphatic chains resulted in a significantly lower incidence of postoperative edema formation following bypass. When the femoral artery is used as the source of inflow for a popliteotibial bypass graft, resection of the saphenous vein through a separate groin incision helps to preserve lymphatic trunks and reduce subsequent edema formation.[25]

Significant leg edema in a postbypass extremity may impede the healing process. Edema can be effectively reduced or prevented by meticulous surgical technique, which helps to preserve lymphatic trunks. In addition, leg elevation in the postoperative period will help reduce excess fluid production from altered capillary hemodynamics following revascularization of an ischemic leg.

Anemia

Although anemia often has been implicated as a cause for poor wound healing, the data to support this concept must be carefully scrutinized. Heughan, Grislas, and Hunt[26] found no significant change in the oxygen economy of experimental wounds in normal rabbits that were made anemic by bleeding and autotransfusion of plasma to restore a normovolemic state. They found that connective tissue synthesis was actually greater at a hematocrit level of 30% compared with a hematocrit level of 40%. Although the red blood cell density was reduced in the anemic group, a decrease in the whole blood viscosity accompanied by an increase in cardiac output appeared to increase the velocity of the red blood cells passing through the wound.[26] In addition, release of oxygen from the erythrocytes to hypoxic tissue becomes more efficient because of an increase in intracellular 2,3-diphosphoglycerate concentration that occurs as a consequence of anemia. Nevertheless, McGinn[27] demonstrated that in both experimental animals and surgical patients, acute blood loss that was insufficient

to cause clinical shock gave rise to impaired wound healing. He demonstrated an increased incidence of both wound dehiscence and incisional hernia. In addition, Taylor, Whamond, and Penhallow[28] examined the effect of compensated oligemia on wound healing. In a normovolemic anemic rat model, they found that the effect on wound healing was more marked in skin than in muscle tissues. The wound healing defect appeared to be an increase in collagen turnover with an increase in collagen reabsorption, rather than a decrease in collagen synthesis.

Compensatory mechanisms exist that enhance oxygen delivery to tissue during the anemic state. Chronic anemia in and of itself, without associated malnutrition, increased blood viscosity, or hypovolemia, is unlikely to be the sole cause of a wound complication. Generally, mild-to-moderate states of anemia (hematocrit level greater than 25%) are well tolerated by most vascular surgery patients. In addition, decreases in blood viscosity accompanying normovolemic anemia actually may improve oxygen delivery to wounds. However, more severe or acute anemic states may lead to impairment in healing of both skin and muscle tissues.

Nutrition

The nutritional status of patients undergoing operations and its effect on wound healing have been of interest to surgeons for some time. It is well known that patients in a poor nutritional state have a higher incidence of wound complications after operation. Casey et al.[29] examined immune and nutritional status parameters in patients undergoing a variety of vascular operations. Wound complications were correlated with defects in the immune system or the nutritional state. A thorough evaluation with anthropometric measurements and serologic testing was used to determine nutritional status. Wound complications were less likely when patients exhibited a serum albumin greater than 3 gm/dl or serum transferrin levels greater than 150 mg/dl. They also found that diabetic patients were more prone to wound problems; however, no stratification was made concerning accuracy of long-term glucose control.[29] Certainly, for elective operations an assessment of nutritional status is necessary. If a nutritional deficiency is demonstrated, it may be reasonable to postpone an elective operation until this deficiency can be corrected. Unfortunately, because of the nature of vascular disease, many operations are performed on an urgent or emergent basis. Under these circumstances an adequate evaluation of the nutritional status cannot be accomplished. Nevertheless, supplementation by total parenteral or enteral nutrition in the immediate postoperative period may help to reduce wound complications as a consequence of alterations in the mechanism of healing.

PREVENTION AND TREATMENT

For the management of prosthetic graft infections, there is likely no truer precept than, "It is much easier to prevent the problem than take care of it." Similarly, the prevention of a wound complication may be much easier than its eventual management, especially if the wound becomes necrotic or infected. As has been mentioned, surgical technique may be one of the most important factors in successfully preventing a wound complication following saphenous vein excision or arterial bypass in the lower extremities. Although no one surgical technique is accepted universally, there are several principles that must be followed if one is to anticipate successful primary wound healing. These universally accepted principles include gentle handling of tissues, meticulous hemostasis, closure of potential dead space, careful apposition of skin edges without undue tension on the wound, and maintenance of sterile technique. In addition, other specific factors that may make a difference in vascular surgery patients include interrupted skin incisions for saphenous vein harvest, careful dissection of arteries with ligation of interrupted lymphatic trunks, the use of autogenous conduits, avoidance of large thigh skin flaps during saphenous vein excision, and subcuticular technique for skin closure. As an adjunct to meticulous surgical technique, prophylactic antibiotics have further reduced the incidence of wound infections following elective vascular operations.

Although prophylactic antibiotics are used almost universally in vascular surgery, there are few studies with hard objective data to support such use. In general, the use of prophylactic antibiotics has been justified because a prosthetic conduit is implanted and the catastrophic nature of a graft infection makes the small risk involved with the preoperative administration of antibiotics seem worthwhile. Most studies that have reported a decreased incidence of wound infections with the use of prophylactic antibiotics in vascular surgery have been retrospective in nature.[5,11,30] However, two prospective, randomized, and double-blind studies have been performed to assess the efficacy of prophylactic antibiotics in reducing the incidence of wound and graft infections in vascular surgery. Kaiser et al.[18] compared cefazolin vs. placebo in a randomized, prospective, double-blind study of 565 arterial reconstructive operations from February 1976 to August 1977. Four hundred sixty-two patients underwent surgery of the abdominal aorta and lower extremity vasculature. Of 237 patients who received placebo, 6.8% developed a wound infection compared with 0.9% of 225 patients who received cefazolin. Four graft infections occurred, all in the placebo group. Pitt et al.[31] performed another prospective, randomized, double-blind study and supported the findings of Kaiser et al.[18] Since the presence of a groin incision is associated with higher rates of infection, only those patients undergoing elective vascular operations in whom a groin incision was planned were eligible for the study. Over a 30-month study period, 217 patients were randomly divided into four treatment groups: group I received no topical or systemic antibiotics; group II had a solution of cephradine instilled in their incisions before closure and did not receive systemic antibiotics; group III received intravenous cephradine prophylactically 1 hour preoperatively and once every 6 hours postoperatively for a total of four doses; group IV had both topical (group II) and intravenous (group III) cephradine prophylaxis. Incisional infections developed in 14 of 62 patients (22.6%) in group I. However, there were no infections in 54 patients in group II nor in 56 patients in group III. Paradoxically, wound infections developed in 3 of 59 patients (5.1%) in group IV receiving both topical prophylaxis and intravenous prophylaxis. Although it is clear from their study that systemic antibiotic prophylaxis was equally as efficacious as topical antibiotics in preventing wound infections, the authors offer no explanation why infections did occur with a combination of both systemic and topical antibiotics.

Prophylactic antibiotics have been shown to be effective in reducing the incidence of wound infections following vascular operations. Although prophylactic antibiotic usage is well accepted, the ideal antibiotic agent for prophylaxis is not known. Moreover, adjunctive antibiotics should not be considered a substitution for meticulous surgical techniques or for consideration of the other etiologic factors that may contribute to wound complications following vascular operations.

If a wound problem occurs, treatment is based on sound surgical principles. Any separation of the wound edges allows entrance of bacteria. Wounds that have separated but are not infected should be carefully dressed with sterile dressings. Fluid drainage from disrupted lymphatic trunks can be reduced by leg elevation. The fluid should be cultured and dry sterile dressings applied. Necrotic wound edges may be left alone if the wound is dry and not suppurative. However, necrosis of the wound that involves wet ischemic tissue should be aggressively débrided. Generally, adequate wound débridement and excision of necrotic tissue will allow for the development of a clean, granulating base. Wound closure by secondary intention will then occur. Delayed primary closure of débrided wounds seldom is appropriate.

In class 3 infections that involve the arterial conduit, more radical techniques are needed. These techniques are covered thoroughly in the chapter on prosthetic graft infections.

REFERENCES

1. Szilagyi DE, Smith RF, Elliott JP, et al. Infection in arterial reconstruction with synthetic grafts. Ann Surg 176:321-333, 1972.
2. Johnson JA, Cogbill TH, Strutt PJ, et al. Wound complications after infrainguinal bypass. Arch Surg 123: 859-862, 1988.
3. Schwartz ME, Harrington EB, Schanzer H. Wound complications after in situ bypass. J Vasc Surg 7:802-807, 1988.
4. Wengrovitz M, Atnip RG, Gifford RRM, et al. Wound complications of autogenous subcutaneous infrainguinal arterial bypass surgery: Predisposing factors and management. J Vasc Surg 11:156-163, 1990.
5. Utley JR, Thomason ME, Wallace DJ, et al. Preoperative correlates of impaired wound healing after saphenous vein excision. J Thorac Cardiovasc Surg 98:147-149, 1989.
6. Angelini GD, Butchart EG, Armistead SH, et al. Comparative study of leg wound skin closure in coronary artery bypass graft operations. Thorax 39:942-945, 1984.
7. Scher LA, Samson RH, Ketosugbo A, et al. Prevention and management of ischemic complications of vein harvest incisions in cardiac surgery—case reports. Angiology 37:119-123, 1986.
8. DeLaria GA, Hunter JA, Goldin MD, et al. Leg wound complication associated with coronary revascularization. J Thorac Cardiovasc Surg 81:403-407, 1981.
9. Baddour LM, Bisno AL. Recurrent cellulitis after coronary bypass surgery. JAMA 251:1049-1052, 1984.
10. Greenberg J, DeSanctis RW, Mills RM Jr. Vein-donor-leg cellulitis after coronary artery bypass surgery. Ann Intern Med 97:565-566, 1982.
11. Lorentzen JE, Nielsen OM, Arendrup H, et al. Vascular graft infection: An analysis of sixty-two graft infections in 2411 consecutively implanted synthetic vascular grafts. Surgery 98:81-86, 1985.
12. Ruoff BA, Cranley JJ, Hannan LA, et al. Real-time duplex ultrasound mapping of the greater saphenous vein before in situ infrainguinal revascularization. J Vasc Surg 6:107-113, 1987.
13. Edwards WH, Martin RS III, Jenkins JM, et al. Primary graft infections. J Vasc Surg 6:235-239, 1987.
14. Cruse PJE, Foord R. A prospective study of 23,649 surgical wounds. Arch Surg 107:206-210, 1973.
15. Verta MJ, Gross WS, Van Bellen B, et al. Forefoot perfusion pressure and minor amputation for gangrene. Surgery 80:729-734, 1976.
16. Goodson WH III, Hunt TK. Wound healing in experimental diabetes mellitus: Importance of early insulin therapy. Surg Forum 29:95-98, 1978.
17. Bagdade JD, Root RK, Bulger RJ. Impaired leukocyte function in patients with poorly controlled diabetes. Diabetes 23:9-15, 1974.
18. Kaiser AB, Clayson KR, Mulherin JL Jr, et al. Antibiotic prophylaxis in vascular surgery. Ann Surg 188:283-289, 1978.
19. Rubin JR, Malone JM, Goldstone J. The role of the lymphatic system in acute arterial prosthetic graft infections. J Vasc Surg 2:92-98, 1985.
20. Liekweg WG Jr, Greenfield LJ. Vascular prosthetic infection: Collected experience and results of treatment. Surgery 81:335-342, 1977.
21. Landreneau MD, Raju S. Infections after elective bypass surgery for lower limb ischemia: The influence of preoperative transcutaneous arteriography. Surgery 90:956-961, 1981.

22. Schubart PJ, Porter JM. Leg edema following femoro-distal bypass. In Bergan JJ, Yao JST, eds. Reoperation Arterial Surgery. Orlando, Fla.: Grune & Stratton, 1986, pp 311-330.

23. Vaughn BF, Slavotinek AH, Jepson RP. Edema of the lower limb after vascular operations. Surg Gynecol Obstet 131:282-290, 1970.

24. Porter JM, Lindell TD, Lakin PC. Leg edema following femoropopliteal autogenous vein bypass. Arch Surg 105:883-888, 1972.

25. Stillman RM, Fitzgerald JF, Varughese G, et al. Edema following femoropopliteal bypass: Etiology and prevention. Vasc Surg 18:354-360, 1983.

26. Heughan C, Grislas G, Hunt TK. The effect of anemia on wound healing. Ann Surg 179:163-167, 1974.

27. McGinn FP. Effects of hemorrhage upon surgical operations. Br J Surg 63:742-746, 1976.

28. Taylor DEM, Whamond JS, Penhallow JE. Effects of hemorrhage on wound strength and fibroblast function. Br J Surg 74:316-319, 1987.

29. Casey J, Flinn WR, Yao JST, et al. Correlation of immune and nutritional status with wound complications in patients undergoing vascular operations. Surgery 93:822-827, 1983.

30. Goldstone J, Moore WS. Infection in vascular prostheses. Am J Surg 128:225-233, 1981.

31. Pitt HA, Postier RG, MacGowan WAL, et al. Prophylactic antibiotics in vascular surgery. Ann Surg 192:356-364, 1980.

IX Amputations

23

Complications in the Management of the Diabetic Foot

Jonathan B. Towne

Diabetic foot problems are a major cause of the morbidity and mortality of the 3 million diabetic patients currently under treatment in the United States. The propensity for the development of foot problems such as ulcers, cellulitis, sepsis, and gangrene in these patients is related to the unique complications of diabetes, including rampant and widespread atherosclerosis often characterized by advanced popliteal and tibial occlusive disease. The coexistence of visual impairment secondary to diabetic retinopathy combined with diabetic neuropathy leaves these patients particularly vulnerable to infection. Abrasions and minor infections that would be recognized and treated in patients with normal sensations often are ignored or not discovered because of visual impairment and, if allowed to progress, become more substantial infections that can result in foot sepsis, septicemia, and occasionally death. The incidence of gangrene in diabetic men is 53 times greater than in their nondiabetic counterparts; in diabetic women the incidence is 71 times greater than in nondiabetic women.[1] At all age levels

the normal male preponderance of atherosclerosis is not present in diabetic patients. In addition to their effect on morbidity and mortality, these lesions have important sociologic implications. A major amputation in an elderly diabetic patient can mean the end of an independent lifestyle and result in the need to enter a nursing home. This chapter outlines the unique pathologic findings found in the diabetic patient and the treatment of the various ischemic and infective complications of the diabetic foot.

ARTERIAL OCCLUSIVE DISEASE

Diabetic arterial occlusive disease can be divided into four categories: (1) the aortoiliac system; (2) the femoral, popliteal, and tibial vessels; (3) the large vessels of the foot—namely, the dorsal pedal, pedal arch, and metatarsal arteries; and (4) the small arteries, arterioles, and capillaries. The aortoiliac system is usually relatively uninvolved in the disease process in diabetic patients and the occlusive disease usually is most severe at the distal superficial femoral, popliteal, and tibial levels. Grossly and microscopically, atherosclerotic disease in diabetic patients is similar to that seen in nondiabetic patients with advanced arteriosclerosis. However, in the diabetic patient it is generally more widespread and often progresses more rapidly with time.[2-4] In a study of limbs amputated for ischemia in both diabetic and nondiabetic patients, there was no difference in the incidence of occlusive disease in the popliteal, tibial, or large vessels in the pedal arch.[5] There was increased calcification deposited adjacent to the internal elastic lamina in the smaller vessels of the foot, including the pedal arch and metatarsal vessels, and a higher incidence of occlusive disease in the metatarsal vessels in the diabetic patients. Sixty percent of diabetic metatarsal arteries had significant occlusive disease compared with only 21% in nondiabetic vessels. There also was more involvement in the digital vessels of diabetic patients: 19% of diabetic digital arteries were obstructed compared with 10% of nondiabetic arteries. The calcification of digital vessels in this series was seen only in diabetic patients and was limited primarily to the proximal digital vessels; atherosclerotic involvement of the digital vessels was seen rarely.

Microangiopathy is a common lesion seen in diabetic patients and histologically appears as intimal thickening. This thickening on electron microscopic examination consists primarily of thickening of the basement membrane. Banson and Lacy[6] found this lesion in 88% of diabetic patients compared with only 23% of nondiabetic persons. Distribution was patchy; normal capillaries often were interspersed with diseased ones. Basement membrane width increased as one proceeded distally in the leg, suggesting an effect of venous hydrostatic pressure in its formation.[3] The thickening usually does not occlude the arterial lumen and its role in selective capillary permeability and its effect on endothelial metabolism are unknown. Some investigators have suggested that it impedes the diffusion of nutrients through the capillary wall and limits the movement of leukocytes into the area of infection.[6] Goldenberg et al.[7] reported endothelial proliferation of such magnitude that it occluded the lumen in the digital and smaller vessels. However, other investigators

have failed to confirm this observation and its importance remains questionable.[2,5,6,8] Thickening of the basement membranes tends to increase with the duration of diabetes mellitus, suggesting that it may be related to carbohydrate intolerance.[9] However, the thickness of the basement membrane does not correlate with the severity or controllability of diabetes; it is seen in patients with both medically controlled diabetes and insulin-dependent diabetes.

Diabetic patients have an increased incidence of coronary artery disease, which is present in more than 50% of such patients aged 40 or older.[10] There is controversy as to whether the incidence of atherosclerosis is higher in diabetic patients compared with that in nondiabetic persons; however, it is very clear that the extent of arterial occlusive disease and its progression are more severe in diabetic patients. The Framingham study demonstrated that both the morbidity and mortality from cardiovascular disease were significantly higher in diabetic patients than in nondiabetic persons and this difference was present in all diabetic subgroups studied.[11]

The severity of atherosclerotic problems in diabetic patients is related primarily to the duration of the clinically apparent disease. Patients who have been treated for diabetes mellitus for more than 10 years have poorer limb salvage than those who have been treated for diabetes for less than 10 years. Steer et al.[8] reported an increased incidence of major amputations (above-knee/below-knee) in patients treated for limb salvage ischemia whose duration of diabetes was greater than 10 years. Duration of diabetes mellitus for less than 10 years did not significantly influence limb salvage. Bendick et al.[12] followed up 274 diabetic patients over a 2-year period to evaluate the progression of lower extremity atherosclerotic occlusive disease and noted that the progression of occlusive disease was related to the presence of preexisting atherosclerotic disease and the duration of the diabetes. The mean duration in patients not noted to have progression of occlusive disease in this 2-year period was 8.1 years compared with 10.6 years in those noted to have significant progression. Abnormalities in nerve conduction indicating diabetic neuropathy were a poor prognostic sign: the median nerve motor velocity was 45.4 m/sec in patients without progression and 42.2 m/sec in the progression group. Sensory nerve conduction and peroneal motor nerve velocities were similarly abnormal in the group with significant atherosclerotic progression. The patients who demonstrated marked progression also had evidence of renal impairment as noted by elevated serum creatinine levels and proteinuria, and a greater prevalence of retinopathy. They concluded that preexisting atherosclerotic disease was the strongest prognostic indicator of disease progression. If measurable disease occurred, it was most likely to have occurred in patients with preexisting occlusive disease and in patients with arterial segments that had initial involvement.

PERIPHERAL NEUROPATHY

Neuropathy is a unique complication of diabetes mellitus that predisposes these patients to foot injury and infection. The nerve lesion is a segmental demyelination that some investigators believe is a defect in the metabolism of the Schwann cell, resulting in delayed nerve conduction velocity.[13] As noted in the capillary, there is a thickening in the basement membrane surrounding the Schwann cell, and in advanced stages there is a breakdown in the medullary sheath into separate concentric conglomerates. Nerves of the distal leg more commonly are affected, with the involvement of both medullated and nonmedullated fibers. There is a diminution of anterior horn cells in the spinal cords of some diabetic patients.[13-15] Degeneration of the dorsal columns also is commonly found and most marked in the lower segments, resulting in scattered destruction and gliosis.[16]

There are probably two causes of nerve dysfunction in a diabetic patient. The mononeuropathies are probably vascular based, caused by an obliteration of the vasovasorum of individual nerves. The other cause is metabolic and is responsible for the development of the symmetric polyneuropathies and autonomic neuropathies. Some researchers suggest that the earliest morphologic change in both the peripheral nerves and sympathetic nervous system is that of axonal degeneration, which appears to preferentially involve the unmyelinated nerve fibers.[17,18] There is a decrease in axonal size and an increase in the density of axoplasmic fibrillar organelles. These changes can be demonstrated in the peripheral nerves in animals with spontaneous or chemically induced diabetes and they can be corrected by careful insulin treatment. It is possible that the diabetic peripheral neuropathy represents disease of the axon and that Schwann cell abnormalities are secondary to changes in the axon that they support. Although the Schwann cell may not be the prime target in diabetic neuropathy, it plays a major role in contributing to the overall process. It not only is responsible for elaboration of myelin, which invests the myelinated fibers, but also is thought to play an important role in energy metabolism of the axons with which it is associated.

When peripheral nerves are examined, the more distal portion of the nerve has greater demyelination than the proximal portion.[14] Neuropathy generally develops slowly, initially consisting of night cramps and paresthesias, progressing to a loss of vibration sense, light touch, pain, and finally, loss of deep tendon reflexes. Since motor nerves also are involved, the following conditions often develop in diabetic patients: weakness in the intrinsic muscles of the feet resulting in pes cavus deformity, hammer toe with extensor subluxation of toes, and concomitant plantar prominence of the metatarsal heads and proximal migration of the metatarsal fat pads. The denervation of the intrinsic muscles of the foot disrupts the normal fine balance between toe flexors and extensors that is necessary for proper weight distribution during walking.[19] The protrusion of the metatarsal head causes a weight-bearing overload on the protruding bony prominences during ambulation. There is also a decrease in the weight bearing performed by the toes, with this weight shifted proximally to the metatarsal area.[20] Instead of weight being distributed over a wide area, the protruding metatarsal heads—primarily the first metatarsal—carry the brunt of the weight during walking.[21] There is a correlation between the site of an ulcer and the point of maximal force during walking. The increase in vertical force seen with abnormal sensation makes the diabetic patient prone to ulceration in this area.

Another effect of the shift in weight bearing is to render these areas more susceptible to bacterial infection. It has been shown experimentally that bacteria localize in areas of compression where their multiplication rates are increased markedly.[22,23] Ischemia with its resultant decrease in arterial flow causes a decreased supply of phagocytes to an infected area. Also, denervation of a limb in the animal model results in increased soft-tissue bacterial growth following inoculation compared with that which occurs in a normally innervated extremity.[24] It is unclear whether this effect is secondary to the presence of edema in the paralyzed extremity or to some other factor. The combination of metatarsal protrusion, the resulting increased load bearing, and neuropathy with this loss of sensation makes a diabetic patient more prone to the development of ulceration and subsequent infection. The pressure points encourage bacterial proliferation and the decreased sensation allows infection to progress without the usual pain normally experienced.

There are obviously many factors that affect the development of digital or forefoot gangrene in the diabetic patient. Of special interest is the deleterious effect of edema secondary to congestive heart failure or venous insufficiency. Lithner and Tornblom[25] noted a closed temporal relationship between the development of edema and the development of gangrene in 66% of 247 patients with gangrene. Patients with edema have increased tissue pressure that makes it more difficult for the collateral flow to reach the tissues. Also, edema secondary to congestive heart failure often is associated with a decrease in cardiac output, which will affect the involved extremity more adversely than other parts of the body. In a more recent publication, Lithner and Tornblom[26] in an update of their series noted that 64% of their patients with gangrenous lesions localized to the feet had edema. A close temporal relationship between the development of edema and the development of foot lesions was observed in 48% of patients. Diabetes had not been diagnosed in several of the patients in their study when they presented with gangrene of the foot, but it developed from 6 months to 6 years later, demonstrating that the complications of diabetes can precede the clinical diagnosis. In these patients hyperglycemia per se was not the cause of the diabetic arterial and nerve complications.

The etiology of autosympathectomy often seen in diabetic patients is related to the decrease in the number of vasomotor nerves in the lower extremity arterioles. Electron microscopic evaluation of the arterioles of diabetic patients demonstrates fewer axons in the arterial smooth muscle when compared with those of similar ischemic legs without diabetes.[6,7] The mechanism of the obliteration of neural fibers is unknown but provides the theoretical basis for the lack of efficiency of lumber sympathectomy in the care of ischemic lesions in the diabetic patient.

INFECTION

There has been a considerable diversity of opinion regarding the diabetic patient's susceptibility to infection. The only clinical problem in which a statistically increased incidence of infection was demonstrated is bacteriuria in female diabetic patients. There are some interesting relationships between bacterial infections and diabetic patients.[27] Smith, O'Connor, and Willis[28] found that 54% of insulin-dependent diabetic adults were nasal carriers of *Staphylococcus aureus* compared with 34% of nondiabetic adults and 35% of noninsulin-dependent diabetic adults. In diabetic children 76% were nasal carriers compared with 44% in nondiabetic children. Also, decreased agglutinating antibodies to *Salmonella typhi, Escherichia coli,* and *S. aureus* and decreased antitoxin antibodies to *S. aureus* and *Corynebacterium diphtheriae* have been reported in the diabetic compared with the nondiabetic patient.[29] Molenaar, Palumbo, and Wilson[30] found that the chemotaxic activity was significantly lower in polymorphonuclear cells of first-degree relatives of patients with juvenile-onset diabetes mellitus when compared with that in other, nondiabetic subjects. Bagdade, Stewart, and Walters[31] tested the adherence of polymorphonuclear cells to nylon fiber columns of ten diabetic patients and found that the adherence was only 53% of normal, which was partially, but not completely, corrected by lowering the blood glucose to normal levels. The decrease in the ability of the polymorphonuclear leukocyte to attach may indicate an adverse effect on its ability to fight infection by interfering with its phagocytic activity. Rayfield et al.[32] studied 241 diabetic patients and noted a correlation between the overall prevalence of infection and elevated mean plasma glucose levels determined at routine visits before the development of infection. Poor diabetic control and the resulting hyperglycemia caused a decrease in white blood cell function. A significant diminution in intracellular bactericidal activity of leukocytes in diabetic groups at 1 and 2 hours of incubation with *S. aureus* and *E. coli* compared with that of the control group was noted. Opsonic activity for both *S. aureus* and *E. coli* was significantly lower in diabetic patients than in control subjects. These data suggest that there was an increase in infection morbidity and a decrease in host-defense capacity when plasma glucose was poorly controlled.

MISCELLANEOUS FACTORS

Two other factors that affect the predisposition of diabetic patients to foot infections are patients' understanding of the disease process and smoking. Patients who understand the problems caused by neuropathy and ischemia are likely to prevent them and, if problems do develop, are more likely to seek medical care earlier, when the process often is easier to treat. Delbridge, Appleberg, and Reeve[33] demonstrated that a good level of patient understanding of the disease process was a significant deterrent to the development of diabetic foot infections. Smoking is an adverse factor in patients with vascular occlusive disease. Because the development of atherosclerosis is a polyfactorial problem with hypertension, lipid metabolism, genetics, and diabetes mellitus all interacting, it is difficult to quantify the deleterious effects of cigarette smoking. Greenhalgh et al.[34] demonstrated the adverse effect of smoking on long-term graft patency. The series of Delbridge, Appleberg, and Reeve[33] also documented that smoking in the diabetic patient was an adverse factor.

CLINICAL EVALUATION

The most important aspect of the evaluation of the diabetic foot is the clinical examination. A careful neurologic examination should be performed to evaluate the vibratory sense, proprioception, and light touch. The proximal extent of the neuropathy should be documented since it is not uncommon for only the forefoot to have significant neuropathy, with the hindfoot and lower leg having relatively normal sensation.

The diabetic patient poses unique problems in the application of noninvasive techniques to quantitate lower extremity arterial flow. Because of increased vessel wall calcification in medium and small arteries, there is difficulty compressing the vessels when arterial segmental limb pressures are measured. This is most marked in long-standing insulin-dependent diabetic patients and results in erroneously high pressures. As noted previously the incidence of calcification of digital vessels is much less than that in the proximal metatarsal, plantar, or tibial vessels, thus allowing the measurement of accurate toe pressures. We use a photoplethysmograph attached to the toe distal to a small pneumatic pressure cuff.[35] Accurate, reproducible pressures can be obtained that correlate well with ankle pressures in patients with compressible vessels. With these techniques we are able to measure digital flow and then calculate toe/brachial and toe/ankle indices. The calculation of these indices gives further insight into the status of the circulation to the whole foot and accurately pinpoints levels of occlusive disease. Toe/ankle indices give a hemodynamic evaluation of the occlusive disease distal to the ankle. Noninvasive tests have the greatest value in assessing the vascular supply to the foot and evaluating the healing potential of local amputation or ulcers. Holstein and Lassen[36] reported successful healing of local amputations when toe pressures were greater than 30 mm Hg. Only 9% of toe amputations healed with a digital pressure of 20 mm Hg or less, whereas all 33 patients with pressures greater than 30 mm Hg healed. Barnes[37] reported successful healing with digital pressures greater than 22 mm Hg. In our own experience we have had patients who heal with pressures greater than 25 mm Hg.[34] In addition to the determination of absolute pressure, evaluation of the foot also is helpful. One of the concepts that is often lost sight of is that having sufficient arterial pressure for healing is only one factor that determines healing. A digital amputation may heal if there is sufficient arterial pressure but not if invasive infection occurs. Studies that have looked only at amputation healing rates do not give proper attention to the role of infection in healing.

All other factors being equal, the pressure necessary for healing is higher in diabetic than nondiabetic patients. This is caused in part by the aggregate effect of occlusive disease in both large and small vessels, which results in greater resistance and lower arterial flow at any given pressure.[38] Toe pressures also have been helpful in evaluating patients who have combined popliteal and tibial occlusive disease and occlusive disease in the smaller vessels of the foot. By quantitating the digital blood pressure, the surgeon can select those patients who will require bypass surgery sooner and avoid unsuccessful attempts at more conservative therapy, thereby shortening the patient's hospital stay. Toe pressures also give an objective measurement of the amount of occlusive disease between the ankle and the toe. However, because of calcified incompressible vessels, falsely elevated ankle pressures, can skew these results. A normal toe/ brachial index is 0.75 and a toe/ brachial index of less than 0.25 represents severe occlusive disease. By calculating the toe/ brachial index and measuring segmental pressures, the surgeon can evaluate the various segments of the vascular tree, from the femoral artery to the digital arteries, and a relative contribution of the arterial obstruction at each level can be quantified.

FOOT PROBLEMS

Diabetic foot lesions can be divided into categories depending on the presence of ischemia and infection. Neurotrophic ulcers in a well-perfused foot without evidence of invasive infection are the mildest problems. Patients in whom infection is the predominant clinical factor include those with septic feet; this is defined as a patient requiring urgent surgical treatment within 24 hours of admission for débridement of infected gangrene, incision and drainage of an abscess, or control of systemic sepsis. The second category associated with infection consists of patients with cellulitis only who do not require urgent surgical intervention and usually are treated initially with systemic antibiotics. The final group consists of patients whose principal problem is ischemia. These patients often have chronic nonhealing ulcers or areas of dry gangrene.

Neurotrophic Ulcers

Initial evaluation consists of obtaining ankle/brachial indices and digital pressures; based on these pressures the patient is assigned to the appropriate group. A patient with neurotrophic ulcers generally has normal vascularity to the skin and good capillary fill, often with the presence of pulses. In a patient who has an ulcer secondary to arterial insufficiency, the ulcers are typically the result of trauma (e.g., striking the lateral malleolus, cutting the soft tissue when trimming the toenails, or malfitting shoes causing blisters). There is usually evidence of occlusive disease, most commonly in the distal superficial femoral, popliteal, and tibial vessels and only occasionally in the iliac segments. Noninvasive evaluation is diagnostic, with toe pressures usually measuring less than 20 mm Hg (occasionally they are undetectable). Classic findings such as delayed capillary filling time, ischemic rubor, and collapsed veins also are found. The treatment of these ischemic ulcers consists of angiography with subsequent distal grafting if a suitable vessel is found.

Patients with ulcers secondary to peripheral neuropathy represent a different problem. They often have palpable dorsal pedal or posterior tibial pulses and the tissues surrounding the ulcer are usually warm and well perfused. The neurologic examination will show a decrease in sensation to light touch and an absence of proprioception, with a dry-warm foot suggesting autosympathectomy. Denervation of the intrinsic muscles is common, with protrusion of the metatarsal heads causing a pes cavus deformity of the foot. The ulcerations are generally over the metatarsal heads, most commonly the first. Treatment begins by assessing the depth of the ulceration to determine whether tendons, bones, or joints are involved. X-ray films of the foot, especially magnification views, are helpful in determining whether osteomyelitis is present. Sinograms also are useful to detect subfascial plantar extension and involvement of the joint space.[39] If the ulcer is limited to the skin and subcutaneous tissue, local care and avoidance of weight bearing are recommended. Because of poor patient compliance, this often is best performed in the hospital setting. If the sinogram demonstrates a sinus tract, it must be unroofed and all necrotic debris excised. Any infected bone adjacent to an ulcer should be removed also. The success of conservative treatment is inversely proportional to the extent of peripheral neuropathy. If neuropathy is minimal, the ulcers heal as in nondiabetic patients. If there is no osteomyelitis and no cellulitis in the surrounding tissues, we do not administer antibiotics to these patients since studies have demonstrated the failure of parenteral antibiotics to influence the bacterial flora in granulation tissue.[40] After successful healing of the ulcers, it is important for patients with severe neuropathy and orthopedic deformation to have special shoes constructed to help distribute the weight as evenly as possible on the plantar surface and to avoid overloading the protruding metatarsal heads. When patients have multiple plantar ulcers or when peripheral neuropathy is limited to the forefoot, consideration should be given to transmetatarsal amputation. This accomplishes two purposes: it removes the area of ulceration and places the insensate skin on the nonweight-bearing surface of the foot as stressed by McKittrick, McKittrick, and Risley.[41] When there is adequate blood supply, these ulcers usually heal without difficulty. Before any operative procedure, precise bacteriology should be obtained so that the patient can be given a preoperative antibiotic that is specific for the infecting organisms.

Griffiths and Wieman[42] have reported excellent results with metatarsal head excision through a dorsal incision for patients with chronic ulcers. Removing the metatarsal head eliminates the pressure point. Use of the dorsal incision eliminates incisions on the weight-bearing portion of the foot. All 25 patients in their series healed at a mean of 2.4 months and none of the ulcers have recurred. Martin et al.[43] also have reported similar excellent results with dorsal excision of the metatarsal head. All patients healed and recurrent ulcers developed in only 18% during the follow-up period.

Septic Foot

The most dreaded complication in the diabetic patient is the development of a septic foot. Often the patients have a long history of inadequately treated plantar ulcers culminating in the extension of the infection into the subplantar space. A second predisposing factor is a superficial abrasion that becomes secondarily infected. The third and most common presentation is the secondary bacterial invasion of gangrenous tissue, most commonly the toe. The combination of vascular insufficiency with peripheral neuropathy allows the infection to progress without causing any significant local symptoms. These patients often present to the emergency department in a septic condition, with their diabetes out of control, and with coexistent congestive heart failure. Treatment must be prompt and aggressive if there is to be any hope of salvaging the patient's limb and to avoid death from septic complications.

Bacteriology

Unlike the nondiabetic patient with infected gangrene, the diabetic patient with foot sepsis usually has an infection caused by multiple organisms, both gram-negative and gram-positive, aerobic and anaerobic. Louie et al.[44] identified an average of 5.8 bacterial species/specimen from an infected diabetic foot, with an average of 2.3 aerobic and 2.6 anaerobic organisms. When the subgroup with cellulitis was studied, an average of 7.3 isolated organisms/specimen was found compared with 4.9 patients with chronic ulcers. The incidence and distribution of the various bacterial species in this series are listed in Table 23-1. The prevalence of anaerobic bacteria in diabetic gangrene was disputed by Sharp and Bessman,[45] who found only a 7.5% incidence in deep wound cultures obtained at amputation.

Table 23-1. Organisms Most Commonly Found in Foot Ulcers in Diabetic Patients*

Organism	%
Gram-negative, aerobic	
Proteus species	55
Escherichia coli	30
Klebsiella species	20
Pseudomonas aeruginosa	15
Gram-positive, aerobic	
Streptococcus faecalis	45
Staphylococcus aureus	35
Streptococci (nongroup A or D)	35
Staphylococcus epidermidis	30
Gram-negative, anaerobic	
Bacteroides fragilis	45
Bacteroides melaninogenicus	35
Gram-positive, anaerobic	
Peptococcus species	80
Clostridium species	35
Proprionibacterium species	25

*Reproduced, with permission, from Louie TJ, Bartlett JG, Tally FP, et al. Aerobic and anaerobic bacteria in diabetic foot ulcers. Ann Intern Med 85:461, 1976.

Table 23-2. Culture Results at Deep and Superficial Sites in Foot Sepsis in Diabetic Patients*

Site	%
Same organisms cultured from both deep and superficial sites	17
No common organism	22
All organisms isolated in superficial sites plus additional organisms in deep sites	16
All organisms isolated in deep sites found in superficial sites plus additional organisms in superficial sites	14
Common organisms and species limited to deep sites alone and superficial sites alone	31
TOTAL	100

*From Sharp CS, Bessman AN, Wagner FW Jr, et al. Microbiology of superficial and deep tissues in infected diabetic gangrene. Surg Gynecol Obstet 149:217, 1979. By permission.

Organisms found on cultures from deep within the wound often differ from those detected on superficial culture. In a study of 58 surgically treated diabetic foot infections for which superficial cultures were obtained before surgery and compared with cultures obtained deep within the wound at surgery, Sharp et al.[46] demonstrated that superficial cultures alone gave imprecise identification of the causative bacteria. An average of 2.3 organisms was found for each superficial site and 2.2 organisms for each deep site (Table 23-2). *Proteus* species and enterococci were the most common organisms cultured from both sites. In the deep wound cultures of 78% of patients, two or more organisms were isolated. The presence of multiple organisms, including both gram-positive and gram-negative and anaerobic bacteria, emphasized the importance of broad-spectrum antibiotic treatment in the diabetic patient with an infected foot. Our preference is to use an aminoglycoside with clindamycin. If enterococci are cultured, ampicillin is added to this regimen. With the development of new antibiotics, other combinations also can give broad-spectrum coverage. These include sulbactam and ampicillin. This combination will not be effective against some *E. coli* and *Pseudomonas* species. Parenteral ciprofloxacin, combined with metronidazole, also will provide broad coverage. It is important to obtain specimens from deep within the wound at the time of surgical débridement or amputation so that specific antimicrobial therapy can be formulated.

Treatment

The diabetic patient with a septic foot represents a surgical emergency. These patients are admitted immediately to the hospital and a regimen of intravenous broad-spectrum antibiotics is initiated. The diabetes is often out of control and on occasion they will present in septic shock. If there is any evidence of septicemia or cardiac instability, a Swan-Ganz catheter is inserted for monitoring fluid resuscitation. Generally 8 to 12 hours are required to prepare the patient for surgery. During this interval hyperglycemia is controlled, any cardiovascular instability is corrected, and adequate blood levels of antibiotics are obtained.

An assessment of the vascular supply of the foot is made. If the patient has diffuse popliteal and tibial occlusive disease and an ischemic hindfoot, a guillotine amputation at the supramalleolar level is performed. The value of a two-stage procedure for dealing with an irretrievable septic foot has been noted by McIntyre et al.[47] and Svoboda and Balaji.[48] The guillotine amputation at the ankle level followed by below-knee amputation when all evidence of infection has cleared has resulted in lower infection and stump revision rates. In patients with good blood supply, (i.e., pedal or posterior tibial pulses) or whose hindfoot is warm with a prompt capillary fill, consideration is given to a foot salvage procedure. The initial procedure consists of extensive débridement of all infected and necrotic tissues, which must be excised without regard for subsequent reconstruction of the foot. Often this will include several digits and metatarsals and occasionally will extend to the level of the tarsal bones. All pockets of purulent material must be opened widely. The amount of devitalized infected tissue is generally much greater than initially appears on examination of the wound. The best indication for extension of the infection above the malleolar level is pain in the calf that is accompanied by crepitus in late cases. At the conclusion of the débridement, all necrotic and devitalized tissues should be removed and all the wound surfaces should be bleeding. In general, I prefer to leave the cartilage intact over exposed bones to prevent the spread of infection into the marrow cavity. The wounds are then reexamined in 24 hours. If there has been any progressive necrosis with new areas of gangrene of the skin edge and particularly of the exposed muscle, we proceed with a below knee amputation. Primary closure of the below-knee amputation usually is possible if there has been no evidence of any spread of the cellulitis to the supermalleolar level. Most wounds in which salvage of the foot is going to be successful develop a granulating base rather promptly and by the third postoperative day, whirlpool treatment is begun to facilitate wound care. When the wounds are granulating well, consideration should be given to secondary closure. Although the wounds generally fill in well,

there is usually a need for additional skin coverage to shorten the period of recovery; this is accomplished most often with the application of split thickness skin grafts. Before the application of skin grafts, we obtain quantitative culture to ensure that the bacterial count is 10^5/gm tissue or less. If the bacterial count is greater than this, we apply amnion dressings or mafenide cream to decrease the surface bacteria count. However, in resistant cases occasionally we will excise the granulation tissue. We do not recommend formal transmetatarsal amputation unless the medial three toes already have been removed.

One technique of obtaining skin coverage is to use the remaining toes as a pedicle graft.[49] The toe is incised on its medial or lateral side, with care taken to protect the neurovascular bundle on its contralateral side. The proximal and distal phalanges are removed and the remaining tissue is used as a full-thickness pedicle graft to cover the defect. It is important that the wound has a good granulating bed and that the appropriate antibiotic coverage is selected. This technique provides a sensate, full-thickness flap that helps close large defects.

When attempting to salvage the foot, the surgeon must be vigilant not to overlook pockets of undrained purulent material. Postoperatively, any purulent material on the dressings generally indicates an incompletely drained abscess pocket that must be incised and widely opened in the operating room. Often pain in the heel or above the ankle will be the only symptom of extension of the infectious process. Occasionally a patient will have an infection that will clear with this treatment but there will not be a sufficient blood supply to heal the resulting wounds. In such patients angiograms are obtained and the appropriate vascular reconstruction is done. We are reluctant to perform bypass grafting even with autogenous vein in patients with active lower extremity sepsis. We believe that a primary amputation is preferable to exposing the patients to the risk of an infected vascular prosthesis. Because of the possibility that we will use a toe as a subsequent flap for closure, we do not amputate a viable digit at the initial procedure even if its metatarsal is excised. On occasion, we will perform a transmetatarsal amputation, usually as a secondary procedure, to facilitate wound closure after control of the initial infection. Often these amputations are variants of the classic procedure since it is not unusual to have several completely resected metatarsals on the medial or lateral aspect of the foot. Failure of wounds to respond to treatment can be traced to two factors. The first is lack of sufficient arterial flow to permit healing; the other is the presence or emergence of bacteria resistant to the administered antibiotics. When wounds fail to respond appropriately, repeat arterial evaluation with toe and ankle pressures should be done to ensure that arterial supply remains adequate. Also, repeat cultures should be obtained to determine the adequacy of the antibiotics.

Ischemic Gangrene

The diabetic patient who presents with non-infected gangrene of the toe or distal portion of the foot requires careful assessment to determine the best treatment. Depending on the blood supply, one of several types of procedures will be done. First, those procedures that require additional inflow into the foot for healing are performed. If there is no suitable vessel, a major amputation, usually below the knee, is performed. Second, procedures that will result in healing of a transmetatarsal or toe amputation are done. Those patients who present with pedal pulses obviously do well with digital amputations but these patients are generally in the minority. Other criteria used to determine the level of amputation include the temperature of the forefoot adjacent to the gangrenous area, the presence of a relatively normal capillary fill time in the forefoot, and the results of noninvasive testing as mentioned previously in this chapter. Toe pressures of 30 mm Hg or more in the adjacent toes generally augur well for a successful toe amputation. If several toes are gangrenous and the distal foot is neurotrophic, transmetatarsal amputation often is preferable. The clinical indications for a transmetatarsal amputation remain similar to those listed by McKittrick, McKittrick, and Risley[41] in 1949. These include gangrene of all or part of one or more toes provided that (1) the accompanying infection is stabilized and the gangrene does not involve the plantar or dorsal aspect of the foot and (2) an open wound involving the distal portion of the foot can be totally excised. Generally lumbar sympathectomy is seldom of value in these patients. In questionable cases we look for evidence of sympathetic activity by placing an occlusive plastic bag around the foot and lower leg for approximately 1 hour and examining sweat gland activity. If sweating is present, a sympathetic block is performed. In those few patients in whom a favorable response is obtained, a lumbar sympathectomy is subsequently performed. This is of limited success in the diabetic patient.

No patient should be denied a conservative amputation solely on the basis of the noninvasive evaluation. The decision for amputation must consider a multitude of factors, including the noninvasive laboratory assessment, clinical examination of the extremity, and the overall status of the patient. Gibbons et al.[50] reported healing of amputations in 38% of patients in whom failure was predicted on the basis of ankle systolic pressure. However, this group did not consider toe pressures, which probably would have increased their diagnostic accuracy. There is no noninvasive evaluation that guarantees successful amputation since patients who have amputations may have secondary progressive infections that further compromise blood supply, resulting in advancing gangrene. The ankle pressure generally believed to be adequate for healing of digital or transmetatarsal amputation is 70 mm Hg or greater.

CLINICAL EXPERIENCE

In an attempt to determine both the short-term morbidity and mortality and the long-term outlook for patients with diabetic foot lesions, we evaluated 117 diabetic patients who presented with 174 foot lesions over a period of several years at the Medical College of Wisconsin.[51] Seven percent presented initially with bilateral extremity involvement (synchronous lesions) and 93% with unilateral involvement. In this latter group, 46% of patients subsequently had lesions of the contralateral extremity (metachronous lesions) during the period of the study. Major amputations (below-knee or above-knee) were required in one third of patients who presented with synchronous lesions, including one patient who required bilateral below-knee amputations. The metachronous lesions occurred from 1 to 95 months (mean, 27 months) after presentation of the original lesion. Major amputations were performed on 18% of the extremities originally affected and 10% of the contralateral extremities; 20% of the patients had bilateral amputations. The risk of major amputation in diabetic patients in whom foot lesions developed was 34%. More important is the fact that 50% of the patients with a lesion in one foot eventually will develop a lesion in the other foot also and 50% of these patients with metachronous lesions will require at least one major amputation. When major amputation is required in at least one leg of a diabetic patient, the risk of amputation for the contralateral leg is 45% if a contralateral lesion develops. The operative mortality for major amputations was 3%.

The diabetic patient who requires vascular reconstruction has results generally comparable with those of the nondiabetic patient. Bergan et al.[52] reported similar patency rates for diabetic and nondiabetic patients for femoropopliteal grafts. Towne et al.[53] did not note a significant difference in cumulative limb salvage in diabetic and nondiabetic patients following profundaplasty for the first 48 months postoperatively although after 4 years diabetic patients did not fare as well. These studies demonstrate that revascularization procedures in a diabetic patient are durable and should be done if technically feasible.

REFERENCES

1. Bell ET. Atherosclerotic gangrene of the lower extremities in diabetic and nondiabetic persons. Am J Clin Pathol 28:27-36, 1957.
2. Guggenheim W, Koch G, Adams AP, et al. Femoral and popliteal occlusive vascular disease. Diabetes 18:428-433, 1969.
3. Levin ME, O'Neal LW, eds. The Diabetic Foot. St. Louis: CV Mosby, 1973, pp 428-433.
4. Semple R. Diabetes and peripheral arterial disease. Lancet 264:1064-1068, 1953.
5. Ferrier TM. Comparative study of arterial disease in amputated lower limbs from diabetics and nondiabetics. Med J Aust 1:5-11, 1967.
6. Banson BB, Lacy PE. Diabetic microangiopathy in human toes. Am J Pathol 45:41-58, 1964.
7. Goldenberg AL, Alex M, Ram AJ, et al. Nonatheromatous peripheral vascular disease of the lower extremity in diabetes mellitus. Diabetes 8:261-273, 1959.
8. Steer HW, Cuckle HS, Franklin PM, et al. The influence of diabetes mellitus upon peripheral vascular disease. Surg Gynecol Obstet 157:64-72, 1983.
9. Williamson JR, Vogler NJ, Kilo C. Regional variations in the width of the basement membrane of muscle capillaries in man and grafts. Am J Pathol 63:359-370, 1971.
10. Bryfogle JW, Bradley RF. The vascular complications of diabetes mellitus. Diabetes 6:159-167, 1957.
11. Garcia MJ, McNamara PM, Gordon T, et al. Morbidity and mortality in diabetics in the Framingham population: Sixteen year follow-up study. Diabetes 23:105-111, 1974.
12. Bendick PJ, Glover JL, Kuebler TW, et al. Progression of atherosclerosis in diabetics. Surgery 93:834-838, 1983.
13. Chopra JS, Hurwith LJ, Montgomery DAD. The pathogenesis of sural nerve changes in diabetes mellitus. Brain 92:391-418, 1969.
14. Dolman CL. The morbid anatomy of diabetic neuropathy. Neurology 13:135-142, 1963.
15. Greenbaum D, Richardson PC, Salmon MJ, et al. Pathological observation on six cases of diabetic neuropathy. Brain 87:201-214, 1964.
16. Olsson Y, Saüe-Soderbergh J, Sourander P, et al. A pathoanatomical study of the central and peripheral nervous system in diabetics of early onset and long duration. Pathol Eur 3:62-79, 1968.
17. Bischoff A. Morphology of diabetic neuropathy. Horm Metab Res Suppl 9:18-28, 1980.
18. Jakobsen J, Malmgren L, Olsson Y. Permeability of the blood-nerve barrier in the streptozotocin-diabetic rat. Exp Neurology 60:277-285, 1978.
19. Sella EJ. Diabetic neurosteoarthropathy of the tarsus. Conn Med 43:70-79, 1979.
20. Lippman HI. Prevention of amputation in diabetics. Angiology 30:649-658, 1979.
21. Ctercteko GC, Dhanondran M, Hutton WC, et al. Vertical forces acting on the feet of diabetic patients with neuropathic ulceration. Br J Surg 68:608-614, 1981.
22. Groth KE. Clinical observations and experimental studies of the pathogens of decubitus ulcers. Acta Chir Scand Suppl 87:207, 1942.
23. Robson MC, Kirzek TJ. The role of infection in chronic pressure ulcerations. In Frederick S, Brody GS, eds. Symposium on the Neurologic Aspects of Plastic Surgery. St. Louis: CV Mosby, 1978, pp 242-246.
24. Robson MC. Difficult wounds: Pressure ulcerations and leg ulcers. Clin Plastic Surg 6:537-540, 1979.
25. Lithner F, Tornblom N. Gangrene localized to the feet in diabetic patients. Acta Med Scand 208:315-320, 1980.

26. Lithner F, Tornblom N. Gangrene localized to the feet in diabetic patients. Acta Med Scand 215:75-79, 1984.

27. Wheat LJ. Infection and diabetes mellitus. Diabetes Care 3:187-197, 1980.

28. Smith JA, O'Connor JJ, Willis AT. Nasal carriage of *Staphylococcus aureus* in diabetes mellitus. Lancet 2:776-777, 1966.

29. Casey JI. Host defense and infections in diabetes mellitus. In Ellenberg M, Ritkin H, eds. Diabetes Mellitus—Theory and Practice, 3rd ed. New Hyde Park, N.Y.: Medical Examination Publishing, 1983, pp 667-674.

30. Molenaar DM, Palumbo PJ, Wilson WR. Leukocyte chemotaxis in diabetic patients with and their diabetic first-degree relatives. Diabetes 25:880-883, 1976.

31. Bagdade JD, Stewart M, Walters E. Impaired granulocyte adherence. Diabetes 27:667-681, 1978.

32. Rayfield EJ, Ault MJ, Keusch GT, et al. Infection and diabetes: The case for glucose control. Am J Med 72:439-450, 1982.

33. Delbridge L, Appleberg M, Reeve TS. Factors associated with development of foot lesions in the diabetic. Surgery 93:78-82, 1983.

34. Greenhalgh RM, Laing SP, Cole PV, et al. Progressive atherosclerosis following revascularization. In Bernhard VM, Towne JB, eds. Complications in Vascular Surgery. New York: Grune & Stratton, 1980, pp 21-40.

35. Vincent DG, Salles-Cunha SX, Bernhard VM, et al. Noninvasive assessment of toe systolic pressures with special reference to diabetes mellitus. J Cardiovasc Surg 24:22-28, 1983.

36. Holstein P, Lassen NA. Healing of ulcers on the feet correlated with distal blood pressure measurements in occlusive arterial disease. Acta Orthop Scand 51:995-1006, 1980.

37. Barnes, RW. In discussion of Gibbons GW, Wheelock FC Jr, Siembeda C, et al. Noninvasive prediction of amputation level in diabetics. Arch Surg 114:1253, 1979.

38. Tenembaum MM, Rayfield E, Junior J, et al. Altered pressure flow relationship in the diabetic foot. J Surg Res 31:307-313, 1981.

39. Robertson C. Diabetic neuropathic foot sinuses. Proc R Soc Med 271-272, 1969.

40. Robson MC, Edstrom LE, Krizek TJ, et al. The efficacy of systemic antibiotics in the treatment of granulating wounds. J Surg Res 16:299-306, 1974.

41. McKittrick LS, McKittrick JB, Risley TS. Transmetatarsal amputation for infection or gangrene in patients with diabetes mellitus. Ann Surg 130:826-842, 1949.

42. Griffiths GD, Wieman TJ. Metatarsal head resection for diabetic foot ulcers. Arch Surg 125:832-835, 1990.

43. Martin JD, Delbridge L, Reeve TS, et al. Radical treatment of mal perforans in diabetic patients with arterial insufficiency. J Vasc Surg 12:264-268, 1990.

44. Louie TJ, Bartlett JB, Tally FP, et al. Aerobic and anaerobic bacteria in diabetic foot ulcers. Ann Intern Med 85:461-463, 1976.

45. Sharp CS, Bessman AN. Microbiology of deep wound cultures in diabetic gangrene. Diabetes 25(Suppl):385, 1976.

46. Sharp CS, Bessman AN, Wagner FW Jr, et al. Microbiology of superficial and deep tissues in infected diabetic gangrene. Surg Gynecol Obstet 149:217-219, 1979.

47. McIntyre KE Jr, Bailey SA, Malone JM, et al. Guillotine amputation in the treatment of non-salvageable lower extremity infections. Arch Surg 116:450-453, 1984.

48. Svoboda JJ, Balaji MR. Open supramalleolar amputation in the infected foot: An underutilized, two-stage procedure. N Y State J Med 2:77-78, 1990.

49. Towne JB. Management of foot lesions in the diabetic patient. In Rutherford RB, ed. Vascular Surgery. Philadelphia: WB Saunders, 1984, pp 661-669.

50. Gibbons GW, Wheelock FC Jr, Hoar CS, et al. Predicting success of forefoot amputations in diabetics by noninvasive testing. Arch Surg 114:1034-1036, 1979.

51. Klamer TW, Towne JB, Bandyk DF, et al. The influence of sepsis and ischemia in the natural history of the diabetic foot. Am Surg 53:490-494, 1987.

52. Bergan JJ, Veith FJ, Bernhard VM, et al. Randomization of autogenous vein and polytetrafluoroethylene grafts in femoral distal reconstuction. Surgery 92:921-930, 1982.

53. Towne JB, Bernhard VM, Rollins DL, et al. Profundaplasty in perspective: Limitations in the long-term management of limb ischemia. Surgery 90:1037-1046, 1981.

24

Complications of Lower Extremity Amputation

James M. Malone   **Jeffrey L. Ballard**

The indications for lower extremity amputation are numerous and include the following: diabetes mellitus (60% to 70%), ischemia with nondiabetic infection (20%), trauma (5%), chronic osteomyelitis (5%), and miscellaneous orthopedic and neurologic problems (5% to 10%).[1] Of the approximately 50,000 to 60,000 major lower extremity amputations performed in the United States each year, more than two thirds are necessitated by complications of diabetes mellitus or peripheral vascular disease. Although the perioperative and operative care of the prospective amputee has improved greatly since the writings of Ambroise Paré (1510-1590), a review of the literature suggests that the mortality rates for below-knee and above-knee amputation are still 4% to 16% and 12% to 40%, respectively.[1-10] A thorough understanding of the medical profile of the prospective amputee and the considerable preoperative preparation, in addition to the appropriate determination of the amputation level, are instrumental in decreasing the morbidity and mortality of lower extremity amputation. Early and late postoperative complications can affect the potential for ultimate recovery and the possibility of bipedal ambulation.

MEDICAL PROFILE OF PROSPECTIVE AMPUTEE

The usual amputee patient is a man in the sixth decade of life. Most series report that 49% to 89% of patients are male.[1,6,11-15] It is noteworthy that the female patients are usually a decade older than their male counterparts. The morbid and nonmorbid complications of amputation surgery are related not only to the advanced age of the patients, but also to the high incidence of associated diseases (Table 24-1).

In a prospective analysis of 188 lower limb amputees, Liedberg and Persson[19] found that diabetes mellitus, smoking, and age were important risk factors in lowering the age at amputation for both men and women. Amputees usually have pansystemic manifestations of atherosclerosis.[4,8,17,20-22] In addition to diabetes mellitus, the incidence of hypertension, previous myocardial infarction, and previous stroke range from 19% to 68%.[5,22-25] Not surprisingly, two thirds of all postoperative deaths are caused by cardiovascular complications, including myocardial infarction, stroke, and congestive heart failure. Further, nearly one third to one half of all early postoperative deaths are caused by myocardial infarction alone.[6,26] Diabetic amputees usually will die as a result of complications of their disease or other cardiovascular diseases within 5 years of their

Table 24-1. Coexistent Diseases Prior to Major Lower Extremity Amputation

Type	%
Smoking-related diseases	50-100
Diabetes mellitus	60-82
Cardiovascular disease	26-77
Hypertension	15-70
Cerebrovascular disease	20-25
Pulmonary disease	5-20
Renal insufficiency	10

Data from references 1, 3, 6, 15-18.

first limb amputation.[1,15,21,27] Also, patients with diabetes mellitus have a 3% to 7% chance per year of becoming a bilateral lower extremity amputee if they do not die of cardiovascular disease in the 5 years following their initial amputation.[1,8,15,21,27]

PREOPERATIVE PREPARATION

The high operative mortality of amputation surgery relative to the technical magnitude of the procedure warrants careful preoperative evaluation for symptoms and signs of immune deficiency, malnutrition, osteomyelitis, soft tissue infection (including impending gangrene), deep vein thrombosis, and neurotrophic ulcers, all of which can affect the primary healing of the most distal amputation possible.[28-33] The risk of skin necrosis occurring between old and new incisions demands that the surgeon be well versed in alternative flap reconstructions. Unless the extremity is unsalvageable, most authorities advocate distal vascular reconstruction to prevent amputation. A carefully planned and performed below-knee amputation will heal in 80% to 85% of cases.[16,34,35] Although primary revascularizations carry operative mortality rates as low as 2.8% to 3.8%,[36-38] controversy remains about whether healing at the below-knee level is compromised by a failed distal bypass.[39-42]

The above data underscore the need for aggressive perioperative medical care of the amputee. Bunt et al.[43] were able to achieve an operative mortality of 0.9% for below-knee amputations and 2.8% for above-knee amputations by adhering to a preoperative management protocol that included the following: (1) noninvasive vascular evaluation and angiography as indicated to assess the need for preamputation revascularization to preserve limb length and to ensure healing of the amputation stump; (2) careful correction of any deficits in preoperative laboratory screening, that is, hydration, transfusion, and stabilization of diabetes; (3) perioperative therapeutic course of antibiotics for limb infections and perioperative prophylactic antibiotics in all amputations; and (4) intensive-care monitoring with aggressive rehydration, Swan-Ganz and arterial pressure monitoring, and cryoamputation with a dry ice boot until maximal cardiopulmonary status was achieved for patients presenting with pedal gangrene, worsening cellulitis, or signs of systemic toxicity. Brinker et al.[44] also found amputation with the patient under cryoanesthesia to be of value in reducing postoperative morbidity, mortality, and length of hospital stay in the acutely ill patient with unreconstructible vascular disease.

AMPUTATION LEVEL DETERMINATION

The balance between better healing at more proximal amputation sites and successful ambulatory rehabilitation following more distal amputation sites must be weighed against 5-year survival rates of 20% for patients undergoing above-knee amputations vs. 40% to 45% for patients with below-knee amputation.[4,21,22,45,46] The advanced degree of extremity ischemia and the generally poor clinical condition of those requiring above-knee amputation play a large part in the survival rates. The clinical variability in patients presenting for possible amputation makes determination of the adequate amputation level one of the most difficult problems facing the amputation surgeon.[45] Although an above-knee amputation may heal without difficulty, the increase in energy expenditure for ambulation is much higher for a unilateral above-knee prosthesis (50% to 70%) than a unilateral below-knee prosthesis (10% to 40%).[47] In addition, successful rehabilitation is achieved in only 10% to 30% of above-knee amputees vs. 70% for below-knee amputees.[1,21,22,48,49]

With the ultimate objective of primary healing at the most distal amputation site, consideration of preexisting joint problems and preoperative activity level will help in determining the appropriate amputation level. Severe knee arthritis or failed total knee replacement may necessitate an above-knee amputation even though there is adequate blood supply for a proposed below-knee amputation site.[50] Rehabilitation potential is limited in patients with hip or knee flexion contractures. Lastly, the appealing presumption of greater mobility in bedridden patients with below-knee amputations does not outweigh the increased risk for knee flexion deformity and stump breakdown.

Above-knee amputations should be performed in patients whose rehabilitation potential is nil.[51]

Certainly, many complications of lower extremity amputation would be avoided if the above-knee level was chosen for virtually every patient. Unfortunately, this would deprive many of a more distal amputation and the potential for bipedal ambulation. Empiric clinical selection of amputation site based on a thorough pulse examination of the affected extremity, skin temperature, and arteriographic correlations has resulted in successful healing of close to 80% of below-knee amputations, 90% of above-knee amputations, but only 40% of below-ankle amputations.[5,16,52-55]

The need for more sensitive, objective methods of preoperative amputation level selection has led to the development of numerous noninvasive techniques including (1) Doppler ankle and calf systolic blood pressures, [56-59] (2) fluorescein dye measurements,[60,61] (3) laser Doppler velocimetry,[62-65] (4) photoelectric skin perfusion pressures,[66-68] (5) isotope measurement of skin perfusion pressures,[69-72] (6) xenon-133 skin blood flow measurements,[35,73-75] (7) skin temperature measurements,[76,77] (8) transcutaneous oxygen measurements ($TcPo_2$),[34,65,78] (9) transcutaneous carbon dioxide measurements ($TcPco_2$),[79-81] and (10) digital or metatarsal photoplethysmographic pressures.[58,82] An overview of the success rates and selection criteria for prediction of healing of toe-level amputations is shown in Table 24-2. Overall, preoperative amputation level selection techniques correctly predicted primary and secondary healing in 116 of 132 toe amputations (88%). Similar data for foot and forefoot amputations are summarized in Table 24-3. Excluding Doppler systolic pressures less than 60 mm Hg and laser Doppler velocimetry measurements, preoperative amputation selection techniques correctly predicted healing in 285 of 340 foot and forefoot amputations (84%). In Tables 24-4 and 24-5, prediction of successful healing was seen overall in 94% of below-knee amputations and 90% of above-knee amputations using various selection techniques.

All of the various techniques for amputation level selection have been well described previously; however, some comments should be made about specific tests relative to the level of the prospective amputation site. At the toe amputation level, Doppler systolic ankle pressures and photoplethysmographic digit/transmetatarsal pressures are comparable. Photoplethysmographic-derived pressures are the most reliable prognosticator, but both are better than the success yield of 75% with empiric criteria alone.[9] Again, with foot and forefoot amputations, Doppler-derived pressures are second line. Accurate objective data can be gathered with the use of fiberoptic fluorometry 99mTc-pertechnetate skin blood pressures or xenon-133 skin clearance techniques, but sophisticated nuclear medicine, computer equipment, and trained technicians are necessary. Newer techniques including transcutaneous oxygen and carbon dioxide measurements ($TcPo_2$, $TcPco_2$), are promising but photoplethysmographic-derived pressures greater than 55 mm Hg are reliable, relatively simple, noninvasive, and inexpensive to obtain. The problem with both Doppler systolic pressures and photoplethysmographic pressures is that the presence of a blood pressure less than a predetermined pressure does not necessarily guarantee failure of amputation healing.

Depending on the equipment and personnel available, comparable rates of successful below-knee amputation healing can be expected using transcutaneous assays, xenon-133 skin blood flow, laser Doppler velocimetry, fiberoptic fluorometry, and photoelectric/radioisotope measurements of skin perfusion pressure. Since empiric selection is met with only 80% success, these preoperative amputation level selection techniques offer improved results and better rehabilitation potential. For above-knee amputations, there are a few preoperative selection techniques that have been able to consistently improve the 90% success rate for empiric selection (Table 24-5). The ability to ensure healing in virtually all appropriately chosen above-knee amputation levels is paramount because the consequences of failure are disastrous and even fatal. Elective lower extremity amputation should not be performed in the absence of objective amputation level testing.

Table 24-2. Preoperative Level Selection: Toe Amputation*

Selection criteria	Total no. of patients	No. successfully healed—primary and secondary	Success (%)
Doppler toe systolic pressure >30 mm Hg	60	47	78
Doppler ankle systolic pressure >35 mm Hg	46	44	96
Photoplethysmographic digit or trans-metatarsal pressure >20 mm Hg	20	20	100
Xenon-133 skin blood flow >2.6 ml/100 gm tissue/min	6	5	83
TOTAL	132	116	88

Data from references 58, 71, 73, 83.
*Modified from Durham JR. Lower extremity amputation levels: Indications, methods of determining appropriate level, technique, and prognosis. In Rutherford RB, ed. Vascular Surgery, 3rd ed. Philadelphia: WB Saunders, 1989, p 1693.

Table 24-3. Preoperative Level Selection: Foot and Forefoot Amputation*

Selection criteria	Total no. of patients	No. successfully healed—primary and secondary	Success (%)
Doppler systolic ankle pressure:			
<40 mm Hg	9[†]	5[†]	56[†]
>40 mm Hg	60[†]	20[†]	33[†]
40-60 mm Hg	5[†]	4[†]	80[†]
>50 mm Hg	21[†]	14[†]	66[†]
>60 mm Hg	91	68	75
>70 mm Hg	93	70	75
Doppler systolic toe pressure >30 mm Hg	5	4	80
Doppler ankle/brachial pressure index >0.45 (nondiabetic) and >0.50 (diabetic)	60	58	97
Photoplethysmographic toe systolic pressure >55 mm Hg	14	14	100
Fiberoptic fluorometry (dye fluorescence index >44)	20	18	90
Laser Doppler velocimetry	6[†]	2[†]	33[†]
I-125 Iodopyrine skin blood flow >8 ml/100 gm tissue/min	18	18	100
Xenon-133 skin blood flow >2.6 ml/100 gm tissue/min	25	23	92
$TcPo_2$ >10 mm Hg (or a >10 mm increase on Flo_2 =1.0)	8	6	75
$TcPo_2$ >28 mm Hg	3	3	100
$TcPco_2$ <40 mm Hg	3	3	100
TOTAL (excluding Doppler systolic ankle pressures <60 mm Hg and laser Doppler velocimetry measurements)	340	285	84

Data from references 55, 56, 63, 71, 79, 82, 84-89.
*Modified from Durham JR. Lower extremity amputation levels: Indications, methods of determining appropriate level, technique, and prognosis. In Rutherford RB, ed. Vascular Surgery, 3rd ed. Philadelphia: WB Saunders, 1989, p 1695.
†Not included in totals.

Table 24-4. Preoperative Level Selection: Below-Knee Amputation*

Selection criteria	Total no. of patients	No. successfully healed—primary and secondary	Success (%)
Doppler systolic ankle pressure >30 mm Hg	70	66	94
Doppler systolic calf pressure			
>50 mm Hg	36	36	100
>68 mm Hg	97	96	99
Doppler systolic thigh pressure			
>100 mm Hg	31	31	100
>80 mm Hg	113	104	92
Fluorescein dye	30	24	80
Fiberoptic fluorometry (dye fluorescence index >44)	12	12	100
Laser Doppler velocimetry	8	8	100
Skin perfusion pressure, 99m Tc-pertechnetate	26	24	92
I-131 or I-125 antipyrine >30 mm Hg	62	60	97
Photoelectric skin perfusion pressure >20 mm Hg	71	60	85
Xenon-133 skin blood flow:			
Epicutaneous >0.9 ml/100 gm tissue/min	15	14	93
Intradermal >2.4 ml/100 gm tissue/min	89	83	93
Intradermal >1 ml/100 gm tissue/min	12	11	92
$TcPo_2 = 0$	3	0	0
>10 mm Hg	80	76	95
>10 <40 mm Hg	7	5	71
>20 mm Hg	26	25	96
>35 mm Hg	51	51	100
$TcPo_2$ index >0.59	17	17	100
$TcPco_2$ <40 mm Hg	8	7	00
TOTAL	864	810	94

Data from references 19, 34, 35, 37, 55, 57, 59, 63, 66-69, 73, 75, 79, 85, 87, 90-96.
*Modified from Durham JR. Lower extremity amputation levels: Indications, methods of determining appropriate level, technique, and prognosis. In Rutherford RB, ed. Vascular Surgery, 3rd ed. Philadelphia: WB Saunders, 1989, p 1700.

Table 24-5. Preoperative Level Selection: Above-Knee Amputation*

Selection criteria	Total no. of patients	No. successfully healed—primary and secondary	Success (%)
Fiberoptic fluorometry (dye fluorescence index >44)	7	6	86
Laser Doppler velocimetry	6	6	100
Photoelectric skin perfusion >21 mm Hg	19	19	100
Skin perfusion pressure (I-131 or I-125 antipyrine)	48	44	92
Xenon-133 skin blood flow intradermal >2.6 ml/100 gm tissue/min	20	20	100
$TcPo_2$			
>10 mm Hg	23	15	65
>20 mm Hg	12	12	100
>23 mm Hg	2	2	100
>35 mm Hg	24	21	88
$TcPco_2$ <38 mm Hg	5	5	100
TOTAL	166	150	90

Data from references 55, 63, 67, 73, 75, 79, 85, 92, 97-99.
*Modified from Durham JR. Lower extremity amputation levels: Indications, methods of determining appropriate level, technique, and prognosis. In Rutherford RB, ed. Vascular Surgery, 3rd ed. Philadelphia: WB Saunders, 1989, p 1707.

POSTOPERATIVE COMPLICATIONS

After deciding on the appropriate amputation level based on clinical findings and objective criteria, the surgeon must remove necrotic, painful, or infected tissue and plan an amputation stump that can be fitted with a prosthesis. Although the surgical techniques for the various amputation levels have been well described,[100,101] some brief points should be made regarding intraoperative considerations to avoid complications. A variety of technical problems such as inadequate beveling of the tibia, inappropriate bone length, a short posterior skin flap, excessive muscle in the posterior flap, incomplete hemostasis, and the presence of foreign materials (i.e., bone wax, multifilament sutures) skin edge necrosis, and dog ears can all lead to stump failure.

The following section addresses major postoperative complications following lower extremity amputation, dividing them into early and late phases with respect to operative procedure.

Early Postoperative Complications
Failure to Heal

Despite changes in perioperative care and surgical technique, major lower extremity amputation continues to be associated with significant morbidity (Table 24-6). The incidence of postoperative nonhealing ranges from 8% to 29%.* In 1986, Keagy et al.[5] reviewed 1028 ma-

*References 1, 6, 14-16, 18, 100, 104, 105.

Table 24-6. Early Postoperative Complications

Description	Incidence (%)
Residual limb pain/phantom pain	5-85
Revision to higher level	0-29
Death	0-35
Failure to heal	3-29
Pulmonary embolus	4-38
Pulmonary complications	8-30
Residual limb infection	0-28
Cardiovascular complications	2-25
Stroke	3-14
Deep vein thrombosis	1-5
Flexion contracture	1-3
Renal insufficiency	1-3

Data from references 3, 6, 7, 11, 12, 14-16, 18, 59, 102, 103.

jor lower extremity amputations in 786 patients and found failure-to-heal rates of 9% and 19% in above-knee and below-knee amputations, respectively. Since nonhealing is a major complication, it is not surprising that the conversion rate of a below-knee amputation to an above-knee amputation for complications caused by failure to heal or infection ranges from 0% to 29%.[1,3,15,16] When the appropriate objective preoperative amputation level technique is used, the literature suggests that the overall failure rate after lower extremity amputation should not be greater than 4% to 9% in a modern amputation program.[1,107] At the Tucson V.A. Medical Center, the early failure rate of wound healing after lower extremity amputation was 1 in 137 (0.7%) in 1986.

In general, failure to heal represents a complication caused by inadequate blood supply at the level selected for amputation, traumatic intraoperative handling of tissue, or prolonged ischemia of marginally vascularized tissue. Additional failures may result from a residual limb hematoma with or without secondary infection, primary residual limb infection, or poor patient nutrition. Serum albumin less than 3.5 gm/dl and lymphocyte count less than 1500/mm³ both have been shown to adversely affect wound healing.[108] In 1988, Hansen, Wethelund, and Skajaa[109] studied the relationship between complication rates and preoperative levels of hemoglobin and hematocrit in 186 consecutive below-knee amputations for incipient gangrene. They found successively higher rates of wound complications with hemoglobin level greater than or equal to 7 gm/dl and hematocrit levels greater than or equal to 40%. Interestingly, they found no such association among diabetic patients, although Bailey et al.[104] in an earlier report suggested that the preoperative hemoglobin level may be an important prognosticator for success or failure in diabetic patients undergoing lower extremity amputation.

Kacy, Wolma, and Flye[110] noted that below-knee stump healing was improved by low hemoglobin levels in diabetic patients with cellulitis but not in diabetic patients without cellulitis. Salvage of marginally ischemic tissues by isovolemic hemodilution has been suggested.[111] but the exact values of hemodilution and its relationship to stump healing in patients with diabetes mellitus are unclear. It has been our experience, and that of others, that there is no significant difference in healing after lower extremity amputation in patients with and without diabetes mellitus.[1,6,14,17,73]

Whether a failed distal bypass compromises healing at the below-knee level is a controversial issue in the literature.[40-42] The incidence of major lower extremity amputation in patients who have undergone prior attempts at arterial reconstruction ranges from 12.5% to 45%.[2,14,60,69,111] Rubin et al.[112] published data in 1985 showing healing problems in only 14.3% (14 of 98) of patients undergoing primary amputation without a prior distal bypass vs. healing problems in 35% (31 of 89) of patients who underwent bypass surgery before amputation (p <.0005). Proponents favoring aggressive distal revascularization point out that limb salvage rates are usually 15% to 20% higher than graft patency rates.[38,113,114] Since patients' attitudes toward impending amputation often are intensely negative, we have remained aggressive in our attempts at more distal bypasses in order to salvage lower limbs with critical ischemia.

Residual Limb Infection

Although the incidence of stump infection following major lower extremity amputation ranges from 0% to 28%,* this complication can be reduced by the appropriate management of preexisting distal extremity infections. Since a significant number of lower extremity amputations are performed specifically for distal limb infections, it is not surprising that there could be a fourfold increase in the incidence of postoperative stump infection in those limbs with preexisting infection over those limbs without preamputation infections.[18] McIntyre et al.[14] reported a statistically significant decrease in the rate of stump infection in patients with pedal sepsis who had undergone a preparatory guillotine amputation (3%) vs. patients who underwent a one-stage amputation (22% p <.01). At the Maricopa Medical Center in Phoenix, we have used cryoamputation with a

---

*References 1, 3, 7, 104, 112, 115.

dry ice boot and tourniquet above the level of infection in preparation for definitive amputation in patients too ill to be taken directly to the operating room. We have not found any significant increase in postoperative infection rates compared with the published data and have noticed a decrease in postoperative morbidity and mortality as a result of better preoperative preparation of the patients.

Residual limb hematoma is also a factor that can increase postoperative stump infection rates. The importance of meticulous hemostasis cannot be emphasized strongly enough since numerous studies have suggested that the use of drains for "wet" wounds in patients undergoing amputations significantly increases the risk of postoperative infection.[3,18] In the event that a drain must be used, a closed suction system is preferable to an open latex drain. The correlation between stump hematoma and stump infection is high enough to make the avoidance of postamputation hematomas highly desirable.

Rubin et al.[112] have suggested that infection in a thrombosed below-knee prosthetic graft after lower extremity amputation is a highly morbid and potentially lethal complication. That group reported an overall incidence of graft infection of 45% (14 of 31) in patients undergoing major lower extremity amputation who had a prior infrapopliteal bypass.[112] In that series local care of the residual limb without graft removal resulted in a high rate of recurrent residual limb infection and significant patient mortality. Similar problems in 4 of 10 patients were reported by Johansen and Zorn.[115] The best management of a noninfected, retained distal bypass graft in a patient undergoing a major lower extremity amputation is unknown; however, simple transection of the graft high in the operative field probably is not appropriate.[112,115] Whether removal of most of the graft (leaving the proximal femoral portion of the graft in place) or removal of the entire graft (with an autogenous vein or artery patch on the femoral arteriotomy) is best is unclear at the present time. A reasonable approach appears to be a cutdown on the graft in an easily accessible place in the midthigh. If the graft appears to be well incorporated and uninfected, it can be transected, its proximal portion obliterated in soft tissue, and its distal portion excised with the amputation. However, if the graft is not well incorporated or there is a question of infection, a portion of the graft should be cultured, and the entire graft should be removed concomitantly with or before amputation.

Broad-spectrum prophylactic antibiotics should be used perioperatively for those patients presenting with cellulitis; necrotic, purulent, or draining ulcers; and wet gangrene. In addition, the patient should be evaluated for occult deep forefoot infection, proximal lymphangitis or inguinal adenopathy, and systemic sepsis, which may not be readily apparent. In a culture study of preamputation extremity wounds, the following organisms were recovered: *Staphylococcus aureus* (22%); *Staphylococcus nonaureus* (9%); fecal coliforms (30%); *Streptococcus faecalis* (15%); *Streptococcus* (3%); and *Pseudomonas* (12%).[116,117] Both aerobes and anaerobes should be well covered. Specifically, in patients with diabetes mellitus, the need for anaerobic covering cannot be overemphasized because the incidence of mixed facultative and obligate anaerobic infections can be as high as 60%.[1] It has been our practice to continue antibiotic administration in these patients for at least 7 to 10 days after performance of the definitive amputation or until satisfactory wound healing is achieved. For those patients who have undergone preparatory ankle guillotine or cryoanesthesia amputation, antibiotic administration is continued for 3 to 5 days following definitive amputation.

The most important factors in achieving a low rate of residual limb infections are proper treatment of preamputation ipsilateral distal extremity infection, good wound hemostasis, avoidance of stump hematoma, perioperative antibiotic therapy, and objective preoperative amputation level selection to validate satisfactory blood flow for primary wound healing. The occurrence of a postoperative stump infection is critical in all amputees but especially in the geriatric patient. Since amputation stump infections usually result in a higher level amputation revision, the conversion of a below-knee to an above-knee amputation can be the difference

between successful ambulation and not walking.[20,103]

Pain

The multifaceted issue of phantom and residual limb pain after major lower extremity amputation, which in recent reports ranges up to 85% of all amputees, is vexing and there is no consensus concerning any aspect of the problem.[1,118-120] Phantom pain is characterized by four major properties: (1) it is persistent, (2) it can be triggered by either proximal or remote stimuli, (3) it is more likely to develop if preamputation pain was present (and may resemble it), and (4) it can be temporarily or permanently abolished by transient changes of somatic input.[121,122] Phantom pain is described as either intense burning or the sensation of an agonizing abnormal or cramped posture. Only a few of the 68 treatment methods currently used for phantom pain management give satisfactory results.[119,123-125]

Phantom pain may be both peripherally and centrally mediated. Treatment must take into account the likelihood of multiple mechanisms working together. Iacono and Linford[126] have stated that the patient's description of the pain is the most important determinant of therapy and should not be overlooked. Patients complaining of a constant dull, burning ache should be started on tricyclic antidepressants or β-blockers. Anticonvulsants are useful for lancinating pain. Spasm may be controlled by baclofen, with or without a β-blocker.[126] As with many other medical problems, patients should be started first on single-agent therapy, and then, depending on the type of pain, combination therapy may be required. Surgical options may be exercised after optimal medical therapy and adequate time duration have failed.

The placement of spinal dorsal root entry zone (DREZ) lesions, deep brain stimulation, spinal cord stimulation (formerly dorsal column stimulation), and direct peripheral nerve stimulation are fairly new neurosurgical procedures that hold promise for the ablation of phantom pain. Part of a recent series of amputees showed that phantom pain could be alleviated in 33% of those with lower extremity amputations at follow-up 6 months to 4 years with DREZ.[127] Deep brain stimulation via stereotaxically implanted electrodes has been successful in 86% of 30 patients in a European cooperative study.[126] In a smaller group, Mundinger and Neumuller[128] showed significant relief of phantom pain in 100% of amputees. Spinal cord stimulation techniques are not destructive and 25% to 100% pain relief has been reported in 55% to 67% of 150 patients in a long-term follow-up by Siegfried and Cetinalp.[129] Lastly, transcutaneous nerve stimulation currently is the benchmark against which newer modalities must be measured. Many series have documented consistent response rates of 45% to 67% in amputees with phantom pain.[95,128,130-132]

The therapy of residual limb pain involves the dynamic interplay of the amputee and a variety of medical and surgical specialties. The impending amputation should be viewed as reconstructive and consideration of pain relief should not wait until after the definitive procedure. Different techniques for nerve transection (cautery vs. scissors, ligature vs. no ligature) do not appear to have a major impact on the incidence of pain after lower extremity amputation. The literature suggests, but is not conclusive, that both a rigid dressing and control of stump edema may be important in decreasing postoperative amputation pain. In those amputation programs that use the immediate postsurgical prosthetic fitting technique coupled with an aggressive postamputation rehabilitation regimen, the incidence of disabling pain problems following major lower extremity amputation is less than 5%.[1,6,14,17,73] Although there is no objective explanation for the difference among reports in the incidence of pain problems after lower extremity amputation, it has been our experience that the incidence of both stump pain and phantom pain is significantly decreased in patients who successfully use their lower extremity prosthesis.

Flexion Contractures

A satisfactorily fitted prosthesis can be the deciding factor in whether an amputee ambulates successfully. Flexion contractures of as little as 10 degrees at the hip or 15 degrees at the knee can affect the ultimate conformity between the amputation stump and prosthesis. The incidence of flexion contracture after major lower extremity amputation is low in general (1% to 3%) but increased in patients over 80 years of age and patients undergoing amputation on the side of a prior stroke.[1,20,103] Every effort should be made to prevent contractures, including intraoperative stabilization of opposing muscle groups, use of rigid postoperative dressings (with or without an immediate postoperative pylon), and aggressive physical therapy. Ideally, a physical therapist should evaluate the prospective amputee before surgery so that range-of-motion and strengthening exercises can begin to help prevent postoperative joint deformities. Regardless of such preoperative training, the new amputee should be referred to the rehabilitation medicine department soon after surgery.

Pulmonary Complications

Since most prospective amputees have a significant smoking history (50% to 100%),[1] it is not surprising that the rate of pulmonary complications, including pneumonia, atelectasis, and sepsis, in patients undergoing lower extremity amputation approaches 8%.[1] For those patients undergoing above-knee amputation, Huston et al.[4] reported a 60% incidence of pneumonia and pulmonary sepsis in their series. Next to myocardial infarction, pulmonary complications are probably the biggest problem facing geriatric patients undergoing lower extremity amputation. Bed rest, inactivity, debilitation, and dehydration all predispose the elderly patient to pulmonary complications. The liberal use of pulmonary function testing, aggressive pulmonary toilet, active exercise, and physical therapy can all help to diminish the rate of pulmonary embarrassment.

Thromboembolic Complications

Since many prospective amputees have undergone prolonged hospitalization and bed rest before amputation, not only are they debilitated and dehydrated, but they also are at a very high risk for venous thromboembolic complications. The incidence of deep vein thrombosis and pulmonary embolism following major lower extremity amputation ranges from 4% to 38% and 1% to 5%, respectively.[1,133] The additive effects of impaired pulmonary function and thromboembolic complications can lead to decreased blood oxygen levels and compromised healing of ischemic tissue in the residual limb. An active rehabilitation program begun on the first postoperative day can help counteract blood stagnation and venous thrombosis.

Adequate perioperative hydration and avoidance of prolonged bed rest are important factors in decreasing thromboembolic complications. Patients undergoing elective major lower extremity amputation in whom there are major risk factors for venous thromboembolic complications probably should receive subcutaneous heparin prophylaxis (5000 U/12 hr). Despite low-dose heparin therapy, thromboembolic complications in patients undergoing above-knee amputation have been reported.[133] In our experience, with the use of low-dose heparin therapy, thromboembolic elastic stockings on the nonamputated extremity, and strict attention to the details of preoperative management, the incidence of pulmonary embolism and deep vein thrombosis is less than 1% in patients undergoing lower extremity amputation.

Local Revision

The actual incidence of revision after major lower extremity amputation in the perioperative period is unknown but should be less than 3%. Some factors that lead to early (first 3 to 4 weeks) local revisions are errors in surgical technique, including failure to bevel the tibia, failure to smooth bone contours, and other technical errors that have been discussed previously. In addition, the surgeon with no experience who applies the immediate postoperative dressing for below-knee amputees may contribute to the residual limb ischemia with a wrap too tight or may miss the opportunity to prevent swelling and external trauma with a dressing that is too loose.[134,135] At the Tucson VA Medical Center, the incidence of early local revision was 0.7% (one patient) in 137 consecutive lower extremity amputations.[1] Careful

attention to surgical details and prosthetic management during the early postoperative period are important in preventing this avoidable complication.

Late Postoperative Complications

Various long-term complications resulting from the patient's general health or inadequate fitting of the prosthesis may occur in the residual limb (Table 24-7). Excessive residual soft tissue may compromise a snug prosthetic fit or lead to uneven pressure distribution within the prosthesis and eventual skin breakdown. Stump lymphatic and venous congestion caused by a poor-fitting prosthesis is thought to cause stump edema. This may result in a "warty-like" appearance of the entire distal stump.[138] Painful callosities can develop at weight-bearing areas and epidermoid cysts or inspissated hair follicles, particularly common in hirsute limbs, and occasionally need to be excised or drained.[138] Osteoporosis from disuse, poor nutrition, and stress shielding by the prosthesis results in an increased fracture risk.

Death

Causes of late death in amputees include cardiovascular complications (60%), acute myocardial infarction (30%), pulmonary complications (6% to 34%), cancer (8%), and gastrointestinal bleeding (1%). The clinical impression that lower limb amputees are more prone to the development of degenerative diseases has been studied recently by numerous investigators. Yekutiel et al.[139] found an increased incidence of ischemic heart disease and diabetes mellitus among 53 lower limb amputees vs. a group of healthy age-matched controls. Rose et al.[140] reported that a significant number of

Table 24-7. Late Postoperative Complications

Description	Incidence (%)
Contralateral limb loss (5 yr)	15-66
Failure of rehabilitation	0-71
Death (5 yr)	25-70
Local residual limb revision	0-3
Abdominal aortic aneurysms	0-6

Data from references 1, 7, 10, 12, 27, 136, 137.

above-knee amputees were obese compared with a group of below-elbow amputees ($p < .05$). Further, they found that excessive maturity-onset weight gain was associated strongly with hypertension, decreased glucose tolerance, and marked hyperinsulinemia.

These data underscore the sobering statistics that predict a limited life expectancy following amputation. Harris et al.[12] found only a 30% 3-year survival rate in geriatric amputees from England and Wales, although their expected 3-year survival rate was 90%. Overall, survival rates after amputation have remained fairly constant over the past 20 years: 70% at 1 year, 60% at 2 years, 50% at 3 years, and 30% at 5 years.[4,122,131] Roon, Moore, and Goldstone[21] reported a 45% overall 5-year survival rate after lower extremity amputation compared with an expected 85% 5-year survival rate for the age-adjusted normal population. Most important, however, was their analysis of the projected 5-year survival rate for diabetic vs. nondiabetic amputees. The projected 5-year survival rate for nondiabetic amputees was almost normal (75%), whereas it was only 39% for amputees with diabetes mellitus.[21] Smith[15] reported similar 5-year survival data for diabetic patients (41%) in his review of lower extremity amputations in diabetic geriatric patients. Decreased survival rates for diabetic amputees primarily reflect increased rates of cardiovascular complications.[11]

Residual Stump Revision

There are few reports in the literature that specifically address the frequency of stump revision in those patients who were successfully discharged from the hospital after lower extremity amputation. Malone et al.[17] reported a series of lower extremity amputees in which there was a 97% rate of primary healing and noted that 88% of amputees followed up for up to 18 months did not need stump revision. In that group of patients, prosthesis use was 100%. The incidence of late local residual limb revision was 2.3% (8 of 351) in a review of patients who underwent major lower extremity amputation at the Tucson VA Medical Center and University of Arizona Medical Center.[107] It is interesting to note that most late revisions

occurred in patients who were ambulatory with their prosthesis. Only with careful prosthetic fitting and diligent long-term postoperative follow-up can the incidence of late revisions be kept to a minimum.

Postamputation Aortic Aneurysm

Vollmar et al.[136] reviewed a series of 545 patients operated on for elective and ruptured infrarenal aneurysms of the abdominal aorta and noted that 5.1% of the patients previously had undergone lower extremity amputation (20 above-knee, eight below-knee). In another report by Vollmar et al.,[137] 5.8% of above-knee amputee veterans of World War II had abdominal aortic aneurysms detected by ultrasound examination as compared with 1.1% of matched nonamputee war veterans. The reason for the increased incidence of abdominal aortic aneurysms (particularly in unilateral above-knee amputees) over the general population (1% to 2%)[141] is not completely understood.

After lower extremity amputation, there is decreased flow in the terminal aorta because of flow diversion into the visceral and renal arteries. This is though to result in a low-flow pattern that favors the development of arteriosclerosis in the infrarenal aorta.[141,142] Above-knee amputations appear to result in greater hemodynamic changes in the terminal aorta than do lower level amputations. In addition, morphologic studies have shown that there is a relative stenosis (even occlusion) of the ipsilateral iliac arteries that can create a vectorial force of counterimpulse and mechanically stress the aortic wall.[136,143] The sum of these forces may lead to early degeneration of elastic elements within the infrarenal aorta and aneurysmal dilatation.[144-147]

Contralateral Limb Loss

The incidence of contralateral limb complications increases throughout the postoperative period. The risk of contralateral limb loss is highest in patients with diabetes mellitus. By 5 years following amputation, significantly more diabetic than nondiabetic patients lost their opposite limb in both a VA series (66% vs. 28%) and a county hospital series (42% vs. 28%).[4]

The incidence of contralateral limb loss ranges from 5% to 13% per year and 15% to 66% over 5 years after major lower extremity amputation.[1,15,27] Up to 2 years after amputation, Mazet et al.[27] found little difference in the percentages (18% to 28%) of diabetic and nondiabetic patients who became bilateral amputees. This underscores the need for diligent long-term follow-up in all amputees, especially diabetic amputees, to avoid the risk of contralateral limb loss.

In a carefully randomized prospective study, Malone et al.[148] recently showed that a simple foot care education program can be instrumental in lowering the rate of contralateral limb loss in diabetic patients. Although there were no significant differences in the medical management or clinical risk factors among the 203 total patients, those with no education program had a significantly higher rate of limb amputation (21 vs. 7 of 177 limbs, $p < .025$). Further, the overall success rate regarding the incidence of infection, ulcer, or amputation was significantly different in those patients who took part in a simple 1-hour educational class (successes in 160 vs. 128 of 177 limbs, $p < .005$). The point is that avoiding amputations is not only beneficial to the patient and family but also may be cost effective since the mean cost for patients undergoing primary below-knee amputation averages $27,255 ± $2896.[149]

REHABILITATION

Successful ambulation after major lower extremity amputation is a bittersweet battle involving such factors as the age of the patient, the level of activity before amputation, and the site of amputation. In general, younger, healthier, and previously active patients tend to have better rates of rehabilitation after amputation. For all patients the incidence of successful rehabilitation after lower extremity amputation ranges from 29% to 98%.* The rates of successful ambulation and rehabilitation after lower extremity amputation should be greater than 90% for the unilateral below-knee amputee, greater than 80% for the bilateral below-knee amputee, probably less than 50% for the unilat-

eral above-knee amputee, and less than 20% for the bilateral amputee with one amputation at the above-knee level.[1,6,14,17,73]

Successful rehabilitation takes time and a great deal of energy from the patient, prosthetist, and members of the rehabilitation medicine department. The reported length of hospital stay after lower extremity amputation (including rehabilitation) ranges from 14 to 384 days.* Malone et al.[6,17] have reported that the average length of stay for postoperative rehabilitation with and without the use of immediate or early postoperative prosthetic fitting is 32 and 125 days, respectively. Interestingly, the projected length of stay of lower extremity amputation (including preoperative days in the hospital and rehabilitation) under diagnosis-related group guidelines is only 25 days.

CONCLUSION

Even in centers with a large volume of amputation surgery, the average mortality rate after lower extremity amputation is approximately 8% to 10%. The incidence of postoperative morbidity ranges considerably but, once again, is significant even in centers treating large numbers of amputees. Careful attention to the selection of an optimal level of amputation that will heal primarily, diligent preoperative preparation, and immediate or early postoperative prosthetic rehabilitation can all help to lessen early postoperative complications. In addition, education of high-risk patients about both the risk of and avoidance of contralateral limb loss and careful long-term follow-up can significantly decrease many of the early and late postoperative complications of major lower extremity amputation.

Familiarity with both prosthetics and rehabilitation is essential for general or vascular surgeons who perform the majority of lower extremity amputations in the United States. This requires that the interested surgeon work closely with his or her orthopedic colleagues or local community prosthetists. Amputation surgery is reconstructive surgery and should not be relegated to an unsupervised junior or inexperienced surgeon. It is the obligation of the sur-

---

*References 1, 6, 7, 14, 16, 17, 27, 73, 107, 144.

*References 1, 3, 6, 14, 17, 73.

geon to participate actively in every aspect of amputation surgery to avoid complications and to ensure the highest degree of success in returning their patients to bipedal ambulation.

REFERENCES

1. Malone JM, Goldstone J. Lower extremity amputation. In Moore WS, ed. Vascular Surgery, A Comprehensive Review. New York: Grune & Stratton, 1983, pp 909-976.
2. Bauer GM, Porter JM, Axthelm S, et al. Lower extremity amputation for ischemia. Am Surg 44:472-477, 1978.
3. Berardi RS, Keonin Y. Amputations in peripheral vascular occlusive disease. Am J Surg 135:231-234, 1978.
4. Huston CC, Bivins BA, Ernst CB, et al. Morbid implications of above-knee amputation. Report of a series and review of the literature. Arch Surg 115:165-167, 1980.
5. Keagy BA, Schwartz JM, Kolb M, et al. Lower extremity amputation: The control series. J Vasc Surg 4:321-326, 1986.
6. Malone JM, Moore WS, Goldstone J, et al. Therapeutic and economic impact of a modern amputation program. Ann Surg 189:798-802, 1979.
7. Moore WS, Hall AD, Lim RC Jr. Below the knee amputation for ischemic gangrene. Am J Surg 124:127-134, 1972.
8. Otteman MG, Stahlgren LH. Evaluation of factors which influence mortality and morbidity following lower extremity amputation for arteriosclerosis. Surg Gynecol Obstet 120:1217-1220, 1965.
9. Porter JM, Bauer GM, Taylor LM Jr. Lower-extremity amputation ischemia. Arch Surg 116:89-92, 1981.
10. Towne JB, Condon RE. Lower extremity amputation for ischemic disease. Adv Surg 13:199-227, 1979.
11. Cranley JJ, Karause RJ, Strasser ES, et al. Below-the-knee amputation for arteriosclerosis obliterans with and without diabetes mellitus. JAMA 98:77-78, 1969.
12. Harris PL, Read F, Eardley A, et al. The fate of elderly amputees. Br J Surg 61:665-668, 1974.
13. Jamieson CW, Hill D. Amputation for vascular disease. Br J Surg 63:683-690, 1976.
14. McIntyre KE, Bailey SA, Malone JM, et al. Guillotine amputation in the treatment of nonsalvageable lower-extremity infections. Arch Surg 119:450-453, 1984.
15. Smith RJ. Amputations in geriatric patients. J Natl Med Assoc 66:108-110, 1974.
16. Lim RC Jr, Blaisdell FW, Hall AD, et al. Below knee amputation for ischemic gangrene. Surg Gynecol Obstet 125:493-501, 1967.
17. Malone JM, Moore WS, Leal JM, et al. Rehabilitation after lower extremity amputation. Arch Surg 116:93-98, 1981.
18. Tripses D, Pollak EW. Risk factors in healing of below knee amputation. Appraisal of 64 amputations in patients with vascular disease. Am J Surg 141:718-720, 1981.
19. Liedberg E, Persson BM. Age, diabetes and smoking in lower limb amputation for arterial occlusive disease. Acta Orthop Scand 54:383, 1983.
20. Kerstein MD, Zimmer H, Dugdale FE, et al. Associated diagnoses complicating rehabilitation after major lower extremity amputation. Angiology 25:536-547, 1974.
21. Roon AJ, Moore WS, Goldstone J. Below-knee amputation. A modern approach. Am J Surg 134:153-158, 1977.
22. Kihn RB, Warren R, Beebe GW. The "Geriatric" amputee. Ann Surg 176:305-314, 1972.
23. Couch NP, David JK, Tilney NL, et al. Natural history of the leg amputee. Am J Surg 133:469, 1977.
24. High RM, McDowell DE, Savrin RA. A critical review of amputations in vascular patients. J Vasc Surg 1:653, 1984.
25. Hunsaker RH, Schwartz JA, Keagy BA, et al. Dry ice cryoamputation: A twelve-year experience. J Vasc Surg 2:812, 1985.
26. Malone JM. Complications of lower extremity amputation. In Moore WS, Malone JM, eds, Lower Extremity Amputation. Philadelphia: WB Saunders, 1989.
27. Mazet R Jr, Schiller FJ, Dunn OJ, et al. The influence of prosthesis wearing on the health of the geriatric patient. Washington, D.C.: Office of Vocational Rehabilitation, DHEW Project 431, March 1963, (unpublished).
28. Bernstein EF. Operative management of acute venous thromboembolism. In Rutherford RB, ed. Vascular Surgery, 2nd ed. Philadelphia: WB Saunders, 1984, pp 1367-1384.
29. Ctercteko GC, Dhanendran M, Hutton WC, et al. Vertical forces acting on the feet of diabetic patients with neuropathic ulceration. Br J Surg 68:608, 1981.
30. LeFrock JL, Joseph WS. Lower extremity infections in diabetics. Infect Surg 5:135, 1986.
31. McKittrick LS, McKittrick JB, Risley TS. Transmetatarsal amputation for infection or gangrene in patients with diabetes mellitus. Ann Surg 130:826, 1949.
32. Sapico FL, Whitte JL, Canawati HN, et al. The infected foot of the diabetic patient: Quantitative microbiology and analysis of clinical features. Rev Infect Dis 6:S171, 1984.
33. Wheat IJ, Allen SD, Henry M, et al. Diabetic foot infections. Arch Intern Med 146:19-35, 1986.
34. Burgess EM, Matsen FA, Wyss CR, et al. Segmental transcutaneous measurements of Po_2 in patients requiring below knee amputation for peripheral vascular insufficiency. J Bone Joint Surg 64A:378-382, 1982.

35. Holloway GA Jr, Burgess EM. Cutaneous blood flow and its relation to healing of below knee amputation. Surg Gynecol Obstet 146:750-756, 1978.

36. Hobson RW, Lynch TG, Jamil Z, et al. Results of revascularization and amputation in severe lower extremity ischemia: A five-year clinical experience. J Vasc Surg 2:174, 1985.

37. Reichle FA, Rankin KP, Tyson R, Finestone AJ, Shuman C. Long-term results of 474 arterial reconstructions for severely ischemic limbs: A fourteen year follow-up. Surgery 85:93-100, 1979.

38. Veith FJ, Gupta SK, Samson RH, et al. Progress in limb salvage by reconstructive arterial surgery combined with new improved adjunctive procedures. Ann Surg 194:386, 1981.

39. Ascer E, White SA, Gutpa SK, et al. Amputation versus revascularization. In Rutherford RB, ed. Vascular Surgery, 3rd ed. Philadelphia: WB Saunders, 1989.

40. Dardik H, Kahn M, Dardik I, et al. Influence of failed vascular bypass procedures on conversion of below-knee to above-knee amputation levels. Surgery 91:64, 1982.

41. Haimovici H. Failed grafts and level of amputation. J Vasc Surg 2:271, 1985.

42. Kazmers M, Satiani B, Evans WE. Amputation level following unsuccessful distal limb salvage operations. Surgery 87:683, 1980.

43. Bunt TJ, Manship LL, Bynoe RPH, et al. Lower extremity amputation for peripheral vascular disease. Am Surg 50:581, 1984.

44. Brinker MR, Timberlake GM, Goff JM, et al. Below-knee physiologic cryoanesthesia in the critically ill patient. J Vasc Surg 7:433-438, 1988.

45. Malone JM, Moore WS. Preparation of the patient and determination of amputation level. In Kempczinski RJ, ed. The Ischemic Leg. Chicago: Year Book, 1985, pp 519-535.

46. Rush DS, Huston CC, Bivins BA, et al. Operative and late mortality rates of above-knee and below-knee amputations. Am Surg 47:36, 1981.

47. Waters RL, Perry J, Antonelli D, et al. Energy cost of walking amputees: The influence of level of amputation. J Bone Joint Surg 58A:42, 1976.

48. Evans WE, Hayes JP, Vermilion BD. Rehabilitation of the bilateral amputee. J Vasc Surg 5:589, 1987.

49. Steinberg FU, Sunwool I, Roettger RF. Prosthetic rehabilitation of geriatric amputee patients: A follow-up study. Arch Phys Med Rehabil 66:742, 1985.

50. Gottschalk FA, Fisher DF Jr. Complications of amputations. In Rutherford RB, ed. Vascular Surgery, 3rd ed. Philadelphia: WB Saunders, 1989.

51. Mooney V. Above-knee amputations. In Mooney V, ed. American Academy of Orthopaedic Surgeons: Atlas of Limb Prosthetics: Surgical and Prosthetic Principles. St. Louis: CV Mosby, 1981, pp 378-382.

52. Cederbert PA, Pritchard DJ, Joyce JW. Doppler-determined segmental pressures and wound-healing in amputations for vascular disease. J Bone Joint Surg 65A:363, 1983.

53. Golbranson FL, Yu EC, Gelberman RH. The use of skin temperature determination in lower extremity amputation level selection. Foot Ankle 3:170-172, 1982.

54. Robbs JV, Ray R. Clinical predictors of below-knee stump healing following amputation for ischemia. South Afr J Surg 20:305, 1982.

55. Silverman DG, Rubin SM, Reilly CA, et al. Fluorometric prediction of successful amputation level in the ischemic limb. J Rehabil Res Dev 22:29, 1985.

56. Baker WH, Barnes RW. Minor forefoot amputations with low ankle pressure. Am Surg 133:331-332, 1977.

57. Barnes RW, Shanik GD, Slaymaker EE. An index of healing in below knee amputation. Leg blood pressure by Doppler ultrasound. Surgery 79:13-20, 1976.

58. Schwartz JA, Schuler JJ, O'Connor RJA, et al. Predictive value of distal perfusion pressure in the healing of amputation of the digits and forefoot. Surg Gynecol Obstet 154:865-869, 1982.

59. Yao JST, Bergan JJ. Application of ultrasound to arterial and venous diagnoses. Surg Clin North Am 54(1):23-38, 1974.

60. McFarland DC, Lawrence PF. Skin fluorescence. A method to predict amputation site healing. J Surg Res 32:410-415, 1982.

61. Silverman DG, Wagner FW Jr. Prediction of leg viability and amputation level by fluorescein uptake. Prosthet Orthot Int 7:69-71, 1983.

62. Holloway GA Jr, Watkins BW. Laser Doppler measurement of cutaneous blood flow. J Invest Dermatol 69:300, 1977.

63. Holloway GA Jr, Burgess EM. Preliminary experiences with laser Doppler velocimetry for the determination of amputation levels. Prosthet Orthot Int 7:63, 1983.

64. Karanfilian RG, Lynch TG, Zirul VT, et al. The value of laser Doppler velocimetry and transcutaneous oxygen tension determination in predicting healing of ischemic forefoot ulcerations and amputations in diabetic and nondiabetic patients. J Vasc Surg 4:511, 1986.

65. Matsen FA, Wyss CR, Robertson CL, et al. The relationship of transcutaneous PO_2 and laser Doppler measurements in a human model of local arterial insufficiency. Surg Gynecol Obstet 159:418, 1984.

66. Holstein P, Trap-Jensen J, Bagger H, et al. Skin perfusion in occlusive disease. Clin Physiol 3:313, 1983.

67. Ovesen J, Stockel M. Measurement of skin perfusion pressure by photoelectric technique: An aid to amputation level selection in arteriosclerosis disease. Prosthet Orthot Int 8:39, 1984.

68. Stockel M, Ovesen J, Brochner-Mortensen J, et al. Standardized photoelectric technique as routine method for selection of amputation level. Acta Orthop Scand 53:875-878, 1982.

69. Holstein P, Lassen NA. Assessment of safe level of amputation by measurement of skin blood pressure. In Rutherford RB, ed. Vascular Surgery. Philadelphia: WB Saunders, 1977, pp 105-111.

70. Holstein P. Distal blood pressure as a guide in choice of amputation level. Scand J Clin Lab Invest 31 (Suppl 128):245, 1973.

71. Holstein P. The distal blood pressure predicts healing of amputations on feet. Acta Orthop Scand 55:227, 1984.

72. Nilsen R, Dahn I, Lassen NA, et al. On the estimation of local effective perfusion pressure in patients with obliterative arterial disease by means of external compression over a xenon-133 depot. Scand J Clin Lab Invest 99(Suppl):29, 1967.

73. Malone JM, Leal JM, Moore WS, et al. The "gold standard" for amputation level selection: Xenon-133 clearance. J Surg Res 30:449-455, 1981.

74. Moore WS, Henry RE, Malone JM, et al. Prospective use of xenon Xe-133 clearance for amputation level selection. Arch Surg 116:86, 1981.

75. Silberstein EB, Thomas S, Cline J, et al. Predictive value of intracutaneous xenon clearance for healing of amputation and cutaneous sites. Radiology 147:227-229, 1983.

76. Goldbranson F. Amputation level determination. Presented at the annual meeting of the American Academy of Orthotists and Prosthetists. San Diego: January 1983.

77. Spence VA, Walker WF. The relationship between temperature isotherms and skin blood flow in the ischemic limb. J Surg Res 36:278, 1984.

78. Spence VA, McCollum PT, Walker WF, et al. Assessment of tissue viability in relation to the selection of amputation level. Prosthet Orthot Int 8:67, 1984.

79. Durham JR, Anderson GG, Malone JM. Methods of preoperative selection of amputation level. In Flanigan, DP ed. Perioperative Assessment in Vascular Surgery. New York: Marcel Dekker, 1987, pp 61-82.

80. Hauser CJ, Shoemaker WC. Use of transcutaneous PO$_2$ regional perfusion index to quantify tissue perfusion in peripheral vascular disease. Ann Surg 197:337, 1983.

81. Malone JM, Anderson GG, Lalka SG, et al. Prospective comparison of noninvasive techniques for amputation level selection. Am J Surg 154:179, 1987.

82. Bone GE, Pomajzl MJ. Toe blood pressure by photoplethysmography: An index of healing in forefoot amputations. Surgery 89:569, 1981.

83. Verta MJ, Gross WS, Van Bellan B, et al. Forefoot perfusion pressure and minor amputation surgery. Surgery 80:729, 1976.

84. Boeckstyns MEH, Jensen CM. Amputation of the forefoot: Predictive value of signs and clinical physiological tests. Acta Orthop Scand 55:224, 1984.

85. Harward TRS, Volny J, Goldbranson F, et al. Oxygen inhalation-induced transcutaneous PO$_2$ changes as a predictor of amputation level. J Vasc Surg 2:220, 1985.

86. Mehta K, Hobson RW II, Jamil Z, et al. Fallibility of Doppler ankle pressure in predicting healing of transmetatarsal amputation. J Surg Res 28:466, 1980.

87. Nicholas GG, Myers JL, Demuth WE. The role of vascular laboratory criteria in the selection of patients for lower extremity amputation. Ann Surg 195:469, 1982.

88. Pinzur M, Kaminsky M, Sage R, et al. Amputations at the middle level of the foot. J Bone Joint Surg 68A:1061, 1986.

89. Welch GH, Leiberman DP, Pollock JG, et al. Failure of Doppler ankle pressure to predict healing of conservative forefoot amputations. Br J Surg 72:888, 1985.

90. Barnes RW, Thornhill B, Nix L, et al. Prediction of amputation wound healing: Roles of Doppler ultrasound and digit photoplethysmography. Arch Surg 116:80, 1981.

91. Cheng EY. Lower extremity amputation level: Selection using noninvasive hemodynamic methods of evaluation. Arch Phys Med Rehabil 63:475, 1982.

92. Christensen KS, Klarke M. Transcutaneous oxygen measurement in healing in leg amputation. J Bone Joint Surg 68B:423, 1986.

93. Gibbons GW, Wheelock FC Jr, Siembrieda C, et al. Noninvasive prediction of amputation level in diabetic patients. Arch Surg 114:1253, 1979.

94. Katsamouris A, Brewster DC, Megerman J, et al. Transcutaneous oxygen tension in selection of amputation level. Am J Surg 147:510, 1984.

95. Klinger D, Kepplinger B. Transcutaneous electrical nerve stimulation (TNS) in the treatment of chronic pain after peripheral nerve lesions. In Siegfried J, Zimmermann M, eds. Phantom and Stump Pain. New York: Springer-Verlag, 1982, pp 103-106.

96. Lepantalo MJA, Haajanen J, Linfors O, et al. Predictive value of preoperative segmental blood pressure measurements in below-knee amputations. Acta Chir Scand 148:581, 1982.

97. Holstein P, Sager P, Lassen NA. Wound healing in below knee amputations in relationship to skin perfusion pressure. Acta Orthop Scand 40:49, 1979.

98. Holstein P, Trap-Jensen J, Bagger H, et al. Skin perfusion pressure measured by isotope washout in legs with arterial occlusive disease. Clin Physiol 3:313, 1983.

99. Ratliff DA, Clyne CAC, Chant ADB, et al. Prediction of amputation wound healing: The role of transcutaneous PO$_2$ assessment. Br J Surg 71:219, 1984.

100. Durham JR. Lower extremity amputation levels: Indications, methods of determining appropriate level, technique, and prognosis. In Rutherford RB, ed. Vascular Surgery, 3rd ed. Philadelphia: WB Saunders, 1989.

101. Moore WS, Malone JM. Lower Extremity Amputation. Philadelphia: WB Saunders, 1989.

102. Burgess EM, Marsden FW. Major lower extremity amputations following arterial reconstruction. Arch Surg 108:655-660, 1974.

103. Reyes RL, Leahey EB, Leahey EB Jr. Elderly patients with lower extremity amputations: Three-year study in a rehabilitation setting. Arch Phys Med Rehabil 58:116-123, 1977.

104. Bailey MJ, Johnston CLW, Yates CJP, et al. Preoperative haemoglobin as predictor of outcome of diabetic amputations. Lancet 28:168-170, 1979.

105. Nagendran T, Johnson G Jr, McDaniel WJ, et al. Amputation of the leg: An improved outlook. Ann Surg 175:994-999, 1972.

106. Sage R, Pinzur MS, Cronin R, et al. Complications following midfoot amputation in neuropathic and dysvascular feet. J Am Podiatr Med Assoc 79:266-280, 1989.

107. Malone JM. Complications of lower extremity amputation. In Bernhard VM, Towne JB, eds. Complications in Vascular Surgery, 2nd ed. New York: Grune & Stratton, 1985.

108. Dickhaut SC, DeLee JC, Pate CP. Nutritional status: Importance in predicting wound-healing after amputation. J Bone Joint Surg 66A:71, 1984.

109. Hansen ES, Wethelund JD, Skajaa K. Hemoglobin and hematocrit as risk factors in below-knee amputation for incipient gangrene. Arch Orthop Trauma 107:92-95, 1988.

110. Kacy SS, Wolma FJ, Flye MW. Factors affecting the results of below-knee amputation in patients with and without diabetes. Surg Gynecol Obstet 155:513-518, 1982.

111. Gatti JE, LaRossa D, Neff SR, et al. Altered skin flap survival and fleuorscein kinetics with hemodilution. Surgery 92:200-205, 1982.

112. Rubin JR, Yao JST, Thompson RG, et al. Management of infection of major amputation stump following failed femoro-distal grafts. Surgery 98:810-815, 1985.

113. Brewster DC, LaSalle AJ, Robinson JG, et al. Femoropopliteal graft failure. Clinical consequences and success of secondary reconstructions. Arch Surg 118:1043, 1983.

114. DeWeese JA, Rob CG. Autogenous venous grafts ten years later. Surgery 82:775, 1977.

115. Johansen K, Zorn R. Amputation stump infection in patients with retained thrombosed prosthetic vascular grafts. Am Surg 47:228-231, 1981.

116. Sonne-Holm S, Boeckstyns M, Menck H, et al. Prophylactic antibiotics in amputation of the lower extremity for ischemia. J Bone Joint Surg 67A:800, 1985.

117. Sonne-Holm S. Correspondence. J Bone Joint Surg 68A:950, 1986.

118. Jensen TS, Brebs B, Nielsen J, et al. Immediate and long-term phantom limb pain in amputees: Incidence, clinical characteristics and relationships to pre-amputation limb pain. Pain 21:267, 1985.

119. Sherman RA, Sherman CJ, Parker L. Chronic phantom and stump pain among American veterans. Results of a survey. Pain 18:83-95, 1984.

120. Sugarbaker PH, Weiss CM, Davidson DD, et al. Increasing phantom limb pain as a symptom of cancer recurrence. Cancer 54:373, 1984.

121. Abramson AS, Feibel A. The phantom phenomenon: Its use and disuse. Bull N Y Acad Med 57:99, 1981.

122. Melzack R. Central neural mechanisms in phantom limb pain. Adv Neurol 4:319, 1974.

123. Sherman RA, Published treatment of phantom pain. Am J Phys Med 59:232-244, 1980.

124. Sherman RA, Sherman CJ. Prevalence and characteristics of chronic phantom limb pain among American veterans–Results of a trial survey. Am J Phys Med 62:227, 1983.

125. Sherman RA, Tippens JK. Suggested guidelines for treatment of phantom limb pain. Orthopedics 5:1595-1600, 1982.

126. Iacono RP, Linford T. Pain management after lower extremity amputation. In Moore WS, Malone JM, eds. Lower Extremity Amputation. Philadelphia: WB Saunders, 1989.

127. Saris SC, Iocono RP, Nashold BS. Dorsal root entry zone lesions for post-amputation pain. J Neurosurg 6:72, 1985.

128. Mundinger F, Neumuller H. Programmed transcutaneous (TNS) and central (DBS) stimulation for control of phantom limb pain and causalgia: A new method for treatment. In Siegfried J, Zimmermann M, eds. Phantom and Stump Pain. New York: Springer-Verlag, 1982, pp 164-178.

129. Siegfried J, Cetinalp E. Neurosurgical treatment of phantom limb pain: A survey of methods. In Siegfried J, Zimmermann M, eds. Phantom and Stump Pain. New York: Springer-Verlag, 1982, pp 148-155.

130. Birkhan J, Carmon A, Meretsky P, et al. Clinical effects of a new TENS using multiple electrodes and constant energy. Proceedings of the Belgian Congress of Anesthesiology, 1982, pp 239-245.

131. Bodily KC, Burgess EM. Contralateral limb and patients' survival after leg amputation. Am J Surg 146:280, 1983.

132. Tamsen A, Hartvig P, Fagerlund C, et al. Patient controlled analgesia: Clinical experience. Acta Anaesthesiol Scand Suppl 74:157, 1982.

133. Williams JW, Eikman EA, Greenberg SH, et al. Failure of low dose heparin to prevent pulmonary embolism after hip surgery or above knee amputation. Ann Surg 188:468-474, 1978.

134. Fisher DF Jr, Valentine RJ. Sympathectomy, amputation, and angioaccess. In McClelland R, ed. Selected Readings in General Surgery, vol. 13. Dallas: University of Texas Southwestern Medical Center, 1986.

135. Mooney V, Harvey JP Jr, McBride E, et al. Comparison of postoperative stump management: Plaster vs. soft dressings. J Bone Joint Surg 53-A:241, 1971.

136. Vollmar JR, Paes EHJ, Pauschinger P, et al. Aneurysma aortae abdominalis und Beinamputation. Zufallige Koinzidenze oder pathogenetische Korrelation? Dtsch Med Wochenschr 188:1795-1800, 1988.

137. Vollmar JF, Paes E, Pauschinger P, et al. Aortic aneurysms as late sequelae of above-knee amputation. Lancet 7:834-835, 1989.

138. Levy SW. Skin Problems of the Amputee. St. Louis: Warren H Green, 1983, p 153.

139. Yekutiel M, Brooks ME, Ohry A, et al. The prevalence of hypertension, ischemic heart disease, and diabetes in traumatic spinal cord injured patients and amputees. Paraplegia 27:58-62, 1989.

140. Rose MG, Schwertr P, Oharoenkul V, et al. Cardiovascular disease risk factors in combat veterans after traumatic leg amputations. Arch Phys Med Rehabil 68:20-23, 1987.

141. Zarins CK, Glasgov S. Aneurysms and obstructive plaques: Differing local responses to atherosclerosis. In Bergman JJ, ed. Aneurysms. Diagnosis and Treatment. New York: Grune & Stratton, 1982.

142. Zarins CK. Hemodynamics in artherogenesis. In Greenhalgh R, ed. Vascular Surgery, 2nd ed. New York: Grune & Stratton, 1986, pp 97-115.

143. Truckenbrodt E. Fluidmechanik, vol 1. Berlin: Springer-Verlag, 1980.

144. Burton AC. Physiologie und Biophysik des Kreislaufs. Stuttgart: Schattauer, 1969, pp 209-210.

145. Landois F, Rosemann HU. In Rosemann HU, ed. Lehrbuch der Physiologies des Menschen. Munich: Urban und Schwarzenberg, 1960, pp 117-119.

146. Latham RD, Westerhof N, Sipkema P, et al. Regional wave travel and reflections along the human aorta: A study with six simultaneous micromanometric pressures. Circulation 72:1257-1269, 1985.

147. Trautwein W, Gauer OH, Koepchen HO, et al. In Gauer OH, Kramer L, Kimg R, eds. Physiologie des Meschen, vol 3. Munich: Urban und Schwarzenberg, 1972, pp 202-205.

148. Malone JM, Snyder M, Anderson G, et al. Prevention of amputation by diabetic education. Am J Surg 158:520-524, 1989.

149. Gupta SK, Veith FJ. Is arterial reconstruction cost effective compared with amputation? In Greenhalgh RM, Jamieson CW, Nicolaides AN, eds. Limb Salvage and Amputation for Vascular Disease. Philadelphia: WB Saunders, 1988, pp 447-452.

25

Skeletal Muscle Ischemia and Revascularization Injury

Malcolm O. Perry

Acute arterial insufficiency most often is the result of an intrinsic obstruction of major arteries by clot. Emboli that originate in the heart frequently are the cause of such obstructions, and patients who have experienced myocardial infarctions, mitral stenosis, or atrial fibrillation are susceptible to the development of intracardiac clots and distal thromboembolism. Arterial emboli usually lodge where the vessels taper and where branches occur; they are found most often in the iliac, femoral, and popliteal arteries. These same arteries are also affected by atherosclerotic narrowing that may cause in situ thrombosis. Any of these events can result in limb loss. Occlusions can be treated effectively by emergency surgical disobliteration, but damage to the nerves and skeletal muscle may occur, particularly if there is a delay in definitive treatment.

PATHOPHYSIOLOGY

The tolerance of the lower extremities to ischemia is difficult to assess because some types of cells are apparently more susceptible to hypoxia than others, presumably as a result of differing oxygen requirements and perhaps also influenced by whether the muscles are at rest or at work. It is clear, however, that peripheral nerves and skeletal muscle have less resistance to hypoxia than skin.

The duration of the ischemic interval is important, although there is no unanimity of opinion regarding how much ischemia skeletal muscle can tolerate. It was originally believed that skeletal muscle could tolerate up to 6 hours of complete ischemia without permanent damage, but recent studies suggest that this view is inaccurate. Shorter periods of ischemia can result in significant changes in the metabolic function of the muscle cell. In patients undergoing aortic reconstruction with temporary aortic occlusion Eklof, Neglen, and Thompson[1] have demonstrated that there is a reduction in the concentration of high-energy phosphate compounds in the muscles of the legs. This metabolic dysfunction was evident for at least 16 hours after the operation. Roberts et al.[2] found that even short periods of partial ischemia can result in alterations in cell membrane electrical potentials, which persist for several hours despite adequate restoration of blood flow. These experimental and clinical studies strongly suggest that partial ischemia is capable of inflicting significant damage to the muscles even if the muscles tolerate the initial ischemic episode. In view of these findings it probably is not reasonable to assume that a period of "safe ischemia" exists.

To properly assess the clinical relevance of experimental research on the pathogenesis of ischemia, it is necessary to observe the differences between hypoxia and ischemia and between infarction and necrosis. Hypoxia alone is compatible with sustained myocardial function, for example, but ischemia almost instantaneously causes loss of cardiac contractility. Ischemia involves not only the inadequate delivery of oxygen, but also the accumulation of metabolic products that may directly or through intermediaries disrupt cellular function. These substances include oxygen-derived free radicals as well as other toxic mediators.

In those situations in which the ischemia is not so prolonged or so severe as to cause cellular necrosis, a period of reperfusion will usually follow the repair. The mechanism of injury in these cases appears to be somewhat different depending on the organ system, and therefore it may be appropriate to deal with ischemia and reperfusion as separate entities.

There is a great deal of evidence to suggest that the outcome following an episode of skeletal muscle ischemia depends not only on tolerance of the cells to hypoxia, but also on local changes that impair the restoration of normal blood flow. This has been called the no-reflow phenomenon.[3] Failure to restore adequate perfusion to the microcirculation after ischemia can increase the ischemic injury, resulting in greater damage than might have been predicted from the observed period of arterial obstruction.

In 1948 Harman[4] produced temporary tourniquet ischemia in the hind limb of rabbits and examined the rate of penetration and elimination of bromphenol blue dye. The vital dye immediately stained normal and mildly ischemic muscle as soon as the tourniquet was released, but when the ischemic interval was longer than 3 hours, the dye was retained within the muscle. If ischemia lasted beyond 6 hours, the dye did not enter the muscle for at least 30 minutes, suggesting that there was stagnation of the circulation. This stagnation was confirmed by histologic findings of dilated capillaries engorged with red blood cells, but no thrombi were seen. Similar phenomena have been observed by Ames et al.[3] in their study of a rabbit cerebral ischemia model; they were unable to reestablish normal blood flow after the ischemic episode. Red blood cells were trapped in narrowed capillaries, but no clots were seen. Swelling of perivascular glial cells occurred and endothelial blebs were noted.

Recent studies of patients with circulatory shock caused by hemorrhage or congestive heart failure have revealed plugging of vessels in the heart, lung, and periphery by leukocytes.[5] A granulocyte is approximately 12 μm in diameter, and even under normal conditions the cells are relatively rigid and slow to deform. A significant delay occurs before they enter small vessels, and if there is endothelial and perivascular cell swelling, the leukocytes can more easily obstruct blood flow. Furthermore, neutrophil adherence to the endothelium can result in activation of the defensive mechanisms within the granulocyte. Proteolytic enzymes, oxygen-derived free radicals, and other toxic products are released, which are capable of causing cell membrane damage. The mediators may also include chemotactic agents such as leukotriene B_4, which attracts additional granulocytes.

The proteolytic enzymes destroy hyaluronic acid and disrupt basement membranes, leading to increased capillary permeability and the accumulation of interstitial fluid.[6] This may present yet another barrier to restoration of normal tissue perfusion, especially when blood viscosity is higher.

REPERFUSION INJURY

The mechanisms of ischemia-reperfusion injury appear to be different in certain organ systems.[7] In the intestine, for example, prolonged periods of ischemia produce direct cell death apparently unrelated to toxic mediators. Lesser degrees of intestinal ischemia cause reversible cell injury that may be the result primarily of the accumulation of toxic agents in the reperfusion period. In contrast, ischemia-reperfusion injury in cardiac muscle appears to be caused by the same mechanisms regardless of the degree of ischemia.

Several experiments have shown that when blood flow to skeletal muscle is interrupted for 30 minutes to several hours, edema formation occurs early in the reperfusion period.[7,8] The amount of edema that develops depends on the duration of ischemia: the longer the period of ischemia, the more interstitial edema. The development of edema is primarily related to changes in vascular permeability. In addition to the activity of the proteolytic enzymes, oxygen-derived free radicals also can increase microvascular permeability.

TOXIC MEDIATORS

It appears that at least some of the tissue damage evident after ischemic episodes is caused by oxygen-derived free radicals and other toxic agents.[9] A free radical is a molecule containing an odd number of electrons, rendering it very chemically reactive. When a free radical reacts with a nonradical, another free radical is produced; thus oxygen-derived free radicals can initiate chain reactions that may be thousands of events long.

Ordinarily 98% of molecular oxygen is completely reduced to water in the process of respiration, but the other 2% can result in the elaboration of potentially toxic free radicals. These toxic species apparently come from "leaky" sites in the mitochondrial electron transport chain.

The primary source of oxygen-derived free radicals in ischemic tissue is the enzyme xanthine oxidase (type O), which is synthesized as xanthine dehydrogenase (type D). Type D accounts for over 90% of the total activity in normal tissue. The conversion of xanthine dehydrogenase to xanthine oxidase (type D–to–type O reaction) is thought to begin because of a decrease in blood flow to the tissue, which limits the availability of adenosine triphosphate (ATP). As the energy charge of the cell is reduced, a proper gradient of calcium cannot be maintained across the cell membrane. Elevation of calcium in the cytosol and activation of a protease that converts the dehydrogenase to the oxidase result. As intracellular ATP is consumed, there is an increase in adenosine monophosphate, which is then catabolized to adenosine, inosine, and then hypoxanthine. Hypoxanthine is a substrate for oxidation by xanthine oxidase, and with the introduction of molecular oxygen (the second substrate required), oxygen-derived free radicals are generated.

The superoxide radical is unstable and spontaneously dismutates to hydrogen peroxide and oxygen. This radical is a weak oxidant and a potent reductant, which can inactivate specific enzymes, but more importantly it acts as a precursor to very reactive free radicals. Hydrogen peroxide is derived from the two-electron reduction of oxygen or the dismutation of superoxide. It is a sluggish but powerful oxidant and can inactivate deoxyribonucleic acid. It can also oxidize sulfhydryl groups, which are essential to the activity of the ATP pump. The superoxide radical and ferric iron can be converted to oxygen and ferrous iron, and when the ferrous iron reacts with hydrogen peroxide, the very toxic hydroxyl radical is produced. This radical is the most reactive of those observed in biologic systems and can react with virtually any organic compound. It causes lipid peroxidation of the cell membrane and can oxidize sulfhydryl groups, inactivate cytochrome enzymes, and alter membrane transport proteins. It appears that the hydroxyl radical is primarily responsible for most of the cellular damage that occurs in reperfusion syndrome.

Although the conversion of xanthine dehydrogenase to xanthine oxidase does not occur readily in skeletal muscle, there is considerable evidence to indicate that these toxic radicals can be produced from the degranulation of leukocytes and perhaps also from endothelial cells.[10,11] As described above, other mediators may be released by the white blood cells as well.

In experiments on the brains of cats, lipid peroxidation has been shown to activate the arachidonic acid pathway.[12] This activation leads to the production of oxygen-derived free radicals as well as other toxic mediators. Although this mechanism has not been demonstrated in skeletal muscle, the presence of these alternative pathways for the production of toxic agents suggests there may be as yet undiscovered mechanisms involved.

Calcium ions also occupy a central role in this mechanism. It has been shown that when the cell energy charge drops, there is a redistribution of calcium ions, causing an increase in calcium content in the cytosol of the cells. This increased calcium content leads to the calcium-triggered proteolytic attack on xanthine dehydrogenase, resulting in the production of xanthine oxidase. In addition to the elaboration of oxygen-derived free radicals, there is strong evidence that direct calcium toxicity can occur in the brain. The calcium overload of neurons can cause cell death. This mechanism has not been observed in skeletal muscle, but the possibility has not been dismissed.

RHABDOMYOLYSIS AND MYOGLOBINURIA

In more severe episodes of ischemia, direct cellular disruption can occur and rhabdomyolysis may follow, with the escape of myoglobin and potassium.[13] With restoration of blood flow these substances are released into the general circulation and are capable of causing direct injury to the lungs and heart. Large amounts of myoglobin can lead to myoglobinuric nephropathy, renal failure, and death. Although these syndromes are unusual, clinical studies have suggested that induction of osmotic diuresis, particularly with the administration of mannitol, offers some protection.[13] Moreover, it has been shown that the administration of mannitol early in evolving compartment syndrome can reduce the extent of muscle injury and death.[14] Initially this effect of mannitol was thought to be the result of osmotic activity, but more recent data show that mannitol is a potent scavenger of the toxic hydroxyl radical.[7]

Surgeons performing vascular reconstructive procedures to salvage ischemic limbs must deal with the aftereffects of ischemia-reperfusion syndrome. There are data suggesting that even asanguineous tourniquet ischemia, thought to be innocuous, can result in mitochondrial damage after as little as 1 hour of tourniquet application.[15] Although no muscle fiber specifically susceptible to this injury has been identified, it may require as long as 1 week for normal levels of muscle power to be regained.

CLINICAL SYNDROMES

Edema is common after reconstructive vascular surgery in the lower extremities and is usually more severe when reconstruction is successful. This finding suggests that reperfusion has an important role in the genesis of edema. Increases in capillary permeability can lead to development of compartmental syndromes (increase in tissue pressure) that eventually disturbs Starling's equilibrium, causing muscle necrosis even in the presence of intact arterial pulses.[15] Early compartmental decompression can reverse this phenomenon, but there may be scattered areas of muscle necrosis, apparently related to direct cellular injury.

Renal failure can occur following lysis of muscle cells and the release of large amounts of myoglobin. Although this myoglobinuria-rhabdomyolysis syndrome can usually be prevented, it remains a threat to any reconstructive vascular surgery performed for limb salvage. Finally, in those limbs in which blood flow cannot be restored, cellular necrosis is widespread.

THERAPEUTIC OPTIONS

It is obviously important to limit ischemia of skeletal muscle. Although skeletal muscle may be capable of tolerating greater degrees of ischemia than the brain, kidney, and liver, recent data suggest that skeletal muscle is susceptible to even short periods of partial ischemia.[1,2] Intraoperative hypothermia and hemodilution have been used to reduce ischemic injury to the cells.[16] It may also be helpful in some cases to drain the initial venous effluent from a severely ischemic extremity in order to remove toxic products that have accumulated in the venous system during ischemia. The red blood cells can be washed, resuspended, and reinfused into the patient.

Recent studies suggest that controlled reperfusion may be of some benefit in these patients. Initial perfusion with reduced blood pressure, a limit in the concentration of oxygen within the perfusate, and the control in some fashion of the concentration and number of white blood cells permitted to initially reenter the reperfused muscle may help to prevent the development of reperfusion syndrome.[16] Although the data supporting these methods are largely experimental, with only a few clinical observations with similar results, it is clear that further investigation to evaluate the effectiveness of these techniques is in order.

These data have led to the consideration that the administration of oxygen-free radical scavengers may also be helpful in reducing the amount of edema and cell damage that occur in the reperfusion period. Recent experiments by Perry and Fantini[9] and by Lindsay, Romaschin, and Walker[17] suggest that the administration of scavengers in certain situations can protect skeletal muscle from injury.

Interest in the use of calcium antagonists and

calcium channel blockers also has emerged as a result of observations of the central role of calcium in cell toxicity.[12,18,19] Preliminary laboratory experiments suggest that some calcium antagonists may be useful, particularly in the treatment of cerebral ischemia, but variations in the experimental models and in the protocols used do not permit a general endorsement other than to indicate that these drugs hold promise.

It therefore appears that there are multiple mechanisms whereby different mediators can damage cells. How these agents are integrated and relate one to another is unclear at this time.[18] Part of the difficulty in separating the possible causes stems from the demonstrated reactions between the agents, such as the calcium-triggered proteolytic attack on xanthine dehydrogenase. Although it is currently not possible to identify the various separate pathogenetic mechanisms, a considerable body of evidence exists that incriminates oxygen-derived free radicals. Attempts to reduce cellular injury by employing agents that interfere with these toxic mediators have been only partially successful, but beneficial effects have been dramatic in some cases.[16] A clear delineation of the pathways leading to cellular injury and death must be completed before effective therapeutic agents can be deployed.

LATE FUNCTIONAL PROBLEMS

Long-term limb disability following ischemia is more often the result of delayed neurologic deficits than failure of the vascular repair.[20] The lack of protective sensation and impaired motor function combine to produce a leg that basically is an "anesthetic post." It is an encumbrance and eventually must be removed, even if the blood supply is adequate.

As the success of acute revascularizations has improved, nerve injury has become the primary cause of dysfunction, although loss of skeletal muscle because of direct cell injury has also been implicated. There are no reliable criteria for predicting functional neurologic recovery in an extremity.[19] In contrast, even if large volumes of skeletal muscle are lost because of ischemia-reperfusion syndromes, newer orthopedic procedures and better prosthetics may allow the limb to retain some useful activity. Direct ischemic injury that subsequently leads to excision of muscle groups often results in unsightly scars and deformity. However, if protective sensation is present, other muscles may be trained to perform some functions or activities that otherwise might be lost.[15]

Damage of proximal nerves (sciatic, peroneal, femoral) by ischemia or other injuries has a worse prognosis than similar damage in more distal nerves. This variation in prognosis apparently is related to the length of nerve regeneration required before muscle reinnervation can occur. Combined injury to muscles and nerves is likely to result in severe disability.

What can be done to reduce the risks? Clearly, early and complete relief of ischemia is the most effective treatment. There is no truly "safe interval." The therapeutic options available are few, and as of yet carefully controlled studies have not been done. Despite this, there is increasing support for the belief that toxic mediators are an important part of this process, and they in turn may be vulnerable to attack.

REFERENCES

1. Eklof B, Neglen P, Thompson D. Temporary incomplete ischemia of the legs induced by aortic clamping in man. Ann Surg 193:89-95, 1980.
2. Roberts JP, Perry MO, Harari RJ, et al. Incomplete recovery of muscle cell function following partial but not complete ischemia. Circ Shock 17:253-258, 1985.
3. Ames A, Wright RL, Kowada M, et al. Cerebral ischemia—The no-reflow phenomenon. Am J Pathol 52:437-444, 1968.
4. Harman JW. The significance of local vascular phenomena in the production of ischemic necrosis in skeletal muscle. Am J Pathol 24:625-630, 1948.
5. Ernst E, Hammerschmidt DE, Bagge U, et al. Leukocytes and the risk of ischemic diseases. JAMA 257:2318-2322, 1987.
6. Korthius R, Granger D, Townsley M, et al. The role of oxygen-derived free radicals in ischemia induced increases in canine skeletal muscle vascular permeability. Circulation 72:599-609, 1985.
7. Buckley CB. Pathophysiology of free radical-mediated reperfusion injury. J Vasc Surg 5:512-513, 1987.
8. Karthius RJ, Smith MK, Carden DC. Hypoxic reperfusion attenuates post-ischemic microvascular injury. Am J Physiol 256(Heart Circ Physiol 25):H315-H319, 1989.
9. Perry MO, Fantini G. Ischemia-reperfusion and cell membrane dysfunction. Microcirc Endothelium Lymphatics 5:241-258, 1989.

10. Korthius RJ, Grisham MB, Granger DN. Leukocyte depletion attenuates vascular injury in post-ischemic skeletal muscle. Am J Physiol 254(Heart Circ Physiol 23):H1068-H1075, 1988.
11. Yokota J, Minei JP, Fantini GA, et al. Role of leukocytes in reperfusion injury of skeletal muscle after partial ischemia. Am J Physiol 257(Heart Circ Physiol 26):H1068-H1075, 1989.
12. White BC, Wiegenstein JG, Winegar CD. Brain ischemic anoxia. Mechanisms of injury. JAMA 251:1586-1590, 1984.
13. Haimovici H. Muscular, renal, and metabolic complications of acute arterial occlusion: Myonephropathic-metabolic syndrome. Surgery 85:461-468, 1979.
14. Buchbinder D, Karmody AM, Leather RP, et al. Hypertonic mannitol. Arch Surg 116:414-420, 1981.
15. Russell WL, Burns RP. Acute upper and lower extremity compartment syndromes. In Bergan JJ, Yao JST, eds. Vascular Surgical Emergencies. Orlando, Fla.: Grune & Stratton, 1987, pp 203-217.
16. Beyersdorf F, Mathus G, Krüger S, et al. Avoiding reperfusion injury after limb revascularization: Experimental observations and recommendations for clinical application. J Vasc Surg 9:757-766, 1989.
17. Lindsay T, Romaschin A, Walker PM. Free radical mediated damage in skeletal muscle. Microcirc Endothelium Lymphatics 5:157-170, 1989.
18. Belkin M, Wright JG, Hobson RW. Iloprost infusion decreases skeletal muscle ischemia-reperfusion injury. J Vasc Surg 11:77-83, 1990.
19. Cronenwett JL, Lee KR, Shlafer M, et al. The effect of ischemia-reperfusion derived oxygen free radicals on skeletal muscle calcium metabolism. Microcirc Endothelium Lymphatics 5:171-187, 1989.
20. Nichols JS, Lillehei KO. Nerve injury associated with acute vascular trauma. Surg Clin North Am 68:837-852, 1988.

X Venous and Lymphatic Surgery

26

Complications of Direct Venous Reconstruction in the Lower Extremity

Robert W. Hobson II

Clinical investigation of the indications and results of direct venous reconstruction performed after trauma or electively because of an obstructed or compromised venous system resulting from previous deep vein thrombosis or extrinsic venous compression has resulted in an increased understanding of the topic over the last 5 years. Although measuring the clinical success of direct venous repair continues to be a challenging issue for vascular surgeons, many researchers have reported improved results and reduced complication rates. For example, earlier concerns regarding an increased incidence of thromboembolism after venous repair as compared with that following venous ligation were unwarranted based on more recent clinical assessments.[1-4] The purpose of this chapter is to update and review reported complications with the performance of direct venous reconstruction after trauma and following elective venous reconstruction.

VENOUS TRAUMA

Historically, the principles and techniques for surgical repair of injured major veins were well established and practiced during the late nineteenth and early twentieth centuries by surgeons including Murphy, Dorfler, Carrel, and Guthrie.[5,6] Early recommendations in favor of venous repair were modified based on clinical observations made during World War I. Makins[7] reported improved limb survival following arterial occlusion or ligation by the performance of concomitant venous ligation. These data also were interpreted as an indication for ligation of major venous injuries until DeBakey and Simeone[8] analyzed clinical reports from World War II that refuted the concept that venous ligation reduced the development of gangrene following arterial ligation. The additional reported association of acute lower extremity edema and in some cases venous gangrene after ligation of major venous injuries, even in the presence of a patent arterial repair, resulted in a more aggressive recommendation for venous repair.[9-11] Furthermore, chronic venous insufficiency developed in some patients when ligation of major injured veins was practiced, particularly at the level of the popliteal and common femoral veins.[11,12]

Stimulated by clinical reports from the Vietnam Vascular Registry, research efforts were directed toward defining the hemodynamic consequences of venous ligation as compared with repair and the implications of venous thrombosis after repair. Several reports have documented the effects of femoral venous occlusion on femoral arterial blood flow, femoral venous pressure, and femoral vascular resis-

tance[13,14] (Fig. 26-1). The gradual improvement in arterial blood flow associated with a reduction in venous pressure and peripheral vascular resistance 48 hours after ligation was caused by an improvement in venous outflow through collateral veins in the canine hindlimb. Consequently, the first 24 to 72 hours were described as the important period of patency for the venous repair. These data supported the recommendation for direct venous repair of major injured veins in an attempt to avoid these adverse hemodynamic consequences, particularly when the venous injury was associated with concomitant arterial injury. However, it is recognized that the presence of venous hypertension in the extremity is the important hemo-

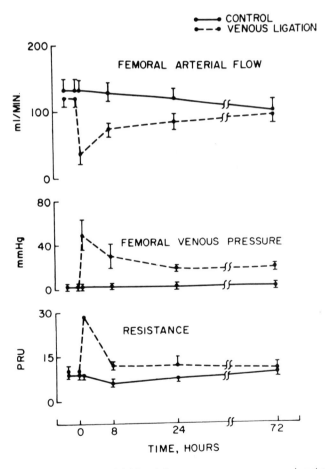

Fig. 26-1. Changes in femoral arterial blood flow, venous pressure, and resistance (mean ± standard error). (From Hobson RW, Howard EW, Wright CB, et al. Hemodynamics of canine femoral venous ligation: Significance in combined arterial and venous injuries. Surgery 78:824, 1973.)

dynamic indication for venous repair (Fig. 26-1). In the absence of acute venous hypertension, repair of the injured vein would appear to have a lesser influence on limb survival and subsequent incidence of chronic venous insufficiency.

Based on these clinical reports and laboratory information, the recommendation for universal repair of major injured veins in the lower extremity has been modified by knowledge of the hemodynamic significance of these injuries and the clinical necessity of performing venous ligation in some cases, particularly when the patient is a multiple trauma victim. Although ligation of upper extremity venous injuries has been well tolerated, routine repair of common femoral and popliteal venous injuries has been recommended by several investigators.[2,4,12,15] Nevertheless, management of these cases also has been tempered during recent years by clinical reports that suggest that there is a lack of major complications when the injuries are ligated as compared with when they are repaired. Mullins, Lucas, and Ledgerwood[16] reported on the results of venous ligation in the lower extremity for venous trauma. No early amputations were required and no instances of massive edema or ulceration were reported. More recently, Timberlake, O'Connell, and Kerstein[17] reported venous injuries managed by ligation that were unassociated with major long-term complications. This series of cases included ligation of 21 of 31 popliteal venous injuries. However, these authors emphasized the importance of elevation of the extremity pending complete resolution of edema and recommended four-compartment fasciotomy based on clinical findings and documentation of elevated compartmental pressures. Although mean follow-up was confined to less than 3 years in these reports, no clinical sequelae were reported during this limited clinical follow-up. However, as emphasized in the Vietnam Vascular Registry, further follow-up is recommended on these patients to define the incidence of chronic venous insufficiency, which may not be apparent until 5 to 10 years after venous ligation. Although the reported incidence of edema after ligation or occlusion of primary femoral venous injuries was 75% in our series at UMDNJ,[4] recommen-

dation for universal venous repair should be modified by the realization that all venous injuries in the lower extremity are not associated with adverse hemodynamic consequences. Therefore the more accurate characterization of these hemodynamic conditions may assist the surgeon in selecting patients for venous repair. This is a topic for potential prospective study in view of its controversial nature and the inherent difficulties of retrospective clinical analysis. One might suspect that ligation would be well tolerated in the subset of patients with satisfactory venous collateralization or anatomic duplication, which would thereby negate the adverse hemodynamic consequences secondary to ligation.

THROMBOSIS OF DIRECT VENOUS REPAIRS OR INTERPOSITION GRAFTS

Thrombosis of direct venous repairs or interposition grafts within the venous system is a major complication; however, several considerations are important in minimizing this complication. Meticulous surgical technique in experimental and clinical venous repairs is a major factor and requires some additional emphasis.[18] Use of interposition grafting, which has not been recommended by all authors,[19,20] constitutes one of the most controversial issues in venous reconstruction. Meyer et al.[19] reported a 59% failure rate with venous grafting and suggested that use of the "usual" arterial reconstructive techniques should have resulted in a much more satisfactory result, approaching 100% patency for arterial repair. Unfortunately, operative venography and hemodynamic studies were not performed to confirm the technical adequacy of the venous reconstructions.

With regard to the technical aspects of venous reconstruction, the margin for error in completion of the venovenous anastomosis is less than that for an arterial anastomosis. Ideally, sutures must be placed loosely to avoid undue tension on the suture line; such tension would result inevitably in narrowing of the anastomosis and the anastomosis would require revision. These lessons have been emphasized in our laboratory experience and subsequent clinical reports.[4,6] Venography is recommended to confirm a successful repair; technically inadequate repairs will result in early venous occlusion. Occlusion of the venous repair in the presence of combined arterial and venous trauma, particularly at the level of the popliteal artery and vein, may be associated with adverse clinical results. Rich, Jarstfer, and Geer[12] have reported venous patency as a major consideration in the high amputation rates for combined popliteal arterial and venous trauma. Reports on the patency of femoral venous reconstruction in both the research laboratory and the clinical arena have been highly variable. This obviously relates to the choice of surgical techniques and the use of various methods for repair of major injured veins (Fig. 26-2). Although the lengthy venous reconstruction should not be performed in the multiple trauma victim, use of interposition grafting can be associated with clinically acceptable results provided certain technical requirements are fulfilled rigorously and adjunctive measurements are used. Recent cases from our clinical experience[4] have confirmed that ligation can be associated with the subsequent requirement for remedial reconstruction. That series has been expanded to more than 50 patients with femoral venous injuries and patency has continued to be in the 75% to 80% range.[21] Symptomatic pulmonary embolism has not occurred in this series; however, approximately 10% of patients have demonstrated tibial venous thrombi on venography. All of these patients were maintained on anticoagulation therapy and edema resolved after 1 week, again without symptomatic pulmonary emboli. Schramek, Hashmonai, and associates[2,22] reported similarly successful results in managing four common femoral injuries, four superficial femoral injuries, and seven popliteal venous injuries in a group of 82 vascular injury cases. Interposition grafts were used in four femoral venous injuries supplemented with distal arteriovenous fistulas. Follow-up venograms in these cases demonstrated patent grafts, prompting the investigators to recommend use of interposition grafts for venous repair as necessary.

Rich et al.[23] reported on 51 autogenous venous interposition grafts for repair of major injured veins: 36 involved the superficial femoral vein; eight, the popliteal vein; and seven, the common femoral vein. They reported a 2% incidence of thrombophlebitis, no pulmonary emboli, and an 11.8% incidence of residual edema in the lower extremity. Recent reports on civilian vascular trauma also have emphasized the value of femoral and popliteal venous repair. Although some investigators[19,20] have reported elevated rates of thrombosis with in-

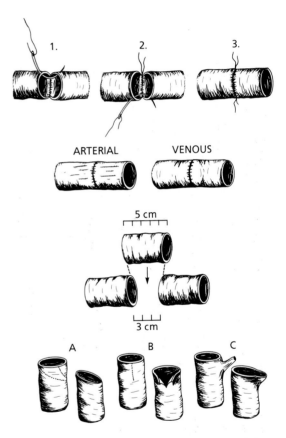

Fig. 26-2. Drawings demonstrating basic principles in performing venous anastomoses. Continuous sutures must be placed loosely in contrast to the usual technique for arterial anastomosis. Grafts in the venous system should be somewhat longer than the defect and of similar diameter. Diagonal cuts **(A)**, "fishmouthing" **(B)**, and use of adjacent branches **(C)** may help prevent stenosis at suture lines. (From Rich NM, Hobson RW, Wright CB, et al. Techniques of venous repair. In Swan KG, ed. Venous Surgery in the Lower Extremity. St. Louis: Warren H. Green, 1974.)

terposition venous grafting and recommended against the use of these repairs, the absence of adjunctive techniques from their protocol may have compromised results. Adjunctive techniques that may improve patency of direct venous repair include the following:

1. Administration of pharmacologic agents, such as intraoperative heparin and post-operative low-molecular-weight dextran
2. Intermittent pneumatic calf compression after popliteal and femoral venous injuries
3. Creation of a distal arteriovenous fistula

In addition, certain technical features at the level of the common femoral vein require use of paneled or spiral vein grafts (Fig. 26-3), which, if not used, would certainly result in a heightened thrombosis rate.

Ultimately, the clinical recommendation for venous repair should be selective and relate to venographic evidence of absence of venous collateralization in the limb or presence of elevated venous pressure. This is particularly true in the area of the superficial femoral vein but perhaps less so in cases of common femoral and popliteal venous injuries, which we have acknowl-

edged as treated preferentially by repair when feasible. The only major exception to this recommendation is the multiple trauma victim, who might be jeopardized by the additional operative time required for venous repair.

ADJUNCTIVE TECHNIQUES TO IMPROVE VENOUS PATENCY

Application of adjunctive techniques will improve the patency of venous repairs after trauma. Various adjunctive methods available are described above. The experimental value of distal arteriovenous fistulas has been well established by several researchers.[24-26] The increased velocity of blood flow and the arterialization of the venous repair should contribute to improved patency. Whether the fistula should be placed immediately adjacent to the venous repair is controversial since a secondary operation might be required for its repair. However, recent techniques involving the construction of smaller fistulas, which can be ligated percutaneously or occluded by use of radiologic intervention, offer innovative clinical options.[27] A more distal placement of the fistula also would allow its ligation or repair without disrupting the venous anastomosis.[26] Although these fistulas have been reported as being an attractive alternative for experimental reasons, clinical application, particularly after trauma, has been limited.[22] However, their use after elective venous reconstruction has been suggested and recommended by others after venous thrombectomy.[28]

The experimental rationale for the use of low-molecular-weight dextran has been reported.[29] Interestingly, postoperative heparinization did not appear to be efficacious. Our current recommendation includes use of intraoperative heparinization and administration of low-molecular-weight dextran that is continued for 48 to 72 hours postoperatively.[4]

Finally, mechanical methods to increase the velocity of blood flow through the deep venous repair by use of intermittent pneumatic compression of the calf would seem to be a useful alternative to the distal arteriovenous fistula.[30] Although the increase in velocity of blood flow would be intermittent with compression boots, this technique has been used by us[4] routinely to

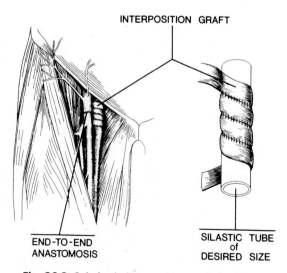

INTERPOSITION GRAFT

END-TO-END ANASTOMOSIS

SILASTIC TUBE of DESIRED SIZE

Fig. 26-3. Spiral vein interposition graft for femoral venous reconstruction. (From Hobson RW, Yeager RA, Lynch TG, et al. Femoral venous trauma: Techniques for surgical management and early results. Am J Surg 146:220, 1983.)

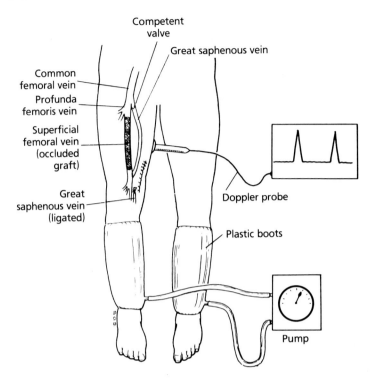

Fig. 26-4. Drawing of the saphenopopliteal bypass performed for femoral venous occlusion with application of pneumatic boots for intermittent calf compressions. The transducer of a Doppler ultrasonic flowmeter has been positioned over the venous bypass. (From Hobson RW, Lee BC, Lynch TG, et al. Use of intermittent pneumatic compression of the calf in femoral venous reconstruction. Surg Gynecol Obstet 159:284, 1984. By permission.)

achieve a reported patency of 74% with femoral venous reconstructions, including use of interposition grafts (Fig. 26-4).

ELECTIVE VENOUS RECONSTRUCTION

Venous valvular reconstruction for chronic venous insufficiency in the lower extremity was recommended in its earliest phases by Kistner.[31] Subsequently, several investigators also have reviewed data suggesting the clinical applicability of valvular reconstruction and repair.[32,33] Overall, complications from venous valvular reconstruction and the more recent valvular transplantation have been few.[32,34] A low incidence of minor venous thrombi has been reported and treated with anticoagulant therapy without adversely affecting the status of the re-

construction. The incidence of symptomatic thromboembolism has been rare. Furthermore, occlusion of these repairs has been unusual and again unassociated with major complications. Although Kistner[31] and Raju and Fredericks[33] have reported clinical success with proximal valvular reconstruction, other authors have suggested that improvement in venous hemodynamic conditions may be temporary and, particularly with valvular transposition, will revert toward a chronic state of venous insufficiency.[35] In addition, the concept that proximal valvuloplasty or other surgical reconstruction to achieve a proximal competent value will be therapeutic has been challenged. Moore, Himmel, and Sumner[36] reported the presence of distal venous incompetence in 67% of limbs with proximal venous incompetence and 57%

of those with proximal valvular competence. These findings have cast some doubt on the value of proximal venous reconstruction. As a result femoral venous valvular repair or venous transposition procedures have not received wide practical application.

However, Kistner's original success stimulated others to use valvular transplantation in an effort to place a competent valve in the deep venous system.[32-34] This concept of improving the physiology of venous blood flow in an extremity by surgical transplantation of a competent axillary venous valve to the popliteal vein has resulted in some clinical success. O'Donnell et al.[32] and Taheri et al.[34] have demonstrated improved results with the use of the axillary venous valve to restore popliteal valvular competency. Shull et al.[37] have reported that the condition and competency of the popliteal valves are the most important factors in determining ambulatory venous pressure and ulceration, lending a physiologic basis for valvular transplantation at the level of the popliteal vein. These authors report occasional wound complications without other morbidity.[32,34] Raju and Fredericks[33] have reported no mortalities and only minimal morbidity following proximal femoral valvuloplasty and valvular transplantation procedures in more than 100 limbs. Deep vein thrombosis occurred in 7% of patients and usually was remote from the site of valvular repair. Symptomatic pulmonary emboli were not observed. Long-term results have been encouraging with the 2-year follow-up, demonstrating that more than 60% of patients have improved after valvuloplasty. Interestingly, the results of valvuloplasty from this group were approximately 20% better than the results for the valvular transplantation patients, although the difference was not statistically significant.

Because of its lower morbidity and mortality, elective venous reconstruction should be evaluated prospectively in the future. Establishing efficacy of operation will require additional clinical follow-up. Newer techniques and multiple valvular reconstructions also may be feasible in the future, contributing to improved results.[34]

REFERENCES

1. Rich NM, Hughes CW, Baugh JH. Management of venous injuries. Ann Surg 171:724, 1970.
2. Schramek A, Hashmonai M, Farbstein J, et al. Reconstructive surgery in major vein injuries in the extremities. J Trauma 15:9, 1975.
3. Rich NM, Hobson RW, Collins GJ, et al. The effect of acute popliteal venous interruption. Ann Surg 183:365, 1976.
4. Hobson RW, Yeager RA, Lynch TG, et al. Femoral venous trauma: Techniques for surgical management and early results. Am J Surg 146:220-224, 1983.
5. Bergan JJ, Yao JST. Venous Problems. Chicago: Year Book, 1978.
6. Hobson RW, Rich NM, Wright CB. Venous Trauma: Pathophysiology, Diagnosis, and Surgical Management. Mt. Kisco, N.Y.: Futura, 1983.
7. Makins GH. Gunshot Injuries to the Blood Vessels. Bristol, England: John Wright & Sons, 1919.
8. DeBakey ME, Simeone EA. Battle injuries of the arteries in World War II. Ann Surg 123:534, 1946.
9. Hughes CW. Acute vascular trauma in Korean War casualties. Surg Gynecol Obstet 99:91, 1954.
10. Spencer FC, Grewe RV. The management of arterial injuries in battle casualties. Ann Surg 141:304, 1955.
11. Rich NM, Hughes CW. Vietnam Vascular Registry: A preliminary report. Surgery 65:218, 1969.
12. Rich NM, Jarstfer BS, Geer TM. Popliteal arterial repair failure: Causes and possible prevention. J Cardiovasc Surg 15:340, 1974.
13. Wright CB, Swan KG. Hemodynamics of venous repair in the canine hindlimb. J Thorac Cardiovasc Surg 65:195, 1973.
14. Hobson RW, Howard EW, Wright CB, et al. Hemodynamics of canine femoral venous ligation: Significance in combined arterial and venous injuries. Surgery 78:824, 1973.
15. Schramek A, Hashmonai M. Vascular injuries in the extremities in battle casualties. Br J Surg 64:644, 1977.
16. Mullins RJ, Lucas CE, Ledgerwood AM. The natural history following venous ligation for civilian injuries. J Trauma 20:737-743, 1980.
17. Timberlake GA, O'Connell RC, Kerstein MD. Venous injury: To repair or ligate, the dilemma. J Vasc Surg 4:553, 1986.
18. Rich NM, Hobson RW, Wright CB, et al. Techniques of venous repair. In Swan KG, ed. Venous Surgery in the Lower Extremity. St. Louis: Warren H. Green, 1974.
19. Meyer J, Walsh J, Schuler J, et al. The early fate of venous repair after civilian vascular trauma. Ann Surg 206:458, 1987.
20. Saroyan RM, Kerstein MD. Role of concomitant venous repair in the management of extremity arterial injuries. In Ernst CB, Stanley JC, eds. Current Therapy in Vascular Surgery—2. Philadelphia: BC Decker, 1991.

21. Manno J, Hobson RW. Unpublished data, 1990.

22. Schramek A, Hashmonai M. Distal arteriovenous fistula for prevention of occlusion of venous interposition grafts to veins. J Cardiovasc Surg (Torino) 15:392, 1974.

23. Rich NM, Collins GJ, Andersen CA, et al. Autogenous venous interposition grafts in repair of major venous injuries. J Trauma 17:512-520, 1977.

24. Levin PM, Rich NM, Hutton JE, et al. Role of arteriovenous shunts in venous reconstruction. Am J Surg 122:183, 1971.

25. Hobson RW, Croom RD, Swan KG. Hemodynamics of the distal arteriovenous fistula in venous reconstruction. J Surg Res 14:483, 1973.

26. Hobson RW, Wright CB. Peripheral side-to-side arteriovenous fistula: Hemodynamics and application to venous reconstruction. Am J Surg 126:411, 1973.

27. Edwards WS. A-V fistula as a complementary or primary procedure for iliac venous occlusion. In Bergan JJ, Yao JST, eds. Surgery of the Veins. New York: Grune & Stratton, 1985.

28. Torngren S, Swedenberg J. Thrombectomy and temporary arteriovenous fistula for iliofemoral venous thrombosis. Int Angiol 7:14-18, 1988.

29. Hobson RW, Croom RD, Rich NM. Influence of heparin and low molecular weight dextran on the patency of autogenous vein grafts in the venous system. Ann Surg 178:773, 1973.

30. Hobson RW, Lee BC, Lynch TG, et al. Use of intermittent pneumatic compression of the calf in femoral venous reconstruction. Surg Gynecol Obstet 159: 284, 1984.

31. Kistner RL. Surgical repair of the incompetent femoral vein valve. Arch Surg 110:1336, 1975.

32. O'Donnell TF, Mackey WC, Shepard AD, et al. Clinical, hemodynamic and anatomic follow-up of direct venous reconstruction. Arch Surg 122:474, 1987.

33. Raju S, Fredericks R. Valve reconstruction procedures for nonobstructive venous insufficiency: Rationale, techniques, and results in 107 procedures with two- to eight-year follow-up. J Vasc Surg 7:301, 1988.

34. Taheri SA, Heffner R, Budd T, et al. Five years' experience with vein valve transplant. World J Surg 10: 935,1986.

35. Johnson ND, Queral LA, Flinn WR, et al. Late objective assessment of venous valve surgery. Arch Surg 116:1461, 1981.

36. Moore DJ, Himmel PD, Sumner DS. Distribution of venous valvular incompetence in patients with the postphlebitic syndrome. J Vasc Surg 3:49, 1986.

37. Shull KC, Nicolaides AN, Fernandez JF, et al. Significance of popliteal reflux in relation to ambulatory venous pressure and ulceration. Arch Surg 114:1304, 1979.

27

Complications of Sclerotherapy

John J. Bergan   **Mitchel P. Goldman**

The varix itself is to be punctured in as many places as circumstances may indicate.

HIPPOCRATES, 500 BC

Hippocrates admonished surgeons not to cut into varicose veins because large ulcers would result. Instead, he advocated multiple punctures of the varices with a slender rod of hot iron. Probably what was achieved was thrombosis of the vein following trauma and obliteration of the vein by subsequent, inevitable infection.

Six centuries later Galen advised tearing out tortuous veins by means of a hook. Further early advances in surgery of varicose veins were made by several physicians, including Paulus Aegineta, who described the Trendelenburg procedure 1200 years before Trendelenburg, and Albucasis who described varicose vein stripping in approximately 1100 AD.

Modern sclerotherapy was introduced as a treatment of varicose veins following the invention of the practical hypodermic syringe. Ochsner and Mahorner[1] in their much quoted monograph credit invention of the hypodermic syringe to Pravaz in 1851. Initially a wide variety of sclerosants were tried including perchloride of iron, iodotannin, iron chloride, and persulfate of iron. More familiar sclerosants used in the twentieth century include carbolic acid, 5% phenol, sodium salicylate (20%, 30%, and 40%), quinine, and urethan. After 1930, morrhuate sodium was the most popular sclerosant, but after 1946 sodium tetradecyl sulfate began to gain favor and was joined in recent years by hypertonic saline solution, polidocanol, and iodinated iodine.

Today, resurgence of interest in sclerotherapy is in part due to the fact that there is a growing belief that superficial venous disease should be treated. Assuming that superficial venous disease should be treated implies that there is a place for both surgery and injection treatment. There is not universal agreement on this point. However, our opinion is that if indications are present for treatment, the largest varicosities and their cause are best treated by surgery, whereas smaller varicosities and telangiectasias can be treated by sclerotherapy.

This chapter reviews the present techniques of sclerotherapy to clarify the causes of complications, to present ways to avoid them, and to offer treatment methods.

TYPES OF SCLEROTHERAPY

Much of the controversy about the role of sclerotherapy in the treatment of venous stasis disease arises from a confusion or lack of agreement about what is being discussed. Sclerotherapy to a gastroenterologist may mean treatment of esophageal varices, to an internist a variety of things, to a surgeon, especially a vascular surgeon, an obsolete treatment no longer in use, and to a dermatologist, the useful ablation of dermal telangiectasias.

In fact, in the treatment of lower extremity venous stasis disease, sclerotherapy has been used successfully to obliterate (1) axial veins including the greater and lesser saphenous veins, (2) clumps of large varicosities arising from tributaries to these two systems of superficial venous drainage, (3) reticular or connecting networks of veins that lie superficial to the membranous fascia, (4) reticular veins identified as the cause of dermal telangiectasia, and (5) superficial venectasias and telangiectasias.

When sclerotherapy is considered as a treatment option, those concerned should be in agreement about which system of veins is involved. Many types of veins are treated by sclerotherapy. A clear understanding of the results that can be achieved with sclerotherapy and its possible complications must be based on the knowledge of the types of veins treated.

Macrosclerotherapy of Axial Veins

Fegan's technique of sclerotherapy[2] has been referred to often in recent years. In brief, his technique, based on 16 years of practicing compression sclerotherapy, is fundamentally different from older methods in that the objective is to produce a short fibrous cord to replace the superficial vein at its junction with the probable perforating vein.[3]

A variation of Fegan's vein injection technique is now described as the French school of sclerotherapy. Tournay[4] has been credited with the development of this technique. The essence of this philosophy is sclerosis of high-pressure inflow points, for example, the greater saphenous vein at the incompetent saphenofemoral valve. This treatment, when successful, is followed by distal sclerotherapy from high to low. Tournay's method is logical in that proximal venous hypertension is cut off. Therefore distal sclerosis of varicose clusters or telangiectasias is more successful. In the United States this technique was advocated by researchers at the Mayo Clinic,[5] by de Takats and Quint[6] in Chicago, and more recently by Schultze-Ehrenburg[7] in Germany, who described a 48% failure rate with this technique at 3 and 5 years.

Sclerosis of Large Varices

Justification for sclerotherapy of large varicosities is based on the opinion that surgical therapy is too traumatic and anticosmetic. This belief is embodied in the remarks of Sigg,[8] the architect of the Swiss school of sclerotherapy:

Injection treatment is the method of choice when all involved veins of every size and location can be sclerosed, because there are few complications or side-effects and the patient can continue to work during the entire treatment. Furthermore, in most cases, surgical treatment necessitates hospitalization for up to one or two weeks and sometimes results in scars which are as troublesome as the original varices.

This, of course, is an outdated viewpoint. The Swiss form of sclerotherapy described in the writings of Dodd and Cockett[9] involves total ablation of varices without particular attention to axial vein reflux or perforator incompetence.

The attitude of most physicians using the various techniques described above is that a very small number of complications occur and results are quite durable. This is too optimistic a view. Prospective trials have now shown that the best results of sclerotherapy for large varicose veins are achieved below the knee where the varices and their cause, the incompetent perforating veins, can be subjected to prolonged, effective compression following accurate sclerosis. These trials have also indicated that incompetence of the long and short saphenous veins and varicosities in the thigh are best treated surgically.[10-12]

As recurrence of varicosities can be considered a complication of sclerotherapy, it should be noted that successful sclerotherapy of the saphenofemoral junction is difficult[13] and results are not durable.

Microsclerotherapy

Modern treatment of telangiectasias began in the early 1930s when Biegeleisen[14] described microsclerotherapy. Physicians who followed Biegeleisen's lead were disappointed with the results of injection with morrhuate sodium. Microsclerotherapy languished until the 1970s, when a spate of publications described better results with the use of different sclerosing solutions.[15-18] Recently treatment outcomes have improved as a result of more accurate cannulation of vascular lesions by disposable, fine-gauge needles and injection of less caustic sclerosing solutions including hypertonic saline solution, diluted sodium tetradecyl sulfate, polidocanol, and chromated glycerin.

With increasing experience it is now recognized that telangiectasias under high pressure are less responsive to sclerotherapy. These include those telangiectasias connected to underlying reticular veins or those that have a rapid refilling time after compression, are red in color, and probably connected to arteriolar loops.[19] Furthermore, some telangiectatic veins of the lower extremity are connected to varicose veins or underlying incompetent deep veins through direct or indirect tributaries. This source of telangiectatic hypertension defeats therapy as has been elegantly demonstrated by Faria and de Moraes[20] of São Paulo.

TECHNIQUES OF SCLEROTHERAPY

Complications of sclerotherapy are linked to technique and solution used (Table 27-1). Complications are minimized by the physician's familiarity with the sclerotherapy technique he uses. In general, large veins are best injected after applying the empty vein technique, in which the vein is emptied of blood by proximal stroking or by leg elevation. In addition, Orbach[21] advocated injecting sclerosant foam rather than sclerosant itself or even clearing the vein by preliminary injection of air. Telangiectasias need no such emptying or clearing.

With regard to sclerosing solutions used, the concentration of solution should be the greatest at the highest point of reflux being treated and in the largest veins being treated. For veins in the proximal and middle thirds of the thigh, 1% sodium tetradecyl is recommended. One milliliter of the solution can be used proximally and 0.5 ml distally.

In microsclerotherapy, a number of principles apply. Preliminary rubbing of the skin with alcohol to cause vasodilatation of the telangiectasia and to enhance visualization by clearing keratin and increasing the refraction index is recommended. Many sclerotherapists use magnifiers of 2.5 to 5 power. Further vasodilatation

can be achieved by having the patient stand before assuming the reverse Trendelenburg position used during injection.

Current practice calls for the use of a disposable No. 30 needle. Finer needles with increased flexibility are available. Sclerosant should be placed within the vessel rather than intradermally. Vessel cannulation is facilitated by stretching the skin, keeping the skin taut, and placing the needle only in the upper dermis within the telangiectasia (Fig. 27-1).

Concentration of solution used for telangiectasias is important. Sodium tetradecyl sulfate, 0.1% to 0.2%, is favored, and, once approved by the Food and Drug Administration (FDA) for use in the United States, polidocanol, 0.25% to 0.5%, can be used. The amount of solution that should be injected varies among authorities. In theory, the amount of fluid injected should not be enough to travel undiluted into the deep venous system. A more practical consideration is limiting the amount of solution to that which can produce an obliteration of the

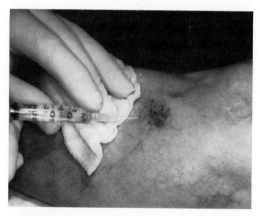

Fig. 27-1. Many of the complications of microsclerotherapy can be prevented with proper technique. This includes injecting dilute solutions through a No. 30 needle, minimizing extravasation by low-pressure injection, discontinuing injection when a skin wheal appears, and limiting the amount of injection placed in any one area. Injection into a telangiectatic mass clearly demonstrates the reticular veins that are associated with the mass and that should be obliterated if a lasting successful result is to be expected.

telangiectasia for a distance of 1 to 2 cm around the point of injection. Another rule is never to use more than 0.5 ml in order to avoid an excessive inflammatory reaction. When hypertonic saline solution is used as a sclerosant, the amount of fluid injected should be limited to 0.1 ml in order to minimize a stinging sensation and muscular cramping.

The final principle is to avoid excessive force while injecting telangiectasias, which may cause fragile vessels to rupture, resulting in extravasation of solution and blood.

COMPLICATIONS AND ADVERSE REACTIONS

As with any interventional therapy, complications and adverse sequelae of sclerotherapy are to be expected (Table 27-1), although they can be minimized.

Pain

Pain is perhaps the most feared and least problematic of the complications of sclerotherapy. Development of disposable fine needles (No. 30) and use of dilute sclerosant solutions, some of which have anesthetic properties, have eliminated pain as a cause of patient dissatisfaction. In fact, three variables enter into the equation of patient pain during sclerotherapy: location of the injection, patient perception of pain, and solution used. Traditionally, several areas have been identified as being subject to more pain than others (ankles, upper medial thigh,

and the anteromedial knee area) and the sclerotherapist can prepare the patient for the possibility of experiencing some pain if the injection is to be made in a pain-sensitive site. However, injection into other sites can unpredictably elicit a painful response.

Patient perception of pain, as all physicians know, is highly variable, quite individual, and totally unpredictable. Apart from psychologic support, presentation of an attitude of confidence, and establishment of proper rapport, there is little that a physician can do to modify this variable.

The third element in the pain equation is the solution used. Hypertonic solutions are notorious for causing pain on injection. Extravascular instillation of hypertonic solution causes stinging, and flow of hypertonic solution into muscular vessels causes cramping. Although it is uncertain exactly what mechanism is invoked with such pain, vascular spasm may play a part. The muscle cramping is dependent on flow of the hypertonic solution into vessels supplying or draining the deep musculature.

Another important factor in pain during sclerotherapy is the presence of cutaneous sensory nerves adjacent to the vessel being penetrated. It is well known that telangiectatic blemishes can produce pain, especially when the patient is subjected to venous hypertension during sitting and standing occupations.[22] It is not surprising then that the needle can produce a painful response as it brushes past or pene-

Table 27-1. Complications of Sclerotherapy

Complication	Sodium tetradecyl sulfate	Hypertonic saline solution	Polidocanol
Pain	Mild	Moderate	None
Edema	Infrequent	Occasional	Infrequent
Urticaria	Occasional	Occasional	Occasional
Angioneogenesis		Related to patient hormonal status	
Pigmentation	Frequent	Occasional	Infrequent
Recurrence		Related to persistent venous hypertension, other factors	
Ulceration	Occasional	Occasional	Rare
Allergic reactions	Rare	None	Very rare
Thrombophlebitis		Dose dependent, affected by technique	
Arterial injection		Determined by location of injection	

trates the cutaneous nerve. Sclerotherapists have noted that a particularly painful blemish, when obliterated by sclerotherapy by a painful injection, will disappear with complete pain relief. The needle caused pain at the cutaneous nerve, which in turn had been stimulated chronically by the blemish.

The pain response to sclerotherapy can be modified by the use of fine-gauge needles, dilute solutions, and avoidance of hypertonic solutions. Furthermore, limiting the volume of injectate to 0.1 to 0.5 ml per injection will prevent vascular overdistention.

Some sclerotherapists add local anesthetic agents to hypertonic solutions to decrease the pain of injection. For example, 2 ml of 2% or 4% lidocaine can be added to 28 ml of 23.4% hypertonic saline solution. This may reduce pain during injection without affecting the sclerosant properties of the solution. However, with this practice there is an increased potential for eliciting an allergic reaction.

Of the sclerosing solutions available, only two can be administered painlessly: polidocanol and sodium tetradecyl sulfate. In fact, sodium tetradecyl sulfate is pain-free only when it is injected into a vessel lumen and when it is very dilute; perivascular injection causes a stinging sensation. In a prospective study of pain response, it was found that patients preferred injection with polidocanol over treatment with other agents.[23]

None of the techniques advocated above decreases the mild posttreatment soreness, which lasts 3 to 7 days following injection. This discomfort has not been particularly troublesome but has been noted in as many as 20% of patients.[24]

Swelling and Edema

Whereas patients fear pain as a consequence of sclerotherapy, physicians fear deep vein thrombosis and pulmonary embolization. Edema, at worst, may be caused by such deep vein thrombosis. In practice, edema is usually the result of prolonged venospasm, which decreases extremity outflow in the posttreatment period.[25] Also, the use of overly concentrated sclerosing solutions or hypertonic solutions causes edema. These solutions increase the postsclero-

therapy inflammatory reaction, which in turn induces histamine release and liberation of vascular mediators, which increase endothelial permeability.

Distal edema occurs in a very small number of sclerotherapy patients, perhaps less than 10%.[26] Some edema is produced by improper bandaging. When tighter compression is applied proximally, a tourniquet effect may be produced; care must be taken to avoid this result. When elastic stockings are used, the tourniquet effect seems to be less of a problem. Distal edema can be decreased by increasing compression time beyond the usual 18 hours to 72 hours.[27]

A second form of tissue swelling, skin wheals, is found after perivascular injection. A small amount of sclerosant solution inadvertently injected perivascularly will induce tremendous fluid inpouring into the area. Such skin wheal edema or swelling can be decreased by the application of a compression dressing and/or a potent topical corticosteroid immediately after sclerotherapy.

Urticaria

Localized itching is a consequence of sclerotherapy and is apparently unavoidable. Assuming that this itching is an allergic reaction is an error: hypertonic saline solution produces this response and it is inconceivable that hypertonic saline solution could produce an allergic reaction.

Common to the use of all sclerosing solutions is the development of an inflammatory reaction. This is inseparably linked to localized urticaria and at the molecular level may be caused by the release of endothelial or platelet-derived factors related in turn to destruction of endothelial cells. This inflammatory reaction may also be caused by stimulation of perivascular mast cells with release of histamine. Although polidocanol is a known anesthetic agent, its use is accompanied by significant urticaria.[28]

Although some have recommended the application of ice to decrease itching and others have advocated the use of corticosteroid creams, simple compression decreases itching sufficiently and is effective in the majority of patients.

Angioneogenesis (Matting)

Although the appearance of new blood vessels following excision of varicose veins in the lower extremities is acknowledged by surgeons, the cause is unknown. A similar phenomenon occurs after sclerotherapy. This complication is understandably disturbing to the patient, who expects treated telangiectasias to disappear and who does not expect the appearance of new unsightly blood vessels.

Because this complication is common, it has been given a number of names, including distal angioplasia, telangiectatic matting,[24] and neoangiogenesis. It has been linked to exogenous estrogen administration and has not been seen in men receiving sclerotherapy. This latter fact is controversial because very few men present for sclerotherapy.[26] The anteromedial aspect of the thighs is an area of predisposition for telangiectatic matting; risk factors include obesity, exogenous use of estrogens, and pregnancy.[27] It may be related to increasing concentration of sclerosant[28] or to the degree of inflammation and intraluminal thrombus formation.[29]

Some have thought that the phenomenon is not true neoangiogenesis but instead a dilation of existing subclinical blood vessels, which then act as collateral flow through arteriovenous anastomoses. Thus it may represent a normal reparative phenomenon, a healing response to trauma, as described by Folkman and Ingber.[30] The hypothesis that telangiectatic matting is actually the opening up of new blood vessels after occlusion of neighboring vessels is viable and coincides with several observations of similar phenomena.[31]

Research on angiogenesis is relevant in areas as varied as tumor growth, diabetic retinopathy, and fundamental formation of the atherosclerotic plaque.[32] If angiogenesis is the actual phenomenon and not simply an opening up of subclinical blood vessels, such research may be pertinent. It is thought that angiogenic factors act either directly on the endothelium or indirectly by mobilization of mast cells and macrophages, which then act as helper cells. If the angiogenic factors act indirectly, then the mast cells and macrophages release endothelial growth factors, new capillaries sprout from the sides of vessels, and endothelial cells degrade the basement membrane. The endothelial cells then migrate towards the angiogenic source, proliferate, form a lumen, and manufacture a new basement membrane. Destruction of outflow, which is, of course, the end result of successful sclerotherapy, is one of the most important factors contributing to this chain of events.[33-35]

Certainly sclerotherapy provides the needed stimulus for neoangiogenesis,[36] and for this reason it is surprising that the incidence of this complication is not higher.

Unfortunately, heparin has been demonstrated to be instrumental in promoting endothelial proliferation in vitro and angiogenesis in vivo. Heparin is important because of its affinity to growth factors and is linked to hypersensitivity reactions in man.[37]

To prevent neoangiogenesis, the angiogenic stimulus should be decreased by limiting as much as possible the degree of inflammation. This may be achieved by decreasing solution concentration and by selecting the most dilute solution possible for each vessel to be treated. In addition, limiting the quantity of the injection may reduce endothelial damage and lessen the stimulus to angiogenesis. Furthermore, the incidence of neoangiogenesis is decreased when the pressure of the injection is minimized and limited to an area 1 cm around the injection site.[38] Not all authorities agree with this concept; some inject as much as 3 ml in each site.[39]

Because estrogens are linked to neoangiogenesis, it might be important to note that spider angiomas develop during pregnancy, resolve after delivery, and are known to occur in patients with hepatic cirrhosis.[40,41] Disappearance of leg telangiectasia has been identified in one patient who was receiving tamoxifen therapy for an estrogen receptor–positive breast carcinoma. However, estrogen receptors have not been demonstrated in biopsies from leg telangiectasia.[42]

Fortunately, neoangiogenesis usually resolves spontaneously over a period of 3 to 12 months. If it persists, pulsed-dye laser therapy can be used.[43] Otherwise, telangiectatic matting is commonly resistant to treatment.

Postsclerotherapy Pigmentation

Pigment deposited in the dermis commonly occurs with skin inflammation. It develops as streaks over veins that have been subjected to thrombophlebitis in the gaiter area in patients with severe chronic venous insufficiency and has been regarded as the indication of a previous episode of inflammation in that area. Because in venous stasis disease the pigment deposited has been shown to be hemosiderin, it has been assumed that postsclerotherapy pigmentation is also hemosiderin and not melanin. Distinction between the two pigmentations is important: hemosiderin pigmentation cannot be treated with bleaching agents, whereas melanin hyperpigmentation may be so treated. Postsclerotherapy pigmentation has been reported in as many as 30% of patients treated with sodium tetradecyl sulfate[44] with a similar frequency in patients treated with hypertonic saline solution[45,46] and in 10% to 30% of patients treated with polidocanol.[26,47]

Some clinical observations relate to the probable cause. Postsclerotherapy hyperpigmentation has been noted to be more frequent in vessels treated below the knee, which leads to the conclusion that presclerotherapy venous hypertension plays a part in causing postsclerotherapy hyperpigmentation. French phlebologists whose practice commonly includes sclerotherapy of the greater saphenous vein to obliterate saphenofemoral reflux have observed that postsclerotherapy hyperpigmentation occurs in vessels that are treated before closure of the saphenofemoral junction, again lending weight to the argument that pretreatment venous hypertension contributes to posttreatment pigmentation[48] (Fig. 27-2).

Further clinical observations suggest that in addition to the gravitational effects of venous hypertension, an increased incidence of pigmentation occurs when blue venectasias are treated as opposed to those that are red.[19]

Predisposition to pigmentation has been

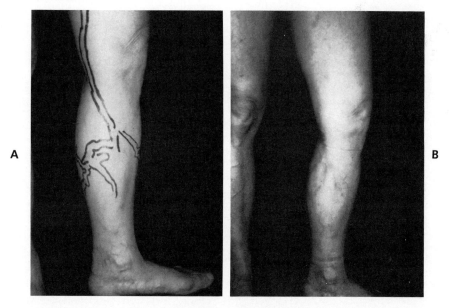

Fig. 27-2. A, Preoperative view of the greater saphenous vein and its varicose tributaries. **B,** Postoperative view. It was elected to limit the amount of operative stripping to the region between the saphenofemoral junction and the joint crease posterior to the knee. The distal remaining varicose veins were then injected. Cutaneous pigmentation following such injection is clearly identified. Although this is an unwanted consequence of the sclerotherapy, such pigmentation can be expected to fade within a period of weeks to months.

noted but not proven in patients who are of Japanese origin, dark haired, and who have red-toned skin, but no accurate data are available in this regard.

Most significant is the fact that pigmentation occurs in association with entrapped blood after sclerotherapy. Blood becomes entrapped when ingress and egress of blood from treated vessels is sealed off by the effects of the sclerotherapy. The remaining, formerly oxygenated blood loses its oxygenation, becomes totally desaturated, and turns blue-black or green in color as red cells leak per diapedesis through the ischemic vascular wall[49] (Fig. 27-3). Many researchers believe that such vessels should be incised and the contained semiliquid coagula expressed externally to decrease postsclerotherapy pigmentation. It is thought that, in the absence of drainage of trapped intravascular blood, the treated vessel will recanalize and reform. Incision and drainage is performed optimally 2 to 4 weeks after treatment, but liquid-entrapped blood can be expressed as late as 4 to 8 weeks following sclerotherapy. Some physicians extract the liquid blood by means of needle aspiration using No. 16 to No. 18 needles. However, this is less efficient than open incision with a No. 11 blade.

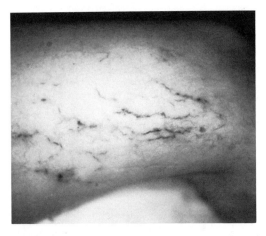

Fig. 27-3. Consequences of sclerosis using undiluted solutions with inadequate compression. The site of entrapped blood and small areas of cutaneous necrosis can be identified. Early pigmentation is apparent where red blood cells have escaped the lumen of vessels per diapedesis or per rhexis.

Histologic study to determine the cause of pigmentation has been fruitful. Two excellent studies have demonstrated that the pigmentation is a complication secondary to hemosiderin deposition. Hemosiderin was found in the superficial dermis and also in the periadnexal and middermal location, especially in the region of the ankle.[50,51] Such studies confirm the fact that pigmentation occurs when red blood cells extravasate into the dermis following escape of the cells per rhexis during injection of the blood vessel or per diapedesis in response to abnormal vascular wall permeability following sclerotherapy.

The natural history of postsclerotherapy pigmentation is important to understand. Despite therapeutic attempts, pigmentation lasts for many months and in some patients for more than a year. It should be recognized that pretreatment pigmentation will persist over the staining produced by sclerotherapy.

Avoidance of postsclerotherapy pigmentation depends on the type of solution used, pressure and amount of injection, and existence of venous hypertension. Polidocanol seems to produce the least pigmentation and sodium tetradecyl sulfate the most, with hypertonic saline solution causing some pigmentation. Chromated glycerin has not been observed to cause pigmentation.

Pressure of injection should be minimized to prevent rupture of the vessel and extravasation of red cells. Postsclerotherapy compression should be applied to diminish efflux of red cells from the treated vessel. A reduction in venous hypertension may be achieved by eliminating proximal escape points either by surgery or sclerotherapy before distal injections are performed. Also, elimination of the reticular veins that feed skin telangiectasias may diminish the chance of pigmentation developing.

Other than avoiding the causes of pigmentation, little can be done once pigmentation occurs. Because the pigmentation is hemosiderin and not melanin, bleaching agents that affect melanocytic function are ineffective. Trichloroacetic acid or phenolate may hasten the apparent resolution of pigmentation by desquamation of skin overlying the pigmentation. This carries a risk of scarring, permanent hypopigmentation, or even postinflammatory hyperpigmentation.

It is possible that topical retinoic acid may enhance resolution of pigmentation, but confirmation of such enhanced fibroblastic removal of hemosiderin has not been obtained histologically. Similarly, chelation of the iron deposition is an attractive possibility. Although success has been reported in use of ointments containing ethylenediaminetetraacetic acid (EDTA), the studies done have been uncontrolled and no confirmatory data are available.

Recurrence

In general, sclerotherapy has achieved a bad reputation because of a high incidence of recurrence of treated vessels. Indeed, the estimated recurrence rate ranges from 20% to 100%.[2] As indicated above, recanalization of initially thrombosed veins is one mechanism that allows return of the lesion being treated.[49] Another cause is inadequate compression, which contributes to thrombus formation, which in turn allows recanalization. The importance of draining postsclerotherapy-entrapped blood has been emphasized by many researchers, including Sigg,[52] Hobbs,[53] and Orbach.[54] Orbach has said that when high recurrence rates are reported following sclerotherapy, the patients were treated with inadequate compression.

Cutaneous Ulceration

Good results in sclerotherapy cannot be achieved if skin ulceration is produced. Such cutaneous necrosis may be caused by extravasation of the caustic sclerosant solution into perivascular tissue or injection of the solution into the arteriolar component of the telangiectatic mass. Related to this latter event is the associated vasospasm affecting the arterial supply to a localized area.

Perivascular injection is an unwanted but unavoidable complication of sclerotherapy. A small quantity of the solution inevitably will find its way into the perivascular tissue, either as a consequence of the injection or as the needle is being withdrawn. Late leakage of solution from the vessel after injection is also a possibility, as is rupture of the vessel during injection if excessive, or even normal, pressure is exerted.

Goldman et al.[55] has used the rabbit ear model to investigate necrosis produced by varying concentrations of commonly used sclerosant solutions. His elegant study revealed that the control agent, bacteriostatic normal saline solution, and polidocanol in concentrations of 0.25%, 0.5%, and 1% did not produce cutaneous necrosis. In contrast, hypertonic saline solution 23.4% and sodium tetradecyl sulfate 0.5% both caused focal dermal necrosis. In addition, hypertonic saline solution produced middermal and adnexal necrosis. The advantage of polidocanol was clearly demonstrated, which confirms its clinical utility already proved by extensive use in Europe.

Various hypertonic solutions have been shown to produce necrosis in the experimental model[55] and the observations described above have been confirmed by other investigators as well.[56,57] Clinical and experimental observations have shown that cutaneous telangiectasias are closely related to dermal arterioles.[58] Histologic observation of skin infarction following sclerotherapy confirms that sclerosants actually reach this dermal arteriole during injection. Wedge-shaped infarcts in the skin have been observed on biopsy.[59] They are inseparably linked to arteriolar thrombosis, which produces the necrosis.

Skin necrosis may be prevented by limiting the concentration of the sclerosant and decreasing the volume injected. Furthermore, careful observation of the injection site for abnormal vasospasm is valuable. When the skin appears to be ivory white, like the appearance of a finger during severe Raynaud's arteriospasm, danger is imminent. If this state is allowed to progress through its natural evolution, a hemorrhagic bulla will appear within 24 hours, which in turn, will eventually develop into an ulceration.

The initial cutaneous reaction is the result of arterial spasm. This may represent the inadvertent filling of a dermal arteriole with the sclerosant solution. Quick infiltration of the area with 1% lidocaine will block the vasospasm. Massage of the affected area will also stimulate vasodilatation.

In addition to noting an ivory white blanching of the peri-injection skin, the detection of a cyanotic appearance of a developing wheal is important. This sign should trigger the alert clinician to infiltrate the area with dilute lidocaine to decrease vasospasm. The cyanotic appearance of the wheal is caused by desaturation of blood as it flows slowly through the area affected by vasospasm.

To a lesser extent, excessive compression also plays a role in the production of cutaneous necrosis. This is avoided by careful bandaging and application of correctly fitted stockings.

Allergic Reactions and Anaphylaxis

A variety of allergic, hypersensitive, anaphylactoid responses may be caused by sclerotherapy. Of these, anaphylaxis is potentially the most serious and the most feared. Anaphylaxis is a systemic hypersensitivity response caused by exposure or re-exposure to a sensitizing substance. It may be IgE-mediated, a mast cell activation reaction, or related to other classes of immunoglobulin such as IgG.[60] The sclerotherapist must be prepared for this reaction simply because the incidence of anaphylaxis increases with repeated exposures to any antigen.[61]

All physicians practicing sclerotherapy should know the principal manifestations of anaphylaxis: airway edema, bronchospasm, and vascular collapse.[62] Anaphylaxis affects areas where mast cell concentrations are the highest: skin, lungs, and gastrointestinal tract. Histamine release is a part of the clinical manifestation; urticaria and abdominal pain are common. Urticaria alone does not constitute an anaphylactoid reaction and should not be treated as such. The earliest manifestations of anaphylaxis are subtle and include anxiety, sneezing, coughing, urticaria, and itching. Angioedema may appear. As bronchospasm develops, wheezing results. Accompanying hoarseness will indicate laryngeal edema.

If anaphylaxis is suspected, the initial treatment is 0.2 to 0.5 ml of 1:1000 epinephrine given subcutaneously. This may be repeated three to four times at 5- to 15-minute intervals to maintain a systolic blood pressure above 90 to 100 mm Hg. An intravenous line should be established and diphenhydramine hydrochloride (50 mg) given with cimetidine (300 mg). Oxygen should be supplied at 4 to 6 L/min and

an endotracheal tube or tracheostomy should be readied. Either of these must be used if upper airway obstruction develops.

Bronchospasm sufficient to produce pronounced wheezing can be treated by intravenous theophylline. A rapid increase in extravascular volume occurs during anaphylaxis and must be replaced intravenously. Colloid is not more effective than crystalloid and rapid administration of 1 to 2 L of Ringer's lactate solution is important in initial therapy. If bronchospasm persists, isoproterenol may be useful as a pure β-adrenergic agonist and bronchodilator. The β_2-adrenergic effects of this drug cause vasodilatation and possible hypotension, especially in those with depleted blood volume.

Administration of corticosteroids should be considered in patients with the most severe reactions, hypotension, and shock. There is no clear evidence that dictates the appropriate dose, but 1 gm of hydrocortisone or its equivalent is appropriate for severe cardiopulmonary collapse. When hypotension is resistant to treatment, sodium bicarbonate, 0.5 to 1 mEq/kg, should be given and acid-base values should be assessed regularly. Needless to say, laryngeal edema is an immediate problem that must be considered and treated before other therapy is instituted.

Thrombophlebitis

In the past, sclerotherapy was referred to as thrombotherapy by wags who noted the frequency of superficial thrombophlebitis after injection of varicose veins. In fact, this complication is no joke. It may be a significant cause of morbidity following sclerotherapy of veins larger than 3 to 4 mm in diameter. The importance of this complication is minimized by sclerotherapists, perhaps because it does not occur frequently following injection of telangiectasias, which is the disease manifestation treated by many sclerotherapists.

Localized superficial thrombophlebitis following sclerotherapy is identical clinically to that which occurs spontaneously, develops following intravenous therapy, or occurs in patients with intravenous substance abuse. It is characterized by inflammation, calor, rubor, tumor, and dolor. Its frequency following sclerotherapy can be diminished by decreasing the concentration of sclerosant, applying effective compression, and avoiding sclerosis of large veins.

Large veins may be an indication for obliteration by injection if they occur in the aged, infirm, or in patients following surgical removal of varices. If large veins are to be injected, proper technique must be followed. Careful bandaging, wrapping, or stocking application is essential. An empty vein after sclerotherapy is not likely to be the site of superficial thrombophlebitis.

Treatment of postsclerotherapy thrombophlebitis is symptomatic and this includes local compression, moist heat, prescription of nonsteroidal anti-inflammatory drugs, and rest. Anticoagulation is unnecessary unless the thrombophlebitis is ascending to a patent saphenofemoral junction. Deep vein thrombosis must be treated with anticoagulation.

If possible, early superficial thrombophlebitis should be aborted by draining entrapped blood from those veins in which fluid blood remains after compression sclerotherapy. This maneuver, followed by a brief period of effective compression, has been found useful in most cases.

Arterial Injection

Though rare, the consequences of sclerosant reaching a peripheral artery can be devastating. Browse, Burnand, and Lea Thomas[63] have described the clinical findings of intra-arterial injection: intense burning pain, paresthesias, extreme pallor followed ultimately by mottling, thrombosis of dermal vessels, and gangrene (Fig. 27-4). In the few cases that have been reported in the literature, this complication most commonly occurs following injections in the region of the medial malleolus, especially in the territory of the posterior tibial artery. Another location where this has reportedly occurred is the saphenofemoral junction following attempts to sclerose the greater saphenous vein. Whereas injections into the posterior tibial artery territory result in malleolar or Syme amputations, injections into the arterial system at the level of the saphenofemoral junction result in above-knee amputation. It is

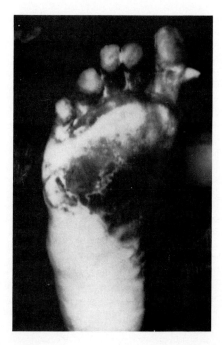

Fig. 27-4. The rare complication of distal gangrene following clear intravenous sclerotherapy at the ankle. Reflux of the sclerosant past the capillary barrier and into the posterior tibial arterial circulation is thought to be the mechanism invoked in this case.

thought that the pathway of sclerosant reaching main arterial flow is through the external pudendal artery, which is in close proximity to the saphenous vein and femoral vein.[63]

REFERENCES

1. Ochsner A, Mahorner H. Varicose Veins. St. Louis: CV Mosby, 1939.
2. Fegan WG. Varicose Veins. Springfield, Ill.: Charles C Thomas, 1967. (Reprinted by Vascular Products, Ltd., Bristol, 1990.)
3. Fegan WG. Treatment of varicose veins by injection-compression: A method practised in Eire. In Hobbs JT, ed. The Treatment of Venous Disorders. Lancaster, England: MTP Press, 1977, pp 99-112.
4. Tournay R, et al. La Sclerose des Varices, 4th ed. Paris: L'Expansion Scientifique Francaise, 1985.
5. Heyerdale WW, Stalker LK. Management of varicose veins of the lower extremities. Ann Surg 114:1042-1049, 1941.
6. de Takats G, Quint H. The injection treatment of varicose veins. Surg Gynecol Obstet 50:545-561, 1930.
7. Schultze-Ehrenburg U. Doppler kontrollierte verodungsbehandlung der Vena saphena magna. Phlebologie Proktologie 13:117-122, 1984.

8. Sigg K. Treatment of varicose veins by injection-sclerotherapy: A method practised in Switzerland. In Hobbs JT, ed. The Treatment of Venous Disorders. Lancaster, England: MTP Press, 1977, pp 113-137.

9. Dodd H, Cockett FB. Pathology & Surgery of the Veins of the Lower Limbs. Edinburgh: E.S. Livingstone, 1956.

10. Hobbs JT. Surgery and sclerotherapy for varicose veins: 10-year result of randomized trial. In Tesi M, Dormandy J, eds. Superficial & Deep Venous Diseases of the Lower Limbs. Milan: Minerva Medica, 1984.

11. Jakobsen BH. Value of different forms of treatment for varicose veins. Br J Surg 66:182, 1979.

12. Neglen P, Einarsson E, Jousson B, et al. Socio-economic benefits of ambulatory surgery and compression sclerotherapy of varicose veins. In Negus D, Jantet G, eds. Phlebology '85. London: John Libbey, 1986.

13. Quill RD, Fegan WG. Reversibility of femorosaphenous reflux. Br J Surg 55:389-393, 1971.

14. Biegeleisen HI. Telangiectasia associated with varicose veins treated by a microinjection technique. JAMA 102:2092-2094, 1934.

15. Foley WT. The eradication of venous blemishes. Cutis 15:665-668, 1975.

16. Alderman DB. Therapy for essential cutaneous telangiectasias. Postgrad Med 61:91-95, 1977.

17. Goldman P. Polidocanol for sclerotherapy of superficial venules and telangiectasias. J Dermatol Surg Oncol 2:204-209, 1989.

18. Shields JL, Jansen GT. Therapy for superficial telangiectasias of the lower extremities. J Dermatol Surg Oncol 8:857-860, 1982.

19. Merlen JF. Telangiectasies rouge, telangiectasies bleues. Phlebologie 22:167-174, 1970.

20. Faria JL, de Moraes IN. Histopathology of the telangiectasias associated with varicose veins. Dermatologia 127:321-329, 1963.

21. Orbach EJ. Sclerotherapy of varicose veins: Utilization of intravenous air block. Am J Surg 66:362-364, 1944.

22. Weiss RA, Weiss MA. Resolution of pain associated with varicose to telangiectatic leg veins after compression sclerotherapy. J Dermatol Surg Oncol 16:333-336, 1990.

23. Carlin MC, Ratz JL. Treatment of telangiectasia: Comparison of sclerosing agents. J Dermatol Surg Oncol 13:1181-1184, 1987.

24. Duffy DM. Small vessel sclerotherapy: An overview. Adv Dermatol 3:221-242, 1988.

25. Wilson MG. A method of treatment of varicose veins. Lancet 1:1273-1275, 1953.

26. Goldman P. Sclerotherapy of superficial venules and telangiectasias of the lower extremities. Dermatol Clin 5:369-379, 1987.

27. Goldman MP, Beaudoing D, Marley W, Lopez L, Butie A. Compression in the treatment of leg telangiectasia: A preliminary report. J Dermatol Surg Oncol 16:322-325, 1990.

28. Norris MJ, Carlin MC, Ratz JL. Treatment of essential telangiectasia: Effects of increasing concentrations of polidocanol. J Am Acad Dermatol 20:643-649, 1989.

29. Ouvry PA, Davy A. Le traitement sclerosant des telangiectasies des membres inferieurs. Phlebologie 35:349-359, 1982.

30. Folkman J, Ingber D. Angiostatic steroids. Ann Surg 206:374-383, 1987.

31. Biegeleisen K. Primary lower extremity telangiectasias: Relationship of size to color. Angiology 38:760-768, 1987.

32. Shing Y, Folkman J, Haudenschild CC, Lund D, Crum R, Klagsbrun M. Angiogenesis is stimulated by tumor-derived endothelial cell growth factor. J Cell Biochem 29:275-287, 1985.

33. Ashton N. Corneal vascularization. In Duke-Elder S, Perkins ES, eds. The Transparency of the Cornea. Oxford: Blackwell, 1960.

34. Haudenschild CC. Growth control of endothelial cells in atherogenesis and tumor angiogenesis. In Altura BM, ed. Advances in Microcirculation, vol. 9. Basel: Karger, 1980, pp 226-251.

35. Folkman J, Klagsbrun M. Angiogenic factors. Science 235:442-447, 1987.

36. Barnhill RL, Wolf JE Jr. Angiogenesis and the skin. J Am Acad Dermatol 16:1226-1242, 1987.

37. Dvorak AM, Mihm MC Jr, Dvorak HF. Morphology of delayed-type hypersensitivity reactions in man. II. Ultrastructural alterations affecting the microvasculature and the tissue mast cells. Lab Invest 34:179, 1976.

38. Mantse L. More on spider veins. J Dermatol Surg Oncol 12:1022-1023, 1986.

39. Lary BG. Varicose veins and intracutaneous telangiectasia: Combined treatment in 1500 cases. South Med J 80:1105-1110, 1987.

40. Bean WB. The vascular spider in pregnancy. In Bean WB, ed. Vascular Spiders and Related Lesions of the Skin. Springfield, Ill.: Charles C Thomas, 1958, pp 59-78.

41. Pirovino M, Linder R, Ross CH, et al. Cutaneous spider nevi in liver cirrhosis: Capillary microscopical and hormonal investigation. Klin Wochenschr 66:298-302, 1988.

42. Sadick NS, Niedt GW. A study of estrogen and progesterone receptors in spider telangiectasias of the lower extremities. J Dermatol Surg Oncol 16:7, 1990.

43. Goldman MP, Fitzpatrick RE. Pulsed-dye laser treatment of leg telangiectasias. J Dermatol Surg Oncol 16:338-344, 1990.

44. Tournay PR. Traitment sclerosant des tres fines varicosites intra ou saous-dermiques. Soc Fran Phlebo 19:235-241, 1966.

45. Bodian EL. Techniques of sclerotherapy for sunburst venous blemishes. J Dermatol Surg Oncol 11:696-704, 1985.

46. Alderman DB. Surgery and sclerotherapy in the treatment of varicose veins. Conn Med 39:467-471, 1975.

47. Cacciatore E. Experience of sclerotherapy with aethoxysklerol. Minerva Cardioangiol 27:255-262, 1979.

48. Chatard H. Discussion de la question of J-C Allart: Pigmentations post-sclerotherapiques. Phlebologie 29:211-216, 1976.

49. Orbach EJ. The importance of removal of postinjection coagula during the course of sclerotherapy of varicose veins. Vasa 3:475-477, 1974.

50. Cuttell PJ, Fox JA. The etiology and treatment of varicose pigmentation. Phlebologie 35:387-389, 1982.

51. Goldman MP, Kaplan RP, Duffy DM. Post-sclerotherapy hyperpigmentation: A histologic evaluation. Dermatol Surg Oncol 13:547-550, 1987.

52. Sigg K. Varizenverodung am hochgelgerten Bien. Deutsches Arzteblatt—Arztliche Mitteilungen. 69. Jahrange, Heft 14, S. 809-818, 6 April 1972, Postverlagsort Koln.

53. Hobbs JT. The management of recurrent and residual veins. Stoke Mandeveille Hospital Symposium. The treatment of varicose veins by injection and compression. Oct. 15, 1971, pp 28-31.

54. Orbach EJ. A new approach to the sclerotherapy of varicose veins. Angiology 1:302-305, 1950.

55. Goldman MP, Kaplan RP, Oki LN, Bennet RG, Strick A. Extravascular effects of sclerosants in rabbit skin: A clinical and histologic examination. J Dermatol Surg Oncol 12:1085-1088, 1986.

56. Reiner L. The activity of anionic surface active compounds in producing vascular obliteration. Proc Soc Exp Biol Med 62:49-54, 1946.

57. Miyake H, Kauffman P, de Arruda Behmer O, et al. Mechanisms of cutaneous necrosis provoked by sclerosing injections in the treatment of microvarices and telangiectasias: Experimental study. Rev Assoc Med Bras 22:112-120, 1976.

58. Blenkinsopp WK. Choice of sclerosant: An experimental study. Angiologica 7:182-186, 1970.

59. Goldman MP, ed. Sclerotherapy: Treatment of Varicose and Telangiectatic Leg Veins. St. Louis: Mosby–Year Book, 1991.

60. Beall GN, Casaburi R, Singer A. Anaphylaxis: Everyone's problem. Specialty conference. West J Med 144:329-337, 1986.

61. Wasserman SI. Anaphylaxis. In Reed CE, Ellis EF, eds. Allergy: Principles and Practice, 2nd ed. St. Louis: CV Mosby, 1983, pp 689-699.

62. Levy JH, Roisen MF, Morris JM. Anaphylactic and anaphylactoid reactions: A review. Spine 11:282-291, 1986.

63. Browse NL, Burnand KG, Lea Thomas M. Diseases of the Veins. London: Edward Arnold, 1988.

28

Vena Cava Interruption: Devices and Results

Lazar J. Greenfield

Considerable progress has been made in the control of pulmonary thromboembolism since the initial approach of operative ligation of the vena cava was introduced. Recognition of the advantages of preserving inferior vena caval blood flow and normal distal venous pressure led to the development of suture plication techniques and external smooth or serrated clips, which are now used only under unusual circumstances. The early transvenous devices, such as the Hunter balloon and the Mobin-Uddin umbrella, either were susceptible to proximal migration or produced unacceptable morbidity from occlusion of the vena cava and have thus been withdrawn from the market. What might be considered as the modern era of transvenous devices, with the development of devices intended to trap emboli while preserving inferior vena caval blood flow and patency, began in 1973 with the introduction of the stainless steel Greenfield filter (MediTech, Inc./Boston Scientific, Watertown, Mass.).[1] This device was designed for operative insertion via either the jugular or femoral vein and has proved to be safe and effective by long-term follow-up evaluation.[2] Since 1984, however, some radiologists have employed percutaneous techniques for insertion of the Greenfield filter and have developed filters of a similar design or alternative types of filters that can be inserted more readily through smaller carrier systems (Fig. 28-1).

Percutaneous insertion of devices designed to provide effective filtration of thromboemboli in the vena cava offers a number of potential advantages for the patient, including less dis-comfort, reduced operative time, and lower costs because the procedure can be performed in the radiology suite rather than in the operating room. This use of percutaneous techniques is made possible by the Seldinger technique, which allows the percutaneous insertion of progressively larger dilators and a sheath over a Teflon-coated guidewire. The usual route of access is the femoral vein but the jugular vein can also be used. Once a guidewire has been inserted, enlargement of the skin incision allows expansion of the track by either balloon or dilators to permit the insertion of a large sheath. A 26 Fr sheath is required for percutaneous insertion of the standard stainless steel Green-field filter (SGF), which uses a 24 Fr carrier system.[1] This approach is customarily employed from the right groin, and although the jugular vein can also be used, it is less desirable because of the risk of air embolism. Several reported series have shown a favorable experience in terms of ease of insertion. However, there seems to be an increased incidence in trauma to the vein; follow-up of these patients has demonstrated a high incidence of venous thrombosis at the insertion site, reported as high as 41% in one series.[2] In view of these problems and the mechanical advantage of a smaller carrier system, a titanium version of the Greenfield filter (TGF; MediTech, Inc./Boston Scientific, Watertown, Mass.) has been developed, which allows the carrier system to be reduced in diameter to 12 Fr.[3] With a carrier system of this size, a 14 Fr sheath is required for percutaneous insertion. Our preliminary experience with this device in 40 patients at

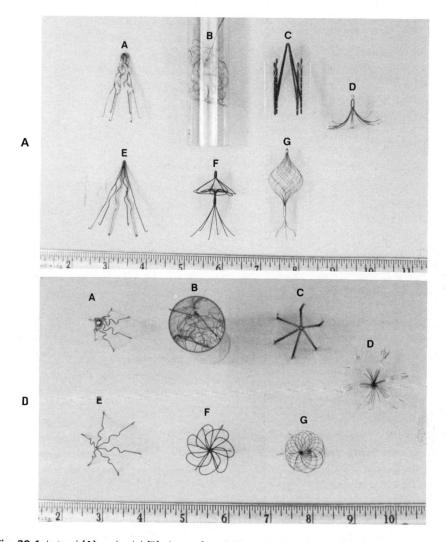

Fig. 28-1. Lateral **(A)** and axial **(B)** views of available and experimental vena caval filter devices. *A*, Standard stainless steel Greenfield filter; *B*, bird's nest filter; *C*, Venatech filter; *D*, Amplatz filter, which is designed to be inserted with the cone inverted; *E*, titanium Greenfield filter; *F*, nitinol filter; *G*, Günther filter, which is also designed to be inserted in an inverted position. (Reprinted with permission from Bergan JJ, Yao JST, eds. Venous Disorders. Philadelphia: WB Saunders, 1991.)

three different institutions indicates that this technique has not been associated with significant insertion-site venous thrombosis.[4] The TGF can also be inserted at the time of laparotomy through either a pursestring suture in the vena cava or a smaller venous tributary. Under these circumstances fluoroscopy is not necessary since the position of the carrier can be determined by palpation and the filter discharged at the appropriate level. Several other devices have been introduced to achieve vena caval filtration using a smaller catheter insertion system, and the status of these devices will be reviewed as well (Fig. 28-1; Table 28-1).

Table 28-1. Comparison of Inferior Vena Caval Filter Devices

Filter device	Clinical experience	No. of patients followed up	Follow-up period	Failures to insert	Misplacement	Tilt	Filter-caval occlusion (%)	Recurrent pulmonary embolism	Proximal migration	Venous stasis
SGF (ref. 2)	469	146	12 yr	3 (0.6%)	12 (2.5%)	8 (1.7%)	2	6 (4%)	0	7 (5%)
Bird's nest (ref. 7)	568	37	6 mo	0	NR	NA	19	12 1 death	5 (16%)	NR
TGF (ref. 4)	52	30	5 mo	1 (2%)	0	1 (2%)	0	2	0	0
Amplatz (ref. 10)	52	42	11 mo	NR	2 (4%)	1 (2%)	21	1	0	NR
Nitinol (ref. 12)	224	65	6 mo	—	—	—	20	4 (1 death)	—	—
Venatech (ref. 13)	100	90	1 yr	2 (2%)	18 (18%)	16 (16%)	8	2 (2%)	4 (4%)	29 (32%)
Modified hook TGF*	122	69	30 d	4	—	—	—	5 (3 deaths)	—	—

NR, not reported; NA, not applicable.
*Unpublished data, 1991.

TITANIUM GREENFIELD FILTER

The TGF is made from a titanium alloy previously described.[5] Its cone shape is similar to that of the SGF, but it is 8 mm wider at the base and 0.5 cm taller (Fig. 28-1). It weighs 0.25 gm as opposed to 0.56 gm for the SGF and can be compressed to a diameter of 0.144 inch. Mechanical properties of the TGF have been tested extensively, and the device shows remarkable resistance to flexion fatigue and induced corrosion.[5] The TGF exerts a force of fixation on the wall of the vena cava that is measurably greater than that of the SGF at diameters over 22 mm but less than that of the SGF at diameters less than 22 mm.

The technique for placement involves the use of a guidewire inserted from either the left or right femoral vein over which a dilator system and attached 14 Fr sheath can be passed. Once the sheath and dilator are in the inferior vena cava at the level of desired filter placement, the dilator is withdrawn and the TGF carrier is then passed to the level of intended insertion under fluoroscopic control. Both the carrier catheter and sheath are retracted as a unit to release the filter. After filter discharge, the carrier and sheath are withdrawn and gentle pressure is applied to the insertion site. An additional advantage to the use of the sheath is the fact that if the filter were prematurely discharged, filter misplacement would occur in the sheath rather than in the patient. Premature discharge is unlikely now that a new control handle has been added that allows no manipulation other than retraction of the carrier for discharge of the filter. The filter is also preloaded into the carrier system, obviating concern about crossed limbs.

In our initial clinical experience, TGFs were inserted successfully in 51 of 52 patients (98%). In one patient previously reported,[4] there was a very tight stricture of the inferior vena cava at the level of the hepatic veins, which prevented operative passage of the carrier catheter. This 56-year-old woman had terminal adenocarcinoma and it was believed that the stricture would prevent massive embolism from occurring. At autopsy 10 days later, there was no evidence of pulmonary thromboembolism. In one other patient, an attempt had been made to insert the SGF operatively via the jugular vein, but thrombosis at the junction of the jugular and subclavian veins prevented its insertion. A TGF was inserted operatively from the right femoral vein. All percutaneous insertions were successful in filter placement.

The indications for filter insertion were a contraindication to anticoagulation in 34 patients (65%), recurrent thromboembolism despite anticoagulation in nine (17%), a complication of anticoagulation in seven (13%), and adjunctive prophylaxis in two patients (4%). Filters were placed below the level of the renal vein in 46 patients (90%) and above the renal vein in five patients (10%).

There were 19 deaths (36%) during follow-up, only one of which could be attributed to recurrent thromboembolism. In this particular patient, previously reported,[4] there was uncontrollable thrombosis involving the subclavian veins and progressive pulmonary hypertension. Although the patient died at home and no autopsy was permitted, it is likely that she died of recurrent thromboembolism. When the subclavian vein thromboses developed, no access was available that would have permitted insertion of a filter in the superior vena cava since both iliac veins were thrombosed and a filter was in position in the inferior vena cava. Recurrent thromboembolism occurred in one other patient, for a rate of 4%.

There were 30 patients who returned for follow-up laboratory examinations at an average interval of 5.2 months. Four patients refused to return for follow-up study. Follow-up duplex examination showed thrombosis in the vein used for insertion in two patients (7%), both of whom were asymptomatic. Although there was no proximal migration, distal migration was evident in nine patients (30%) for distances of 9 to 64 mm (average, 23 mm), usually with an increase in limb diameter. Eight filters had a slight tilt at the time of insertion varying from 4 to 30 degrees. At follow-up, 12 filters were tilted, with an angulation from 5 to 23 degrees. Penetration of the filter beyond the wall of the vena cava was suspected in nine patients (30%) and the follow-up CT scan was confirmatory in the four patients in whom a CT scan was obtained. Significant mobility of the

TGF was noted with respiration, particularly in the suprarenal position, where it is likely that diaphragmatic motion added direct pressure. In one patient, caval wall perforation by the apex of the filter occurred at the time of insertion via the left femoral vein when it was not appreciated that the apex of the filter was impinging on the wall of the vena cava. At the time of discharge it was noted that the filter did not open, so a second TGF was placed below it via the right common femoral vein at the level of L3. No sequelae followed this misplacement, and at follow-up examination 4 months later the filters were stable and the vena cava was patent. No adverse sequelae resulted from the penetrations, tilting, or distal migration; however, the frequency of migration makes this device unacceptable for widespread use.

The present carrier used for the SGF is large enough to occasionally cause mechanical problems during both introduction into the vein and passage through the eustachian valve at the atriocaval junction or into the vena cava from the pelvis. Reducing the diameter of the carrier system from 24 Fr to 12 Fr has facilitated both entry and positioning and has completely eliminated bleeding during percutaneous filter insertion. The mobility of the TGF, however, suggests that it has less initial purchase on the wall of the vena cava than the SGF despite the measured greater lateral forces. There is still no evidence that the TGF will migrate proximally or that it will fail to remain secure after entrapping a thromboembolus. In order to correct the problems of migration and caval wall penetration, the hook has been redesigned to a recurved form with an 80-degree hook (Fig. 28-2). In experimental studies and current clinical trials, this modified TGF appears to be stable and has shown no significant caval wall penetration.[6]

In a multi-institutional study of the modified hook TGF a total of 118 filters were placed out of 122 attempts (97%) (L.J.G., unpublished data, 1991). The four patients in whom filter placement was unsuccessful had anatomic constraints that prevented positioning of the carrier system. Follow-up data at 30 days were available for 69 patients, of whom 17 patients demonstrated filter movement of a mean 12 mm,

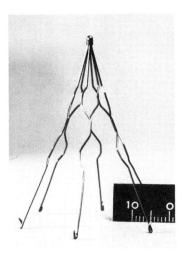

Fig. 28-2. Lateral view of the titanium Greenfield filter with modified hook design. The recurved and 80-degree angle hook appears to limit caval wall penetration and distal migration in preliminary clinical trials.

which is within the range of normal respiratory variation in filter position. An increase in filter base diameter was seen in nine patients for a mean 9 mm, but actual limb penetration occurred in only one patient. Recurrent pulmonary embolism occurred in five patients and was fatal in three. In comparison with the standard hook TGF, there was a 59% decrease in the incidence of migration and a 95% decrease in the incidence of caval wall penetration. Further follow-up studies are anticipated, but it would appear that the modified hook design has adequately addressed the problems with migration and penetration seen with the standard hook TGF.

BIRD'S NEST FILTER

Results with the bird's nest filter (Cook, Bloomington, Ind.) were initially reported in 1984 and a larger series of 568 patients was reported in 1988.[7,8] The device is constructed of four stainless steel wires, each of which is 25 cm long and 0.18 mm in diameter. The wires are preshaped with nonmatching bends and each wire end is attached to a strut that ends in a hook for fixation to the vena caval wall (Fig. 28-1). One strut is Z-shaped so that a pusher wire can be screwed into it. The original model

was preloaded into an 8 Fr Teflon catheter, but in 1986 the struts were modified with the addition of a stiff wire measuring 0.46 mm in diameter in an attempt to improve fixation and prevent the proximal migration that occurred with the original design. The broader struts required an increase in the diameter of the preloaded catheter to 12 Fr. The insertion procedure consists of pushing the first set of hooks into the wall of the vena cava and then extruding the wire in an effort to pack the loops of wires closely in the vena cava. The second pair of hooks is then pushed into the vena caval wall. The pusher wire is rotated to free it and allow removal of the catheter. The intention is to pack the wires into an approximately 7 cm length of the vena cava in order to provide multiple barriers to the passage of emboli.

Follow-up information on the bird's nest filter is limited because only 37 of the 481 patients in whom the filter had been in place for 6 months or more were objectively evaluated by means of venacavography or ultrasound.[8] Seven of the patients (19%) had caval occlusion. Pulmonary angiograms were performed in three symptomatic patients for recurrent pulmonary thromboembolism, which was confirmed in one patient, although there were 12 patients with recurrent embolism in the total experience. In addition to problems with thrombosis, the bird's nest filter has demonstrated migration proximally following what appeared to be secure placement. This has been seen both experimentally and clinically, with reports of proximal migration in five patients and one death. In the patient who died, the bird's nest filter was found with a massive embolus in the pulmonary artery 10 days after placement. It was this experience that led to modification of the struts to prevent inversion in the vena cava. In a subsequent report from the University of Arkansas, their experience with three cases of filter migration out of 32 placements was described.[9] In two cases filter migration was recognized within 24 hours of filter insertion and the partially migrated filter was successfully retrieved percutaneously by retraction of the filter to the intrahepatic segment of the inferior vena cava. The third case of migration was not detected for 6 months, at which time the filter was imbedded in the right atrium and ventricle and could not be recovered. This experience occurred before the change in hook design. Additional clinical studies of the modified filter are in progress.

AMPLATZ FILTER

The Amplatz filter (William Cook, Europe; Bjaeverskov, Denmark) was introduced in 1984 and clinical experience has been reported in 52 patients.[10] This filter is also cone shaped and made from a stainless steel alloy, but it is designed to be inserted in an inverted position in the vena cava, with pronged loops designed to limit caval wall penetration to 2 mm in order to avoid injury to pericaval structures (Fig. 28-1). A loop has also been added at the apex to allow for repositioning or retrieval. In one patient in this series the filter was repositioned from a suboptimal position immediately after insertion, and of the eight patients who were considered candidates for retrieval because of their short-term high risk for anticoagulation, retrieval was actually performed in five patients at 1 to 16 days after insertion. After retrieval, two patients demonstrated intramural abnormalities suggesting local hemorrhage. The follow-up experience (mean, 11 months) showed one insertion-site venous thrombosis (3%). Distal migration occurred in one patient, and tilting of the filter was observed in another patient. Thrombi in the apex of the filter cone were demonstrated in 9 of 34 patients (25%) at vena-cavography, but the researchers believed that these were not likely to produce embolism despite the fact that they were on the unprotected side of the filter. Larger thrombi trapped by the filter were seen in 4 of 34 patients (12%) and in two of these patients, there was propagation through the filter. The third patient had thrombus propagating through the filter with a benign course, but a fourth patient with thrombus on both sides of the filter was found to have pulmonary embolism at autopsy. Overall, 9 of 42 patients (21%) had thrombosed vena cavas at follow-up examination. Two patients required Greenfield filter placement above the original Amplatz filter. The researchers believe that the denser arrangement of wire results in greater clot-trapping efficiency but at the expense of a

higher rate of filter and vena caval occlusion. Of particular concern is the tendency for trapped thrombi to propagate through this particular device. Retrievability is also of only marginal benefit since a filter that has remained patent during the period of risk should not pose any long-term risk to the patient.

NITINOL FILTER

Nitinol is a nickel-titanium alloy that can exist as a pliable straight wire when cooled but rapidly transforms into a previously imprinted rigid shape when warmed. Although a filter made of this material was described in 1977 (Simon nitinol filter; Nitinol Technologies, Woburn, Mass.), clinical experience with the device has been reported only recently.[11] The filter design includes a 28 mm dome with eight overlapping loops; below, the wire is shaped into six diverging legs with terminal hooks to engage the vena caval wall in the configuration of a cone (Fig. 28-1). The preliminary report on the clinical experience with this device indicated that it was inserted in 103 patients in 17 participating centers.[11] Detailed information, however, was available on only 44 patients. The insertion procedure uses iced normal saline solution infused through a 9 Fr delivery catheter. The filter wire is advanced rapidly with the feeder pump and then discharged from the storage tube. The nitinol filter is said to then expand instantly into the appropriate shape and lock into place. In the multicenter study, for the brief period of follow-up there were three cases of recurrent pulmonary embolism and seven cases of confirmed vena caval occlusion, with two additional suspected occlusions on the basis of clinical findings. In five of 18 patients studied by ultrasound, thrombosis was evident at the site of insertion. Of the 44 patients followed up, 10 were studied at 3 months but only four completed the 6-month follow-up. Within this group, six occlusions of the vena cava and two additional suspected occlusions were documented, for an occlusion rate of 18%. Edema developed in an additional five patients with signs of thrombus within the filter. In one of the three patients with recurrent pulmonary embolism, a proximal propagating thrombus above the filter was identified by venacavography. Migration of one of the filters was mentioned in an addendum to the report.

A more recent update on the clinical experience shows that 224 patients have received nitinol filters, 102 are being followed up, and 65 have completed 6-month follow-up.[12] There were four patients who sustained recurrent pulmonary embolism with one fatality and 20 documented caval occlusions to which the author added three deaths associated with massive caval thrombosis. The high rate of vena caval thrombosis in this series with very short follow-up suggests that the filter material and/or design may be thrombogenic.

VENATECH FILTER

In 1986, another cone-shaped filter with added stabilizing struts on each limb was developed in France and introduced as the LGM filter (L.G. Medical, Chassenveil, France).[13] It is currently being marketed in the United States as the Venatech filter and is designed for percutaneous introduction. The filter is made of Phynox, which is similar to Elgiloy used in temporary cardiac-pacing wires. The Venatech filter is a stamped, six-pronged device with hooked stabilizers with sharp ends intended to center and fix the device (Fig. 28-1). It is inserted through a 12 Fr single-use catheter system, preferentially via the right internal jugular vein. A guidewire is used and the filter is ejected after it has been passed through the full length of the catheter.

The initial reported experience is from France and consists of 100 attempted insertions resulting in 98 filters discharged, 82 of which were positioned correctly. Eight filters had a 15-degree or more tilt, five opened incompletely, and an additional three were both incompletely opened and tilted. All of the filters were implanted via the jugular route. Nine of the filters were observed to migrate distally and four in a cephalad direction, for a 13% migration rate. The follow-up experience is limited to 1 year, at which time there were seven occlusions, resulting in a 92% patency rate. Recurrent pulmonary embolism was seen in two patients, both of whom had incompletely opened filters. At the end of 1 year, 13 filters were observed to have migrated, nine to the

iliac vein and four to the renal veins. Twenty-nine patients had lower limb edema despite the use of elastic support hose; seven had vena caval thrombosis.

Another study reported a 13% rate of tilting or partial opening and a caudal migration rate of 13%. Caval occlusion was seen in 8% at follow-up and there was a 2.5% incidence of recurrent embolism.[14] There have been isolated reports of breakage of the stabilizer struts, and it is surprising that the incidence of tilting has been so high in a device that was designed to prevent a tilt.

GÜNTHER FILTER

The Günther filter (William Cook, Europe) was described in 1987 as a percutaneous removable filter consisting of a helix of wires with an inverted cone above[15] (Fig. 28-1). It has been tested in Europe but is not available in the United States. No long-term follow-up information is available on the device, but preliminary results indicate a 7% caval thrombosis rate and a disturbing caudal migration rate of 70%.[16] In addition, caval wall penetration by the struts occurred in 20% and perforation by the retrieving hook in 78%. Proximal migration of the device into the right ventricle has also been reported,[17] which raises concern regarding its ability to trap thromboemboli safely.

CONCLUSION

Considerable ingenuity is apparent in the number of devices now available for clinical trial as vena caval filters. The primary objective to provide a safe, effective device for permanent implantation should lead to continued evolution of materials and design. The issue of retrievability, however, is overrated since any implanted device should not represent a long-term risk to the patient and the assumption that thromboembolism can be predicted as a short-term risk is incompatible with the unpredictability of the disorder. The standard for comparison should remain the Greenfield filter, with a recurrent embolism rate of 4% and a long-term patency rate at 12-year follow-up of 98%. The present concern regarding the percutaneous insertion of the SGF overlooks the fact that it can be inserted quite safely at operation with the patient under local anesthesia with minimal morbidity. It seems clear that advances in percutaneous techniques will make this approach the obvious choice for insertion of vena caval devices in the future, but the safety and efficacy of the conical design of the Greenfield filter suggest that a new design may not be needed for use via the percutaneous approach.

REFERENCES

1. Tadavarthy SM, Castaneda-Zuniga WR, Salomonowitz E, et al. Kimray-Greenfield vena cava filter: Percutaneous introduction. Radiology 151:525-526, 1984.

2. Kantor A, Glanz S, Gordon DH, Scalfani SJA. Percutaneous insertion of the Kimray-Greenfield filter: Incidence of femoral vein thrombosis. AJR 149:1065-1066, 1987.

3. Burke PE, Michna BA, Harvey CF, Crute SL, Sobel M, Greenfield LJ. Experimental comparison of percutaneous vena caval devices: Titanium Greenfield filter vs. bird's nest filter. J Vasc Surg 6:66-70, 1987.

4. Greenfield LJ, Cho KJ, Pais SO, Van Aman M. Preliminary clinical experience with the titanium Greenfield vena caval filter. Arch Surg 124:657-659, 1989.

5. Greenfield LJ, Savin MA. Comparison of titanium and stainless steel Greenfield vena caval filters. Surgery 106:820-828, 1989.

6. Greenfield LJ, Cho KJ, Tauscher JR. Evolution of hook design for fixation of the titanium Greenfield filter. J Vasc Surg 9:345-353, 1990.

7. Roehm JOF Jr, Gianturco C, Barth MH, Wright KC. Percutaneous transcatheter filter for the inferior vena cava: A new device for treatment of patients with pulmonary embolism. Radiology 150:255-257, 1984.

8. Roehm JOF Jr, Johnsrude IS, Barth MH, Gianturco C. The bird's nest inferior vena cava filter: Progress report. Radiology 168:745-749, 1988.

9. McCowan TC, Ferris EJ, Keifsteck JE, Lin GC, Baker ML. Retrieval of dislodged bird's nest inferior vena caval filters. J Intervent Radiol 3:179-183, 1988.

10. Epstein DH, Darcy MD, Hunter DW, Coleman CC, Tadavarthy SM, Murray PD, Castaneda-Zuniga WR, Amplatz K. Experience with the Amplatz retrievable vena cava filter. Radiology 172:105-110, 1989.

11. Simon M, Athanasoulis CA, Kim D, Steinberg FL, Porter DH, Byse BH, Kleshinski S, Geller S, Orron DE, Waltman AC. Simon nitinol inferior vena cava filter: Initial clinical experience. Radiology 172:99-103, 1989.

12. Dorfman GS. Percutaneous inferior vena caval filters. Radiology 174:987-992, 1990.

13. Ricco JB, Crochet D, Sebilotte P, Serradimigni A, Lefebvre JM, Barisson E, Geslin P, Virot P, Vaislic C, Gallet M, Biron Y, Lefant D, Dosmarq JM, DeLaFaye D. Percutaneous transvenous caval interruption with the "LGM" filter: Early results of a multicenter trial. Ann Vasc Surg 3:242-247, 1988.

14. Maquin P, Fajadet P, Railhac N, Bloom E, Brunet M, Railhac JJ. LM and Günther: Two complementary vena cava filters [abstr]. Radiology 173(P):476, 1989.

15. Günther RW, Schild H, Hollman JP, Vorwerk D. First clinical results with a new caval filter. Cardiovasc Intervent Radiol 10:104-108, 1987.

16. Fobbe F, Dietzel M, Korth R, et al. Günther vena caval filter: Results of long-term follow-up. AJR 151:1031-1034, 1988.

17. Johnson SG, Pickford M, Wilkins RA. Migration of a Günther caval filter to the right ventricle. J Intervent Radiol 3:33-36, 1988.

29

Lymphatic Problems and Revascularization Edema*

Peter Gloviczki   R. Thomas Bergman

Problems with the lymphatic circulation caused by insufficiency of lymph transport or injury to the lymph vessels or lymph nodes can be challenging and require the special expertise of the vascular surgeon. Developmental abnormality of the lymphatic system and congenital or acquired obstruction of the lymph vessels and lymph nodes result in accumulation of protein-rich interstitial fluid.[1] In some cases "leaky" capillaries, usually with the limb in a dependent position, result in high lymphatic load and lead to swelling of the extremity.[2] The edema may reverse if (1) sufficient collateral lymphatic circulation develops, (2) the limb is elevated, or (3) overproduction of protein-rich interstitial fluid stops. In chronic lymphedema all of the possible compensatory mechanisms, such as collateral lymphatic circulation, the proteolytic activity of the tissue macrophages, and spontaneous lymphovenous anastomoses, are exhausted.[1,3,4] Secondary tissue fibrosis and chronic inflammatory changes in these patients may cause irreversible changes in the subcutaneous tissue. Treatment is necessary to decrease the volume of the extremity and prevent and treat infectious complications although in this stage cure of this frequently incapacitating disease seldom is possible.[5]

Since the lymph vessels usually run parallel with arteries and veins, and major groups of lymph nodes are in close proximity to major vessels, some injury to the lymphatic system during vascular reconstructions is almost unavoidable. Regeneration of transected or ligat-ed lymphatics with reestablishment of normal lymphatic transport is frequent, and minor leaks from transected lymph vessels also usually cease. Significant lymphatic injury during vascular reconstruction may cause edema of the extremity[2,6-11] or may result in lymphatic fistula[12,13] or lymphocele.[14-20] In the abdomen injury to the mesenteric lymph vessels or the cysterna chyli may lead to the development of chylous ascites.[17,21-35]

In this chapter we review problems encountered with microvascular reconstructions of obstructed lymph vessels to treat chronic lymphedema. We discuss the different theories of the pathomechanism of postrevascularization edema and suggest methods to avoid it. We also present our approach to the diagnosis and management of lymphatic complications of vascular procedures such as lymphatic fistula, retroperitoneal and groin lymphoceles, and chylous ascites.

PROBLEMS WITH MICROSURGICAL TREATMENT FOR CHRONIC LYMPHEDEMA

The development of improved microsurgical techniques has enabled surgeons to perform successful anastomoses of vessels less than 2 mm in diameter. Lymphatic microsurgery has introduced techniques to bypass the obstructed superficial or deep lymphatic system of the upper or lower extremities (Figs. 29-1 and 29-2). Two different microsurgical methods have been developed to treat chronic obstructive lymphedema: lymphovenous anastomoses and lymphatic grafting. Although clinical improve-

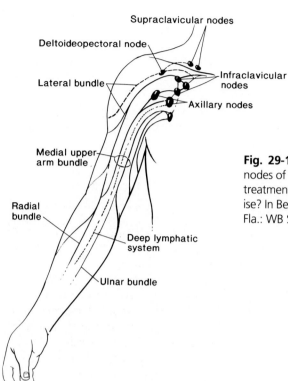

Supraclavicular nodes

Deltoideopectoral node

Lateral bundle

Infraclavicular nodes

Axillary nodes

Medial upper-arm bundle

Radial bundle

Deep lymphatic system

Ulnar bundle

Fig. 29-1. Anatomy of major lymph vessels and lymph nodes of upper extremity. (From Gloviczki P. Microsurgical treatment for chronic lymphedema: An unfulfilled promise? In Bergan JJ, Yao JST, eds. Venous Disorders. Orlando, Fla.: WB Saunders, 1991.)

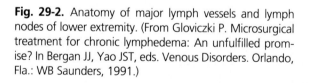

Fig. 29-2. Anatomy of major lymph vessels and lymph nodes of lower extremity. (From Gloviczki P. Microsurgical treatment for chronic lymphedema: An unfulfilled promise? In Bergan JJ, Yao JST, eds. Venous Disorders. Orlando, Fla.: WB Saunders, 1991.)

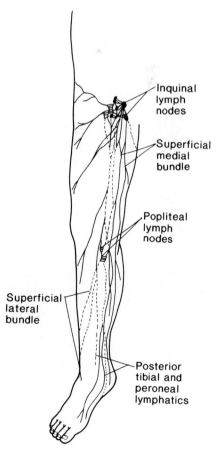

Inquinal lymph nodes

Superficial medial bundle

Popliteal lymph nodes

Superficial lateral bundle

Posterior tibial and peroneal lymphatics

ments with both techniques have been reported, the effectiveness of these procedures has not yet been confirmed by several independent surgical teams. Indeed, doubts, not entirely unfounded, about the merit of these operations have been raised.[36]

Lymphovenous Anastomoses

Experimental and initial clinical experiences with lymphovenous anastomoses (Fig. 29-3) to treat chronic obstructive lymphedema began in the 1960s.[37-40] In the last 30 years, a number of studies on lymphovenous anastomoses demonstrated patency in experiments[41-43] and claimed success in patients.[44-55] However, there are several aspects of this operation that have been controversial. The first question raised concerns the microsurgical technique: Can patent anastomoses with lymph vessels be performed? The second issue debated is: Does the late patency of lymphovenous anastomoses warrant their performance? The third problem concerns lymphodynamics: Is there lymphatic flow through the anastomosis despite the higher pressure in the venous system? Also, do patent and functioning lymphovenous anastomoses reverse the secondary tissue changes that have

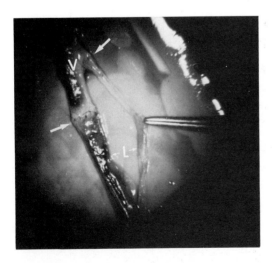

Fig. 29-3. Lymphovenous anastomoses (original magnification ×2) between two major lymph vessels *(L)* and bifurcated tributary of the greater saphenous vein *(V)*. Arrows indicate anastomoses.

already developed in chronic obstructive lymphedema? Finally, are the methods of evaluating the postoperative results satisfactory to claim the effectiveness of the operation and prove late patency and function of the anastomoses?

Each of these issues is examined separately although satisfactory answers to all of the questions raised are not available at present.

Microsurgical Techniques

Several experimental studies have proved that with fine microsurgical technique, adequate magnification, needles of small diameter (50 µm), and 10-0 to 12-0 suture material, lymphovenous anastomoses can be performed with excellent (80% to 100%) early patency.[39,41,43,56] In our experiments most failures occurred in those animals who were operated on in the first half of the experiments. This too suggests the importance of perfect technique in lymphatic microsurgery.

Late Patency: Experimental and Clinical

A patency rate of 50% to 70% at 3 to 8 months has been documented in several experiments[39,41-43]; however, similar results have not been obtained by other investigators. Carefully conducted studies by Puckett et al.[56] failed to demonstrate patency of lymphovenous anastomoses after 3 weeks in an experimental model of chronic lymphedema. In our experiments[43] a 50% patency rate could be achieved up to 8 months after operation. Patency of the anastomoses that were performed between normal deep femoral lymph vessels and a tributary of the femoral vein was documented by lymphangiography. Scanning electron microscopy showed complete endothelial coverage of the anastomotic line by 4 weeks (Fig. 29-4). In our clinical experience,[55] we noted improvement in only 5 of 14 patients who were operated on for chronic lymphedema. Lymphovenous anastomoses were performed between superficial lymph vessels and superficial veins on both the upper and lower extremities. Of the seven patients who had secondary obstructive lymphedema, four experienced improvement. The mean follow-up of these patients was 46.2 months. However, we could not obtain objective evidence of late patency of lymphovenous anastomoses in patients.

A recent report from Australia[57] provided long-term follow-up on 90 patients who underwent lymphovenous anastomoses for chronic lymphedema. Although 38 patients underwent excisional operations also, significant clinical benefit could be documented even in the group with lymphovenous anastomoses only: 73% showed subjective improvement, 42% had decrease in the volume of the limb, and 74% of all patients were able to discontinue elastic compression treatment. Although these clinical data show improvement in the operated patients, lymphangiography to provide objective evidence of late patency of the anastomoses was not performed.

Lymphodynamics

Lymph flow is low and intermittent. Lower extremity lymph flow in humans is estimated to be normally 120 ml/24hr.[58] Patients in the early stage of lymphedema have a high lymphatic load and an elevated lymphatic flow. This helps maintain patency of lymphovenous anastomoses. Unfortunately, as lymphedema is decompressed by the lymphovenous anastomoses, lymphatic flow decreases accordingly.[56] In our experiments, however, we could demonstrate patency of the lymphovenous anastomoses despite low lymphatic flow. The amount of lymph flow in the normal canine hindlimb is indeed low; in one study it measured 0.233 ± 0.077 ml/hr/100 ml tissue fluid volume.[59]

Pressure in the lymph vessels at rest is somewhat lower than venous pressure. However, lymphatic pressure is high during muscular exercise. In experiments Olszewski[58] was able to demonstrate intermittent intralymphatic pressure as high as 50 mm Hg. The intermittent elevated intralymphatic pressure is the propulsive force to forward lymph toward a higher pressure venous system. In addition to muscular exercise, additional extrinsic factors that influence propulsion of the lymph include arterial pulsation, gravity, and positive abdominal and negative intrathoracic pressures.[60] The main intrinsic force determining the rate of lymph flow is the spontaneous intrinsic contraction of the smooth muscle in the wall of the lymph

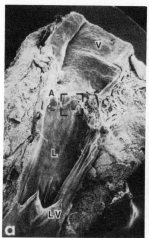
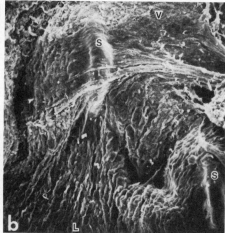

Fig. 29-4. a and **b**, Scanning electron micrographs of patent anastomosis 4 weeks after operation. Endothelial cells cover suture line. *A,* anastomosis; *L,* lymph vessel; *LV,* lymphatic valve; *S,* suture; *V,* vein. (**a**, original magnification ×10; **b**, original magnification ×200.) (From Gloviczki P, Hollier LH, Nora FE, Kaye MP. The natural history of microsurgical lymphovenous anastomoses: An experimental study. J Vasc Surg 4:148-156, 1986.)

vessel.[1] Unfortunately, it has been demonstrated that compliance of the lymph vessels increases significantly in the late phase of chronic lymphedema.[1] If secondary tissue changes, chronic inflammation and fibrosis of the subcutaneous tissue decrease interstitial pressure, then the effective driving force of lymph flow is diminished. This problem is discussed in detail by Clodius, Piller, and Casley-Smith.[3] The chances of lymphovenous anastomoses staying open and functioning in the late stage of chronic lymphedema are truly diminished.

Another problem that can decrease late patency and function of a lymphovenous anastomosis is valvular incompetence in the lymphatic system. This not only decreases the chance of forward lymphatic flow, but also allows for reflux of blood into the anastomosis, which, at least in the early postoperative period before endothelialization of the anastomosis is completed, may lead to thrombosis. Fortunately, complete valvular loss of the lymphatics is observed only in the very severe form of lymphedema or in patients who have lymphangiectasia. Also, if there is a competent valve on the venous side of the anastomosis, reflux of blood can be prevented completely. Nieuborg[61] reported that in more than 150 lymphovenous anastomoses performed for postmastectomy lymphedema, retrograde flow during the procedure was noted in only two cases. The avoidance of limb dependency and the increase of interstitial pressure with elastic compression also improve chances of patency and function of lymphovenous anastomoses.

Problems With Reporting Standards

Criteria by which clinical success was claimed in the published series include measurements of circumference and volume, patient satisfaction, episodes of cellulitis, or, more recently, lymphoscintigraphy.[44-55,57] Unfortunately, the volume measurements, even if expressed as percent reduction of excess volume of the extremity, are not always accurate.[57] Many patients have only a mild decrease in excess volume but have a softer extremity and more pliable skin. No surgical study has used a control group of unoperated patients who have undergone a correct regimen of conservative treatment with elastic stockings or intermittent pneumatic compression treatment. As predicted, most of the operated patients were encouraged to gain better control of the extremity and most were probably more conscientious in wearing elastic stockings because of regular postoperative surveillance. Because of the low number of good surgical candidates for this procedure, the feasibility of a randomized study is limited at present.

Currently the only available method to objectively document patency of lymphovenous anastomoses is cinelymphangiography. Spot films taken during contrast lymphangiography are not always satisfactory. Since the Ethiodol is lipid soluble, the contrast droplets are taken away immediately by the venous bloodstream when they pass through the lymphovenous anastomoses into a large vein. In experiments we demonstrated late patency of lymphovenous anastomoses with contrast cinelymphangiography.[43]

Concerns about the use of contrast lymphangiography in patients with chronic lymphedema have been raised.[5,57,62] Because of the severely damaged lymph transport, residual contrast is seen frequently in the lymph vessels and lymph nodes of these patients several weeks or even months after the test. In one of our patients inspissated contrast was found in the lymph vessels 6 months after lymphangiography during exploration to perform lymphovenous anastomoses. Contrast lymphangiography is invasive and worsening of the lymphedema has been described following lymphangiography.[5,62] In one review of 51 patients who underwent lymphangiography for chronic lymphedema, one third of the patients experienced an increase in the volume of the extremity following the test.[62] Therefore none of the clinical studies has used lymphangiography to document late patency of lymphovenous anastomoses. Now our routine diagnostic test for lymphedema is lymphoscintigraphy[63] and we use lymphangiography only in patients with presumed lymphangiectasia or if malignancy cannot be excluded by other tests. Lymphoscintigraphy, however, provides only indirect evidence of patency of lymphovenous anastomoses.[55]

Direct objective proof of late patency of lymphovenous anastomoses in patients is not available at present. The data provided by the most recent publication of O'Brien et al.[57] are in strong support of continuing our efforts in this field. For the first time late clinical improvement in a large, well-documented group of surgical patients was reported.

Lymphatic Grafting

The technique to bypass the obstructed lymphatic system with lymphatic grafts has been developed by a group in Germany.[64-66] Baumeister and associates[64] reported 100% patency of lymphatic grafts in experiments and recently published convincing data on the clinical effectiveness and late function of lymphatic grafts.[66] The operation is performed on the upper extremity for postmastectomy lymphedema or in the lower extremity for unilateral chronic obstructive lymphedema. The operation on the lower extremity is similar to the Palma procedure used for iliac vein obstruction. Our own experience is limited to five patients (Fig. 29-5, *A* to *D*) and early lymphoscintigraphic evidence of patency and function of the lymphatic grafts was demonstrated in only two patients (Fig. 29-6). Two to three superficial lymph vessels are dissected first on the normal lower extremity. The lymph vessels are divided above the knee and tunneled subcutaneously in the suprapubic space to the contralateral groin. There end-to-end lympholymphatic anastomoses are performed between the large collecting lymph vessels of the swollen extremity and the lymphatic grafts.

For bypassing obstructed axillary lymph vessels, lymphatic grafts are removed from the thigh and interposed as free lymphatic grafts between superficial or deep lymphatics of the arm and larger lymph collectors in the supraclavicular space. Baumeister and Siuda[66] showed with lymphoscintigraphy that patency of the functioning lymphatic grafts can be confirmed.

Fig. 29-6 shows early filling of an inguinal lymph node contralateral to the swollen extremity following suprapubic bypass. Colloid was injected into the swollen right lower extremity only and inguinal nodes noted preoperatively were not visualized even on late images.

Baumeister and his group are the only surgeons at present who have significant experience with this procedure. In their recent report on 55 surgical patients, a decrease in the volume of the extremity was documented in 80% of the patients with follow-up over 3 years.[66] They also studied 30 patients by lymphoscintigraphy and documented late improvement in lymphatic transport index measured by semiquantitative evaluation of the lymphoscintigrams. Although several patent grafts were imaged by lymphoscintigraphy, unfortunately, a patency rate of the implanted grafts was not provided by the authors.

One potential problem that can complicate this procedure is development of lymphedema in the donor extremity. Therefore a lymphoscintigram always should be performed on the donor limb for evidence of normal lymphatic transport. It was reassuring that lymphedema of the donor lower extremity did not develop in any of Baumeister and Siuda's patients.

Since lymph is less coagulable than blood and platelets are not present in peripheral lymph, the chances of occlusion of lympholymphatic anastomoses are probably less than of the lymphovenous anastomoses. Also, the higher venous pressure that may play a role in the failure of lymphovenous anastomoses is not a factor in lymphatic grafting.[66,67] However, surgical technique of lymphatic grafting is even more meticulous and more demanding than that of lymphovenous anastomosis. The possibility of secondary changes in the lymphatic grafts also is unknown and data on late patency are not available.

Although this operation may be more promising than lymphovenous anastomoses, results will have to be confirmed by several surgical teams and compared with those obtained with currently practiced standard conservative regimens.

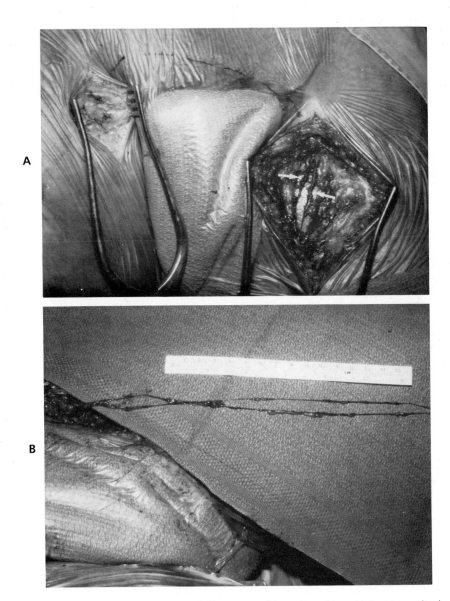

Fig. 29-5. A, Exposure of lymph vessels for suprapubic transposition. Note two major lymph vessels of the left thigh that will be used for grafting (arrows). **B,** Two lymphatic grafts divided at the distal thigh are prepared for lymphatic grafting.

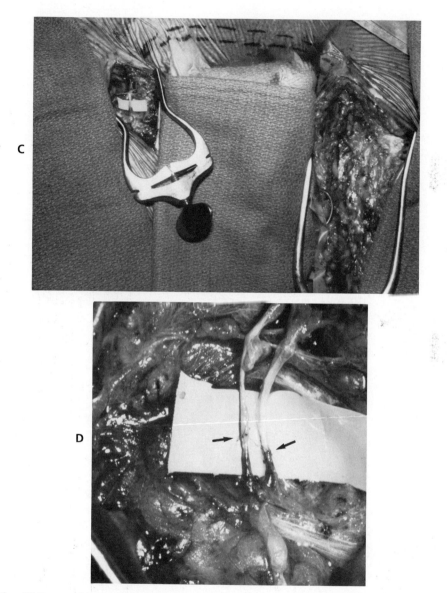

Fig. 29-5, cont'd. C, Completed suprapubic lymph grafting with two lympholymphatic anastomoses at right groin. Broken line indicates position of suprapubic lymphatic grafts. **D,** Magnified photograph of two end-to-end lympholymphatic anastomoses (arrows) performed with 11-0 interrupted monofilament sutures.

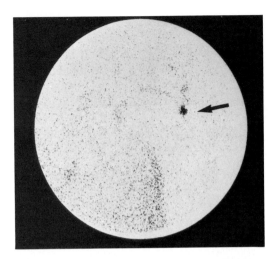

Fig. 29-6. Lymphoscintigram at 3 months confirms early filling of left inguinal lymph node (arrow). Colloid was injected into the right foot only. Preoperative lymphoscintigram showed no inguinal nodes.

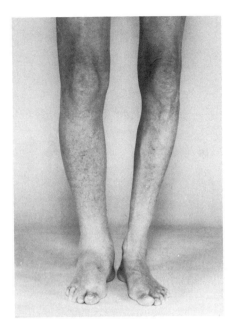

Fig. 29-7. Postrevascularization edema in 65-year-old man 6 weeks after in situ femoropopliteal bypass graft and profundaplasty. Two years later the patient still has persisting edema.

LYMPHATIC COMPLICATIONS OF ARTERIAL RECONSTRUCTIONS
Postrevascularization Edema

Some edema occurs in most, if not all, patients who undergo infrainguinal revascularization for chronic ischemia; only rarely is this problem seen after aortoiliac reconstruction.[2] Postrevascularization edema in patients with chronic ischemia differs in several aspects from ischemic and reperfusion injuries observed in patients with acute limb ischemia.[68] Although there are some similarities between the two syndromes (endothelial injury, hyperemia, increased permeability), they differ in cause, presentation, treatment, and prognosis.

In patients who undergo successful femoropopliteal or femorotibial bypass for chronic ischemia, leg swelling usually becomes evident when the patient resumes ambulation (Fig. 29-7). The pitting edema normally subsides within 2 to 3 months. During this period normal ambulation may be impaired and wound healing delayed. In a significant number of patients the edema becomes chronic and even incapacitating, requiring elastic stockings and avoidance of leg dependency. These few patients may become functionally impaired despite a patent bypass graft.

The cause of leg swelling following bypass for chronic ischemia has been a topic of much investigation historically. Several mechanisms have been implicated and in most instances the cause is multifactorial. If revascularization is not successful, edema almost never occurs. The lymphatic system plays the most important role in the development of edema in two ways. First, there is an overproduction of interstitial fluid following revascularization, which results in high lymphatic load, and edema may develop as a result of a "high-output" lymphatic failure. Second, injury to the lymph vessels and lymph-conducting elements of the lymph nodes results in reduced lymphatic transport capacity and "low-output" lymphatic failure. If lymphatic transport capacity decreases to a critical level, edema develops.

Postbypass Edema: A High-Output Lymphatic Failure?

Lymphedema develops if the rate of production of protein-rich interstitial fluid exceeds the rate of removal. In high-output lymphatic failure, even increased lymphatic transport is insufficient to cope with the excessive lymphatic load. Factors responsible for increased production of lymph include elevated arterial pressure following revascularization, alterations in regulation of the microcirculation, probable endothelial injury from chronic ischemia, and increased permeability to protein or solute components of the plasma.[2]

Myhre and Dedichen[69] observed edema in 46 of 154 patients following femoropopliteal bypass and supported the hypothesis that the sudden increase in distal pressure alters the responsiveness of the vascular wall. Simeone and Husni[70] first suggested in 1959 that edema after revascularization was the result of "hyperemia" caused by decreased arterial and arteriolar smooth muscle tone. Restoration of normal smooth muscle tone was believed to occur from 1 to 9 weeks after revascularization when edema resolved in the majority of patients. Increased capillary filtration caused by distention of the weakened arterial wall was implicated as a causative factor by other authors also.[71]

[125]I-labeled serum albumin clearance studies in a small group of patients with postrevascularization edema showed significant increase in lymphatic flow. Albumin kinetics and its relation to edema formation was studied by Campbell and Harris,[72] who demonstrated reduction of plasma albumin and increase in extremity albumin content following femoropopliteal bypass. Decreased colloid osmotic pressure was postulated to contribute to edema formation. Edema developed in 11 of 13 patients after femoropopliteal bypass, corresponding with a large quantity of albumin sequestered in the interstitial fluid as a result of altered capillary permeability following bypass. Of importance was the observation of a threefold increase in albumin content in limbs revascularized with femoropopliteal bypass compared with those with aortoiliac grafts.[72]

It appears that a combination of elevated distal arterial pressure, loss of arteriolar constriction to limb dependency, loss of microcirculatory autoregulation, endothelial injury, and smooth muscle atrophy all result in increased production of interstitial fluid following revascularization (Fig. 29-8). These changes are accompanied by increased permeability to proteins and large molecules, which increases lymphatic load and results in high-output lymphatic failure.

Postbypass Edema: A Low-Output Lymphatic Failure

Transection, ligation, or obstruction of lymph vessels during exposure of the femoral or popliteal vessels or dissection of the saphenous vein decreases the transport capacity of the lymphatic system. If the number of functioning major lymph collectors decreases to a critical level, lymphedema develops. Vaughan, Slavotinek, and Jepson[6] found that after femoropopliteal bypass the average number of patent superficial lymph vessels was reduced to 1.7/patient as compared with the normal average of 9.5. In addition, extravasation of contrast and interruption of lymph vessels were noted on lymphangiograms performed in patients following revascularization. Improvement of lymphedema occurred after several weeks when lymphatic collaterals developed. Schmidt et al.[10] supported this observation in their series of 37 patients; if more than three lymph vessels remained intact postoperatively, the increase in the circumference of the extremity was always less than 2 cm. Others also have demonstrated that postoperative edema is limited to the subcutaneous tissues, supporting the role of lymphatic injury in the pathogenesis of postoperative edema.[73]

In a recent report, AbuRahma, Woodruff, and Lucente[11] examined the involvement of the lymphatic system in the pathomechanism of edema formation in 72 patients who underwent femoropopliteal bypass grafting. Forty percent of the patients developed edema following revascularization. Leg swelling developed in 85% (17 of 20) of the patients who had conventional

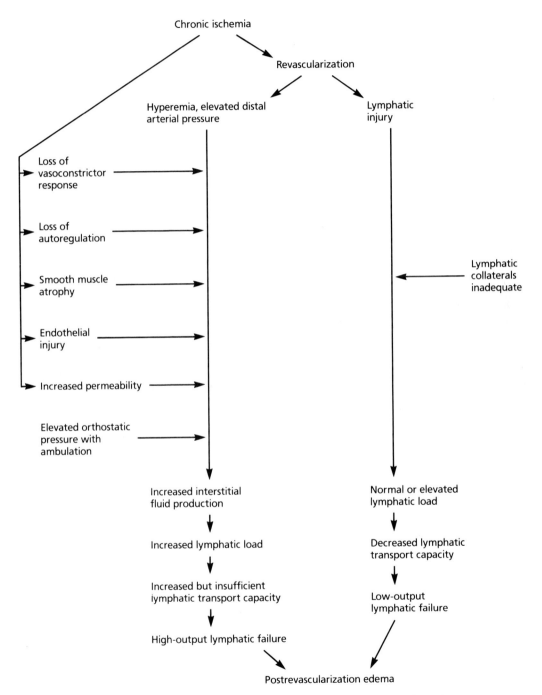

Fig. 29-8. Pathomechanism of lymphatic failure in postrevascularization edema.

dissection of the femoropopliteal arteries. However, if careful exposure of the femoropopliteal arteries was performed preserving lymphatics, the incidence of edema was only 10% (2 of 20 patients). Lymphangiograms showed normal anatomy in six of the eight patients with no edema and mild disruption was noted in only two patients. However, severe injury to the lymphatic system was present in all eight patients with edema who underwent contrast lymphangiography.

Venous Thrombosis

Some investigators presumed venous thrombosis to be the major cause in the development of postoperative edema.[74] Hamer[75] performed venography in patients following femorotibial bypass and found a surprisingly high incidence of acute deep vein thrombosis as indicated on the venograms of 7 of 12 patients. The incidence of venous thrombosis was less if the distal anastomosis was performed above the knee. He concluded that if the increase in the extremity circumference postoperatively was less than 1.5 cm, deep vein thrombosis was rare. However, if the increase in calf circumference was greater than 4.5 cm, thrombosis of tibial and popliteal veins was most likely.

Clinical studies by Husni,[71] however, confirmed normal venous hemodynamics and morphology in 41 of 45 patients with postoperative edema; Myhre and Dedichen[69] demonstrated deep vein thrombosis in only 8% of patients with postbypass edema. In one series the incidence of deep vein thrombosis following femoropopliteal bypass graft was similar in patients with edema (7%) and in those without edema (10%).[11]

We agree with Schubart and Porter[2] that deep vein thrombosis plays a minor role in postbypass edema in most patients. However, it is important to remember that deep vein thrombosis can occur in some patients following infrainguinal revascularization. In our practice all postoperative patients with moderate-to-severe swelling, or with any swelling, if associated with cyanosis or unusual postoperative pain, undergo evaluation for deep vein thrombosis. If duplex scanning or contrast venography confirms this diagnosis, treatment with heparin is started.

Postbypass Edema: Prevention and Treatment

Multiple factors contribute to the development of postrevascularization edema, including lymphatic injury, alterations in capillary function and permeability, disturbances in microcirculatory regulation, and rarely venous thrombosis. The type of graft and the severity of preoperative ischemia do not appear to be important. Of all the possible causes, lymphatic injury is the primary contributing factor in most patients. Meticulous, lymphatic-preserving surgical dissection is needed to minimize postbypass edema. Dissection of the femoral artery may damage both the superficial and deep lymphatic systems. Extensive dissection of the profunda femoris artery injures additional deep lymph vessels. To preserve patency of lymph vessels and integrity of lymph nodes, a vertical groin incision slightly lateral to the femoral pulse should be made. The inguinal lymphatics should be retracted medially and a vertical incision made in the femoral sheath to dissect the femoral arteries. The tissue between the artery and the vein or around the femoral vein itself is never dissected. Even if an in situ bypass is performed, attempts should be made to preserve as much lymphatic and adipose tissues between the saphenofemoral junction and the femoral artery as possible. A skin bridge is always left between the groin incision where the proximal greater saphenous vein is dissected and the incision in the thigh made to dissect the remaining portion of the greater saphenous vein. Multiple short skin incisions to dissect the saphenous vein will preserve more superficial lymphatics.[11]

The popliteal artery also should be dissected carefully; the vascular sheath should be opened longitudinally without dissection of the popliteal vein or the posterior tibial nerve in the neurovascular bundle. The fibroadipose tissue, which contains the deep lymphatics in the popliteal fossa, also should be left intact. Postoperatively, mild edema of the extremity requires frequent elevation of the limb and some restriction of ambulation. Cardiac failure also should be treated if present. If deep vein thrombosis is suspected, duplex scanning or contrast venography is performed. Moderate-to-severe postrevascularization edema is treated with elastic stockings; the degree of compression depends on the location of the bypass (superficial vs. deep) and the site of the distal anastomosis. In general, we suggest a custom-made, firm elastic stocking with a compression of 30 to 40 mm Hg. In patients with below-knee in situ bypass or any bypass to the distal tibial or pedal arteries, management is individualized to avoid direct compression and occlusion of a subcutaneous vein graft.

Lymphatic Fistula

Lymph drainage most often arises from groin incisions following dissection of the femoral vessels. The diagnosis usually is made clinically with the observation of persistent, clear, yellowish drainage from the wound. Lymphatic division at surgery and inadequate wound closure contribute to fistula formation. Early diagnosis and correct management are especially important if a prosthetic graft has been implanted.

When a lymphatic fistula is suspected, lymphoscintigraphy can be used to confirm the diagnosis.[13] We do not advocate a fistulogram if lymphatic leak occurs in the early postoperative period. If there is any sign of graft infection, if the fluid resembles chyle, or if a lymphatic fistula develops several months to years after operation, computed tomography is performed. This is important to diagnose graft infection or confirm the presence of retroperitoneal lymphocele draining through a fistula at the groin.

In the past such fistulas often were treated conservatively with limb elevation and pressure dressings. Similar to Kwaan, Bernstein, and Connolly,[12] we advocate early operative closure of persistent fistulas to prevent the development of wound infection and dehiscence and to prevent graft infection. In the operating room under sterile conditions, we inject 5 ml of Lymphazurine dye subcutaneously into the first and third interdigital spaces (Fig. 29-9).

The incision then is opened and the site of the lymphatic injury that is stained by the dye is oversewn. The wound is closed in multiple layers.

Injury to the terminal portion of the thoracic duct may cause significant lymphatic leak with persistent high output, which can be milky in appearance. Thoracic duct injury may occur during dissection of the proximal portion of the subclavian artery, or during carotid-subclavian bypass when the graft is tunneled behind the left internal jugular vein. In neglected cases malnutrition, lymphocytopenia, and anemia can be observed, similar to that seen in patients with chylous ascites, which is discussed later in this chapter. Again, we prefer early operation and make every attempt to perform lateral closure of the thoracic duct with 7-0 or 8-0 nonabsorbable monofilament sutures. Since the confluence of the thoracic duct with the jugular-subclavian venous junction is frequently a network of several larger lymphatic trunks, ligation of a leaking duct should be done if lateral closure is not successful. The incision then is closed after placement of a subcutaneous drain. Early closure of lymphatic fistulas reduces hospital stay, facilitates wound healing, and reduces the risk of prosthetic graft infection.

Lymphocele

Lymphocele, a localized collection of lymphatic fluid, develops after injury to major lymph vessels or lymph nodes. Following arterial reconstruction, lymphocele can occur at sites where the arteries were exposed or in the bed of the saphenous vein dissected for distal bypass (Fig. 29-10).

Groin Lymphocele

Because of the rich lymphatic network at the groin, lymphoceles are most frequent following dissection of the femoral vessels. Since disastrous consequences can be associated with infection of a prosthetic graft, early diagnosis and correct management of a groin mass following vascular reconstruction are mandatory. The diagnosis of lymphocele can be obvious on physical examination: localized collection of

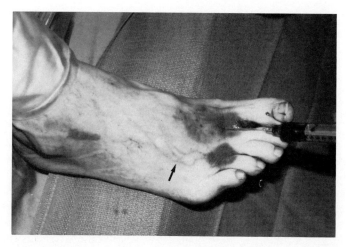

Fig. 29-9. Male patient, 58 years of age, in whom lymphocele developed following femoral artery dissection during open heart surgery. Lymphazurine dye was injected into first and third interdigital spaces subcutaneously to identify the site of lymphatic injury at groin. Arrow indicates stained superficial lymph vessels on the dorsum of the foot.

subcutaneous fluid in the early postoperative period, occasionally with intermittent drainage of clear lymph through a cutaneous fistula. Physical examination may disclose other abnormalities also: infection (draining pus), incarcerated hernia (painful mass, rarely with strangulated viscus with peritonitis), or pulsatile mass with or without bruit (pulsatile hematoma, false aneurysm). Ultrasound examination distinguishes solid and cystic lesions.

Computed tomography is performed selectively in the early postoperative period. However, it is always performed if lymphocele develops in the late follow-up. As mentioned earlier it can suggest graft infection or could identify an occasional retroperitoneal lymphocele, which may be continuous with a lymphocele at the groin.

In the early postoperative period, lymph collects between tissue planes; later a true pseudocapsule develops (Fig. 29-11). In contrast to a seroma, the lymphocele has a well-localized connection with one or more of the injured lymphatic channels, which can be confirmed by lymphoscintigraphy.[16]

Similar to treatment of lymphatic fistula, we

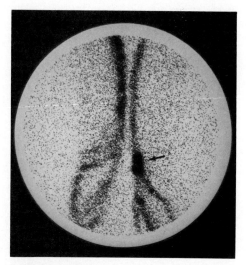

Fig. 29-10. Lymphoscintigram demonstrating small lymphocele in 60-year-old man following femoro-popliteal in situ saphenous vein bypass graft. Arrow indicates accumulation of lymph at the knee.

suggest early operation in these patients, especially if there is a prosthetic graft in the groin. We inject Lymphazurine dye into the foot, oversew the site of the lymphatic leak, and, if present, excise the pseudocapsule of the lymphocele (Fig. 29-11). Closure in multiple layers is then performed.

Retroperitoneal Lymphocele

Although some injury to mesenteric and aortoiliac lymphatics occurs frequently during aortic reconstructions, symptomatic retroperitoneal lymphoceles are rare. In an excellent review of retroperitoneal lymphoceles, Garrett et al.[20] found an incidence of 0.1% after 4000 aortic reconstructions. Together with the two cases we have observed recently (Figs. 29-12 and 29-13), there are now 11 patients reported in the English literature who are known to have retroperitoneal lymphoceles (Table 29-1). However, the number of asymptomatic or unreported cases undoubtedly is high.

The cause of retroperitoneal lymphocele is iatrogenic injury to the aortoiliac, ascending lumbar or mesenteric lymphatic trunks, or the cysterna chyli (Fig. 29-14) during retroperitoneal exposure of the aorta and its branches. There is no apparent difference whether the operation is performed for aneurysmal or occlusive disease. However, 9 of the 11 patients had a bifurcated graft placed and a large lymphocele developed in another patient following thoracoabdominal aneurysm repair, suggesting that there is a higher incidence if extensive dissection during vascular reconstruction is needed.

Eight of the 11 retroperitoneal lymphoceles were diagnosed between 2 months and 8 years after graft placement. Distention, nausea, vague abdominal pain, or an abdominal or flank mass was present in 6 of 11 patients, but in five patients the initial sign was a groin mass. Further workup in these patients showed the presence of retroperitoneal lymphocele with communication to the groin. Four patients had ureteral compression and hydronephrosis.

The diagnosis of retroperitoneal lymphocele can be considered in the rare patient who has milky, odorless discharge resembling chyle from a groin fistula following aortofemoral reconstruction. Rarely, a large abdominal or flank mass is palpable in a similar patient. Lymphoscintigraphy confirms the presence of a lymphocele, and the risk of graft infection with late, persistent perigraft fluid collection is significant. Computed tomography in these pa-

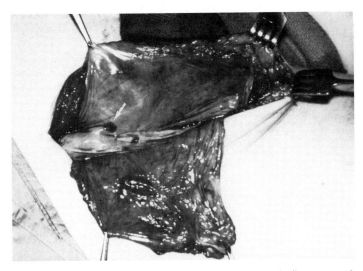

Fig. 29-11. Large sac of lymphocele opened at right groin. Arrow indicates opening of feeding lymph vessel into lymphocele, stained by Lymphazurine dye. The orifice was oversewn and the sac of lymphocele was excised.

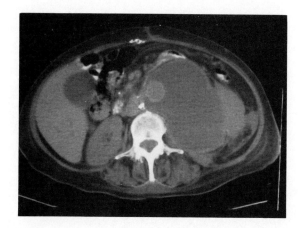

Fig. 29-12. CT scan of large retroperitoneal lymphocele in 69-year-old woman 2 months after repair of a thoracoabdominal aortic aneurysm. The lymphocele was reduced with percutaneous aspiration and is stable in size 2 years later.

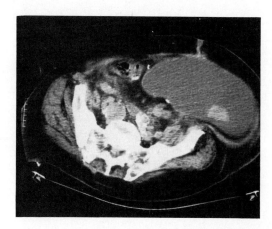

Fig. 29-13. CT scan demonstrating retroperitoneal lymphocele in 79-year-old man 3 weeks after repair of an abdominal aortic aneurysm with an aortobiiliac graft. Percutaneous aspiration confirmed clear lymph and resulted in resolution of the symptoms.

Fig. 29-14. Anatomy of the mesenteric and ascending lumbar lymphatic trunks and cysterna chyli.

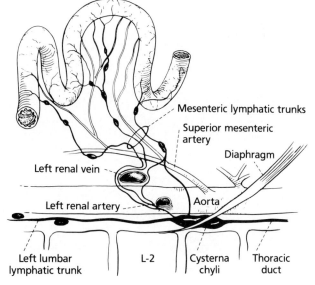

Table 29-1. Retroperitoneal Lymphocele After Aortic Reconstruction

Author	Age/sex of patient	Surgical indication	Operation performed	Postoperative presentation; interval	Treatment	Outcome
Dillon and Postlethwait[14] (1970)	51/M	AAA	Aortobi-iliac bypass	Abdominal mass; 1 wk	Aspiration (failed); surgical closure	Resolved at 2 yr
Fitzer et al.[15] (1980)	63/F	AIO	Aortobifemoral bypass	Right flank mass, ureteral obstruction	Surgical drainage (×2)	Resolved
Puyau et al.[19] (1985)	64/F	AIO	Aortobifemoral bypass	Bilateral groin mass, right hydronephrosis; 8 mo	Surgical closure	Stable small lymphocele at 1 yr
Jensen et al.[17] (1986)	70/M	AAA	Aortobi-iliac bypass	Abdominal pain, mass on CT scan; 5 yr	Aspiration	Resolved at 3 mo
Pardy et al.[18] (1986)	55/M	Renal artery occlusion	Aortorenal bypass	Abdominal pain, mass on CT scan; 10 wk	Multiple aspirations	Stable small lymphocele at 8 mo
Garrett et al.[20] (1989)	58/M	AAA	Aortobifemoral bypass	Right groin mass, hydronephrosis; 2 yr	Irrigation-drainage	Graft infection requiring removal; cysterna ligated
	57/F	AIO	Aortobifemoral bypass	Bilateral groin mass, hydronephrosis; 4 yr	Irrigation-drainage	Graft infection requiring removal; cysterna ligated
	65/M	AIO	Aortobifemoral bypass	Bilateral groin mass; 8 yr	Surgical drainage, muscle flap	Resolved at 4 mo
	58/M	AIO	Aortobifemoral bypass	Bilateral groin mass; 3 yr	Aspirations (failed); bilateral obturator bypasses with cysterna ligation	Resolved at 18 mo
Gloviczki (1990)*	69/F	Thoracoabdominal aortic aneurysm	Thoracoabdominal tube graft	Abdominal pain, mass on CT scan; 2 mo	Aspiration	Stable lymphocele unchanged at 2 yr
	79/M	AAA	Aortobi-iliac bypass	Abdominal pain, mass on CT scan; 3 wk	Aspiration	Small stable lymphocele at 1 mo

AAA, abdominal aortic aneurysm; AIO, aortoiliac occlusion.
*Unpublished data.

tients should be performed routinely. Except in the early postoperative period, we perform a labeled white cell scan and search for further evidence of infection. Small, asymptomatic retroperitoneal fluid collections are observed with computed tomography at 3-month intervals. If the volume of fluid collection is increasing, is large at first detection, or the patient has gastrointestinal or urinary symptoms, needle aspiration under computed tomography or ultrasound guidance is performed. This is both diagnostic and therapeutic.

Previous experience indicates that the placement of any irrigation-drainage system has a high risk of infection.[20] Repeated aspiration also carries a risk of infection. Therefore if the lymphocele recurs or enlarges after aspiration, operation to ligate or oversew the site of the lymphatic injury is suggested. In patients with nonchylous retroperitoneal lymphocele, we inject Lymphazurine dye into the foot of the corresponding side to identify the site of the lymphatic injury. The lymphocele is unroofed and if the graft is exposed, it is covered by retroperitoneal tissue or omentum. If aspiration of the lymphocele confirms chyle, a nasogastric tube is placed preoperatively and 24 oz of cream is given through the tube 4 hours before the operation. The site of the leak in the mesenteric lymphatic trunks or in the cysterna then is easily identified during exploration. The leaking mesenteric trunk is ligated but if the cysterna is injured, lateral closure is attempted.

Prevention of retroperitoneal lymphatic injury is essential during aortic reconstruction. Lymph vessels should be ligated before division and any visible leak should be controlled immediately by ligation or suture. Since patients with lymphatic injury have a high risk of graft infection, such preventive measures and careful surgical technique may save not only the limb but also the life of the patient.

Chylous Ascites

The development of chylous ascites is a rare but potentially grave complication of aortic surgery, with mechanical, nutritional, and immunologic consequences. It is more frequent following operation for abdominal aortic aneurysm than for aortoiliac occlusive disease

although this complication, similar to retroperitoneal lymphocele, most probably is underreported. A review of the English literature shows that of 17 patients with this complication, 14 underwent repair of an abdominal aortic aneurysm (Table 29-2). The development of chylous ascites was noted within 6 weeks of the operation in all but one patient. Signs and symptoms include progressive abdominal distention, dyspnea, nausea, and vague abdominal pain. The presentation can be similar to that of retroperitoneal lymphocele although malnutrition usually is more prominent. In patients whose treatment has been delayed for several weeks, hypoproteinemia, lymphocytopenia, and anemia may be significant. Ultrasound or computed tomography will demonstrate peritoneal fluid but the diagnosis is confirmed by paracentesis. The milky abdominal fluid stains positively for fat, has no unpleasant odor, and contains many lymphocytes. The amount of fat in the chyle ranges from 0.4 to 4 gm/dl and its protein content is above 3 gm/dl.[27] The specific gravity of the chyle is greater than 1.012 gm/ml and it is a sterile alkaline fluid.[35]

The cause of chylous ascites following aortic surgery is iatrogenic injury to the mesenteric lymphatic trunks, the cysterna chyli, or the abdominal thoracic duct. The cysterna chyli usually is located posterior and to the right of the aorta at the level of the second lumbar vertebra. In 50% of patients the thoracic duct arises from a lymphatic plexus rather than the cysterna. The cysterna chyli, if present, is formed mainly by the right and left lumbar and the mesenteric lymphatic trunks. A somewhat less known description of the anatomy of the mesenteric lymphatic trunks has been provided by Servelle and Nogues[76] (Fig. 29-14). This explains why lymphatic trunks filled with milky fluid frequently are found during dissection of the neck of an infrarenal aortic aneurysm. Several mesenteric lymphatic trunks course distal to the left renal vein before joining the cysterna chyli behind the upper abdominal aorta. Any injury to these lymphatics during aortic dissection should be treated immediately by ligation, or if it is the cysterna, by lateral closure with 6-0 or 7-0 Prolene sutures.

Table 29-2. Chylous Ascites After Aortic Reconstruction

Author	Age/sex of patient	Surgical indication	Operation performed	Postoperative presentation; interval	Treatment	Outcome
Bradham et al.[22] (1970)	71/M	AAA	"Repair" of AAA	Ascites; 3 wk	Multiple paracenteses, surgical closure	Resolved
Klippel and Hardy[24] (1971)	68/M	Ruptured AAA	"Repair" of AAA	Ascites; 2 wk	Multiple paracenteses with reinfusion	Resolved
DeBartolo and Etzkorn[23] (1976)	67/M	AAA	"Repair" of AAA	Ascites; 3 wk	Multiple paracenteses	Resolved after 6 mo
Lopez-Enriquez et al.[26] (1979)	72/M	AAA	"Repair" of AAA	Ascites; 4 wk	Paracentesis low-fat diet	Died 3 wk later of pulmonary embolus
Meinke et al.[27] (1979)	65/M	Ruptured AAA	"Repair" of AAA	Ascites; 6 wk	Total parenteral nutrition	Resolved
Stubbe and Terpstra[32] (1979)	72/M	AAA	Aortobifemoral bypass	Ascites; 2 wk	Diuresis, medium-chain triglyceride diet	Resolved
McKenna and Stevick[29] (1983)	59/M	AIO	Aortobifemoral bypass	Ascites; 2 wk	Total parenteral nutrition (failed); lateral suture of cysterna	Resolved
Savrin and High[31] (1985)	66/M	AAA	Aortobifemoral bypass	Ascites; 3 wk	Total parenteral nutrition	Resolved
Jensen et al.[17] (1986)	54/M	AIO	Aortobifemoral bypass	Ascites; 16 wk	Multiple paracenteses	Died 5 wk later from sepsis
Sarazin and Sauter[33] (1986)	56/M	Ruptured AAA	Tube graft	Ascites; 4 wk	Diet (failed); peritoneovenous shunting	Resolved
Fleischer et al.[30] (1987)	71/F	AAA	"Repair" of AAA	Ascites; 3 wk	Total parenteral nutrition (failed); peritoneovenous shunting	Resolved
Schwein et al.[28] (1987)	60/M	AAA	Tube graft	Ascites; 2 wk	Paracentesis, total parenteral nutrition	Resolved
Williamson and Provan[34] (1987)	65/M	AIO	Aortobifemoral bypass	Ascites; 4 wk	Diuresis and medium-chain triglyceride diet (failed); cysterna ligated	Resolved

	Age/Sex	Diagnosis	Procedure	Presentation	Treatment	Outcome
Boyd et al.[21] (1989)	54/M	Ruptured AAA	Tube graft	Ascites; 20 d	Total parenteral nutrition and paracentesis (failed); peritoneovenous shunting	Resolved at 6 mo
Heyl and Veen[25] (1989)	62/M	AIO	Aortobifemoral bypass	Abdominal pain; 1 wk	Laparotomy (x2), cysterna ligated	Resolved
Ablan et al.[35] (1990)	65/M	AAA	Aortoiliac graft	Ascites; 1 wk	Paracentesis, low-fat, medium-chain triglyceride diet	Resolved
	59/M	AAA	Aortoiliac graft	Ascites; postoperative	Paracentesis, low-fat, medium-chain triglyceride diet	Died

AAA, abdominal aortic aneurysm; AIO, aortoiliac occlusion.

Although chylous ascites that develops in patients with abdominal malignancies carries a poor prognosis, occurrence after aortic surgery generally means a better chance for a successful outcome. However, 3 of the 18 reported patients died in the early postoperative period. The causes of death were malnutrition in one patient, pulmonary embolus in another, and sepsis following multiple paracenteses in the third patient. Most patients, however, could be successfully managed nonoperatively with paracentesis and aggressive nutritional support. Since only long-chain triglycerides are absorbed by the mesenteric lymphatics, several patients responded well to a high-protein, low-fat, medium-chain triglyceride diet. To decrease the total volume of chyle, total parenteral nutrition and bowel rest also may be needed. Surgical treatment was required in 7 of the 18 patients. In three cases leaking mesenteric trunks or cysterna were ligated and in one patient lateral closure of the cysterna was performed. Peritoneovenous shunts were placed with good results in three additional patients. Because of the possibility of infectious complications associated with peritoneovenous shunting, we would perform reexploration if elemental diet or total parenteral nutrition failed. Preoperative preparation of the patient is similar to that described for patients with chylous retroperitoneal lymphocele. The ideal surgical treatment of chylous ascites, as suggested by McKenna and Stevick,[29] is lateral closure of the injured cysterna chyli. Since collateral circulation usually is sufficient, ligation or oversewing of the site of the lymphatic leak also should be effective. As pointed out in a recent editorial,[77] surgical treatment for chylous ascites following abdominal surgery is rarely needed.

REFERENCES

1. Olszewski W. Pathophysiological and clinical observations of obstructive lymphedema of the limbs. In Clodius L, ed. Lymphedema. Stuttgart: Thieme, 1977, pp 79-102.
2. Schubart PJ, Porter JM. Leg edema following femorodistal bypass. In Bergan JJ, Yao JST, eds. Reoperative Arterial Surgery. Orlando, Fla.: Grune & Stratton, 1986, pp 311-330.

3. Clodius L, Piller NB, Casley-Smith JR. The problems of lymphatic microsurgery for lymphedema. Lymphology 14:69-76, 1981.

4. Gloviczki P. Treatment of acquired lymphedema—Medical and surgical. In Ernst CB, Stanley JC, eds. Current Therapy in Vascular Surgery-II. Philadelphia: BC Decker, 1991, pp 1030-1036.

5. Casley-Smith JR, Foldi M, Ryan TJ, Witte MH, Witte CL, Cluzan R, Partsch H, Jamal S, O'Brien B. Lymphedema: Summary of the 10th International Congress of Lymphology working group discussions and recommendations, Adelaide, Australia, August 10-17, 1985. Lymphology 18:175-180, 1985.

6. Vaughan BF, Slavotinek AH, Jepson RP. Edema of the lower limb after vascular operations. Surg Gynecol Obstet 133:282-290, 1970.

7. Porter JM, Lindell TD, Lakin PC. Leg edema following femoropopliteal autogenous vein bypass. Arch Surg 105:883-888, 1972.

8. Storen EJ, Myhre HO, Stiris G. Lymphangiographic findings in patients with leg oedema after arterial reconstructions. Acta Chir Scand 140:385-387, 1974.

9. Stillman RM, Fitzgerald JF, Varughese G, et al. Edema following femoropopliteal bypass: Etiology and prevention. Vasc Surg 18:354-360, 1983.

10. Schmidt KR, Welter H, Pfeifer KJ, Becker HM. Lymphographic investigations of oedema of the extremities following reconstructive vascular surgery in the femoropopliteal territory. ROFO 128:194-202, 1978.

11. AbuRahma AF, Woodruff BA, Lucente FC. Edema after femoropopliteal bypass surgery: Lymphatic and venous theories of causation. J Vasc Surg 11:461-467, 1990.

12. Kwaan JHM, Bernstein JM, Connolly JE. Management of lymph fistula in the groin after arterial reconstruction. Arch Surg 114:1416-1418, 1979.

13. Stolzenberg J. Detection of lymphaticocutaneous fistula by radionuclide lymphangiography. Arch Surg 113:306-307, 1978.

14. Dillon ML, Postlethwait RW. The management of an abdominal mass recurring after resection of abdominal aortic aneurysm. Surg Clin North Am 50:1021-1029, 1970.

15. Fitzer PM, Sallade RL, Graham WH. Computed tomography and the diagnosis of giant abdominal lymphocele. Vasc Med 107:448-449, 1980.

16. Patel BR, Burkhalter JL, Patel RB, Raju S. Interstitial lymphscintigraphy for diagnosis of lymphocele. Clin Nucl Med 10:175-176, 1985.

17. Jensen SR, Voegeli DR, McDermott JC, Crummy AB, Turnipseed WD. Lymph vessels: Lymphatic disruption following abdominal aortic surgery. Cardiovasc Intervent Radiol 9:199-201, 1986.

18. Pardy BJ, Harris P, Mourad K, Cunningham J. Case reports: Upper abdominal lymphocele following urgent aortorenal bypass grafting. J R Soc Med 79:674-676, 1986.

19. Puyau FA, Adinolfi MF, Kerstein MD. Lymphocele around aortic femoral grafts simulating a false aneurysm. Cardiovasc Intervent Radiol 8:195-198, 1985.

20. Garrett HE, Richardson JW, Howard HS, Garrett HE. Retroperitoneal lymphocele after abdominal aortic surgery. J Vasc Surg 10:245-253, 1989.

21. Boyd WD, McPhail NV, Barber GC. Case report: Chylous ascites following abdominal aortic aneurysmectomy: Surgical management with a peritoneovenous shunt. J Cardiovasc Surg 30:627-629, 1989.

22. Bradham RR, Gregorie HB, Wilson R. Chylous ascites following resection of an abdominal aortic aneurysm. Am Surg 36:238-240, 1970.

23. DeBartolo TF, Etzkorn JR. Conservative management of chylous ascites after abdominal aortic aneurysm repair: Case report. Mo Med 73:611-613, 1976.

24. Klippel AP, Hardy DA. Postoperative chylous ascites. Mo Med 68:253-255, 1971.

25. Heyl A, Veen HF. Iatrogenic chylous ascites: Operative or conservative approach. Neth J Surg 41:5-7, 1989.

26. Lopez-Enriquez E, Gonzalez A, Johnson CD, Perez C. Chylothorax and chyloperitoneum: A case report. Bol Asoc Med P R 71:54-58, 1979.

27. Meinke AH, Estes NC, Ernst CB. Chylous ascites following abdominal aortic aneurysmectomy. Ann Surg 190:631-633, 1979.

28. Schwein M, Dawes PD, Hatchuel D, Decker GAG. Postoperative chylous ascites after resection of an abdominal aortic aneurysm: A case report. S Afr J Surg 25:39-41, 1987.

29. McKenna R, Stevick CA. Chylous ascites following aortic reconstruction. Vasc Surg 17:143-149, 1983.

30. Fleischer HL, Oren JW, Sumner DS. Chylous ascites after abdominal aortic aneurysmectomy: Successful management with a peritoneovenous shunt. J Vasc Surg 6:403-407, 1987.

31. Savrin RA, High R. Chylous ascites after abdominal aortic surgery. Surgery 98:866-869, 1985.

32. Stubbe LTHFL, Terpstra JL. Chylous ascites after resection of an abdominal aortic aneurysm. Arch Chir Neerlandicum 31:111-113, 1979.

33. Sarazin WG, Sauter KE. Chylous ascites following resection of a ruptured abdominal aneurysm. Arch Surg 121:246-247, 1986.

34. Williamson C, Provan JL. Chylous ascites following aortic surgery. Br J Surg 74:71-72, 1987.

35. Ablan CJ, Littooy FN, Freeark RJ. Postoperative chylous ascites: Diagnosis and treatment. Arch Surg 125:270-273, 1990.

36. Bergan JJ, Yao JST. Discussion of Baumeister RG, Siuda S, Bohmert H, Moser E. A microsurgical method for reconstruction of interrupted lymphatic pathways: Autologous lymph-vessel transplantation for treatment of lymphedemas. In Bergan JJ, Yao JST, eds. The Year Book of Vascular Surgery 1988. Chicago: Year Book, 1988, pp 241-242.

37. Jacobson JH. Discussion of Danese C, Bower R, Howard J. Experimental anastomoses of lymphatics. Arch Surg 84:9, 1962.

38. Laine JB, Howard JM. Experimental lymphatico-venous anastomosis. Surg Forum 14:111-112, 1963.

39. Yamada Y. The studies on lymphatic venous anastomosis in lymphedema. Nagoya J Med Sci 32:1-21, 1969.

40. Nielubowicz J, Olszewski W. Surgical lymphaticove-nous shunts in patients with secondary lymphoedema. Br J Surg 55:440-442, 1968.

41. Gilbert A, O'Brien BMcC, Vorrath JW, Sykes PJ. Lymphaticovenous anastomosis by microvascular technique. Br J Plast Surg 29:355-360, 1976.

42. Gloviczki P, LeFloch P, Hidden G. Anastomoses lymphatico-veineuses experimentales. J Chir (Paris) 116:437-443, 1979.

43. Gloviczki P, Hollier LH, Nora FE, Kaye MP. The natural history of microsurgical lymphovenous anasto-moses: An experimental study. J Vasc Surg 4:148-156, 1986.

44. Degni M. New technique of lymphatic-venous anasto-mosis (buried type) for the treatment of lymphedema. Vasa 3:479-483, 1974.

45. O'Brien BM, Chait LA, Hurwitz PJ. Microlymphatic surgery. Orthop Clin North Am 8:405-424, 1977.

46. O'Brien BMcC, Shafiroff BB. Microlymphaticove-nous and resectional surgery in obstructive lymphede-ma. World J Surg 3:3-15, 1979.

47. Huang GK, Ru-Qi H, Zong-Zhao L, Yao-Liang S, Tie-De L, Gong-Ping P. Microlymphaticovenous anastomosis for treating lymphedema of the extremi-ties and external genitalia. J Microsurg 3:32-39, 1981.

48. Jamal S. Lymphovenous anastomosis in filarial lymph-edema. Lymphology 14:64-68, 1981.

49. Krylov V, Milanov N, Abalmasov K. Microlymphatic surgery of secondary lymphoedema of the upper limb. Ann Chir Gynaecol 71:77-79, 1982.

50. Nieuborg L. The Role of Lymphaticovenous Anasto-moses in the Treatment of Postmastectomy Oedema. Alblasserdam, Netherlands: Offsetdrukkerij Kanters BV, 1982.

51. Gong-Kang H, Ru-Qi H, Zong-Zhao L, Yao-Liang S, Tie-De L, Gong-Ping P. Microlymphaticovenous anastomosis in the treatment of lower limb obstructive lymphedema: Analysis of 91 cases. Plast Reconstr Surg 76:671-685, 1985.

52. Ingianni G, Holzmann T. Clinical experience with lympho-venous anastomosis for secondary lymphede-ma. Handchirurgie 17:43-46, 1985.

53. Campisi C, Tosatti E, Casaccia M, et al. Microchirur-gia dei linfatici. Minerva Chir 41:469-481, 1986.

54. Zhu JK, Yu GZ, Liu JX, Pang SF, Lao ZG, Tang HY. Recent advances in microlymphatic surgery in China. Clin Orthop 215:32-39, 1987.

55. Gloviczki P, Fisher J, Hollier LH, Pairolero PC, Schirger A, Wahner HW. Microsurgical lymphove-nous anastomosis for treatment of lymphedema: A critical review. J Vasc Surg 7:647-652, 1988.

56. Puckett CL, Jacobs GR, Hurvitz JS, Silver D. Evalua-tion of lymphovenous anastomoses in obstructive lymphedema. Plast Reconstr Surg 66:116-120, 1980.

57. O'Brien BMcC, Mellow CG, Khazanchi RK, Dvir E, Kumar V, Pederson WC. Long-term results after microlymphatico-venous anastomoses for the treat-ment of obstructive lymphedema. Plast Reconstr Surg 85:562-572, 1990.

58. Olszewski WL. Physiology and microsurgery of lym-phatic vessels in man. Lymphology 14:44-60, 1981.

59. Miller GE, Smathers JB, Hightower D, Seale J, Hood D. Lymphatic clearance of radioactive sulfur colloid. Lymphology 13:24-29, 1980.

60. Wolfe JHN. The pathophysiology of lymphedema. In Rutherford RB, ed. Vascular Surgery, 3rd ed. Philadel-phia: WB Saunders, 1989, pp 1648-1656.

61. Nieuborg L. Diskussion. Stellungnahme zur Verof-fentlichung von RGH Baumeister. Mikrochirurgie des lymphgefass Systems. Chirurg 55:353-354, 1984.

62. O'Brien BMcC, Das SK, Franklin JD, Morrison WA. Effect of lymphangiography on lymphedema. Plast Reconstr Surg 68:922, 1981.

63. Gloviczki P, Calcagno D, Schirger A, Pairolero PC, Cherry KJ, Hallett JW, Wahner HW. Noninvasive evaluation of the swollen extremity: Experiences with 190 lymphoscintigraphic examinations. J Vasc Surg 9:683-690, 1989.

64. Baumeister RG, Seifert J, Wiebecke B. Homologous and autologous experimental lymph vessel transplanta-tion: Initial experience. Int J Microsurg 3:19-24, 1981.

65. Baumeister RG, Siuda S, Bohmert H, Moser E. A microsurgical method for reconstruction of interrupt-ed lymphatic pathways: Autologous lymph-vessel transplantation for treatment of lymphedemas. Scand J Plast Reconstr Surg 20:141-146, 1986.

66. Baumeister RG, Siuda S. Treatment of lymphedemas by microsurgical lymphatic grafting: What is proved? Plast Reconstr Surg 85:64-76, 1990.

67. Gloviczki P. Microsurgical treatment for chronic lymphedema: An unfulfilled promise? In Bergan JJ, Yao JST, eds. Venous Disorders. Orlando, Fla.: WB Saunders, 1991, pp 344-359.

68. Haimovici H. Metabolic complications of acute arte-rial occlusions and related conditions: Role of free radicals (myonephropathic-metabolic syndrome). In Haimovici H, ed. Vascular Surgery. Norwalk, Conn.: Appleton & Lange, 1989, pp 386-408.

69. Myhre HO, Dedichen H. Hemodynamic factors in the oedema of arterial reconstructions. Scand J Thorac Cardiovasc Surg 6:323-326, 1972.

70. Simeone FA, Husni EA. The hyperemia of reconstruc-tive arterial surgery. Ann Surg 150:575, 1959.

71. Husni EA. The edema of arterial reconstruction. Circulation (Suppl) 35:169-173, 1967.

72. Campbell H, Harris PL. Albumin kinetics and edema following reconstructive arterial surgery of the lower limb. J Cardiovasc Surg 26:110-115, 1985.

73. Scott DJA, Allen MJ, Bell PRF, McShane M, Barnes MR. Does oedema following lower limb revascularisa-tion cause compartment syndromes? Ann R Coll Surg Engl 70:372-376, 1988.

74. Taylor GW. Arterial grafting for gangrene. Ann R Coll Surg Engl 31:168-186, 1962.

75. Hamer JD. Investigation of oedema of the lower limb following successful femoral popliteal bypass surgery: The role of phlebography in demonstrating venous thrombosis. Br J Surg 59:979-982, 1972.

76. Servelle M, Nogues C. Anatomy of the lymphatics of the small intestine. In Servelle M, Nogues C, eds. The Chyliferous Vessels. Paris: Expansion Scientifique Francaise, 1981, pp 1-9.

77. Savrin RA, High R. Chylous ascites after abdominal aortic surgery [Discussion]. In Bergan JJ, Yao JST, eds. The Year Book of Vascular Surgery 1987. Chicago: Year Book, 1987, pp 78-79.

XI Upper Extremity Vascular Surgery

30

Complications of Vascular Access

Mark B. Adams   **Christopher P. Johnson**   **Allan M. Roza**

Currently 80,000 patients are maintained on chronic hemodialysis in the United States. Approximately 8000 other patients undergo acute dialysis or hemofiltration for the treatment of a variety of conditions ranging from acute renal failure to drug overdose.[1] Obtaining vascular access, temporary or permanent, in order to institute treatment in these patients involves the implementation of prosthetic devices, requires specific knowledge, and demands careful monitoring. Many of the complications related to vascular access are specific to the access technique, device, and site.

TEMPORARY ACCESS

Temporary access techniques use external prosthetic devices such as Scribner shunts that are not intended to be used on a permanent basis. Scribner shunts were originally the only available form of vascular access for chronic hemodialysis. These shunts are placed after surgical dissection of an appropriate artery (usually radial or posterior tibial) and an accompanying vein. Using a cutdown technique, the surgeon cannulates and joins the vessels with externally positioned Silastic tubing. A cumbersome arrangement of cannulas, adapters, and tubing is required. Scribner shunts have fallen into disuse because of the associated high incidence of thrombotic and infectious complications. In addition, their use often precludes permanent access at the same site, although it may be possible to convert the site into a fistula.

The most common form of temporary vascular access currently in use is the percutaneous subclavian or femoral dialysis catheter. Femoral catheters are not used as often as subclavian catheters because they are associated with a high rate of infection and are difficult to immobilize. Femoral catheters are frequently placed at the beginning of each dialysis treatment and removed at the end. Their use may lead to an increased incidence of iliofemoral venous thrombosis, with its attendant risk of pulmonary embolism, and may also be the cause of significant retroperitoneal hemorrhage. The major advantage of using femoral catheters is the avoidance of risks associated with subclavian and jugular punctures.

Subclavian venous catheters are currently

the most popular choice for temporary access. Subclavian catheters are introduced using standard subclavian technique over a guidewire. These catheters are usually double lumen, with the two lumens separated by 3 to 4 cm. The double-lumen catheter allows the patients to be dialyzed using the standard two-needle machine technique. Single-lumen catheters require a different technique, which generally gives a lower clearance rate and causes an increased recirculation effect.

Both types of catheters are available in a variety of models but have several characteristics in common. They must be of sufficient caliber to support the high flow rates required for adequate hemodialysis (greater than 200 cc/min) and be rigid enough to prevent collapse when drawing pressures become high.[2] The most commonly used temporary catheter is the Quinton-Mahukar polyurethane double-lumen catheter (Quinton Instrument Co., Seattle, Wash.).

With careful nursing and patient management, these catheters may be left in place for 4 to 6 weeks, which is usually sufficient time to construct a permanent fistula.

Complications
Infection

Infection represents the most common complication of temporary vascular access and requires the removal or replacement of the catheter. Infection will eventually occur in most percutaneously placed temporary access catheters. The clinical impact of infection related to the catheter can be minimized by early removal whenever signs of fever, pericatheter exudate, or erythema appear. In situations in which the access site is of great clinical importance and another access site would be difficult to obtain, replacement of the catheter over a guidewire and careful observation with antibiotic coverage frequently allows continued use of the site.

As an additional barrier to infection, some subclavian dialysis catheters are manufactured with a proximal cuff (e.g., PermCath; Quinton Instrument Co., Seattle, Wash.). The cuff becomes incorporated into the subcutaneous tissue and retards the migration of bacteria along the catheter surface. The incidence of infection appears to be reduced with this modification, but these catheters remain prone to thrombosis and failure as a result of fibrin sheath formation at the tip. In general, their use is limited to patients in whom all other routes for permanent vascular access have been exhausted or in patients in whom permanent access will not be usable for 6 to 8 weeks. The presence of a cuffed catheter minimizes the risk of infection and usually provides reliable access for at least the time necessary until a permanent access site can be developed. These catheters have also been advocated for permanent access use. In our hands, they have not worked well in this role. Other reports are more optimistic.[3]

Cuffed subclavian dialysis catheters are often placed percutaneously using large dilators and peel-away sheaths. The size (20 Fr) and rigidity of these sheaths are troublesome, however. Subclavian disruption and/or superior vena caval disruption have occasionally occurred. We have had good results with the direct placement of cuffed catheters through either the internal or external jugular veins with the patient under local anesthesia.

The way in which a subclavian dialysis catheter is cared for and flushed will, in most cases, determine its useful life span. Temporary subclavian catheters should be handled in an aseptic manner and flushed routinely with high-dose heparin solution (5000 U/ml). Care must be taken to aspirate the residual heparin before using the catheter for any purpose other than dialysis. Often the patient or a relative can handle flushing of the catheter, but in most cases qualified medical personnel should be responsible for the dressing change since this requires knowledge and practice of sterile technique.

Bleeding

The surgeon performing vascular access will undoubtedly become involved in situations in which uremic patients experience excessive and prolonged bleeding. Most commonly this occurs following percutaneous placement of access catheters.

Bleeding is more likely with temporary hemodialysis catheters than with other central venous catheters because of their size, rigidity, and the manipulation that inevitably occurs. Bleeding can be minimized by careful handling of the catheter during dialysis. When bleeding is experienced, it can usually be controlled by local pressure and correction of any coagulation abnormalities.

Uremic patients have a well-known tendency for increased bleeding.[4,5] The precise derangements are not entirely understood but predominantly relate to primary hemostasis (i.e., platelet-vessel interaction and platelet aggregation). The single best test that quantitatively measures this platelet dysfunction is the skin bleeding time. Other hemostatic defects that have been identified include abnormally increased prostaglandin I_2 production by the uremic vessel wall, decreased platelet thromboxane A_2 production, changes in the von Willebrand factor (vWf) molecule, and decreased platelet factor III.

Presumably, the platelet dysfunction in uremia allows improved patency of vascular access. Observations that support this theory include the well-known propensity of fistulas to clot following renal transplantation and the generally accepted difficulty of maintaining vascular access in preuremic individuals.

Platelet transfusions will have little beneficial effect in these circumstances since in the uremic milieu normal platelets acquire the characteristics of uremic platelets. Cryoprecipitate is a plasma derivative and is a good source of factor VIII and vWf. Infusion of cryoprecipitate shortens the bleeding time of uremic patients, with the peak effect seen 4 to 6 hours after infusion. Because of the risk of transmissible diseases, however, cryoprecipitate is not the agent of choice for correction of uremic bleeding.

Desmopressin (DDAVP) is a synthetic derivative of an antidiuretic hormone and acts to increase plasma concentrations of vWf by releasing it from storage sites.[6] Administration of DDAVP intravenously (0.3 µg/kg) temporarily corrects prolonged bleeding time and has a more rapid onset of action (peak effect, 1 hour) than cryoprecipitate. DDAVP can also be given intranasally or subcutaneously at ten times the intravenous dose.

Conjugated estrogens can normalize bleeding time for 3 to 10 days in patients with chronic renal failure. The mechanism of this effect is unknown but may relate again to an alteration of vWf. A single oral dose of estrogen (Premarin 25 mg) or intravenous doses (3 mg/kg) divided over 5 consecutive days may be effective and long lasting.[7]

Whenever bleeding occurs that is not easily controlled by pressure, the possibility of major vessel injury and/or coagulopathy should be considered. A bleeding time, prothrombin time, and partial thromboplastin time should be obtained and corrected with appropriate therapy. Most patients on dialysis have a significant qualitative platelet defect. Even if platelet counts are adequate, DDAVP or cryoprecipitate will often reduce bleeding that is otherwise difficult to control. Heparinized patients usually respond to protamine. As in other surgical situations, however, it is unwise and unsafe to attribute ongoing bleeding to coagulopathy alone. If bleeding fails to come under control and the patient is in jeopardy, operation is indicated.

Major hemorrhage related to vessel injury is rare and most often occurs as a complication of venous perforation. Catheter removal, application of pressure, and correction of coagulation defects is the usual treatment. If the bleeding is vigorous and the catheter has been in place for some time, the possibility that erosion into an artery has occurred should be considered. Several units of blood can easily be lost into the pleural space or retroperitoneum with few outward signs. Rarely, these patients require surgery for control of arterial or venous lacerations. Operation should not be delayed if bleeding cannot be readily controlled.

Pneumothorax/Hemothorax

Hemothorax and pneumothorax are relatively uncommon complications of subclavian placement of temporary access when the procedure is performed by experienced physicians.[8] When performed by those with little experience, it is doubly dangerous because these complications are not only more likely to occur, but also are often not immediately recognized. A postplacement chest x-ray film should be obtained both to locate the catheter and to rule out hemorrhage and pneumothorax. These complications should be suspected whenever a patient complains of shortness of breath and/or hypotension develops after catheter placement.

The diagnosis can be difficult since many of these catheters are placed just before the initiation of dialysis and patients may experience brief episodes of hypotension during hemodialysis as a result of reactions to materials in the dialysis system or fluid shifts. The chance of a major hemorrhage is also increased in this setting because the patient is often systemically anticoagulated during dialysis. When hemothorax or pneumothorax is suspected, it should be treated by removal of the catheter and placement of a chest tube. X-ray film documentation should not delay appropriate treatment.

Catheter perforation of the superior vena cava is best treated by placing the patient in an upright position, inserting a chest tube, and removing the catheter. Hypotension should be rapidly corrected before placing the patient in an upright position since this position change can be dangerous in the hypovolemic patient.

Thrombosis

Catheter thrombosis. Thrombosis of the catheter is a frequent problem encountered in patients with temporary central venous access. It can be treated by aggressive flushing with normal saline solution, enzymatic digestion with streptokinase or urokinase, or reestablishment of a lumen with a large guidewire. If these measures fail, the catheter can be replaced over a guidewire unless signs of infection at the insertion site are present.

Subclavian thrombosis. Subclavian thrombosis is not uncommon in patients with temporary access because of the size and mechanical properties of these catheters. If subclavian thrombosis occurs, the catheter should be removed and another route of dialysis used. The administration of anticoagulation therapy (heparin) in this setting is controversial. Pulmonary embolism in dialysis patients appears to be extremely rare. Patients with massively swollen arms may benefit symptomatically from a short course of heparin.

Replacement of the subclavian catheter on the opposite side may be unwise in such situations since occlusion of both subclavian veins may lead to a superior vena cava syndrome. Also, bilateral subclavian thrombosis severely limits future choices for the site of permanent access, but unfortunately this may be unavoidable. When repeated thromboses occur, a primary hypercoagulable state should be suspected (e.g., antithrombin III deficiency or protein C or S deficiency). Such individuals frequently have associated heavy proteinuria.[9] Antithrombin deficiencies can be effectively treated by administering fresh frozen plasma to correct the deficiency at the time of access placement and until conversion to long-term warfarin (Coumadin) therapy is complete.

With the increased use of subclavian dialysis catheters for initial vascular access in the patient presenting for dialysis, the incidence of subclavian thrombosis has increased, which may be as high as 30%. Creation of an arteriovenous fistula (AVF) distal to an occluded subclavian vein usually results in marked edema of the extremity and the eventual necessity of fistula takedown. Since in most patients currently referred for permanent access placement, subclavian dialysis catheters have been used previously, the access surgeon must document that the subclavian vein is patent before proceeding with fistula formation. Verification of patency is most easily accomplished with color Doppler ultrasonography and can also be obtained with venography. The importance of this step cannot be overemphasized in the current milieu of ready placement of subclavian access.

Pulmonary Embolism

Pulmonary embolism appears to be rare in uremic patients because of their platelet dysfunction but should be suspected in any patient with a long-standing indwelling central venous or femoral catheter who experiences symptoms such as dyspnea or chest pain. Pulmonary embolism should also be suspected when thrombectomy of venous access catheters or a Scribner shunt is associated with dyspnea, hemoptysis, or deteriorating pulmonary function. The small size of these emboli makes death from a single embolus unlikely. However, repeated declottings can produce a total volume of embolus sufficient to produce chronic pulmonary hypertension.

PERMANENT ACCESS

Permanent vascular access is any type of access used frequently and repeatedly for an extended or indefinite period of time. Forms of permanent access include both autogenous AVFs and fistulas constructed with prosthetic material (polytetrafluoroethylene [PTFE], umbilical vein, Dacron).[10]

Even in patients undergoing peritoneal dialysis, an autogenous AVF should be constructed. Patients on peritoneal dialysis may have episodes of peritonitis or other complications, which temporarily interrupts their treatment. In addition, since patients are spending increasing periods of time in end-stage renal failure, cephalic veins are frequently used for intravenous therapy, often resulting in thrombosis. The best time for fistula placement is when the patient initially presents with renal failure.

With more patients in renal failure presenting without adequate vessels available for autogenous fistula construction, the use of synthetic material has increased. The most common synthetic materials currently in use for access are PTFE (Gore-Tex—W.L. Gore & Associates, Inc, Elkton, Md.; Impra—Impra, Inc., Tempe, Ariz.), tetrafluoroethylene (Medtronic, Minneapolis, Minn.), and tanned human umbilical vein (Biograft). Dacron has not proved useful because of the associated high rate of infection and pseudoaneurysm formation.

These materials are readily available and most vascular surgeons have experience with them in peripheral vascular reconstruction. Such fistulas have the advantage of being large and therefore easily palpated and cannulated. They can also be used almost immediately following placement.[11,12] This is particularly useful when a patient with advanced uremia is referred for urgent access, which has increasingly become the case. Synthetic grafts have their own significant and somewhat unique problems, however.[13]

Choice of Access Location and Type

Permanent access is preferably placed at the wrist in the nondominant arm. This allows the patient use of the dominant arm during dialysis and may lessen the chance of trauma to the fistula during daily activities. Unfortunately, in many patients the cephalic vein on one or both wrists is unavailable for use, usually as the result of injudicious placement of intravenous lines, by the time the patients are seen by a vascular surgeon. In these patients obtaining quality vascular access becomes a challenge.

If neither wrist has a patent cephalic vein, the antecubital space is the next best site. An AVF at this site is constructed between the brachial artery and the cephalic vein or between the brachial artery and a connecting branch such as the median antecubital vein. It is important to disconnect the new fistula from the deep venous system by ligation of deep veins going into the forearm to prevent the subsequent development of venous hypertension.

Fistulas constructed between the brachial artery and the basilic vein or another deep vein are doomed to failure since dialysis personnel cannot consistently gain access to the deep venous system. In addition, because the vein is adjacent to the brachial artery, cannulation carries a significant risk of arterial injury.

Occasionally, the basilic vein in the upper arm can be exteriorized by dissecting it out for a distance of 10 to 15 cm and then bringing it into a superficial position, where it is easy to cannulate. This procedure frequently leads to wound complications (seroma, hematoma, arm swelling) because of the extent of dissection required and the rich lymphatic network around the brachial and axillary arteries.

When there are no usable veins in the arms for fistulas, the decision must be made whether to continue to pursue autogenous access or to construct access with prosthetic material. Although it is almost always easier to use prosthetic grafts, their useful life is rarely comparable to that of autogenous tissue.

Excellent autogenous access can usually be constructed using the saphenous vein, when available. It can be mobilized completely to the knee and then looped subcutaneously on the anterior surface of the thigh and anastomosed to the superficial femoral artery just distal to the bifurcation of the common femoral artery. Alternately, in a thin patient, the saphenous vein can be left in situ and anastomosed end to side to the distal superficial femoral artery at the level of the adductor canal. It is unnecessary to ligate venous branches since their presence only increases the venous outflow from the fistula. This particular procedure can easily be accomplished with the patient under local anesthesia and provides good length for easily accessible cannulation sites in the thin patient. The saphenous vein can also be harvested and transplanted to the arm for use as autogenous fistula graft material.

In the event an autogenous fistula cannot be constructed, most surgeons prefer PTFE for prosthetic material. PTFE has generally outperformed most other prosthetic materials in terms of long-term patency. Many different grafts are currently available including straight, tapered, stepped, and externally reinforced grafts. No single form of PTFE has demonstrated clear superiority. Thick-walled grafts are preferable because of their increased durability with repeated cannulations.

Forearm constructions include straight grafts (radial artery to antecubital vein) and loops (brachial artery looping back into antecubital vein). Loop grafts have the theoretical advantage of higher flow because of the larger artery on which they are based. However, this is a theoretical consideration and loop grafts have not been proved to be superior over straight grafts.

Straight grafts have the advantage in that in the event of infection, graft removal is safer since the radial artery can almost always be ligated without placing the hand in jeopardy. Ligation of the brachial artery may result in tissue loss, especially in diabetic patients with extensive peripheral vascular calcification.

Upper arm loop prosthetic fistulas are based on the more proximal brachial artery and generally return into the basilic or deep venous system. Sites as low as possible in the forearm should be selected first, since with each successive access placement, the vein distal to the arteriovenous anastomosis is ligated to prevent venous hypertension. Therefore an upper arm loop generally precludes further attempts distally in the ipsilateral extremity.

When an upper arm loop PTFE fistula is being created, it is generally easier to perform both venous and arterial anastomoses at the same level (through the same incision medially on the upper arm). We usually do this with the venous anastomosis directed toward the heart and the arterial anastomosis situated deep to it. There may be some advantage in performing end-to-end venous anastomoses, although this has not been proved.

In general, it is unwise to cross joints with prosthetic graft material. Prolonged flexion at the joint, such as that which occurs during sleep, may lead to graft occlusion. However, use of spiral-wrapped reinforced PTFE can help to prevent kinking.

If access cannot be obtained in either upper extremity, more exotic maneuvers will need to be undertaken. It behooves the surgeon performing access to frequently remind his colleagues of the importance of preserving cephalic veins in those patients with renal disease because once the cephalic vein is lost, obtaining good autogenous access becomes difficult.

Complications
Problems Associated With Cannulation

Because the technique for cannulation of synthetic grafts is different from that of autogenous AVFs, dialysis units with less experienced personnel have a high rate of perigraft hematomas, pseudoaneurysm formation, and graft infection.

Perigraft hematoma results from cannulation with the needle entering parallel to the graft, severing a portion of the graft wall. Graft infection occurs when less than ideal aseptic technique is used during cannulation and dialysis. Proper technique involves puncturing the graft perpendicular to the long axis and then changing the angle of the needle once its tip has entered the graft lumen. It is important to avoid repeated punctures at the same site since extensive damage to the graft wall will eventually result in pseudoaneurysm formation and/or localized infection.

Perigraft hematomas should be treated conservatively unless signs of infection appear; if infection occurs, incision and drainage are required. Infected perigraft hematomas usually necessitate graft revision or removal. It is wise to avoid the use of a fistula with a large perigraft hematoma; temporary access should be used until the hematoma has resolved.

Once a fistula has been successfully constructed, the surgeon has an ongoing responsibility to the patient to ensure that the fistula lasts as long as possible. To maximize fistula longevity, the surgeon must consider three important points. First, the new fistula should not be used until it has had sufficient time to mature. Maturation of autogenous fistulas usually takes 4 to 6 weeks. In most cases the fistula can be easily palpated and could be cannulated before this time; however, the vein wall requires 4 to 6 weeks to sufficiently enlarge and arterialize. Early use frequently results in hematoma formation around the fistula, which eventually progresses to scarring and stenosis and markedly shortens the useful life of the fistula. Fistulas constructed with prosthetic material usually require 10 to 14 days for sufficient incorporation of the foreign material. Premature puncture of the graft commonly leads to perigraft hematoma formation with a high likelihood of subsequent infection.

Second, the surgeon needs to ensure that dialysis personnel use proper aseptic technique at the time of cannulation and that they rotate puncture sites. Continual cannulation of a single site leads to degeneration of the vessel or prosthetic graft wall, with pseudoaneurysm formation and/or infection. This is a matter of education and communication, which is the surgeon's, as well as the nephrologist's, responsibility. It is also important to avoid cannulation in the vicinity of the anastomotic sites to prevent cutting a suture and causing disruption.

Third, the dialysis nurses and technicians should be informed of the need to contact the surgeon whenever a problem with the fistula occurs. Early detection of changes in the hemodynamic characteristics of the fistula such as high venous pressures, which frequently precede thrombosis, is vital. Correction of the abnormality before the fistula clots will markedly improve the useful life of the access site.

Thrombosis

Thrombosis is the most common problem with permanent AVFs. The majority of patients on hemodialysis will need revision or thrombectomy of the fistula at some time during their time on dialysis. Once thrombosis occurs, performance of a fistulogram is useless. Early exploration yields the highest salvage rates. At exploration, a careful search will usually determine the cause of thrombosis. Unless the cause is discovered and corrected, thrombectomy will be unsuccessful in reestablishing a usable fistula. This cannot be overemphasized.

In most cases the existing fistula can be salvaged with thrombectomy and revision. AVFs that have been clotted longer than 24 to 48 hours have a lower rate of salvage, probably because of the intimal damage that occurs when clot is present in the vessel lumen. Even in patients who present late following thrombosis of an AVF, an attempt at thrombectomy or reconstruction should usually be made.

Thrombosis of synthetic AVFs occurs frequently enough that many surgeons view it as a routine part of management of patients with fistulas made with synthetic material. In most cases, such grafts can be successfully thrombectomized if both arterial and venous connecting vessels are patent and thrombectomy is accomplished before clot has propagated and occluded the proximal venous runoff or before extensive intimal damage has occurred in the runoff vessels. Recently placed grafts are easy to thrombectomize. Older grafts may accumulate thick layers of pseudointima, which is difficult to remove. When this is the situation, it usually is better to excise and replace the graft or to place another fistula elsewhere.

It is important to remove all thrombus from the arterial and venous ends of the fistula. Visualization of the arterial end can be difficult once blood flow is restored. One way to obtain a good look at the arterial anastomosis is to temporarily occlude arterial flow with a proximal sterile tourniquet, which allows complete inspection and calibration of the arterial anastomosis with a minimal amount of blood loss. Calibration can be performed with a balloon catheter or coronary dilator. Both anastomoses should be directly visualized. When there is less than a clear, strong, palpable thrill proximally in the fistula, an operative fistulogram should be obtained.

The most common cause of graft thrombosis with synthetic materials is stenosis at the venous anastomosis. This probably represents a form of the pseudointimal hyperplasia often seen in PTFE peripheral arterial reconstructions. Correction requires angioplasty, bypass, or movement of the anastomosis to another outflow vein.

Assessment of what constitutes adequate venous runoff is probably the single most difficult decision when creating permanent venous access. Calibration of the outflow tract with coronary artery dilators is useful. Free passage of anything smaller than a No. 3 coronary dilator is probably insufficient. If the graft or vein has a strong pulse but no thrill, venous outflow obstruction is present.

USE OF DIALYSIS HISTORY AND PHYSICAL EXAMINATION
Arterial or Inflow Stenosis

Arterial or inflow stenosis may be diagnosed by noting that before occlusion the fistula was not providing adequate inflow into the dialysis machine (frequent "negative pressures"). On physical examination before occlusion, the fistula usually appears somewhat collapsed. Such inflow stenoses are most common in radial artery–based fistulas. Treatment usually involves revision of the fistula with anastomosis to a more proximal area of the radial artery. If there is no associated venous stricturing, the cephalic vein can be thrombectomized and will provide excellent outflow. Because the vein is already arterialized, such a fistula can be used immediately following revision.

Venous or Outflow Stenosis

This situation is diagnosed by noting that before occlusion high venous (or "return") pressures were present. In autogenous fistulas, venous stenoses are usually caused by premature cannulation of an inadequately arterialized vein or by repeated punctures at the same site. Occasionally, it is possible to revise the anastomosis or bypass the area of stenosis. However, in many cases the stenoses are multiple and cannot be bypassed, and the fistula must be moved to another site. In PTFE fistulas, neointimal hyperplasia at the distal venous anastomosis is the common cause and is best treated by patch angioplasty or revision to bypass the area of stenosis.

Hypotension

Patients undergoing hemodialysis frequently experience episodes of hypotension as a result of extracellular fluid being removed during dialysis or occasionally from sepsis. AVFs may thrombose during these events. If the fistula was functioning well before thrombosis, thrombectomy is frequently successful. As noted earlier, it is wise to carefully evaluate both arterial and venous limbs at the time of thrombectomy to rule out mechanical obstruction as a predisposing factor.

Hypercoagulable State

Hypercoagulable states are not uncommon in dialysis patients and should be considered in two situations: (1) when a well-functioning fistula suddenly thromboses and cannot be salvaged even though the thrombectomy or revision seems adequate intraoperatively and (2) when a patient on chronic hemodialysis presents with a history of repeated unsuccessful attempts at obtaining vascular access by competent vascular surgeons.

Any patient in whom a technically adequate AVF has failed to remain patent should be suspected of having a hypercoagulable state. Technically adequate is defined as the operative documentation of a palpable thrill or postoperative presence of a clearly audible bruit in the AVF. If an adequate thrill and bruit are present but are subsequently lost in the immediate postoperative period, the patient should be evaluated for a coagulation abnormality.

The two most common abnormalities resulting in hypercoagulability and access failure are antithrombin III deficiency and heparin-induced platelet aggregation.[9] Patients with antithrombin deficiency can usually be managed by perioperative infusion of fresh frozen plasma to supply the missing factors, followed by Coumadin therapy. Patients with heparin-induced platelet aggregation often have a history of frequent blockage of dialysis coils by clots. If hemodialysis is the only means for maintenance dialysis, these patients can usually be dialyzed without the use of heparin; however, this situation presents difficulties for most dialysis units. The majority of such patients will eventually require peritoneal dialysis.

Erythropoietin

When erythropoietin is administered to hemodialysis patients, they are usually not as anemic as previously. Anemia contributes to impaired coagulation in uremic patients and thus promotes patency of AVFs.[14] Vigorous correction of anemia using erythropoietin therapy may therefore serve to potentiate thrombosis. It has been our experience that patients on erythropoietin therapy in whom the fistula thromboses have a technical abnormality to explain the incident. A higher hematocrit level probably accelerates access loss, however.

Pseudoaneurysm Formation

Pseudoaneurysms occur commonly in AVFs that have been used for vascular access over a prolonged period of time. They occur in both autogenous and prosthetic fistulas. They result from improper technique in graft cannulation coupled with the nonhealing nature of the material. If pseudoaneurysms erode through overlying skin, the result may be life-threatening hemorrhage. Once diagnosed, correction can be performed by bypassing or replacing the involved segment with new material or, when the pseudoaneurysm involves an anastomosis, by reconstructing that portion of the AVF.

Occasionally, a pseudoaneurysm is so large and complex that it requires the sacrifice of the fistula. The principal risks of pseudoaneurysm are continued enlargement with thrombosis, rupture, or distal embolization. Dialysis personnel should be cautioned to avoid repeated cannulations of areas of pseudoaneurysm because of the risk of skin breakdown and rupture.

Infection

Infection can occur in any fistula but is more common with vascular access using synthetic graft material. It is usually related to lack of proper aseptic technique at the time of cannulation.[15] Repeated cannulations at the same site and poor sterile technique (e.g., poor skin preparation, touching the prepared site with an ungloved finger) also place the fistula at a higher risk of infection. Such infections can occasionally be managed by excision of the involved segment if the graft has been well incorporated before onset of the infection and the infected area does not involve an anastomosis to a host vessel.

More often, infection in prosthetic material involves one or both anastomoses and the whole graft must be removed. Before a wound with a suspected prosthetic graft infection is opened, a proximal tourniquet should be readily available. At the time of removal, a rim of prosthetic material may be left attached to the artery to provide a secure closure. Infected wounds are best left open and allowed to heal secondarily.

Infection that occurs in an autogenous fistula is usually the result of a secondary infection of a hematoma surrounding the fistula caused by repeated cannulation of the same segment of vein.

When prosthetic materials are inserted, perioperative coverage with systemic antibiotics is recommended. A single dose of an antibiotic with gram-positive coverage (first-generation cephalosporin, nafcillin, or vancomycin) is probably sufficient. The surgeon should try to anticipate when prosthetic material might be used so that antibiotics can be administered before the skin incision.

Infection involving a major artery, such as the brachial artery at its bifurcation or the superficial femoral artery, may place a limb in jeopardy. With synthetic grafts placed in the groin, the arterial anastomosis should be made to the superficial femoral artery and not to the common femoral artery. In this way if graft infection should occur and ligation of the donor vessel becomes necessary, it may be done with a lesser chance of limb loss. In general, it is better to avoid placing any prosthetic material in the groin for vascular access if alternate sites are available in the upper body.

Venous Hypertension

Venous hypertension results from either high flow into a venous bed distal to the AVF or proximal venous occlusion.[16] Occasionally both conditions may be present. Patients usually present with edema of a hand or arm, and stasis ulcers may actually develop. Other signs of venous stasis include rapid capillary filling time, cyanosis, brawny edema, and ecchymosis. If the AVF is placed at the wrist, there are usually prominent pulsatile veins palpable through the edema on the dorsum of the hand. When an antecubital fistula is the source of venous hypertension, patients more commonly present with edema of the hand and forearm and a vigorous thrill at the site of the fistula extending distally into the forearm.

Attention to detail at the time of initial access placement can usually avoid postoperative venous hypertension. Distal venous branches from the fistula should be ligated unless such branches allow for filling of vessels that will be needed for access. The most common example of this situation is the lateral ulnar vein on the dorsum of the forearm, which in some cases will fill through a branch off the distal cephalic vein proximal to the fistula. In the case of an antecubital AVF, the distal cephalic vein extending to the forearm may provide excellent sites for cannulation and should be preserved. However, venous branches going deep into the forearm and proximally along any major arteries should be ligated. Even though there is no apparent flow at the time of fistula construction, as veins dilate, venous valves may become incompetent, resulting in distal flow and venous hypertension.

When an AVF is being created with deep veins in the antecubital fossa, care should be taken to ligate the distal side of the venous tributary (toward the hand). Otherwise, venous flow may reverse, producing significant venous hypertension in the hand, which will necessitate a second operation to ligate the responsible venous branch.

If a patient with a previously functioning AVF suddenly presents with venous hypertension, deep venous occlusion should be suspected. This serious situation can only be resolved by takedown of the fistula on the affected side. If the fistula is patent at the time, it may be possible to secure new access elsewhere before taking down the fistula that is causing the venous hypertension. Delay in takedown in this situation may put the patient at risk for subsequent skin necrosis.

Fistulogram

A fistulogram is a radiographic contrast study of the AVF to define arterial and venous anatomy. Although noninvasive techniques such as color duplex ultrasound scanning can provide similar information, a fistulogram provides the precise anatomic information that the surgeon requires. A fistulogram may play an important role in diagnosing and treating venous hypertension and the failing fistula. It aids in both locating venous branches supplying the distal venous bed and documenting the presence or absence of proximal deep venous occlusion.

The technique is simple and can be done without formal arteriography. A needle is placed into a vein connecting with the AVF or into the prosthetic graft itself, and a blood pressure cuff is placed high on the upper arm and inflated above systolic pressure. Intravascular contrast (usually full-strength) is injected into the needle, which will fill both veins and arteries supplying the fistula. More than a single view may be necessary to demonstrate the relevant anatomy. The fistulogram is rarely of use in the evaluation of a thrombosed fistula and its use in this situation should be abandoned.

Immediately following thrombectomy and/or revision, the surgeon may wish to perform an intraoperative arteriogram. This often proves useful because unsuspected stenoses may be identified and corrected before the next episode of thrombosis occurs. It is rarely necessary to perform angiography. Venography is occasionally of use in evaluation of veins preoperatively in obese patients in whom physical examination alone is inconclusive.

Steal Syndromes

Steal syndromes occur most often in diabetic patients with advanced peripheral atherosclerosis involving the arteries of the upper extremities. Patients at high risk have skin changes typical of diabetes and at operation have heavily calcified atherosclerosis of even 2 to 3 mm vessels. These patients can usually be identified preoperatively by careful palpation of the radial artery and/or by the examination of x-ray films of the forearms for vascular calcifications. Attempts at obtaining vascular access for hemodialysis are often unsuccessful in these patients. However, some individuals with calcified vessels can still undergo successful fistula placement. A more precise approach is the use of vascular laboratory measurements of finger pressures on both sides. The side with the least severe disease can be chosen for placement of the fistula. In extremities with finger pressures less than 90 mm Hg, the results will predictably be poor. Any fistula placed in a patient with arterial insufficiency of the limb places distal tissue at risk and should be avoided. Some patients may not have an acceptable site for vascular access and will need to have peritoneal dialysis.

If the access has already been placed and ischemic changes of the hand or fingers develop, the fistula should be taken down urgently. Once ischemic neuropathy or gangrene develops, many of these patients will eventually require amputation of fingers and, on occasion, a hand.

THE FAILING FISTULA

Many episodes of access failure can be prevented if the surgeon, nephrologist, and dialysis personnel work in concert to identify and correct access problems before thrombosis occurs. This same principle has been shown to apply in peripheral arterial bypass surgery.[17] The role of noninvasive vascular imaging techniques in the evaluation of fistulas used for vascular access is unclear. Rather, the best evaluation is to determine the hemodynamic functioning of the access during dialysis and to perform a careful physical examination of the access.

Vascular surgeons are frequently called to evaluate patients with "failing fistulas," that is, AVFs that previously provided adequate sites for cannulation and flow on dialysis for prolonged periods of time but are becoming difficult to cannulate or are not providing enough flow for adequate dialysis. In these situations it is important to speak directly with the dialysis nurse or technician to determine the exact nature of the problem in addition to performing a careful physical examination since a number of different situations may exist to cause this problem. With a dialysis history and physical examination, a fistulogram will rarely provide useful information.

High Venous Pressure

The AVF may have developed high venous resistance to the reinfusion of blood. For this reason, extra pressure is required to reinfuse blood into the patient, resulting in ultrafiltration. A rising venous pressure over a period of weeks to months should be a clue that proximal venous obstruction is developing and revision should be undertaken before the access fails completely.

A fistulogram is often useful in this setting to delineate the site of stenosis. If the area of venous stenosis is single and is located near a radiocephalic anastomosis, in most cases it is possible to reconstruct the fistula proximal to the stenosis. This will usually provide a number of sites for cannulation. If the area causing the problem is some distance from the anastomosis and is too proximal to readily bypass, it may be possible to perform an angioplasty or to resect the area of stenosis. Often there are several stenotic areas with surrounding scar and a new AVF will need to be constructed at another site.

Venous stenosis occurring proximal to the venous anastomosis of a PTFE graft may occur at one site or at multiple sites. The single-site stenosis can be corrected by bypassing it or by performing patch angioplasty. Balloon angioplasty of venous stenoses have been reported; but, in our limited experience, they have rarely been successful. Problems on the venous side of a fistula are usually more serious than arterial problems in terms of maintaining adequate vascular access in the same general area.

Poor Arterial Inflow

The second type of problem occurs when there is insufficient or failing arterial inflow to the dialysis machine. Useful access requires arterial inflow of at least 200 cc/min. Problems with arterial inflow present with collapse of the arterial segment of the dialysis circuit because the inflow pressure becomes negative with respect to the dialysis pump. Here, as in the case when there is a high venous pressure, a fistulogram will usually provide useful information regarding the location of the problem.

The radiologist should be informed that special attention needs to be paid to the arterial segment of the fistula. Occasionally, additional films will be required to demonstrate the full arterial anatomy separate from overlying veins. Unless the patient is diabetic, the stenosis most often occurs in the vicinity of the anastomosis and can be corrected by reconstructing the fistula proximal to the original site.

If the problem is extensive atherosclerosis, it usually will be necessary to create a new fistula at another site. The hemodynamic effects of sequential stenoses are greater than the severity of any single stenosis would suggest.[18]

Difficulty in Cannulation

The final problem that occurs in the dialysis unit and causes a "failing fistula" is increased difficulty with cannulation. This is more common in units with less experienced personnel or with an uncooperative or obese patient. It is important to carefully examine the involved extremity. Not infrequently, the problem is progressive scarring around a site that has been used for an extended period of time. There are often additional viable sites proximal to the favored one.

If, in fact, the fistula is patent but cannot be reliably cannulated, a new one will need to be constructed, usually at a different site. A fistula that can only be cannulated with difficulty by the most experienced nurse or technician is inadequate, regardless of its hemodynamic characteristics once cannulated. Before another fistula is constructed, a concerted attempt should be made to use the existing access site. The performance of a fistulogram may be useful, followed by a cannulation demonstration of the access site by the surgeon or nephrologist and/or their marking of new access sites for dialysis personnel.

Congestive Heart Failure

Congestive heart failure is a rare complication of an AVF created for hemodialysis access.[19] A well-developed AVF may obligate as much as 10% to 15% of the cardiac output, which ordinarily is 300 to 500 cc/min. Rarely, flow through a large antecubital or femoral loop fistula can develop to greater than 2 L/min. If the patient is small or has significant organic heart disease, this can result in high output cardiac failure. The diagnosis is only missed when it is not considered. Confirmatory evidence consists of the usual x-ray film and laboratory data and observation of a drop in heart rate with temporary occlusion of the fistula. The diagnosis can be more difficult in patients taking large doses of β-blockers in whom the heart rate response to fistula occlusion is muted. Thermodilution cardiac output measurements may be useful in unusual situations.

If vascular access is still required, two alternatives exist: either the fistula may be ligated after usable access (either temporary or permanent) is obtained or the flow through the existing access site may be decreased by reconstructing the fistula as one of a smaller size. This can be done by direct reconstruction of the anastomosis or by banding the outflow vein to a smaller diameter. It is difficult to adequately judge the degree to which the fistula can be diminished without causing thrombosis and is one situation in which flow probes may be of use. The best intraoperative information supporting adequate diminution of flow is a significant decrease in heart rate.

Takedown of Arteriovenous Fistulas

If the AVF is no longer needed (resolution of renal failure, permanent peritoneal dialysis, successful renal transplant), takedown of the AVF may be indicated. This may be done either for cosmetic reasons or because of the possibility of hemorrhage from minor trauma.

In general, fistula takedown following renal transplant should not be considered until renal function has been stable for at least 1 year without significant complications relating to immunosuppression or recurrent renal disease. A patient's history of vascular access should be considered when deciding to remove a fistula. Patients in whom it has been difficult to obtain and maintain vascular access usually should not have the fistula removed.

AVF takedown can easily be done as an outpatient procedure with the patient under local anesthesia. A pneumatic tourniquet should be in place, but it should be deflated proximal to the fistula because fistula veins can be thin walled and easily injured. Ligation of outflow veins will accomplish takedown. Arterial flow to the hand should be preserved by reconstruction or preservation of the artery. Alternately, venovenous reanastomosis and arterial reconstruction may preserve the vein and artery for future use and requires little extra time or effort.

Following fistula takedown or ligation, the large venous conduit becomes relatively stagnant and thrombosis with rather pronounced phlebitis frequently occurs. The treatment for this condition is heat plus anti-inflammatory medications, and the patient should be reassured that the problem will resolve.

Preservation of Cephalic Veins

In any patient with abnormal renal function or a disease process likely to lead to renal failure, all cephalic veins should be carefully preserved. This is often difficult to accomplish since the cephalic veins are the most readily accessible intravenous sites. Often by the time the surgeon has been consulted regarding vascular access, both cephalic veins are thrombosed because of ill-advised placement of intravenous sites. Obtaining an AVF in this situation becomes more difficult. It is important to constantly remind those taking care of patients with any renal abnormality, or with the potential for it, that the need for quality permanent vascular access requires preservation of all cephalic veins.

Neurologic Sequelae

The patient should be informed that the position of the radial cutaneous nerve puts it at high risk for injury during fistula formation or takedown. Injury results in a small area of decreased sensation on the back of the thumb. Careful preservation of the radial cutaneous nerve at operation will minimize the risk of this complication. This nerve is more often injured during takedown than during formation of AVFs, probably because of the scar tissue created by the original operation through which the takedown dissection must proceed.

Rarely, a patient with marked distal arterial insufficiency caused by the AVF will present with palsy of the radial or median nerve. Nerve conduction studies will demonstrate abnormalities that cannot be related to the operative site and that occur at close to the same level for both nerves. When nerve palsy occurs, the fistula must be taken down urgently and another form or site of dialysis undertaken.

Carpal Tunnel Syndrome

Carpal tunnel syndrome occurs more commonly in hemodialysis patients than in the general population for unknown reasons. Since the syndrome occurs as commonly on the side without the fistula, it probably is not related to its presence.

Treatment of carpal tunnel syndrome in a wrist with a functioning fistula requires planning. Since carpal tunnel syndrome is best treated surgically under tourniquet hemostasis, attention must be given to preservation of the fistula. We handle this problem by injecting the fistula with heparin before inflation of the tourniquet. Using this technique, we have not lost a fistula even with up to 20 minutes of tourniquet occlusion.

CONCLUSION

Complications common to all areas of vascular surgery occur frequently in vascular access patients. Morbidity rarely involves limb loss as it does in peripheral reconstructive surgery but represents significant problems nevertheless. Because these vessels or grafts are routinely cannulated, sometimes under less than ideal conditions, infection and pseudoaneurysm formation are not uncommon.

The usable life of any vascular access site depends to a large extent on how it is handled by personnel in the dialysis unit. The vascular surgeon's responsibility to the patient continues beyond the point at which usable vascular access is obtained. It is important to continually remind dialysis personnel of the rules in handling and cannulating AVFs and to remind physicians caring for these patients not to use any cephalic veins for intravenous sites. A well-constructed and cared-for autogenous fistula can last 10 years or more.

REFERENCES

1. Shrier RW, Gottschalk CW. Diseases of the Kidney, 4th ed. Boston: Little, Brown, 1988, p 1526.
2. Bour ES, Weaver AS, Yang HC, Gifford RRM. Experience with the double lumen Silastic catheter for hemoaccess. Surg Gynecol Obstet 171:1, 33-39, 1990.
3. Schwab ST, Buller GL, McCann RL, Bollinger RL, Stickel DL. Prospective evaluation of a Dacron cuffed hemodialysis catheter for prolonged use. Am J Kidney Dis 11:166-169, 1988.
4. Castaldo PA. Homeostasis and kidney disease. In Tatnoff OD, Forbes CD, eds. Disorders of Hemostasis. Orlando, Fla.: Grune & Stratton, 1984, pp 473-483.
5. Livio M, Benigni A, Remuzzi G. Coagulation abnormalities in uremia. Semin Nephrol 5:82-90, 1985.
6. Mannucci PM, Remuzzi G, Pusiner F, Lombardi R, Valsecchi C, Mecca G, Zimmerman TS. Deamino-8-D-arginine vasopressin shortens the bleeding time in uremia. N Engl J Med 308:8, 1983.
7. Liu KY, Kosfeld RE, Marcum SG. Treatment of uremic bleeding with conjugated oestrogen. Lancet 2:887-890, 1984.
8. Kappes S, Towne JB, Adams MB, Kauffman HM, Maierhofer W. Perforation of the superior vena cava: A complication of subclavian dialysis. JAMA 249:2232-2233, 1983.
9. Kauffman HM, Ekbom GA, Adams MB, Hussey CV. Hypercoagulability: A cause of vascular access failure. Proc Clin Dialysis Transplant Forum 9:28, 1979.
10. Giacchino JL, Geis P, Buckingham JM, Vertumo VL, Bansal VK. Vascular access: Long-term results, new techniques. Arch Surg 114:403-409, 1979.
11. Anderson CB, Etheredge EE, Sicard GA. One hundred polytetrafluoroethylene vascular access grafts. Dialysis Transplant 9:1980.
12. Tellis VA, Kohlberg WI, Bhat DJ, Driscoll B, Veith FJ. Expanded polytetrafluoroethylene graft fistula for chronic hemodialysis. Ann Surg 189:101-105, 1979.
13. Morgan AP, Dammin GJ, Lazarus JM. Failure modes in secondary vascular access for hemodialysis. Am Soc Artif Int Organs 1:44-52, 1978.
14. Livio M, Gotti R, Marchesi D, Mecca de Gaetano G. Uremic bleeding: Not of anemia and beneficial effect of red cell transfusions. Lancet 2:1013-1015, 1982.
15. Appel GB. Vascular access infections with long-term hemodialysis. Arch Intern Med 138:1609-1610, 1978.
16. Wilson SE. Complications of vascular access procedures. In Wilson SE, Owens ML, eds. Vascular Access Surgery. Chicago: Year Book, 1980, pp 185-207.
17. Bandyk DF, Schmitt DD, Seabrook GR, Adams MB, Towne JB. Monitoring functional patency of in situ saphenous vein bypasses: The impact of a surveillance protocol and elective revision. J Vasc Surg 9:286-296, 1989.
18. Beckmann CF, Levin DC, Kubicka RA, Henschke CI. The effect of sequential arterial stenoses on flow and pressure. Radiology 140:655-658, 1981.
19. Fee HJ, Levisman JE, Doud RB, Golding AL. High-output congestive failure from femoral arteriovenous shunts for vascular access. Ann Surg 183:321-323, 1976.

31

Complications of Surgery for Thoracic Outlet Syndrome

Gary R. Seabrook

The thoracocervicobrachial passage, bound by a rigid configuration of bones, muscles, and ligaments through which neurovascular structures traverse to connect the upper extremity with the trunk, is called the thoracic outlet. Thoracic outlet syndrome describes a complex of symptoms resulting from the abnormal compression of the neurovascular structures in this region. Originally symptoms were attributed to an abnormal first rib or the presence of a cervical rib impinging on the subclavian vessels.[1,2] Thoracic outlet syndrome now is associated more frequently with nerve compression from hypertrophied anterior and middle scalene muscles, congenital bands extending around and even through the brachial plexus, or narrowing of the costovertebral angle. In the absence of an anatomic deformity, it has been postulated that a chronically contracted anterior scalene muscle may elevate the first rib to compress the brachial plexus against the inferior border of the clavicle, suggesting that resection of the anterior scalene muscle is appropriate treatment.[3]

Symptoms include compression of the brachial plexus with paresthesia and dysesthesia, subclavian vein obstruction and associated effort thrombosis, and, rarely, subclavian artery stenosis or occlusion with distal ischemia.

The differential diagnosis of thoracic outlet syndrome is extensive, including carpal tunnel syndrome, cervical disc degeneration, and tendinitis of the shoulder and paraspinal muscles. The patient may require detailed neurologic examination to precisely define the cause of the symptoms. Most patients are managed with conservative therapy involving exercise programs, physical therapy, muscle relaxants, and analgesics. A variety of surgical procedures and approaches has been developed to rectify these anatomic anomalies and structural defects of the musculoskeletal system. These include resection of cervical and first thoracic ribs, anterior scalenectomy, and disruption of fibrous bands extending from the cervical vertebrae to the thoracic rib cage and shoulder girdle.

Patient selection and determination of the proper indications for surgery may be the most important factors in reducing the incidence of surgical complications associated with the procedure. The purpose of this chapter is to identify and discuss surgical complications that occur following the surgical treatment of thoracic outlet syndrome, identifying specific complications that may be associated with a given surgical approach; however, it is not intended to be a debate on the relative merits of various operative techniques.

ANATOMY OF THE THORACIC OUTLET

The thoracic outlet is composed of the musculoskeletal structures enclosing the nerves and blood vessels that supply the arm. In addition to anatomic variations in the bones and muscles composing the thoracic outlet, the presence of cervical ribs, costovertebral ligaments, tendinous insertions, and nonradiopaque fibrous bands investing the arteries and nerves may contribute to symptoms of neurovascular compression.

The thoracic outlet should be visualized as a triangle in the sagittal plane of the body. The base of the outlet is composed of the first rib. Posteriorly, the middle scalene muscle extends from the cervical spine to the first rib. Superiorly, the clavicle courses tangentially from the scapula to the sternal notch. Traversing across this triangular space, the anterior scalene muscle divides the thoracic outlet into two triangles: the scalene triangle containing the brachial plexus and the subclavian artery, and the costoclavicular space containing the subclavian vein.

Approximately 0.5% of the population have cervical ribs; however, less than 10% of these persons are symptomatic. Fifty percent of cervical ribs are bilateral. The cervical rib originates from the transverse tubercle of the seventh cervical vertebrae and connects to various locations along the upper border of the first thoracic rib, occasionally extending anteriorly to the sternal manubrium. Frequently ossification of the cervical rib is incomplete, with cartilage forming the connecting band to the first rib or sternum. The presence of a cervical rib narrows the space through which the subclavian artery and brachial plexus traverse. The anterior scalene muscle will distribute its insertions over a cervical rib, further impinging on the neurovascular structures. If the subclavius muscle becomes hypertrophied, it encroaches within the costoclavicular triangle, narrowing the space for the subclavian vein. The endothoracic fascia extends over the pleural cap from the medial border of the first rib to the transverse process of the seventh cervical vertebra and invests the subclavian vessels and brachial plexus. To liberate the neurovascular structures that are compromised as they pass through these triangular passages, operative therapy for thoracic outlet syndrome may require resection or disruption of two sides of an anatomic triangle.

SURGICAL PROCEDURES

First rib resection is accepted as the definitive surgical treatment for thoracic outlet syndrome.[4] Detaching the insertion of the anterior scalene muscle from the first rib will further release lateral compression on the subclavian artery and the upper roots of the brachial plexus. Complete mobilization of the first rib requires that the middle scalene muscle be transected for exposure of the neck of the rib at the costovertebral junction. This eliminates posterior compression of the brachial plexus. Cervical rib excision and removal of the attached fibrotendinous bands become part of the surgical procedure when these structures are present. Supraclavicular, transaxillary, and posterior intercostal approaches have been described for obtaining access to perform first rib resection.

The anterior supraclavicular approach allows access to the subclavian artery and brachial plexus as they traverse over the first rib.[5] The neurovascular bundle must be carefully mobilized and retracted while the rib is being excised. Exposure of the posterior segment of the first rib and mobilization of the middle scalene muscle may be compromised with the supraclavicular approach. Resection of the midportion of the clavicle may be required to better expose the subclavian artery should it require reconstruction for occlusive disease or poststenotic aneurysmal dilatation. The transaxillary approach provides wide exposure of all of the osseous and ligamentous structures attaching to the first rib, facilitating the resection.[6] Arterial reconstruction may be awkward through this approach. The combination of the supraclavicular and transaxillary approaches may provide improved exposure for resection of a large anterior scalene muscle and first thoracic rib.[7-9] A parascapular thoracotomy provides an alternative posterior exposure to the muscular and fibrotendinous bands that attach to the first rib. This approach exposes the brachial plexus without considerable manipulation and may be the most effective surgical technique for patients requiring reoperation on the thoracic outlet.[10] However, access to the subclavian vessels may be limited. Following transaxillary or transthoracic approaches, evacuation of a pneumothorax may be required and placement of an extrapleural closed suction drain is recommended to prevent fluid accumulation that may produce inflammatory reactions adjacent to the pleura and enhance scar formation in the operative field.

COMPLICATIONS

Complications associated with operation in the thoracic outlet may involve the vascular, nervous, pulmonary, and lymphatic systems.

Vascular System

During surgery, particularly with recurrent surgery in the thoracic outlet, plans for proximal vascular control should be in place in the event of inadvertent injury to the subclavian artery. Access is available to the proximal subclavian artery via the transaxillary approach at the anterior aspect of the incision through the third intercostal space with inferior displacement of the lung. Control of the right subclavian artery can be obtained through a supraclavicular incision. The subclavian artery, with its elastic characteristics, is at risk for injury during dissection of the scalene muscles and exposure of the first rib. Small side branches must be carefully identified and ligated without injury to the adjacent brachial plexus. The subclavian artery is at particular risk when the insertion of the anterior scalene muscle is being divided through the transaxillary approach because the artery lies directly behind the area of dissection yet is poorly visualized. It may be awkward to achieve optimal illumination. Fibrous bands may attach the subclavian artery to the scalene muscle and care must be taken to protect the artery while the muscle fibers are being lifted forward before division. Following first rib resection careful inspection should be made to ensure that bony spicules will not lacerate the artery with subsequent shoulder motion.

The transverse scapular artery usually arises from the posterior aspect of the subclavian artery and may be divided inadvertently as the artery is being dissected. Because it traverses between the artery and brachial plexus, caution must be used in controlling the vessel with clamps and electrocautery should be avoided.

Injury to the subclavian vein by the transaxillary approach may be better repaired by applying tamponade to the vein and then repairing the injury after removal of the first rib to gain better exposure. Control of an injured vein approached through the supraclavicular technique may require an infraclavicular incision to gain control of the vessel.

Air embolus can be successfully prevented by positioning the patient so that the level of the operative field is above the right atrium and by allowing backfilling of the venous conduit, following repair of a venotomy.

Subclavian vein thrombosis in a patient with a history of thoracic outlet surgery may be caused by residual obstruction of the vessel. The obstruction may be opened with intravenous infusion of fibrinolytic agents, and venography will allow precise identification of anatomic compression on the vein.[11] In the absence of residual external compression, a fibrosed venous valve or web may be identified and can be excised successfully through venotomy.

Nervous System

Traction injuries to the brachial plexus represent the most frequent neurologic complication following surgery involving the thoracic outlet[12,13] (Table 31-1). As dissection is performed adjacent to the brachial plexus, traction on the cords may result in injury that most frequently affects the C8 and T1 nerve roots. With the transaxillary approach the brachial plexus may be stretched by excessive elevation of the arm in an attempt to gain better exposure. Retraction of the brachial plexus as the middle and anterior scalene muscles are mobilized from the first rib may result in a neurapraxia. The amount of tension tolerated without symptoms by these nerve roots and cords will vary from patient to patient.

Table 31-1. Nerve Injury Following Operation for Thoracic Outlet Syndrome*

Neurologic deficit	Incidence (%)
Brachial plexus	1-3
Long thoracic nerve	1
Intercostal brachial nerve	20-35
Phrenic nerve	7
Transient	
Permanent	0.5

*Data from Graham GG, Lincoln BM. Anterior resection of first rib for thoracic outlet syndrome. Am J Surg 126:803-805, 1973; Sanders RJ, Monsour JW, Gerber WF, et al. Scalenectomy versus first rib resection for treatment of the thoracic outlet syndrome. Surgery 85:109-121, 1979.

Other neurologic injuries may result from the injudicious use of electrocautery during dissection. In addition to the brachial plexus, the long thoracic nerve, intercostal brachial nerve, and musculocutaneous nerve must be protected during dissection. The long thoracic nerve innervates the serratus anterior muscle and will result in elevation or winging of the scapula if injured. The symptoms of traction injury to this nerve usually resolve within several months. The long thoracic nerve traverses within the belly of the middle scalene muscle and exits along its lateral border. The nerve is at particular risk for injury during mobilization of the posterior segment of the first rib.

The intercostal brachial nerve provides cutaneous innervation of the medial aspect of the arm. It exits the nerve trunk through the second intercostal space through a fat pedicle and usually is outside the operative field during first rib resection. However, traction on the nerve root frequently is associated with transient complaints of numbness or hypoesthesia of the medial aspect of the arm.[14,15]

Sensory deficits observed postoperatively usually resolve within 2 to 4 months. Persistent, severe causalgia, often described as an intense, burning pain, may occur years after surgery.[12] The condition may be treated with nerve block or may require surgical neurolysis or resection of a neuroma. Cervical sympathectomy may be performed at the time of reexploration.

The phrenic nerve, which courses over the anterior surface of the anterior scalene muscle in a lateral-to-medial direction, is at significant risk for traction injury or inadvertent transection during surgery in the thoracic outlet. When the phrenic nerve lies on the lateral rather than the medial edge of the anterior scalene muscle, manipulation and neurapraxia from traction are more common.[5] Loss of phrenic nerve function results in paralysis of the hemidiaphragm on the affected side, resulting in serious postoperative pulmonary complications with atelectasis and respiratory insufficiency. Phrenic nerve palsy may require months for diaphragmatic function to return completely.

Pulmonary System

The pleural space may be entered during the dissection of fibrous bands connecting the anterior scalene muscle and the pleural cap or during the removal of intercostal attachments to the first rib. During first rib resection the pleural cap should be bluntly dissected free from the surrounding structures down to the level of the superior border of the second rib. Bony spicules from the resected rib must be removed because normal respiratory action will push the pleural cap into the adjacent space. Pneumothorax can be diagnosed by flooding the operative field with saline solution before wound closure and directing the anesthesiologist to forcefully inflate the lungs. Presence of air bubbling into the saline solution–filled wound or drainage of the saline solution into the pleural cavity dictates the need for tube thoracostomy to treat the pneumothorax. Several investigators have advocated aspirating residual pneumothoraces with a syringe and plastic catheter introduced over a needle, precluding the need for a thoracostomy tube and closed suction system.[3,9] Pneumothorax is unexpected when the supraclavicular approach is used since there is no planned entry of the thoracic cavity. Therefore particular vigilance is necessary and an upright chest x-ray film should be obtained in the immediate postoperative period to identify a pneumothorax, if present. Twenty-four hours of closed drainage by tube thoracostomy is usually adequate treatment for a pneumothorax. In the course of dissection, subcutaneous emphysema may occur, with an occult injury to the pleural space. Air can be evacuated from any residual dead space by filling it with saline solution before wound closure.

Lymphatic System

The left supraclavicular approach for decompression places the thoracic duct at risk. The duct ascends adjacent to the vertebral column to the right of the aorta and then courses to the left side behind the esophagus at the level of T5 or T6. It traverses behind the left subclavian vein but in front of the left sympathetic trunk, left vertebral artery, left phrenic nerve, and anterior scalene muscle, entering the venous system near the junction of the left internal jugular and subclavian veins. The jugular and subclavian trunks of the thoracic duct also occupy the space in front of the site in which the anterior scalene muscle attaches to the first rib posterior to the subclavian vein.

Should injury to the thoracic duct become apparent by the wound filling with lymph fluid, the duct should be identified and ligated to prevent postoperative lymphocele or chylothorax. Should an injury to the thoracic duct *not* be apparent, persistent lymphocele may require reexploration, with suture ligature of the lymph leak. Chylothorax may require treatment with tube thoracostomy and modification of the diet to lower lymph flow.

REOPERATION

Recurrence of symptoms can result from regeneration of bone from the stump of a resected cervical or first rib.[16] Scarring may involve C5, C6, and C7 roots. Complete removal of the rib at the costovertebral junction may obviate this problem. Subperiosteal rib resection can possibly result in regeneration of bony spicules along the tract of the retained periosteum, which can be diagnosed by speckled calcifications on x-ray films. This calcified tissue may provide an anchor for the adherence of scar tissue.

Scarring may involve Sibson's fascia, covering the apex of the pleura, and entrap the subclavian artery and vein. Scarring adjacent to the middle scalene muscle will impinge on the C8-T1 nerve roots. If the original procedure involved dividing the anterior scalene muscle without first rib resection, residual muscle fibers may reattach through bands of scar tissue to the first and second ribs.[17] Reoperation requires complete extirpation of the scalene muscle tissue. Scar formation involving the upper roots of the brachial plexus (C5-C7) may result in facial pain or a feeling of fullness behind the eye, stuffiness of the ear, discomfort of the jaw or cheek with mastication, or irritation of the skin adjacent to the nose. Complaints that the neck is "tight" or "bound" may be associated with pain radiating into the trapezius or rhomboid muscle complexes.

Scarring may occur between residual congenital bands going through the brachial plexus from the anterior to middle scalene muscles.[7] Treatment involves complete neurolysis. The nerve bundles then should be covered with a pedicle of fat to better protect them from further scarring. A fat pedicle can be fashioned from the upper flap of the incision, which is sewn to the prevertebral fascia beneath the neurovascular bundle. When adipose tissue is not available, use of an expanded polytetrafluoroethylene patch has been recommended as a covering for the brachial plexus to retard the invasion of scar tissue. Long-term efficacy of this technique has not been established.[18]

Scarring can be minimized by the prevention of hematoma, which causes an inflammatory reaction adjacent to the pleural cap. Premature return to physical activity involving the arm may contribute to the collection of lymphatic fluid or formation of a hematoma, which predisposes the patient to scar formation. Some surgeons advise patients to refrain from significant physical activity, particularly repetitive motion, for 6 to 8 weeks postoperatively with the hope of minimizing scar tissue formation adjacent to the liberated structures from the operation.[16,17]

When reoperation is necessary, high posterior thoracoplasty incisions may be preferable. This approach allows better exposure of the vessels, permits careful dissection of the nerves without undue tension, and provides better visualization of the vessels that are scarred in the wound. Severing the tendon of the pectoralis minor muscle will further enhance exposure. A nerve stimulator is useful to differentiate the nerve bundles within dense scar tissue. Nerve conduction testing may indicate if recurrent symptoms are from scarring or compression of the brachial plexus; however, nerve conduction velocities will not distinguish traction injuries from compression on the nerves.[16,19]

In reoperative surgery in the thoracic outlet, performance of cervical sympathectomy may be considered to relieve symptoms or anticipated symptoms of causalgia. The sympathetic chain can be identified at the T2 or T3 level outside the previously operated field and followed superiorly.

REFERENCES

1. Coote H. Exostosis of the left transverse process of the seventh cervical vertebrae, surrounded by blood vessels and nerve: Successful removal. Lancet 1:360-361, 1861.
2. Bramwell F. Lesion of the first dorsal nerve root. Rev Neurol Psych 1:235, 1903.
3. Ochsner A, Gage M, DeBakey M. Scalenus anticus (Naffziger) syndrome. Am J Surg 28:669-693, 1935.
4. Clagett OT. Presidential address: Research and prosearch. J Thorac Cardiovasc Surg 44:153-166, 1962.
5. Sanders RJ, Raymer S. The supraclavicular approach to scalenectomy and first rib resection: Description of technique. J Vasc Surg 2:751-756, 1985.
6. Roos DB. Transaxillary approach for first rib resection to relieve thoracic outlet syndrome. Ann Surg 163:354-358, 1966.
7. Qvarfordt PG, Ehrenfeld WK, Stoney RJ. Supraclavicular radical scalenectomy and transaxillary first rib resection for thoracic outlet syndrome. Am J Surg 148:111-116, 1984.
8. Cikrit DF, Haefner R, Nichols WK, Silver D. Transaxillary or supraclavicular decompression for the thoracic outlet syndrome: A comparison of the risks and benefits. Am Surg 55:347-351, 1989.
9. Sanders RJ, Pearce WH. The treatment of thoracic outlet syndrome: A comparison of different operations. J Vasc Surg 10:626-634, 1989.
10. Johnson CR. Treatment of thoracic outlet syndrome by removal of first rib and related entrapments through posterolateral approach: A 22 year experience. J Thorac Cardiovasc Surg 68:536-545, 1974.
11. Sanders RJ, Haug C. Subclavian vein obstruction and thoracic outlet syndrome: A review of etiology and management. Ann Vasc Surg 3:397-410, 1990.
12. Horowitz SH. Brachial plexus injuries with causalgia resulting from transaxillary rib resection. Arch Surg 120:1189-1191, 1985.
13. Graham GG, Lincoln BM. Anterior resection of first rib for thoracic outlet syndrome. Am J Surg 126:803-805, 1973.
14. Sanders RJ, Monsour JW, Gerber WF, Adams WR, Thompson N. Scalenectomy versus first rib resection for treatment of the thoracic outlet syndrome. Surgery 85:109-121, 1979.
15. Daskalakis MK. Thoracic outlet compression syndrome: Current concepts and surgical experience. Int Surg 68:337-344, 1983.
16. Urschel HD, Razzuk MA. The failed operation for thoracic outlet syndrome: The difficulty of diagnosis and management. Ann Thorac Surg 42:523-528, 1986.
17. Sessions RT. Reoperation for thoracic outlet syndrome. J Cardiovasc Surg 30:434-444, 1989.
18. Reilly LM, Stoney RJ. Supraclavicular approach for thoracic outlet decompression. J Vasc Surg 8:329-334, 1988.
19. Dawson DM, Krarup C. Perioperative nerve lesions. Arch Neurol 46:1355-1360, 1989.

XII Interventional Radiologic Techniques

32

Complications of Percutaneous Transluminal Angioplasty of Peripheral Arterial Occlusive Disease

K. Wayne Johnston   **Kenneth W. Sniderman**

Most vascular surgeons now recognize percutaneous transluminal angioplasty (PTA) as an important treatment modality for managing selected patients with peripheral arterial occlusive disease. The risks of the procedure are quite low but include potential systemic and radiologic complications, consequences of PTA failure, inadequate clinical and/or hemodynamic improvement following PTA, and late failure. This chapter reviews these complications of PTA and discusses approaches that can reduce the risks and improve the long-term results.

Data in this chapter are based on the results of a prospective study carried out at the University of Toronto.[1] Between July 1978 and July 1986, 984 PTAs performed in 902 patients at the Toronto General Hospital for the management of peripheral arterial occlusive disease were studied prospectively. The complications were recorded, as were the variables believed to be important in predicting long-term re-

sults. The results were determined using a combination of clinical and vascular laboratory criteria (see box). The vascular characteristics of the patient population are presented in Table 32-1.

CRITERIA USED FOR DEFINING SUCCESS OF PTA

Clinical grade improved by at least one level:
  Asymptomatic
  Mild claudication
  Disabling claudication
  Ischemic night pain or rest pain
  Ulceration or gangrene
One or more of the following vascular laboratory
  measurements improved:
  ABI increased by at least 0.1
  Monophasic Doppler frequency analysis
    recordings became biphasic or triphasic
  Doppler pulsatility index increased >20%
  Treadmill exercise distance at least doubled

Table 32-1. Characteristics of Patient Population in the University of Toronto Series*

Characteristic	%
Indications for PTA	
Mild claudication (i.e., more than 2-block walking distance)	5
Disabling claudication	79.4
Limb salvage	8
Other indications	2.5
Site of PTA	
Aortoiliac segment	69.5
Femoropopliteal segment	25.7
Other sites	4.8
Severity of stenosis	
Stenosis	80.9
Occlusion	19.1
Number of sites dilated	
One	82.8
Two or more	17.2
Runoff (i.e., runoff of the arterial segment just distal to the site of the PTA)	
Normal	50
<50% stenosis or one tibial artery occluded	10.7
>50% stenosis or two tibial arteries occluded	17.5
Complete arterial occlusion or three tibial arteries occluded	21.8
Diabetes	
None	80.3
Diet-controlled	5.1
Oral hypoglycemic drug	6.1
Insulin	8.5

*A total of 984 procedures were performed in 902 patients; average age was 60.4 ± 10.2 years.

MORTALITY AND SYSTEMIC COMPLICATIONS

Four of the 902 patients (0.4%) died during their hospital stay; three of myocardial infarction and one from bleeding from a ruptured iliac artery. This low mortality was achieved by very experienced angiographers; however, as illustrated by the results for renal PTA reported by Bennicke et al.,[2] mortality may be as high as 6% if the radiologists are not well trained. In high-risk patients, especially those in whom PTA is indicated for limb salvage, the 30-day mortality rate may be 2% to 3%.[3-5]

Although renal failure was not observed in our series, transient abnormalities of renal function may have been overlooked because the period of hospitalization was short. Contrast-induced renal failure has been reported in 4% of tibioperoneal dilatations.[6] Renal toxicity is prevented by adequately hydrating the patient and limiting the dose of contrast agent.[7,8] Although nonionic dyes were originally thought to be less nephrotoxic, recent clinical trials have not supported this observation.[9]

LOCAL COMPLICATIONS

As detailed in Table 32-2, local complications occurred in 9.2% of the 984 procedures performed in the University of Toronto series. Emergency surgery was necessary in 1.2% of cases, major complications that delayed expected hospital discharge occurred in 3.4%, and minor complications were recorded in 4.6%. The overall complication rate was similar to that of Gardiner et al.,[10] who reported 59 complications in 453 percutaneous angioplasties (13%). Brewster et al.[11] reported a 6% incidence of major complications with iliac PTA. With tibioperoneal PTA, significant complications (death, emergency bypass surgery, or distal embolization) occurred in 3% in the series reported by Dorros et al.,[6] and Bakal et al.[12] reported three serious complications and 20 minor complications in 57 procedures. However, Schwarten and Cutcliff[13] have reported excellent results with few complications.

Bleeding

In our series arterial rupture occurred in one case, resulting in death. Gardiner et al.[10] reported arterial rupture in 0.4%. A ruptured artery is usually the result of significant overdilatation or PTA of a weakened aneurysmal artery. Most often the complication is recognized by evidence of contrast extravasation on a subsequent angiogram or continuing pain and hypotension. Although surgical repair is usually necessary, treatment by balloon tamponade without surgery may be appropriate in selected cases.[14-16]

Puncture-site bleeding and/or hematoma was the most common complication, occurring in 5.8% (57 cases). Fortunately, emergency surgery was necessary in only five cases. Significant hematomas occurred more often after femoropopliteal PTA (5.1%) than iliac PTA (2.6%).

Table 32-2. Local Complications in the University of Toronto Series (984 PTAs)

Complication	Severity		
	Surgery required	Major	Minor
Bleeding			
Ruptured artery	1	—	—
Puncture site	1	26	29
Ischemic limb			
Thrombosis	8	7	—
Distal emboli	—	—	6
False aneurysm	1	—	—
Arteriovenous fistula	1	—	—
Miscellaneous			
Arterial dissection	—	—	3
Dye extravasation	—	—	3
Other	—	—	5
TOTAL	12 (1.2%)	33 (3.4%)	46 (4.6%)

Ischemia

Significant limb ischemia caused by thrombosis at the puncture site or PTA site was observed in 1.5%. In the series reported by Gardiner et al.[10] acute arterial thrombosis occurred in 2%. Because of the age of the thrombus, fibrinolytic therapy is effective treatment for acute thrombosis at the site of the PTA, provided a significant dissected plaque is not present.[17] If acute thrombosis occurs following iliac PTA, it may be possible to open the artery by extracting the dissected atherosclerotic plaque using a Fogarty catheter passed upwards from the femoral artery,[18] thus avoiding more major arterial reconstructive surgery.

Distal emboli did not prove to be a major cause of limb ischemia. The incidence in our series was similar to the 1.5% incidence reported by Gardiner et al.[10]; however, with tibioperoneal PTA, Dorros et al.[6] noted an incidence of 4%.

Cholesterol embolization may complicate any angiographic procedure, but fortunately this complication is rare.[19,20] Occlusion of arterioles in the skin by cholesterol crystals and atheromatous debris produces acute, painful, blotchy discoloration. The prognosis depends on the severity of visceral involvement. No specific treatment is possible, although anti-platelet drugs, anticoagulants, or dextran is often used.

False Aneurysm and Arteriovenous Fistula

In our study false aneurysm and arteriovenous fistula were rare (two cases). The development of an aneurysm at the site of PTA is rare. Gehani et al.[21] reported a popliteal aneurysm that developed 9 months after PTA, which was complicated by subintimal dissection and was associated with the use of fibrinolytic therapy and long-term oral anticoagulants.

Other Complications

Other complications such as arterial dissection, intimal tear, and dye extravasation may cause thrombosis but alone do not prove to be significant. In the series of Gardiner et al.[10] subintimal passage of the guidewire or catheter occurred in 2% and arterial dissection in 1%. The placement of a balloon-expandable intraluminal stent may be useful for treating a severely dissected artery after PTA.[22]

Consequences of Failure of PTA

In an earlier analysis of our data,[23] 198 of 631 dilatations were considered failures. The consequences of failure of iliac and femoropopliteal PTA were analyzed separately.

When an iliac dilatation failed, the clinical grade became worse in 10.3% and the ankle/brachial index (ABI) fell by more than 0.2 in 9.5%. Amputations were necessary in 4.3% of the failed cases, but in each of these cases, dilatation was performed for limb salvage and the patients were not considered surgical candidates.

After failure of a femoropopliteal dilatation, the clinical grade was worse in 8.5% and the ABI was lower in 4.9%. Amputation was necessary in 15.8% of the failed cases, but in these cases PTA was indicated for limb salvage, and vascular reconstruction was not possible.

After failure of PTA, at 6-month follow-up 46.5% had no further treatment, 19.8% had repeat dilatation, 25% had vascular surgery, 7.8% had amputation, and 0.9% had other treatment.

Inadequate Improvement After PTA

In order to determine if a successful PTA completely relieved patient symptoms and/or normalized vascular laboratory measurements, we studied the improvement after successful PTA in two groups of patients with normal distal vessels who would be expected to show maximal symptomatic and objective benefit.[24] After successful PTA involving 207 iliac dilatations with normal distal vessels, 79% of the patients were asymptomatic and 21% had persistent, albeit mild, claudication. The ABI increased significantly in all cases and was normalized in 43% and remained abnormal in 57%. Similar results were obtained in a group of 65 patients who underwent successful femoropopliteal procedures. Sixty-two percent were asymptomatic but 28% had persistent symptoms. The ABI was normal in 44% and abnormal in 56%.

In other words, following successful dilatation in these ideal patients with no distal disease, mild persistent symptoms were frequent and the ABI often remained abnormal.

FAILURE OF PTA
Overall Results

The overall results for the 984 PTAs in the University of Toronto series are presented in

Table 32-3. Overall Results of PTA in the University of Toronto Series (n = 984)

Time of follow-up	Cumulative success (%)* (mean ± 1 SE)
1 mo	88.6 ± 1
1 yr	70.7 ± 1.5
2 yr	61 ± 1.7
3 yr	56.5 ± 1.8
4 yr	52.5 ± 2
5 yr	48.2 ± 2.3

*Calculated by the Kaplan-Meier method.

Table 32-3, which lists the cumulative percentage of success vs. time of follow-up. Note that 48.2% (± 2.3%) of the PTA sites remained successful at 5 years.

Individual Predictive Variables

To determine if an individual variable was predictive of long-term success, the statistical significant difference between survival curves was determined by the generalized Wilcoxon (Breslow) test and the log-rank (Mantel-Cox) test. Variables were analyzed separately in terms of their relationship to the success of the procedure. For each variable, the success rates at 1 month, 1 year, 3 years, and 5 years were determined (Table 32-4). These data should be compared to the results summarized by Casarella.[25]

Indication

Patients with mild or disabling intermittent claudication had a better PTA success rate than those with limb salvage (50.2% ± 2.4% vs. 33.1% ± 6.4%).

Site of PTA

Results with iliac PTA were better than those with femoropopliteal PTA. When the data were analyzed further, it was apparent that the difference in results between the two groups resulted primarily from the higher success rate for common iliac PTA. Thus the 5-year success rate for common iliac PTA (58.8% ± 3.5%) was higher than that for external iliac (46.5% ± 4.7%) and femoropopliteal PTA (37.9% ±

Table 32-4. Success Rates for PTA in Relationship to Individual Variables

Variable	No. of procedures	Success (%) (±1 SE)*			
		1 mo	1 yr	3 yr	5 yr
Indications					
Claudication	826	91.4 ± 1	74 ± 1.6	58.9 ± 2	50.2 ± 2.4
Salvage	127	70.9 ± 4	46.1 ± 5	37.2 ± 5.7	33.1 ± 6.4
Site					
Common iliac	373	90.9 ± 1.5	78.5 ± 2.2	64.8 ± 2.8	58.8 ± 3.5
External iliac	220	90.9 ± 1.9	73.2 ± 3.2	51.1 ± 4.3	46.5 ± 4.7
Femoropopliteal	253	88.9 ± 2	62.5 ± 3.2	50.6 ± 3.6	37.9 ± 4.5
Severity					
Stenosis	792	92.2 ± 1	74.4 ± 1.6	59.6 ± 2	50.5 ± 2.6
Occlusion	187	73.3 ± 3.2	55 ± 3.8	43.6 ± 4.1	38.5 ± 4.6
Runoff					
Good	577	91 ± 1.2	75.5 ± 1.9	61.6 ± 2.3	54.1 ± 2.7
Poor	373	84.5 ± 1.9	62.7 ± 2.7	46.9 ± 3.3	35.3 ± 4.4
Number sites dilated					
One	810	89.9 ± 1.1	72.3 ± 1.7	58 ± 2	49.2 ± 2.5
Two or more	169	82.3 ± 2.9	62.8 ± 4	49.1 ± 4.6	41.8 ± 5.2
Diabetes					
Absent	830	89.5 ± 1.1	72.8 ± 1.6	58 ± 2	50.6 ± 2.4
Present	144	84 ± 3.1	58.9 ± 4.4	47.9 ± 5	31.7 ± 7.2
Occurrence of complication					
No	884	89.8 ± 1	72.1 ± 1.6	58 ± 1.9	49.3 ± 2.4
Yes	94	76.6 ± 4.4	57.1 ± 5.5	41.6 ± 6.2	37.4 ± 6.8

*Calculated by the Kaplan-Meier method.

4.5%). Cole et al.[26] reported 5-year cumulative patency rates of 72% for iliac PTA and 53% for femoropopliteal PTA.

Severity of Lesion

Arterial stenoses were dilated more successfully than occlusions.

Runoff

Patients with good runoff had a higher PTA success rate than those with poor runoff.

Number of Sites Dilated

PTA results were better when only one site was dilated than when there were multilevel dilatations.

Diabetes

Nondiabetic patients (i.e., patients with no diabetes or with diabetes controlled by diet alone) had better PTA results than patients in whom diabetes was controlled by oral hypoglycemics or insulin. These results are in agreement with data reported by Stokes et al.[27]

Occurrence of the Complication

If the patient did not have a complication when PTA was performed, the long-term success rate was higher.

Other Variables

It should be noted that the following variables were not predictive of long-term success ($p > .05$): age, sex, limb, early vs. late experience of the radiologist, specialty of the referring physician, repeat PTA, pre-PTA pressure gradient, post-PTA pressure gradient, and ABI.

Multiple-Variable Analysis

In order to achieve improved late results of PTA, it is important to select patients who are most likely to benefit from the procedure.

Hence, it is essential to determine which combination of variables is predictive of success. The results of multivariate analysis are discussed below.

PREVENTION OF COMPLICATIONS AND FAILURE
Collaboration

PTA should be carried out only by an experienced angiographer in a center where appropriate surgical backup and hospital facilities are available for the management of complications. The radiologist should be well trained, continually involved in the performance of PTA, and have a low complication rate. There must be close collaboration and cooperation between the radiologist and referring physicians. Ideally, a vascular surgeon should see all patients in consultation before the procedure, since in most cases he is in the best position to establish the therapeutic plan based on knowledge of the natural history of peripheral arterial occlusive disease and based on an understanding of the risks and benefits of alternative therapies including conservative treatment, interventional radiology, and surgery. The experienced angiographer is in the best position to choose among alternative interventional procedures (PTA, stents, laser angioplasty, and/or atherectomy) and evaluate the risks.

Use of Meticulous Radiologic Technique

Complications are minimized by the use of precise radiologic technique by an experienced angiographer. Usually, the diagnostic angiogram is performed as a separate procedure because the surgeon and the radiologist are then allowed time for consultation. With improved duplex Doppler systems, it may be possible through the use of noninvasive studies to select patients who are likely candidates for PTA and thus perform diagnostic angiography and dilatation at the same time.[28,29]

We have previously described the details of the PTA technique used at the Toronto General Hospital.[30] Intravenous fluids are started to ensure that the patient is adequately hydrated. A narcotic sedative is administered. Enteric-coated aspirin (325 mg b.i.d.) and dipyridamole (50 mg t.i.d.) are administered for 3 or 4 days before the procedure and for 1 month afterwards. Since the arterial endothelium is damaged, the subendothelial and medial connective tissues are exposed, and on occasion the contents of atherosclerotic plaques are released during PTA, these drugs may minimize the risk of early thrombosis. In addition, antiplatelet agents may be of value in reducing platelet aggregation at the site of PTA, thereby lowering the restenosis rate.[31] Although long-term oral anticoagulants are used routinely in some centers,[32] we believe their risks outweigh the benefits except in patients with poor outflow in whom their use may improve early patency.

During the procedure the tissues are anesthetized and the femoral artery is entered using the Seldinger method. The femoral artery is usually punctured on the same side as the vessel to be dilated, but if necessary, the catheter can be passed from the contralateral side to treat a distal external iliac, common femoral, or profunda femoris artery lesion.[33] After the catheter has passed through the stenosis, 5000 units of heparin is administered. Pressure gradients are measured, the guidewire is reinserted, and the angiographic catheter is replaced by a Gruntzig balloon dilating catheter of appropriate length and diameter. After PTA, a follow-up angiogram is obtained and the residual pressure gradient is measured across the stenosis. The patient is observed for approximately 6 hours and, in selected cases, discharged home.

For lesions at the common iliac origin, a "kissing" or tandem balloon technique is used to prevent contralateral embolization and to buttress the bifurcation for better dilatation.[34] Originally, the catheters for PTA were 7 to 9 Fr but now 5 Fr or smaller catheters can be used for all dilatations. With a smaller size catheter there is less damage to the arterial wall during passage of the catheter, and with a smaller puncture hole the incidence of local complications is lower. Steerable guidewires allow the radiologist to negotiate the stenoses more safely. For dilatation of tibial vessels, the use of a balloon on a guidewire has been described.[35] Sheaths are used if several catheter exchanges are to be made, scar tissue is present at the puncture site, or the artery is easily damaged (e.g., axillary artery).

Appropriate Patient Selection

Patients should be considered for the procedure only if they have significant symptomatic arterial occlusive disease, the arterial disease is localized (i.e., the lesion is less than 10 cm in length and the adjacent vessels are relatively free of disease), and there is a good chance of long-term success of PTA.

The Cox proportional hazard model[36] was used to determine which variables were associated with success of PTA and to estimate the chances of success for all combinations of significant variables. From the results calculated by the Cox regression analysis, the following combination of variables was found to be associated with the long-term success of PTA: (1) indication for the procedure (i.e., claudication vs. salvage); (2) site of PTA (i.e., common iliac vs. external iliac or femoropopliteal segments); (3) severity of lesion (i.e., stenosis vs. occlusion); and (4) runoff (i.e., good vs. poor) (Table 32-5).

Reducing Late Failures

The causes of late failure following PTA include an inadequate initial angioplasty, progression of atherosclerotic disease, and/or development of intimal hyperplasia. Most of the studies that have attempted to determine the efficacy of alternative methods of treatment have examined PTA in the coronary circulation. Since these results may also be relevant to PTA of peripheral arteries, they are summarized in the following sections.

Improve Results of Initial PTA

The value of using an oversized balloon to improve the initial dilatation has been studied in the coronary circulation. When the ratio of the balloon diameter to the arterial diameter was greater than 1, the incidence of acute complications was found to be very high.[37] In a recent experimental study of atherosclerosis induced in rabbits,[38] the use of an oversized balloon with a high inflation pressure was associated with significant acute arterial wall damage including dissection, medial necrosis and mural thrombus, and the development of extensive intimal hyperplasia. Nonetheless, in

Table 32-5. Probability of Successful PTA Based on Four Significant Predictive Variables

Predictive variables				Success (%)*			
Indication	Site	Severity	Runoff	1 mo	1 yr	3 yr	5 yr
Claudication	Common iliac	Stenosis	Good	94	81	70	63
			Poor	91	74	59	51
		Occlusion	Good	90	72	56	48
			Poor	86	61	43	33
	Femoropopliteal and external iliac	Stenosis	Good	91	75	62	53
			Poor	88	66	49	40
		Occlusion	Good	87	63	46	36
			Poor	81	51	31	22
Salvage	Common iliac	Stenosis	Good	91	73	58	50
			Poor	87	63	45	36
		Occlusion	Good	86	61	42	32
			Poor	80	48	28	19
	Femoropopliteal and external iliac	Stenosis	Good	88	65	48	38
			Poor	82	53	34	24
		Occlusion	Good	81	50	30	21
			Poor	73	36	17	10

*Calculated by Cox regression analysis.

clinical practice mild overdilatation and the use of high-pressure balloons may be necessary with very dense plaques.

Several techniques are being evaluated that may improve the late results of PTA. Although hot-tip laser recanalization and angioplasty have demonstrated acceptable results, it is clear that the late results with current technology are no better than those with PTA alone.[39,40] Furthermore, it does not appear that a hot-tip laser is able to penetrate a femoropopliteal occlusion more frequently than a guidewire and catheter alone.[41] Future laser developments may provide new treatment opportunities. The placement of balloon-expandable intraluminal stents consisting of a tube of flexible metallic mesh may improve the early results and reduce the incidence of restenosis.[42,43] Stents should be considered for lesions that do not respond to conventional PTA, especially if the artery is occluded or an eccentric or severely ulcerated plaque is present. Atherectomy devices such as the Simpson device remove atherosclerotic plaque and thrombotic material; preliminary results using such contemporary technology are encouraging.[44] However, although these exciting new approaches are under investigation, at the present time no appropriate studies have clearly demonstrated improved long-term results compared to PTA or defined the indications for the procedures.

Control Progression of Atherosclerosis

In order to improve the late results of PTA, attempts to control the progression of atherosclerosis by controlling the risk factors (smoking, hypertension, hyperlipidemia, and diabetes) are prudent. Currently no studies have been carried out that demonstrate the benefit of risk factor control in improving the late results of PTA.

Control Progression of Intimal Hyperplasia

Intimal hyperplasia is an important cause of late failure of PTA. The mechanism responsible for producing successful PTA also causes significant acute arterial injury and activates mechanisms that lead to the development of intimal hyperplasia and arterial occlusion. The acute pathologic changes associated with PTA include loss of endothelium, exposure of intimal and medial connective tissue as a consequence of the circumferential splitting of the plaque from the vessel wall, and damage to the remaining cells in the arterial wall. Immediately after the dilatation, healing of the artery is associated with adherence and activation of platelets, deposition of fibrin, and reendothelialization. Subsequently, growth factors and chemotactic substances are released from platelets, white blood cells, and the cells in the arterial wall, which causes smooth muscle cells to proliferate, produce extracellular matrix and fibers, and migrate into the intima. Thus the arterial wall heals by the formation of fibrocellular tissue containing smooth muscle cells, collagen fibers, and extracellular matrix.

There have been several studies to determine if drugs will interfere with this cellular response and prevent intimal hyperplasia. Most of the studies have been carried out following coronary PTA. In Europe, long-term warfarin (Coumadin) administration is common practice, based on the rationale that it reduces the incidence of late failure. When coronary PTA was assessed by repeat angiography, there was no statistical difference in the incidence of restenosis between patients receiving warfarin vs. those receiving aspirin.[45,46] It has been shown that following injury to a rabbit artery, smooth muscle cells proliferate and migrate into the intima, produce intimal hyperplasia, and cause luminal stenosis and eventual occlusion. Furthermore, in animals, heparin administration can retard smooth muscle cell proliferation and migration into the intima.[47,48] In a preliminary clinical report, 18 to 24 hours of heparin infusion at the time of coronary PTA did not improve the late results in comparison with a control group.[49]

Animal studies have demonstrated that antiplatelet drugs reduce platelet adhesion at the time of angioplasty and reduce the incidence of restenosis following PTA. However, human studies have not shown a reduction in the incidence of restenosis after coronary angioplasty.[50] When compared with a group of patients taking a placebo, patients taking aspirin and dipyridamole did not have a reduced incidence of coronary restenosis as determined by angiography. The administration of calcium channel blockers has been advised since they may reduce arterial vasospasm and the incidence of restenosis, particularly in the coronary circulation. However, neither nifedipine nor diltiazem have been shown to be of benefit in preventing restenosis in a prospective clinical study.[51] In animal studies the administration of corticosteroids reduces the incidence of restenosis, perhaps by inhibiting the production of growth factors by the endothelial cells, macrophages, and smooth muscle cells. However, a randomized clinical study concluded that steroids did not reduce the rate of restenosis after coronary PTA.[52]

The incidence of atherosclerosis is lower in populations that have a high dietary content of fish oils (Ω-3 fatty acids). These fats have multiple effects and may reduce the cellular response to arterial injury produced by PTA. In a study of the effect of Ω-3 fatty acid therapy on early restenosis after coronary PTA, the group receiving conventional antiplatelet treatment had a 36% incidence of coronary restenosis. In the patient group receiving Ω-3 fatty acids, restenosis was significantly reduced to 16%.[53]

CONCLUSION

The relatively low incidence of serious complications associated with PTA makes it an attractive alternative in the treatment of selected patients. When a physician is determining whether PTA is indicated, the advantages and disadvantages of the procedure should be considered. Since it is associated with a low morbidity and mortality, PTA can be used in patients with high anesthetic risk or short life expectancy. PTA is also an option in obese patients, in patients in whom the risk of infection is high, or in patients in whom a saphenous vein is not available. If dilatation fails, the procedure can usually be repeated and does not preclude future vascular reconstructive surgery.

On the other hand, the morbidity of PTA can be quite high if the radiologist is not experienced with the technique, and the extent of symptomatic and objective improvement following successful PTA is less dramatic than that following surgery.

In our experience, PTA is an alternative to surgery in approximately 25% of the patients presenting to our vascular surgery service. Patients should be considered for the procedure only if they have significant symptomatic arterial occlusive disease, the arterial disease is localized (i.e., the lesion is less than 10 cm in length and the adjacent vessels are relatively free of disease), the angiographer is experienced with the technique, and the risk-benefit ratio of PTA is favorable relative to conservative therapy on one hand and surgery on the other. The risks of PTA have been identified in the prospective University of Toronto study: the mortality was 0.4%, serious complications requiring operation occurred in 1.2%, and the incidence of major complications delaying hospital discharge was 3.4%. The benefits of PTA (i.e., the chances of success as measured in the University of Toronto study by clinical and vascular laboratory improvement) can be predicted from knowledge of four interrelated variables: indication for the procedure, site of the PTA, severity of the lesion, and degree of runoff. Results are best if the patient has claudication, common iliac artery stenosis, and good runoff. After a successful PTA, even in the ideal patient with no distal disease, mild persistent symptoms are frequent and the ABI often remains abnormal.

There are no proven methods for reducing the incidence of late failure following PTA. To correct an inadequate initial PTA, new technology such as lasers and atherectomy devices offer exciting prospects but remain unproven. Reducing the progression of atherosclerosis by controlling risk factors is prudent but its effect on PTA remains unproven. Drug therapy to counteract the development of intimal hyperplasia has not been of benefit, at least when assessed in the coronary circulation. Specifically, antiplatelet drugs, warfarin, heparin, calcium channel blockers, and corticosteroids have not reduced the incidence of restenosis. However, Ω-3 fatty acids have shown promise in a recent study.

The authors wish to acknowledge the assistance of Ms. P. Purdy in the preparation of the manuscript.

REFERENCES

1. Johnston KW, Rae M, Hogg-Johnston SA, Colapinto RF, Walker PM, Baird RJ, Sniderman KW, Kalman P. 5-year results of a prospective study of percutaneous transluminal angioplasty. Ann Surg 206:403-413, 1987.
2. Bennicke K, Ladefoged SD, Ulrich I, Sorensen K. Results and complications of balloon dilatation of renal artery stenosis in patients with renovascular hypertension. Ugeskr Laeger 151:557-560, 1989.
3. Rush DS, Gewertz BL, Lu CT, Ball DG, Zarins CK. Limb salvage in poor-risk patients using transluminal angioplasty. Arch Surg 118:1209-1212, 1983.
4. Glover JL, Bendick PJ, Dilley RS, Becker GJ, Richmond BC, Yune HY, Holden RW. Balloon catheter dilation for limb salvage. Arch Surg 118:557-560, 1983.
5. Milford MA, Weaver FA, Lundell CJ, Yellin AE. Femoropopliteal percutaneous transluminal angioplasty for limb salvage. J Vasc Surg 8:292-299, 1988.
6. Dorros G, Lewin F, Jamnadas P, Mathiak LM. Below-the-knee angioplasty: Tibioperoneal vessels, The acute outcome. Cathet Cardiovasc Diagn 19:170-178, 1990.
7. Gomes AS, Baker JD, Martin-Paredero V, Dixon SM, Takiff H, Machleder HI, Moore WS. Acute renal dysfunction after major arteriography. AJR 145:1249-1253, 1985.
8. Martin-Paredero V, Dixon SM, Baker JD, Takiff H, Gomes AS, Busuttil RW, Moore WS. Risk of renal failure after major angiography. Arch Surg 118:1417-1420, 1983.
9. Schwab SJ, Hlatky MA, Pieper KS, Davidson CJ, Morris KG, Skelton TN, Bashore TM. Contrast nephrotoxicity: A randomized controlled trial of a nonionic and an ionic radiographic contrast agent. N Engl J Med 320:149-153, 1989.
10. Gardiner GA Jr, Meyerovitz MF, Stokes KR, Clouse ME, Harrington DP, Bettmann MA. Complications of transluminal angioplasty. Radiology 159:201-208, 1986.
11. Brewster DC, Cambria RP, Darling RC, Athanasoulis CA, Waltman AC, Geller SC, Moncure AC, Lamuraglia GM, Freehan M, Abbott WM. Long-term results of combined iliac balloon angioplasty and distal surgical revascularization. Ann Surg 210:324-330, 1989.
12. Bakal CW, Sprayregen S, Scheinbaum K, Cynamon J, Veith FJ. Percutaneous transluminal angioplasty of the infrapopliteal arteries: Results in 53 patients. AJR 154:171-174, 1990.
13. Schwarten DE, Cutcliff WB. Arterial occlusive disease below the knee: Treatment with percutaneous transluminal angioplasty performed with low-profile catheters and steerable guide wires. Radiology 169:71-74, 1988.
14. Villarica J, Gross RC. Treatment of angioplasty-related iliac-artery rupture without bypass surgery (case report). AJR 147:389-390, 1986.
15. Joseph N, Levy E, Lipman S. Angioplasty-related iliac artery rupture: Treatment by temporary balloon occlusion. Cardiovasc Intervent Radiol 10:276-279, 1987.
16. Ashenburg RJ, Blair RJ, Rivera FJ, Weigele JB. Renal arterial rupture complicating transluminal angioplasty: Successful conservative management. Radiology 174:983-985, 1990.
17. Katzen BT. Technique and results of "low-dose" infusion. Cardiovasc Intervent Radiol 11(Suppl):S41-47, 1988.
18. Train JS, Dan SJ, Mitty HA, Dikman SH, Harrington EB, Miller CM, Jacobson JH. Occlusion during iliac angioplasty: A salvageable complication. Radiology 168:131-135, 1988.
19. Wolter M, Marsch WC. Pampiniform livedo—An acute cardinal symptom of a cutaneous cholesterol embolism. Dtsch Med Wochenschr 115:452-455, 1990.
20. Dahlberg PJ, Frecentese DF, Cogbill TH. Cholesterol embolism: Experience with 22 histologically proven cases. Surgery 105:737-746, 1989.
21. Gehani AA, Ashley S, Kester RC, Brooks SG, Davies GA, Rees MR. Aneurysm formation after dynamic catheter-assisted balloon angioplasty. Clin Radiol 41:283-285, 1990.
22. Becker GJ, Palmaz JC, Rees CR, Ehrman KO, Lalka SG, Dalsing MC, Cikrit DF, McLean GK, Burke DR, Richter GM. Angioplasty-induced dissections in human iliac arteries: Management with Palmaz balloon-expandable intraluminal stents. Radiology 176:31-38, 1990.
23. Kalman PG, Johnston KW. Outcome of a failed percutaneous transluminal dilatation. Surg Gynecol Obstet 161:43-46, 1985.
24. Morin J-F, Johnston KW, Rae M. Improvement after successful percutaneous transluminal dilatation treatment of occlusive peripheral arterial disease. Surg Gynecol Obstet 163:453-457, 1986.
25. Casarella WJ. Noncoronary angioplasty. Curr Probl Cardiol 11:141-174, 1986.
26. Cole SE, Baird RN, Horrocks M, Jeans WD. The role of balloon angioplasty in the management of lower limb ischaemia. Eur J Vasc Surg 1:61-65, 1987.
27. Stokes KR, Strunk HM, Campbell DR, Gibbons GW, Wheeler HG, Clouse ME. Five-year results of iliac and femoropopliteal angioplasty in diabetic patients. Radiology 174:977-982, 1990.
28. Jager KA, Phillips DJ, Martin RL, Hanson C, Roeder-er GO, Langlois YE, Ricketts HJ, Strandness DE Jr. Noninvasive mapping of lower limb arterial lesions. Ultrasound Med Biol 11:515-521, 1985.

29. Langsfeld M, Nepute J, Hershey FB, Thorpe L, Auer AI, Binnington HB, Hurley JJ, Peterson GJ, Schwartz R, Woods JJ Jr. The use of deep duplex scanning to predict hemodynamically significant aortoiliac stenoses. J Vasc Surg 7:395-399, 1988.

30. Colapinto R, Harries-Jones E, Johnston KW. Percutaneous transluminal dilatation and recanalization in the treatment of peripheral vascular disease. Radiology 135:583-587, 1980.

31. Faxon DP, Sanborn TA, Haudenschild CC, Ryan TJ. Effect of antiplatelet therapy on restenosis after experimental angioplasty. Am J Cardiol 53:72c-76c, 1984.

32. Gruntzig A, Kumpe DA. Technique of percutaneous transluminal angioplasty with the Gruntzig balloon catheter. AJR 132:547-552, 1979.

33. Bachman DM, Casarella WJ, Sos TA. Percutaneous iliofemoral angioplasty via the contralateral femoral artery. Radiology 130:617-621, 1979.

34. Tegtmeyer CJ, Kellum CD, Kron IL, Mentzer RM Jr. Percutaneous transluminal angioplasty in the region of the aortic bifurcation. The two-balloon technique with results and long-term follow-up study. Radiology 157:661-665, 1985.

35. Tegtmeyer CJ. Guide wire angioplasty balloon catheter: Preliminary report. Radiology 169:253-254, 1988.

36. Hopkins A. Survival analysis with covariates: Cox models. BMDP Statistical Software, 1983, pp 576-594.

37. Roubin GS, Douglas JS Jr, King SB III, Lin S, Hutchison N, Thomas RG, Gruntzig AR. Influence of balloon size on initial success, acute complications, and restenosis after percutaneous transluminal coronary angioplasty: A prospective randomized study. Circulation 78:557-565, 1988.

38. Sarembock IJ, LaVeau PJ, Sigal SL, Timms I, Sussman J, Haudenschild C, Ezekowitz MD. Influence of inflation pressure and balloon size on the development of intimal hyperplasia after balloon angioplasty. A study in the atherosclerotic rabbit. Circulation 80:1029-1040, 1989.

39. Seeger J, Abela GS. Current status of laser angioplasty. Surg Annu 22:299-315, 1990.

40. Cragg AH, Gardiner GA Jr, Smith TP. Vascular application of laser. Radiology 172:925-935, 1989.

41. Jeans WD, Murphy P, Hughes AO, Horrocks M, Baird RN. Randomized trial of laser-assisted passage through occluded femoro-popliteal arteries. Br J Radiol 63:19-21, 1990.

42. Rees CR, Palmaz JC, Garcia O, Roeren T, Richter GM, Gardiner G Jr, Schwarten D, Schatz RA, Root HD, Rogers W. Angioplasty and stenting of completely occluded iliac arteries. Radiology 172:953-959, 1989.

43. Palmaz JC, Garcia OJ, Schatz RA, Rees CR, Roeren T, Richter GM, Neoldge G, Gardiner GA Jr, Becker GJ, Walker C, Stagg J, Katzen BT, Dake MD, Paolini RM, McLean GK, Lammer J, Schwarten DE, Tio FO, Root HD, Rogers W. Placement of balloon-expandable intraluminal stents in iliac arteries: First 171 procedures. Radiology 174:969-975, 1990.

44. Dorros G, Lewin RF, Sachdev N, Mathiak L. Percutaneous atherectomy of occlusive peripheral vascular disease: Stenoses and/or occlusions. Cathet Cardiovasc Diagn 18:1-6, 1989.

45. Thornton MA, Gruntzig AR, Hollman J, King SB III, Douglas JS. Coumadin and aspirin in prevention of recurrence after transluminal coronary angioplasty: A randomized study. Circulation 69:721-727, 1984.

46. Urban P, Buller N, Fox K, Shapiro L, Bayliss J, Rickards A. Lack of effect of warfarin on the restenosis rate or on clinical outcome after balloon coronary angioplasty. Br Heart J 60:485-488, 1988.

47. Clowes AW, Karnovsky MJ. Suppression by heparin of injury-induced myointimal thickening. J Surg Res 24:161-168, 1978.

48. Clowes AW, Clowes MM. Kinetics of cellular proliferation after arterial injury. IV. Heparin inhibits rat smooth muscle mitogenesis and migration. Circ Res 58:839-845, 1986.

49. Ellis SG, Roubin GS, Wilentz J, Douglas JS Jr, King SB III. Effect of 18- 24-hour heparin administration for prevention of restenosis after uncomplicated coronary angioplasty. Am Heart J 117:777-782, 1989.

50. Schwartz L, Bourassa MG, Lespérance J, Aldridge HE, Kazim F, Salvatori VA, Henderson M, Bonan R, David PR. Aspirin and dipyridamole in the prevention of restenosis after percutaneous transluminal coronary angioplasty. N Engl J Med 318:1714-1719, 1988.

51. Schlant RC, King SB III. Usefulness of calcium entry blockers during and after percutaneous transluminal coronary artery angioplasty. Circulation 80:IV88-IV92, 1989.

52. Pepine CJ, Hirshfeld JW, Macdonald RB, Henderson MA, Bass TA, Goldberg S, Savage MP, Vetrovec G, Cowley M, Taussig AS, et al. A controlled trial of corticosteroids to prevent restenosis after coronary angioplasty. M-Heart Group. Circulation 81:1753-1761, 1990.

53. Dehmer GJ, Popma JJ, van den Berg EK, Eichhorn EJ, Prewitt JB, Campbell WB, Jennings L, Willerson JT, Schmitz JM. Reduction in the rate of early restenosis after coronary angioplasty by a diet supplemented with n-3 fatty acids. N Engl J Med 319:733-740, 1988.

33

Complications Associated With Intravascular Instrumentation: Endoscopy, Atherectomy, Lasers, and Dilatation Devices

Rodney A. White

Complications of intravascular instrumentation encompass a broad spectrum. Many of the devices used in endovascular procedures can cause similar types of complications, such as vessel wall perforation, dissection, or embolization, whereas some devices can cause problems unique to that instrument, such as thermal injury by lasers. The complication rates are potentially high as a result of the number of new devices that are in an early development phase. Indications for many instruments have not yet been determined, and therefore the use of an instrument to treat lesions beyond the capabilities of the device increases the potential for adverse outcome.

Complications during the procedure may lead to immediate failure or may compromise the long-term durability of the repair. Even though immediate vessel recanalization may be accomplished, long-term patency is frequently limited by imprecise instrument guidance during recanalizations and inadequate removal of the lesions. In addition, intravascular interventions and the concomitant complications are directly affected by the skill and training of the instrument operator. A learning curve is experienced by almost all investigators during the initial procedures, particularly if the interventionalist is inexperienced with endoluminal methods. Other variables, including the quality of ancillary equipment such as fluoroscopy and imaging devices, significantly affect the success of intravascular procedures.

This chapter addresses the most frequently encountered complications common to all endovascular procedures and devices as well as those that are related to particular instruments or selected interventions. Appropriate forms of therapy and methods to help avert problems are described.

PROCEDURE-RELATED COMPLICATIONS

Intravascular surgical procedures may be performed by either percutaneous or open-incision surgical techniques. Percutaneous insertion of devices is used both in radiology and cardiology suites and in the operating room. Outside of the operating room the percutaneous route is used in the majority of procedures, whereas in the operating room a higher percentage of the interventions are done through an open surgical incision to accommodate the introduction of larger devices or to combine an intravascular procedure with a conventional operation. Aside from balloon angioplasty catheters, many new intravascular devices are difficult to use percutaneously because of size limitations. As interventional devices are developed, percutaneous adaption occurs following miniaturization of the instruments.

Passage of devices along the lumen of a vessel theoretically enhances thrombogenicity of the vessel wall by causing endothelial denudation, which can predispose the vessel to the long-term development of hyperplastic lesions

420

caused by concomitant fracture of the internal elastic lamina of the artery.[1] During endovascular procedures, multiple insertions and withdrawals of devices compound the potential risk of this complication. Fluid overload is possible during procedures in which repeated contrast dye examinations and anticoagulant fluid irrigations are used to avert thrombogenesis and to clear the field of view for angioscopic examinations. Contrast media volumes should be minimized during difficult procedures in which repeated imaging is required. Blood loss must also be closely monitored in prolonged cases, particularly if an open operative approach is used or in cases in which undetected bleeding can occur.

Introducer sheaths that have a hemostatic valve at the instrument introduction port and additional ports for infusion of fluids and contrast dyes are extremely useful in reducing the trauma to vessel walls and in controlling blood loss (Fig. 33-1). Newer intraluminal access devices for use during both percutaneous and open-incision approaches are being devel-

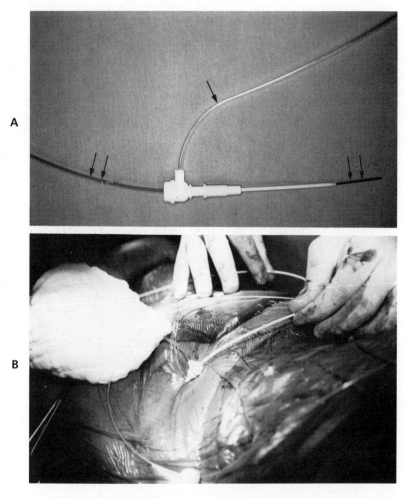

Fig. 33-1. A, Hemostatic 8 Fr introducer sheath with sideport (single arrow) for infusion of fluids or contrast media. A 1 mm angioscope is passed through the instrument port (double arrows). **B,** Intraoperative application of the percutaneous introducer for antegrade femoral artery angioplasty. A 7 Fr catheter containing an 800 μm angioscope is passed through the hemostatic valve of the 8 Fr introducer sheath for angioscopic inspection of the vessel lumen.

oped to decrease vessel trauma, provide better hemostasis, and facilitate removal of intravascular material. The Fogarty expandable access device (Intimax; Applied Vascular Devices, Inc., Laguna Hills, Calif.) illustrates a novel approach by providing an expandable sheath that is initially low profile for safe intraluminal introduction and then enlarges to conform to the arterial wall, limiting trauma and enhancing hemostasis. A large-diameter (9 to 15 Fr) iris-type valve on the instrument introduction port accommodates large-diameter devices and minimizes blood loss because it allows ease of introduction of devices and demonstrates sealing characteristics (Fig. 33-2).

Percutaneous Procedures

Percutaneous procedures are limited to those that can be performed using low-profile catheters (less than 8 to 10 Fr) and to proce-dures in which a segment of patent vessel proximal to the interventional site is available for introduction of the instruments. Introduction of percutaneous devices is usually accomplished using the conventional Seldinger technique. Percutaneous vascular access is gained by inserting a beveled needle through the arterial wall via a small skin incision to facilitate subsequent insertion of vessel dilators and instruments. The needle is slowly withdrawn until pulsatile arterial blood flow is achieved, signifying that the needle tip is in the arterial lumen. A guidewire is then introduced through the lumen of the needle and is positioned under fluoroscopic control. For many procedures an introducer sheath is threaded over the guidewire after passage of a vascular dilator. The diameter of the sheath is determined by the size of the device that will be passed through the sheath lumen into the artery.

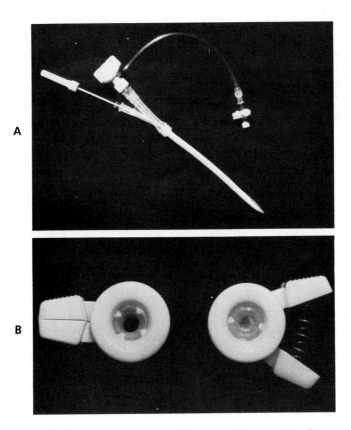

Fig. 33-2. A, Intimax access device. **B,** Iris hemostatic valve.

Passage of needles, introducers, and instruments through the arterial wall predisposes to dissection and formation of intimal flaps. Acute arterial occlusion may occur from dislodged or embolized intimal lesions. Perforations of vessels caused by smaller diameter interventional devices in most cases do not require repair, particularly if the perforations are in previously occluded or thrombosed vessels. In this situation there is usually little blood loss and the perforation seals by rethrombosis of the segment. In addition, arterial venous fistulas often close spontaneously following reversal of anticoagulation. Rarely, perforations may continue to bleed, requiring surgical control. The most common site for such perforations is in intraperitoneal vessels or in the external iliac artery above the inguinal ligament when attempts are being made to facilitate antegrade access to the femoral vessels. This approach is associated with a risk of hemorrhage into the retroperitoneum.

Intimal flaps usually require operative repair if they cause flow restriction. Microembolization of thrombus or atheromatous material is in most cases of no consequence if it is limited and there is no evidence of distal ischemia. If occlusion develops in a larger artery, percutaneous aspiration thrombectomy or open surgical embolectomy is required to restore flow.[2] Intra-arterial thrombolytic therapy may also be effective in dissolving fresh thrombus.[3] Massive embolization of small (20 to 200 µm diameter) particles can cause diffuse necrosis of tissues, producing devastating clinical consequences such as a "trash limb."

The majority of complications of percutaneous procedures associated with long-term failures (in particular, recurrence of lesions) are common to the use of all endovascular devices. False aneurysms or pseudoaneurysms at the puncture site in the arterial wall are unique to the percutaneous introduction sites, and the frequency with which they occur increases with increasing size of the cannulas and endovascular instruments. False aneurysms frequently become apparent at a relatively short time after the procedure and require surgical repair to prevent bleeding or embolization.

Intraoperative Applications of Endovascular Devices

Intraoperative application of endovascular devices permits use of a larger variety of instruments as either primary therapy or as an adjunct to another vascular procedure. A key factor in accomplishing successful angioplasty in the operating room is adequate radiologic imaging. High-resolution images significantly enhance the precision with which procedures can be performed; the lack of availability of high-resolution imaging is a limiting factor in many institutions. Digital subtraction techniques have increased contrast-imaging sensitivity, allowing detection of low levels of iodinated materials. Many digital units have freeze-frame and road-mapping features that permit superimposition of a subtracted contrast image of a vessel on a live fluoroscopic visualization. The quality of equipment available for radiologic imaging of procedures varies from conventional C-arm fluoroscopes to sophisticated image-intensifiers and TV monitoring systems. Immediate image-replay systems can improve the accuracy of information and enhance the safety of interventions. Recent advances in computerized image-processing systems extend the advantages of digital imaging technology to C-arm fluoroscopy by enabling the modular addition of contrast enhancement, image holding, and road-mapping during angiographic procedures using available equipment.[4]

Intraoperative percutaneous use of devices is accomplished by the methods described previously. Many patients have significant vascular occlusive disease near a possible insertion site, which precludes safe passage of a percutaneous introducer. In these cases surgical incisions provide the best access to the vessel. Introduction of intravascular instruments through an open surgical incision has several advantages compared to percutaneous methods. Open incisions permit inspection of intravascular anatomy, such as the orifices of adjacent branch vessels, and helps decrease the incidence of vessel wall dissection during device introduction. Control of blood flow from collateral vessels by conventional operative methods also

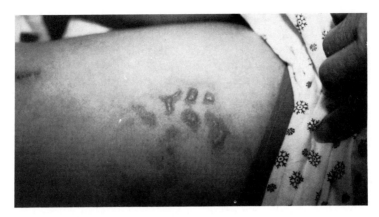

Fig. 33-3. Skin discoloration and blistering overlying the site of a laser thermal probe perforation. (From White RA, White GH. Laser angioplasty: Development, current status, and future perspectives. Semin Vasc Surg 2:123-142, 1989.)

expedites angioscopic intraluminal visualization.

Once an arteriotomy has been fashioned, it is advantageous to work through a hemostatic introducer sheath with a sideport similar to ones used for percutaneous procedures. In this way trauma to the blood vessel wall by repeated introduction and withdrawal of devices is prevented, hemostasis at the introduction port can be provided, and a port for injection of contrast dye is available. Introducer sheaths must be used very carefully because it is easy to injure the luminal surface of the artery during placement of the sheath, particularly when it is inserted some distance into the artery. If a vessel is too diseased to accommodate an introducer sheath, hemostasis can be maintained with Roumel tourniquets or by passing the endoluminal devices carefully through the controlled area.

Introduction of instruments through surgical incisions also permits continuation of anticoagulant therapy throughout the procedure and postoperatively if the wound is drained to prevent hematoma formation. Continuation of anticoagulation postoperatively has been shown to help prevent acute thrombosis of difficult recanalizations in the open-incision surgical technique; in percutaneous procedures anticoagulation is reversed and pressure is applied to the wound following removal of the intra-

luminal device to ensure hemostasis. An obvious liability of the open-incision technique is the risk of wound infection, particularly if a patch material or prosthetic is used in the repair. The incidence of wound infection has been shown to be higher using the open-incision technique during endovascular procedures.[5]

An additional wound problem that has been noted sporadically following endovascular procedures using access through the groin is skin discoloration, blistering, and variable-thickness skin loss over the anterior thigh (Fig. 33-3). This complication was initially thought to be caused by thermal injury from perforations with laser thermal devices, but it is most likely caused by embolization. This complication has been noted with both the percutaneous route and the surgical-incision route and with devices other than lasers.

DEVICE-RELATED COMPLICATIONS
Introduction Catheters and Guidewires

A variety of introducers are used to provide access to the vascular lumen for guidewires and angioplasty devices. The main complications of the introducers are disruption of the vascular surface, producing intimal flaps or embolization, and formation of thrombus on catheter

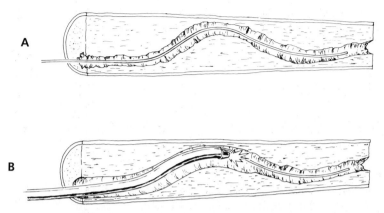

Fig. 33-4. A, Placement of a guidewire through the meandering, eccentric lumen of an atherosclerotic vessel. **B,** The ability of a device passed over the guidewire is limited in its ability to adequately remove the lesion without causing vessel-wall perforation because the device is maintained in the eccentric position by the guidewire.

surfaces when they are positioned in low blood-flow areas without anticoagulation. Some catheters incorporate anticoagulants in the catheter surface to decrease thrombogenicity, but systemic anticoagulation is required in most instances to prevent thrombosis.

The complications related to introducer sheath placement can be reduced by accurately judging the appropriate diameter and length of the device for the vascular segment being treated. Many diseased vessels have segmental narrowings or friable luminal surfaces that can easily be disrupted. If intimal flaps result, a localized endarterectomy can sometimes be performed, although an otherwise successful angioplasty procedure can be disrupted by introducer complications, which frequently require a vascular reconstruction to bypass the segment.

Guidewires are extremely useful for introducing intravascular devices and helping to maintain intraluminal guidance. Stiffer wires with less flexible tips have a greater tendency to produce intimal lesions, dissections, and perforations. Some of the newer flexible-tip wires and catheters have a hydrophilic polymer coating, which aids in atraumatic passage through stenotic or occluded vessel segments. Although introduction of angioplasty devices over guidewires can be used to help prevent complications, the obligatory off-center positioning of the guidewire through eccentric atherosclerotic obstructions prevents complete debulking of lesions without affecting adjacent vessel walls that have minimal or no involvement (Fig. 33-4). Alleviation of this problem awaits improved guidance systems to provide concentric alignment of the device within the arterial lumen. Combined intraluminal ultrasound and angioscopic-guided angioplasty catheter delivery systems are promising in this regard.

Angioscopy

Angioscopy, the intraluminal inspection of vessels, is not a new idea. Recent improvements in instrumentation have led to a resurgence of interest and use. Angioscopy is used to determine etiology, establish diagnosis, evaluate technical accuracy of reconstructions, and visualize intraluminal instrumentation.[6] Several investigators have reported that angioscopy reveals clinically important information that is not apparent by extraluminal inspection, probing, or angiography in 20% to 30% of vascular procedures. Angioscopic findings have altered the choice of surgical therapy in a significant number of these cases. Additional benefits of angioscopy are the ability to visually inspect and assist introduction and manipulation of intraluminal instrumentation. Observation of the completeness of valvulotomy in in situ vein bypasses; use in angioscopic-assisted thrombectomy; and inspection, guidance, and post-procedure evaluation of angioplasties are current applications.

At present, angioscopy offers an alternative to angiography, with the advantage of providing repeatable three-dimensional intraluminal views before blood flow is restored (Fig. 33-5). Potential complications of angioscopy include fluid overload from excessive administration of irrigation and the creation of intimal lesions. Inspecting vessels that approximate or are smaller than the diameter of the angioscope can cause spasm and possible thrombosis. The clarity of angioscopic images is usually excellent, but learning how to obtain adequate clearance of blood flow from collateral and distal vessels by fluid infusion and how to center the device for examinations requires an initial learning curve. These factors are frequently implicated in the limitation of visualization, but adequate examinations can be performed in approximately 85% of cases.

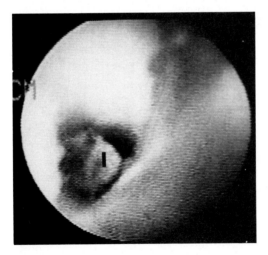

Fig. 33-5. Intraluminal lesion *(l)* that remains after laser-assisted balloon angioplasty of a superficial femoral artery. (From White RA, White GH. Angioscopy in the management of infrainguinal occlusive arterial disease. In Ernst CB, Stanley JC, eds. Current Therapy in Vascular Surgery-2. Philadelphia: BC Decker, 1990.)

Atherectomy Catheters

Atherectomy devices are designed to remove atherosclerotic plaque from the vessel by cutting, drilling, or pulverizing atheroma; they produce a luminal surface quite different from that produced by balloon dilatation or surgical endarterectomy.[7] Some of the currently available atherectomy devices have mechanisms for extracting the fragments of ablated plaque, whereas others reduce the plaque to microparticles, which are circulated within the bloodstream and are removed by the lung and reticuloendothelial organs.

Most current atherectomy devices are suitable for short stenotic lesions only and are inserted over a guidewire. If the stenotic arterial lesion is not sufficiently enlarged after a successful atherectomy procedure, adjunctive balloon dilatation is often performed. As a corollary, angioplasty complications, such as dissection or acute occlusion following balloon dilatation, or an inadequate vessel recanalization may be improved by subsequent passage of an atherectomy catheter. Complication rates for transluminal atherectomy are less than 5% to 10% in most studies, with vessel perforation, thrombosis, and embolization being the most common short-term limitations. Hemoglobinuria and hemolysis have been reported with several devices. The systemic effects of microembolization have yet to be determined, although embolization to distal tissues in the leg has not been a serious clinical problem in preliminary studies.

Indications for atherectomy have not been defined, and its role in the management of vascular disease will be determined by further developments and clinical experience. Although initial successes have been achieved with several atherectomy devices, restenosis has been a problem in some studies, particularly when the amount of plaque removed may have been inadequate. Preliminary data suggest that adequate removal of lesions to <20% residual stenosis and control of the level of removal within the arterial wall improve follow-up patency and hemodynamic results.[8] If this finding is substantiated, development of the debulking principle could dramatically improve the results of endovascular recanalizations, enabling more widespread application of the technology.

Lasers

Lasers have been investigated as a method to recanalize and debulk atherosclerotic occlusions for less than a decade. These devices more than any other have undergone rapid development and application. In this regard, controversy concerning the use of lasers as angioplasty devices highlights the problems and discussions relevant to the use of all endovascular surgical instruments.

The initial laser devices used available energy sources such as the continuous-wave argon and Nd:YAG lasers. Preliminary attempts to recanalize lesions using fiberoptic delivery from these continuous-wave, thermal sources resulted in a high incidence of vessel perforation and thermal damage. To capture the thermal energy and in an attempt to prevent perforations, ovoid metal tips were placed on the ends of the fibers. Although there were enthusiastic preliminary reports based on treatment of stenotic lesions and short occlusions using the laser thermal devices plus balloon angioplasty compared with balloon angioplasty alone,[9] application of this technology to longer lesions that conformed to surgical indications for therapy is associated with higher complication and failure rates.[5,10] Even when obstructions are successfully recanalized, the long-term patency is quite disappointing. Newer devices include a hybrid instrument with partial emission of laser energy combined with the thermal effect, pulsed high-energy laser devices for precise ablation of tissue, and guided laser angioplasty systems. At this time the current role of these devices is undetermined and depends on whether future evolution of the instruments can eliminate some of the present limitations.

The most frequent complication of laser angioplasty is vessel-wall perforation. Regardless of the device, if the probes are used in lesions through which a guidewire cannot be initially passed, perforations are a frequent limiting factor. In most situations perforations are of no consequence because only a small hole is made tangentially through the lesion in the arterial wall, which subsequently rethromboses. Arteriovenous fistulas usually close readily once anticoagulation is reversed (Fig. 33-6), but rarely venous trauma may lead to vein thrombosis, which requires anticoagulant therapy (Fig. 33-7).

A theoretical problem related to the laser thermal devices is thermal injury to surrounding tissues. It has been considered as a possible cause of early reocclusion of successful vessel recanalizations. In another respect, it has been suggested that thermal injury may retard smooth muscle proliferation, enhancing long-term patency. Thus the utility of thermal angioplasty devices has yet to be determined.

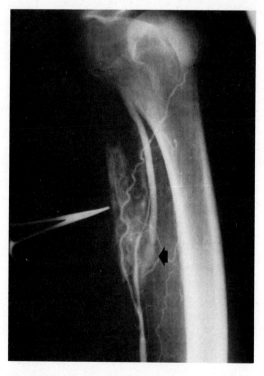

Fig. 33-6. Angiographic appearance of a laser thermal perforation (arrow) of the superficial femoral artery and concomitant arteriovenous fistula. (From White RA, White GH. Laser thermal probe recanalization of occluded arteries. J Vasc Surg 9:594-604, 1989.)

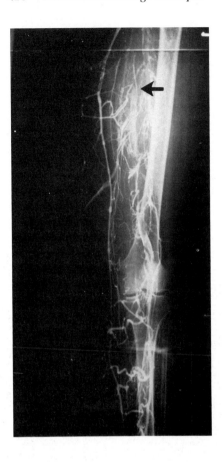

Fig. 33-7. Deep vein thrombosis subsequent to laser thermal perforation. It was speculated that the perforation resulted from intraluminal vein thermal damage. Arrow marks the approximate site of the suspected laser thermal perforation. (From White RA, White GH. Laser angioplasty: Development, current status and future perspectives. Semin Vasc Surg 2:123-142, 1989.)

Laser angioplasty has been used widely in its early evolution, which has accentuated the problems associated with guidance of endovascular devices.[11] The guidance issue is pertinent because (1) most atherosclerotic lesions are positioned eccentrically within the vessel lumen and (2) failures, including perforations, dissections, and short-term reocclusions, are caused by inaccurate guiding and debulking of lesions[12] (Fig. 33-8).

An additional complication of laser angioplasty, which is related to imprecise delivery of energy to normal or minimally diseased artery, is the development of lesions in previously unaffected sites adjacent to the treated segment (Fig. 33-9). The most evident presentation of this complication occurs in patients who were previously treated for short stenoses or occlusions and who return with long segments of reoccluded vessels. This limitation stresses the importance of treating only well-defined lesions that can be precisely ablated with current devices. It also emphasizes that treatment of minimal disease, such as claudication, should be reserved for interventionalists who have technical excellence, vast experience, and optimal systems available to treat these lesions.

Intravascular Stents

Vascular stents or intraluminal splints were first investigated by Dotter[13] in 1969, when he placed nonexpanding stainless steel coils in canine femoral arteries. His work prompted studies by other investigators using a variety of stent designs. Early prototypes suffered from many problems including bulky configurations, unpredictable expansion of the stent, migration, abrupt thrombosis, and gradual restenosis from intimal hyperplasia.

Currently, there are three basic designs: stainless steel spring-loaded stents, thermally

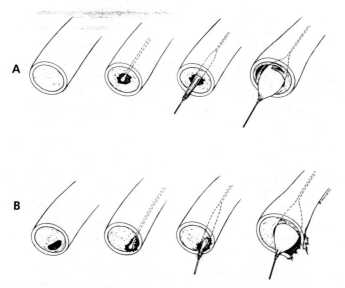

Fig. 33-8. A, Favorable result with concentric recanalization. **B,** Enhanced potential for perforation of eccentric lesions. (From White RA, White GH. Laser thermal probe recanalization of occluded arteries. J Vasc Surg 9:594-604, 1989.)

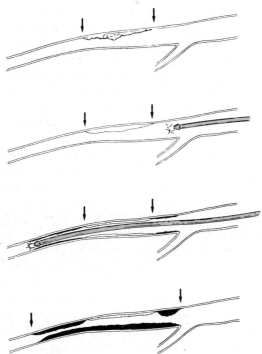

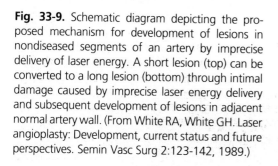

Fig. 33-9. Schematic diagram depicting the proposed mechanism for development of lesions in nondiseased segments of an artery by imprecise delivery of laser energy. A short lesion (top) can be converted to a long lesion (bottom) through intimal damage caused by imprecise laser energy delivery and subsequent development of lesions in adjacent normal artery wall. (From White RA, White GH. Laser angioplasty: Development, current status and future perspectives. Semin Vasc Surg 2:123-142, 1989.)

expanded memory metal stents, and balloon-expandable stents. The balloon-expandable stent is the most popular type because it can be inserted at the time of concomitant balloon angioplasty. In animal studies intra-arterial stents can prevent elastic recoil of the vessel wall and maintain luminal diameter by plaque compression following angioplasty. Although stents do become incorporated in the vessel wall and are covered by endothelium, preliminary histologic studies performed several months following placement reveal that the stented segments show thinning of the media and neointimal proliferation over the stent.[14]

Stents currently are most beneficial clinically in large-diameter high-flow vessels. Stenting of lesions in iliac arteries and veins and superior vena caval stenoses has been particularly useful. Their application in medium-caliber vessels of lower velocity such as the femoral and popliteal arteries is unknown. Stents may be most useful in the treatment of acute reclosure of angioplasties, either from residual thrombotic material, flaps, and dissections or from recoil of the vessel wall. Preliminary clinical evaluation of these devices has demonstrated a benefit in patients who experience abrupt closure of coronary balloon angioplasties by restoring patency and preventing myocardial infarctions.[14] Similar benefits have been shown in the treatment of residual stenoses, intimal flaps, dissections, and recoil of large-vessel angioplasties. Prevention of restenosis by stent therapy remains to be demonstrated; thus use of stents for this indication remains controversial, particularly in terms of risks of chronic thrombosis, dislodgement and migration, or embolization.

RESOLVING CURRENT LIMITATIONS

To resolve the current limitations and complications of endovascular surgical procedures and devices, the problems related to guidance of angioplasty instruments and restenosis subsequent to initial recanalization must be addressed. The guidance issue is particularly relevant since most atherosclerotic lesions are eccentrically positioned within the vessel wall. Many of the failures, including initial perforations and dissections and short-term reocclu-sions, are caused by inaccurate guidance of angioplasty devices and inadequate debulking of lesions. For this reason, major emphasis is being directed toward development of precise guidance methods for endoluminal instruments.

Several interesting devices are being developed and tested to address the guidance problem. Target-specific laser angioplasty may become possible by analysis of emitted fluorescence patterns (laser-induced fluorescence) from the vessel wall.[15] An interesting prototype that uses spectroscopic guidance for controlled activation of a multifiber catheter has been developed and is being evaluated.[16] When argon laser radiation is used to excite both normal and atherosclerotic vessels, distinct patterns of fluorescence from each tissue can be disseminated from a 19-fiber array by a multichannel spectral analyzer. The spectra and images that are produced permit selective identification of lesions and ablation in individual quadrants around the circumference of the arterial wall. Although the concept is appealing, current devices require frequent calibration to adjust signal sensitivity and are expensive to purchase and maintain.

Other prototype delivery systems for angioplasty devices incorporate multiple modalities, that is, spectroscopy, angioscopy, or intravascular ultrasound, to enhance the precision of initial vessel recanalizations. Intravascular ultrasound promises to be the most user-friendly and accurate way to accomplish this goal in occluded vessels. This technology is available as a component of the tip of 3 to 8 Fr catheters and produces a detailed image of the thickness of the blood vessel wall[17,18] (Fig. 33-10).

Lesion recurrence caused by thrombosis and organization of residual debris or restenosis from smooth muscle cell proliferation of recanalized lesions remains the most troublesome problem limiting the effectiveness of endoluminal surgery devices, particularly once the guidance issues permitting precise direction of devices are solved. Minimal progress has been made in defining either the etiology or the control of this phenomenon. The concepts regarding the etiology and development of recurrent lesions are confused and are based on

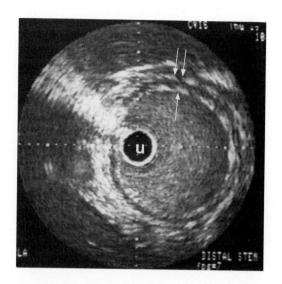

Fig. 33-10. Intraluminal ultrasound image of a human iliac artery demonstrating luminal (single arrow) and adventitial surface (double arrows). An echolucent media is apparent between the two structures. *u*, ultrasound probe.

poorly controlled studies of angiographic measurements of one- or two-dimensional angiographic images of lesions before and after interventions. Accurate data regarding the intraluminal dimensions of treated lesions before and after angioplasty and the types of tissue components that have been ablated or displaced are not available in the reported studies. Without controlled studies to evaluate these parameters, little progress can be expected regarding control of lesion recurrence.

Combined approaches to disobliterate occluded arteries using thrombolysis, luminal dilatation, and tissue ablation or removal all offer unique potentials if improved guidance and delivery systems become available. Future angioplasty device delivery catheters may combine angioscopy for visual inspection of the lumen, spectroscopy for characterization of the tissue elements, and ultrasound for determining the vessel wall and lesion dimensions. Improved intraluminal ultrasound devices will provide not only improved visualization of cross-sectional vessel anatomy, but also three-dimensional longitudinal reconstruction of the

vasculature by storing a sequence of ultrasound images. Improved guidance of angioplasty catheters will help eliminate the primary causes of failure of recanalizations and recurrence of lesions: vessel wall perforation and inadequate debulking of lesions. This advance is required as the first step toward solving the limitations of current technology. Further improvement will occur as the fundamental processes responsible for restenosis of lesion are elucidated and methods of control become available.

REFERENCES

1. Clowes A. Theories of atherosclerosis. In White RA, ed. Atherosclerosis and Arteriosclerosis: Human Pathology and Experimental Animal Methods and Models. Boca Raton, Fla.: CRC Press, 1989, pp 3-15.
2. White RA, White GH. Percutaneous aspiration thromboembolectomy. In Ernst CB, Stanley JC, eds. Current Therapy in Vascular Surgery-2. Philadelphia: BC Decker, 1990, pp 598-600.
3. Montarjeme A. Thrombolytic therapy in arterial occlusion and graft thrombosis. Semin Vasc Surg 2:155-178, 1989.
4. White RA, Kopchok GE, Hsiang Y, Guthrie C, Colman P, Rosenbaum D, White G. Perspectives for development of angioplasty guidance systems. In White RA, Grundfest WS, eds. Lasers in Cardiovascular Disease: Clinical Applications, Alternative Angioplasty Devices and Guidance Systems, 2nd ed. St. Louis: Mosby-Year Book, 1989, pp 207-217.
5. White RA, White GH, Mehringer CM, Chaing FL, Wilson SE. A clinical trial of laser thermal angioplasty in patients with advanced peripheral vascular disease. Ann Surg 212:257-265, 1990.
6. White GH, White RA, eds. Angioscopy: Vascular and Coronary Applications. St. Louis: Mosby-Year Book, 1989.
7. Ahn SS. Peripheral atherectomy. Semin Vasc Surg 12:143-154, 1989.
8. Graor RA, Whitlow P, Bartholomew J, Olin J, Ruschhaupt WF, Young JR. Directional atherectomy for occlusive peripheral vascular disease. J Vasc Surg (in press).
9. Sanborn TA, Cumberland DC, Greenfield AJ, Motarjeme A, Schwarten DE, Leachman DR, Ferris EJ, Myler RK, McCowan TC, Tatpati D, Ginsburg R, White RI. Peripheral laser-assisted balloon angioplasty: Initial multicenter trial in 219 peripheral arteries. Arch Surg 124:1099-1103, 1989.
10. Seeger JM, Abela GS, Silverman SH, Jablonski SK. Initial results of laser recanalization in lower extremity arterial reconstruction. J Vasc Surg 9:10-17, 1989.
11. White RA, White GH, eds. Color Atlas of Endovascular Surgery. London: Chapman & Hall, 1990.

12. White RA, White GH, Vlasak J, Fujitani RM, Kopchok GE. Histopathology of human laser thermal angioplasty recanalizations. Lasers Surg Med 8:469-476, 1988.

13. Dotter CT. Transluminally placed coil-spring endoarterial tube grafts, Long-term patency in canine popliteal artery. Invest Radiol 4:329-332, 1969.

14. Penn IM, Levine SL, Schatz RA. Intravascular stents as an adjunct to endovascular intervention. In Moore WS, Ahn SS, eds. Endovascular Surgery. Philadelphia: WB Saunders, 1989, pp 258-277.

15. Murphy-Chutorian D. Laser angioplasty and endarterectomy: Present status and future potential. In Veith FJ, ed. Current Critical Problems in Vascular Surgery. St. Louis: Quality Medical Publishing, 1989, pp 188-194.

16. Hoyt CC, Richards-Kortum RR, Costello B, Sacks BA, Kittrell C, Rattiff NB, Kramer JR, Feld MS. Remote biomedical spectroscopic imaging of human artery wall. Lasers Surg Med 8:1-9, 1988.

17. White RA. Intravascular ultrasound. In Kadir S, ed. Current Practice of Interventional Radiology. Philadelphia: BC Decker (in press).

18. Bom N, Roelandt J, eds. Intravascular Ultrasound: Techniques, Developments, Clinical Perspectives. Dordrecht, The Netherlands: Kluwer, 1989.

34

Complications of Thrombolytic Therapy

Michael Belkin   **Thomas F. O'Donnell, Jr.**

The practice of pharmacologically lysing thrombus has naturally been accepted enthusiastically by vascular surgeons and interventional radiologists. As experience with various fibrinolytic agents has increased, however, this enthusiasm has been tempered by our recognition of the many possible complications of thrombolytic therapy. These complications range from mild allergic reactions to life-threatening hemorrhage (see box). The incidence and variety of complications vary with mode of administration (systemic vs. local), indication for treatment, and experience of the clinician. The experience of the clinician is an especially important factor when employing intra-arterial thrombolytic therapy. A dedicated team consisting of a vascular surgeon, interventional radiologist, and support personnel is essential for safe and effective therapy. Proper selection of patients to receive thrombolytic therapy requires an understanding of the realistic goals of therapy, success rates that can be anticipated, and complications that occur.

In this chapter we will review the major indications and results of thrombolytic therapy. The complications of this therapy including the incidence, etiology, management, and factors in prevention are addressed.

INDICATIONS AND RESULTS

The most common application of thrombolytic therapy employed by vascular surgeons involves intra-arterial infusion. This is generally employed for acute arterial thrombosis (either spontaneous or post–balloon angioplasty) or for thrombosis of arterial bypass grafts (vein or prosthetic). The results from several studies employing intra-arterial thrombolytic therapy are shown in Table 34-1. In general, success rates of approximately 75% can be expected for lysis of occlusions in the arterial circulation. In our experience, as in those of others, urokinase (UK) has demonstrated superior success over streptokinase (SK) in achieving lysis. UK has resulted in successful lysis in 80% to 100% of cases compared with 43% to 63% of cases with SK. Despite its increased expense, the improved efficacy and decreased incidence of complications associated with UK have made it the preferred agent for intra-arterial use.

More recently several authors have begun to report their experiences with intra-arterial recombinant human tissue-type plasminogen activator (t-PA) infusions. Unlike UK, which converts plasminogen to plasmin within the blood, t-PA is thought to bind specifically to

---

COMPLICATIONS OF THROMBOLYTIC THERAPY

Hemorrhage
  Catheter site
  Gastrointestinal
  Retroperitoneal
  CNS
  Adrenal
  Transgraft
  Occult
  Other
Allergic reaction
  Anaphylaxis
  Fever

Embolism
  Arterial
  Pulmonary
Stroke
  Embolic
  Hemorrhagic
Reperfusion syndrome
  Myoglobinuria
  Renal failure
  Compartment
    syndrome

Table 34-1. Results of Intra-arterial Thrombolytic Therapy

Series	Drug	Maintenance dose	Mean duration (hr)	No. of cases	Success rate (%)	No. of bleeding episodes (%)
Belkin et al.[1]	UK	40,000 IU/hr	46	10	100	3 (25)
	SK	5000 IU/hr	44	22	50	12 (55)
O'Donnell et al.[2]	UK	12,000 IU/hr	21	17	82	0 (0)
	SK	40,000 IU/hr	31	16	44	3 (19)
Gardiner et al.[3]	UK	60,000 IU/hr	26	22	77	1 (5)
	SK	5000 IU/hr	47	22	41	5 (23)
van Breda et al.[4]	UK	40,000-60,000 IU/hr	22	24	80	(8)
	SK	5,000-10,000 IU/hr	14	24	63	(33)
McNamara and Fischer[5]	UK	60,000 IU/hr	18	93	89	6 (7)
Graor et al.[6]	t-PA	0.05-0.1 mg/kg	<8	22	88	9 (41)
Meyerovitz et al.[7]	t-PA	5 mg/hr	—	16	50	5 (31)
	UK	60,000 IU/hr	—	16	38	2 (13)

UK, urokinase; SK, streptokinase; t-PA, tissue-type plasminogen activator.

fibrin and to convert plasminogen that is complexed with fibrin to plasmin. Thus t-PA offers the theoretical advantage of forming plasmin and activating fibrinolysis at the clot surface. The early results have not demonstrated any clear superiority of t-PA over UK. Graor et al.[6] reviewed their experience with intra-arterial infusion of t-PA for thrombosed bypass grafts and reported successful lysis in 29 out of 33 infusions (88%). In another small (n = 32) randomized prospective comparison of t-PA vs. UK for intra-arterial therapy, success rates were similar (50% for t-PA and 38% for UK); however, t-PA resulted in faster clot lysis.[7]

The vast majority of studies on intra-arterial therapy are short-term evaluations that judge success or failure by the radiologic demonstration of clot lysis and early clinical improvement. It should be stressed that thrombolytic infusion is seldom sufficient therapy and that it usually serves a diagnostic function to identify the lesion responsible for thrombosis. This lesion must be corrected either surgically or by angioplasty to prevent recurrent thrombosis. Unfortunately, even after a successful elimination of thrombus by thrombolytic therapy followed by surgical or radiologic interventional therapy, the long-term patency rates achieved are often

poor. We reviewed the long-term results of 22 occluded vein grafts that were successfully lysed and then followed by correction of the defects presumed to be responsible for thrombosis. Unfortunately, there was a high recurrent thrombosis rate, resulting in patency rates of only 37% and 23% at 1 and 3 years, respectively.[8] In a second study of 20 thrombosed PTFE grafts we found similar results. Of 17 grafts undergoing successful thrombolysis and revision, only 37% remained patent at 2 years.[2] Thus a realistic evaluation of the risks and benefits of intra-arterial thrombolytic therapy must consider the long-term results and recognize the temporizing nature of much of this therapy.

Systemic infusion of fibrinolytic agents has been employed for the management of pulmonary emboli and deep vein thrombosis. The Urokinase Pulmonary Embolism Trial (UPET)[9] and the Urokinase-Streptokinase Pulmonary Embolism Trial (USPET)[10] have demonstrated that after 24 hours of therapy, patients with pulmonary emboli receiving thrombolytic therapy demonstrate improved pulmonary angiograms, lung scans, and pulmonary hemodynamics compared with similar patients receiving heparin. There was no difference in mortality, however, and by 7 days following therapy lung scan improvements were similar in the heparin-treated patients. In an interesting follow-up study that examined pulmonary vascular function by measuring pulmonary capillary blood volume and diffusing capacity, patients receiving thrombolytic therapy showed persistent improvements compared with those receiving heparin.[11] Patients with massive pulmonary emboli seemed to derive particular benefit from fibrinolytic infusion. More recent studies that have employed t-PA in the management of pulmonary emboli have demonstrated short-term benefits similar to those found with other fibrinolytic agents.[12,13]

The role of systemic thrombolytic therapy in the management of deep vein thrombosis remains controversial. The main goals of therapy are the prevention of both pulmonary emboli and postthrombotic syndrome. Adequate anticoagulation with heparin followed by the administration of warfarin (Coumadin) has proved effective in the prevention of pulmonary emboli, and comparative studies have not demonstrated any benefit of fibrinolytic agents in this regard. It has been estimated from early studies that in as many as 80% of patients suffering deep vein thrombosis, postthrombotic sequelae will eventually develop. The associated edema, induration, dermatitis, and skin ulceration are attributable to the loss of venous valve function. It has been theorized that thrombolytic therapy may lead to rapid clot lysis before venous valve destruction, thereby preventing postthrombotic syndrome. Goldhaber et al.[14] have reviewed six randomized trials comparing SK to heparin in the management of deep vein thrombosis. They found that thrombolytic therapy was 3.7 times more likely to achieve phlebographically documented clot lysis than heparin. Despite the universal recognition of improved early clot lysis with fibrinolytic infusion, it is unclear whether this therapy will translate into a decreased incidence of long-term sequelae. Several investigators have addressed the long-term sequelae of acute deep vein thrombosis following thrombolytic therapy, principally with SK. Arnesen and Hoseth[15] compared patients who received SK to those who underwent conventional heparin therapy

for acute deep vein thrombosis and found a lower incidence of edema, pigmentation, and ulcer in those patients treated with SK. Elliot et al.[16] observed a reduced incidence of both edema and pigmentary changes in patients treated with SK. There was no difference, however, in the incidence of venous ulcer between the heparin-treated and SK-treated groups. In both Elliot's and Arnesen's studies the incidence of normal-appearing legs was approximately 60% to 80% in the SK-treated group. In a randomized study of patients receiving either SK or heparin, Kakkar et al.[17] followed up patients for 2 years after the initial episode of acute deep vein thrombosis. Limbs were evaluated by noninvasive hemodynamic assessment rather than by clinical criteria. Kakkar failed to show any difference in the incidence of normal, moderate, or severe hemodynamic impairment between the two groups. However, his use of hemodynamic rather than clinical criteria as an end-point, as well as the short follow-up period, have been criticized.

HEMORRHAGIC COMPLICATIONS OF SYSTEMIC AND INTRA-ARTERIAL THROMBOLYTIC THERAPY

Given the therapeutic goal of thrombolytic therapy, the dissolution of intravascular thrombus, it is to be expected that the most common, most feared, and potentially serious complication of thrombolytic therapy is hemorrhage.

Etiology

When thrombolytic therapy is administered intravenously for deep vein thrombosis or pulmonary embolus, a systemic lytic state is established. Although the systemic increase in plasmin is partially controlled by systemic antiplasmins (α_2-antiplasmin, α_2-macroglobulin), plasmin formed at clot surfaces actively leads to fibrin breakdown. Obviously, physiologic hemostatic fibrin plugs are just as susceptible to lysis as pathologic intravascular thrombi. Therefore the majority of bleeding complications occur as a result of trauma to the vasculature from diagnostic and therapeutic procedures.[3,5,9] Occult bleeding, which results in a drop in the hematocrit value or hemodynamic instability, is usually from unrecognized GI lesions or the retroperitoneum. Unfortunately, bleeding may occur anywhere vascular integrity is compromised, resulting in CNS hemorrhage (less than 1%),[18] urinary tract bleeding, epistaxis, vaginal bleeding, aortic aneurysmal bleeding, and almost any other imaginable source.[3,9,19-21] Similarly, when the fibrin ingrowth into the interstices of Dacron grafts (usually knitted) is lysed, transgraft extravasation of blood may occur.[22,23] Transgraft hemorrhage has also been rarely reported with polytetrafluoroethylene (PTFE) grafts.[3] Fortunately, transgraft contrast extravasation noted during arteriography usually does not result in clinically severe bleeding.

Intra-arterial administration of thrombolytic therapy, by definition, requires continuous cannulation of the arterial system with an infusion catheter. Bleeding around the indwelling catheter site or from the back wall of an arterial puncture site is by far the most common etiology of hemorrhage with intra-arterial therapy.

The proteolytic properties of plasmin are not specific to fibrin. Fibrinogen; clotting factors V, VIII, IX, and X; and other plasma proteins are also substrates for plasmin's proteolytic actions. Breakdown and consumption of these factors can result in acquired coagulopathy. This coagulopathy may result in hemorrhagic complications that are not directly related to clot lysis, which may explain the observation that many bleeding complications occur after cessation of thrombolytic therapy when active clot lysis has stopped.[1,16,24] Numerous authors have noted that hypofibrinogenemia is associated with an increased incidence of bleeding complications.[1,25-27]

Incidence

The incidence of bleeding complications from thrombolytic therapy varies with mode of administration, fibrinolytic agent employed, and length of infusion. The incidence of bleeding complications with systemic intravenous therapy ranges from 3.3% to 63.6% (Table 34-2). This includes local bleeding (cannulation sites) in 3.3% to 50% of cases and systemic bleeding in 0% to 63.6% of cases.

Table 34-2. Results of Systemic Intravenous Thrombolytic Therapy

Series	Drug	Maintenance dose	Duration	No. of cases	Total no. of bleeding episodes (%)	No. of local bleeding episodes (%)	No. of systemic bleeding episodes (%)
van de Loo et al.[20]	UK	1100 IU/kg/hr	3 d	11	3 (27.3)	0 (0)	3 (27.3)
	UK	2200 IU/kg/hr	3 d	11	2 (18.2)	0 (0)	2 (18.2)
	SK	100,000 IU/hr	3 d	11	7 (63.6)	0 (0)	7 (63.6)
Graor et al.[19]	UK	4400 IU/kg/hr	24-48 hr	30	1 (3.3)	1 (3.3)	0 (0)
	SK	100,000 IU/hr	48-106 hr	30	5 (16.7)	0 (0)	5 (16.7)
USPET[10]	UK	2000 IU/lb/hr	12 hr	59	31 (52.5)	24 (40.7)	7 (11.9)
	UK	2000 IU/lb/hr	24 hr	54	29 (53.7)	27 (50)	2 (3.7)
	SK	100,000 IU/hr	24 hr	54	17 (31.5)	12 (22.2)	5 (9.2)
Verstraete et al.[28]	t-PA	0.75 mg/kg	1 hr	60	15 (25)	15 (25)	0 (0)
	SK	1,500,000 IU	1.5 hr	60	29 (48.3)	29 (48.3)	0 (0)
TIMI Trial[29]	t-PA	80 mg	3 hr	114	56 (49)	49 (43)	7 (6)
	SK	1,500,000 IU	3 hr	112	64 (57)	53 (47)	11 (10)

UK, urokinase; SK, streptokinase; t-PA, tissue-type plasminogen activator.

Perhaps of greater concern to the vascular surgeon are the hemorrhagic complication rates associated with intra-arterial thrombolytic therapy. In our experience bleeding has occurred in 19% to 55% of cases with SK and 0% to 25% of cases with UK.[1,2] As shown in Table 34-1, similar results have been reported by others. The increased hemorrhagic complication rate with SK is consistent with the observation that SK has a more profound effect on the systemic coagulation system than UK.[1,10] In a review of studies comparing results with SK vs. those with UK, decreases in systemic fibrinogen to less than 100 mg/dl occurred in approximately 70% of patients receiving SK and 13% of patients receiving UK.[30]

Tissue plasminogen activator is theoretically activated only at the surface of thrombus. Despite these theoretical "clot-specific" properties, significant bleeding complications have occurred with t-PA. In a series of 22 patients who received intra-arterial t-PA for thrombosed arterial bypass grafts, bleeding and/or hematomas developed at the catheter entry site that did not require transfusion or cessation of therapy in eight patients (36%). One additional patient suffered anastomotic hemorrhage, requiring surgical evacuation and transfusion.[6] In a small (n = 32) randomized comparison of results with intra-arterial t-PA to results with UK, there were major bleeding complications in 31% of t-PA infusions vs. 13% of UK infusions.[7] Interestingly, in this study systemic fibrinogen levels during infusion were decreased more significantly with t-PA than UK. Despite the theoretical clot specificity of t-PA, infusions of this agent have been found to decrease fibrinogen levels and to induce systemic lysis. More experience with t-PA and other clot-specific agents such as pro-urokinase and anisoylated plasminogen-streptokinase activator complex (APSAC) is necessary to determine their ultimate roles in thrombolytic therapy.

Management

Since the majority of bleeding complications of thrombolytic therapy are local phenomena at venipuncture sites or around indwelling catheters, most can be managed with local compres-

sion. We have seldom found it necessary to transfuse or curtail therapy for this type of hemorrhage.

When a patient receiving thrombolytic therapy suffers a major bleeding episode (e.g. retroperitoneal or GI hemorrhage) that results in a falling hematocrit value and hemodynamic instability, emergent intervention is required. Immediate cessation of thrombolytic therapy followed by volume resuscitation with infusion of crystalloid and packed red blood cells should be undertaken. Systemic clotting factors should be replaced with fresh frozen plasma, and fibrinogen should be repleted with cryoprecipitate. When there is life-threatening hemorrhage, the plasmin inhibitor, $\in$-aminocaproic acid (EACA), may be infused to arrest fibrinolysis. However, the half-life of UK is only 12 minutes, and the supportive measures described above are almost always adequate to maintain the patient through the active fibrinolytic phase. In our experience EACA infusion has never been necessary and we believe it is seldom, if ever, indicated. Concomitant heparinization to prevent pericatheter thrombosis is a standard part of most intra-arterial thrombolysis protocols. Cessation of heparin and, if necessary, reversal with protamine should be instituted when bleeding is severe.

Prevention

The absolute and relative contraindications to systemic lytic therapy are reviewed in the box on p. 438. We have safely employed local intra-arterial therapy with many of these relative contraindications. Certain safety guidelines and important technical aspects are fundamental in the application of intra-arterial thrombolytic therapy. Patients should be carefully selected to include only those who are cooperative and who are able to endure the prolonged bed rest (24 to 36 hours) with minimal movement. The importance of this bed rest should not be underestimated, as the most frequent patient complaint during intra-arterial thrombolytic therapy is severe back pain from absolute bed rest in the supine position. The practice of minimizing invasive procedures and needle punctures should be adopted. When thrombolytic therapy is anticipated, we prefer, when

---

CONTRAINDICATIONS TO SYSTEMIC THROMBOLYTIC THERAPY

Absolute
   Active bleeding source
   CVA within 2 months or other intracranial
      process
Relative (major)
   Recent major surgery or organ biopsy (within 2
      weeks); postpartum status (within 10 days of
      delivery)
   Recent GI bleeding
   Recent trauma
   Severe hypertension (>200 mm Hg systolic)
Relative (minor)
   Recent minor trauma (including CPR)
   Left heart thrombus
   Bacterial endocarditis
   Coagulation deficits
   Pregnancy
   Hemorrhagic retinopathy
   Active peptic ulcer disease
   Recent SK infusion (SK only)
   Previous allergic reaction to SK (SK only)

CVA, cerebrovascular accident; SK, streptokinase.

---

technically feasible, to puncture and cannulate through the contralateral groin to minimize bleeding around the catheter insertion site. We have adopted the infusion protocol of McNamara and Fischer,[5] which involves direct intra-thrombus administration of UK at 4000 IU/min for 2 to 4 hours to establish antegrade flow through the thrombus. The dose is then decreased to 1000 IU/hr and repeat angiography is performed at 8- to 12-hour intervals until clot lysis is complete. Patients receive concomitant heparinization through an intra-arterial coaxial catheter. Heparinization does not seem to increase bleeding complications appreciably and is essential to prevent pericatheter thrombosis. Patients are monitored in an ICU for vascular status, bleeding, and other complications during intra-arterial therapy. Serial hematocrit values as well as coagulation parameters are evaluated every 8 to 12 hours. Although prolongation of coagulation values does not correlate with efficacy, depletion of systemic fibrinogen below 100 mg/dl does correlate with

the occurrence of bleeding complications. Naturally, the risk of bleeding complications increases as the duration of thrombolytic therapy increases. We therefore generally stop therapy when thrombolysis fails to progress over a 12-hour period between angiograms.

ALLERGIC REACTIONS

SK is a foreign protein derived from β-hemolytic streptococci. As a result, hypersensitivity reactions caused by acquired antistreptococcal antibodies develop in 12% of patients receiving SK.[31,32] These reactions may be either immediate (IgE-mediated) or delayed (IgG-mediated) and usually consist of a fever, rash, musculoskeletal pain, headache, nausea, pruritis, mild hypotension, or frank anaphylaxis (2%). These reactions have been severe enough to limit the therapeutic course in approximately 3% of cases.[18] In addition to hypersensitivity reactions, antibodies to SK may decrease the drug's efficacy by directly binding to and deactivating the SK molecule. van Breda et al.[4] measured SK antibody titers in patients receiving intra-arterial SK. Patients with high titers had only a 22% clot lysis, whereas those with normal titers had a much better response. The levels of antistreptococcal antibodies tend to rise after a week of therapy and remain elevated for 4 to 6 months. Reinfusion of SK within 6 months of a prior infusion is therefore relatively contraindicated.

Other second- and third-generation fibrinolytic agents that are based on SK such as APSAC are associated with allergic reactions in approximately 2% of cases.[33] Research is currently being focused on attempts to bind fibrinolytic agents to antifibrin antibodies in order to improve their clot specificity. Since these antifibrin antibodies are not derived from humans, similar reactions to these agents can be anticipated.

Unlike SK, UK and t-PA are human proteins derived from tissue culture and recombinant technology, respectively. As such, allergic reactions to these agents rarely if ever occur. Nonetheless, adverse reactions may arise. For example, nausea, vomiting, and other nonspecific problems have occurred in up to 40% of patients receiving t-PA.[34]

COMPLICATIONS OF INTRA-ARTERIAL THROMBOLYTIC THERAPY

There are numerous complications that may develop during intra-arterial thrombolytic therapy as a result of its invasive character. Accordingly, there are several absolute and relative contraindications that apply specifically to intra-arterial therapy (see box). Patients with profound ischemia characterized by pallor, paresis, and decreased sensation are unable to tolerate the time necessary for a course of thrombolytic therapy and are best treated with emergent surgical intervention. Although intra-arterial UK has been demonstrated to increase the salvage of acutely ischemic skeletal muscle in an experimental model, thrombolytic therapy in the setting of acute ischemia introduces certain potential complications.[35] Myonephropathic syndrome (acidosis, hyperkalemia, and myoglobinuria), compartment syndrome, and hemorrhagic necrosis may result when profoundly ischemic tissue is reperfused after thrombolysis.

Occasional complications of arteriography and arterial cannulation such as arterial wall injury, mural dissection, or thrombosis must be anticipated. Similarly, allergic reactions and renal injury may occur with the repetitive contrast loads that are essential during the course of intra-arterial thrombolytic therapy. We attempt to minimize contrast loads by employing digital subtraction arteriography and by doing only limited follow-up studies during the fibrinolytic infusion. These studies are generally conducted directly through the infusion catheter.

As intra-arterial thrombus is lysed and blood flow is restored through the vessel, embolization of clot into the distal vasculature may occur. In our experience the incidence of distal embolization has varied from 16% to 65%.[1,2] We have characterized the resulting clinical picture as "the storm before the calm" since these patients usually suffer an acute worsening of their ischemic symptoms that almost always resolves with continued thrombolytic infusion. Thus, when the patient suffers a sudden clinical deterioration and distal embolization has occurred, the reflex to discontinue therapy should

---

CONTRAINDICATIONS TO INTRA-ARTERIAL THROMBOLYTIC THERAPY

Absolute
    Severe ischemia with neurologic changes
    Devitalized limb with irreversible ischemic damage
Relative
    Thrombosis of new Dacron graft
    Acute postoperative graft failure (<30 days)

---

be resisted. Arteriography may be useful in documenting the presence and significance of distal emboli. Thrombolytic infusion at the aortic level may result in significant embolization both distally and into the visceral vessels.[36]

The direct instillation of thrombolytic agent into distal arterial thrombus requires the presence of long intra-arterial infusion catheters. Pericatheter thrombosis remains a significant clinical problem when the patient does not receive concomitant heparinization. This may lead to increased ischemia, distal embolization, retained thrombus, or total vessel occlusion. In our early experience before heparin administration was used, pericatheter thrombus occurred in 36% of cases, but that incidence has decreased to less than 5% since the practice of routinely administering heparin was instituted.[1] We infuse heparin as necessary to maintain the partial thromboplastin time at 75 seconds or more during intra-arterial thrombolytic infusion. Similar positive experiences with heparin have been noted by others.[5] When significant pericatheter thrombosis does occur, it can usually be managed by pulling back the infusion catheter proximal to the thrombus and continuing the infusion.

CONCLUSION

Thrombolytic therapy is an important tool for the vascular surgeon and interventional radiologist. In some cases it may play an essential diagnostic or therapeutic role in contributing to limb salvage. In other instances it may represent only an expensive temporizing measure that places the patient at excessive risk. Effective and safe application of thrombolytic therapy requires experience and a realistic understanding of the risks and potential benefits of therapy.

REFERENCES

1. Belkin M, Belkin B, Bucknam CA, Straub JJ, Lowe R. Intra-arterial fibrinolytic therapy. Arch Surg 121:769-773, 1986.
2. O'Donnell TF, Coleman JC, Sentissi J, et al. Comparison of direct intra-arterial streptokinase to urokinase infusion in the management of failed infrainguinal ePTFE grafts. In Veith FJ, ed. Current Critical Problems in Vascular Surgery, vol. 1. St. Louis: Quality Medical Publishing, 1989.
3. Gardiner GA, Koltun W, Kandarpa K, et al. Thrombolysis of occluded femoropopliteal grafts. AJR 147:621-626, 1986.
4. van Breda A, Katzen BT, Deutsch AS. Urokinase versus streptokinase in local thrombolysis. Radiology 165:109-111, 1987.
5. McNamara TO, Fischer JR. Thrombolysis of peripheral arterial and graft occlusions: Improved results using high-dose urokinase. AJR 144:769-775, 1985.
6. Graor RA, Risius B, Young YR, et al. Thrombolysis of peripheral arterial bypass grafts: Surgical thrombectomy compared with thrombolysis. J Vasc Surg 7:347-355, 1988.
7. Meyerovitz MF, Goldhaber SZ, Reagan K, et al. Recombinant tissue-type plasminogen activator versus urokinase in peripheral arterial and graft occlusions: A randomized trial. Radiology 175:75-78, 1990.
8. Belkin M, Donaldson MC, Whittemore AD, et al. Observations on the use of thrombolytic agents for thrombotic occlusion of infrainguinal vein grafts. J Vasc Surg 11:289-294, 1990.
9. The Urokinase Pulmonary Embolism Trial: A national cooperative study. Circulation 47 (Suppl II):1-108, 1973.
10. Urokinase-Streptokinase Pulmonary Embolism Trial—Phase 2 results. JAMA 229:1606-1613, 1974.
11. Sharma GVRK, Burleson VA, Sasahara AA. Effect of thrombolytic therapy on pulmonary-capillary blood volume in patients with pulmonary embolism. N Engl J Med 303:842-845, 1980.
12. Goldhaber SZ, Vaughan DE, Markis JE, et al. Acute pulmonary embolism treated with tissue plasminogen activator. Lancet 2:886-888, 1986.
13. Goldhaber SZ, Heit J, Sharma GVRK, et al. Randomised controlled trial of recombinant tissue plasminogen activator versus urokinase in the treatment of acute pulmonary embolism. Lancet 2:293-298, 1988.
14. Goldhaber SZ, Buring JE, Lipnick RJ, et al. Pooled analysis of randomized trials of streptokinase and heparin in phlebographically documented acute deep venous thrombosis. Am J Med 76:393, 1984.
15. Arnesen H, Hoseth A. Streptokinase or heparin in the treatment of deep venous thrombosis: Follow-up results of a prospective study. Acta Med Scand 211:65-68, 1982.
16. Elliott MS, Immelman EJ, Jeffery S, et al. A comparative randomized trial of heparin versus streptokinase in the treatment of acute proximal venous thrombosis: An interim report of a prospective trial. Br J Surg 66:838-843, 1979.
17. Kakkar VV, Flanc C, Howe CT, et al. Treatment of deep vein thrombosis. A trial of heparin, streptokinase, and Arvin. Br Med J 1:806-810, 1969.
18. Thayer CF. Results of postmarking surveillance program on streptokinase. Curr Ther Res 30:129-140, 1981.
19. Graor RA, Young JR, Risius B, et al. Comparison of cost-effectiveness of streptokinase and urokinase in the treatment of deep vein thrombosis. Ann Vasc Surg 1:524-528, 1987.
20. van de Loo JCW, Kriessmann A, Trubestein G, et al. Controlled multicenter pilot study of urokinase-heparin and streptokinase in deep venous thrombosis. Thromb Haemost 50:660-663, 1983.
21. Zimmermann R, Epping J, Rasche H, et al. Urokinase and streptokinase treatment of deep vein thrombosis. Results of a randomized study. Haemostasis 16:9, 1986.
22. Hargrove WC, Barber CF, Berkowitz HD, et al. Treatment of acute peripheral arterial and graft thromboses with low-dose streptokinase. Surgery 92:6, 1982.
23. Rabe FE, Becker GJ, Richmond BD, et al. Contrast extravasation through Dacron grafts: A sequelae of low-dose streptokinase therapy. AJR 138:917, 1982.
24. Fessinger JN, Vayssiairat M, Juillet Y, et al. Local urokinase in arterial thromboembolism. Angiology 31:715, 1980.
25. Sicard GA, Schier JJ, Totty WG, et al. Thrombolytic therapy for acute arterial occlusion. J Vasc Surg 2:65, 1985.
26. Berni GA, Bandyk DF, Zierler RE, et al. Streptokinase treatment of acute arterial occlusion. Ann Surg 198:2, 1983.
27. van Breda A, Robinson JC, Feldman L, et al. Local thrombolysis in the treatment of arterial graft occlusions. J Vasc Surg 1:103, 1984.
28. Verstraete M, Bernard R, Borey M, et al. Randomised trial of intravenous recombinant tissue-type plasminogen activator versus intravenous streptokinase in acute myocardial infarction. Lancet 1:842-847, 1985.
29. The Thrombolysis in Myocardial Infarction (TIMI) Trial—Phase one findings. N Engl J Med 321:932-936, 1985.
30. Bell WR, Sasahara AA. Adverse Events in Review of Thrombolytic Therapy and Thromboembolic Disease. Glenview, Ill.: Physicians and Scientists Publishing, 1989.

31. Nazari J, Davison R, Kaplan K, et al. Adverse reactions to thrombolytic agents—Implications for coronary reperfusion following myocardial infarction. Med Toxicol 2:247-286, 1987.

32. Rutkowski DM, Burkle WS. Advances in thrombolytic therapy. Drug Intell Clin Pharmacol 16:115-121, 1982.

33. Anderson JL. Development and evaluation of anisoylated plasminogen streptokinase activated complex (APSAC). A second generation thrombolytic agent. J Am Coll Cardiol 10:22B-27B, 1987.

34. Sobel BE. Safety and efficacy of tissue-type plasminogen activator produced by recombinant DNA technology. J Am Coll Cardiol 10(Suppl B):40B-44B, 1987.

35. Belkin M, Valeri R, Hobson RW. Intra-arterial urokinase increases skeletal muscle viability after acute ischemia. J Vasc Surg 9:161-168, 1989.

36. Wood WA, Tisnado J, Cho SR. Visceral embolization during low dose fibrinolysis of aortic graft occlusion. AJR 141:1055, 1983.

35

Stroke as a Complication of Noncerebrovascular Surgery

Gregory L. Moneta   **Robert DeFrang**   **John M. Porter**

Although improvements in perioperative care are resulting in the generally safe performance of increasing numbers of complex operations in elderly, high-risk patients, serious complications continue to occur in this group. With the exception of death, stroke is doubtless the most feared postoperative complication. Although it occurs infrequently, postoperative stroke following noncerebrovascular surgery is associated with devastating disability and very high mortality.[1] All surgeons who operate on elderly, high-risk patients must understand the risk factors for stroke, the incidence of postoperative stroke associated with various procedures, and variables that may be modified to reduce the risk of perioperative stroke.

ETIOLOGY

The etiology of strokes is diverse but the large majority share the common feature of being related to a vascular event of some type. Presently it is estimated that a vascular event is the cause of more than 90% of acute neurologic deficits.[2] Although the frequency of various vascular-related neurologic deficits varies from report to report, overall the underlying cause is subarachnoid hemorrhage in about 8% of cases, intracerebral hemorrhage in 12%, and central thromboembolism in 70%; the remaining 10% result from cerebral hypoperfusion, venous thrombosis, arteritis, and other uncommon causes.[2] Less than one half of thromboembolic events appear to originate from the extracranial cerebrovascular system and thus may be amenable to potential preoperative surgical correction.[2-4]

DEMOGRAPHICS

Throughout the 1970s and early 1980s, a clear decrease in stroke mortality occurred in the United States, Canada, and western Europe. This decrease extended to both sexes and all age groups. Interestingly, over the same period stroke mortality actually increased in eastern European countries.[5] Although the decline in stroke mortality rates in the United

443

States is encouraging and we now have the lowest rates in the industrialized world, recent evidence suggests that the fall in stroke rates has stabilized and may even be rising once again.[6] Stroke is currently the third leading cause of death in the United States.[7] Approximately 1% of persons between 65 and 75 years of age die of stroke annually. The overall annual stroke mortality for all Americans more than 65 years of age is 2.3%, clearly indicating a greater prevalence in the elderly population. Recent data suggest that about half of all strokes occur in persons more than 75 years of age.[6,8,9]

Worldwide, stroke mortality remains consistently higher in men than women. The age-standardized stroke mortality rate/100,000 population in 1985 for U.S. men was 45.4 compared with 35.1 for U.S. women.[5] In addition to mortality, stroke remains a major source of disability. Stroke accounts for one half of all patients hospitalized for neurologic disease. At any time there are an estimated 2 million stroke survivors in the United States, many of whom have moderate-to-severe permanent neurologic deficits.[10]

RISK FACTORS

In 1984, the Subcommittee on Risk Factors and Stroke of the Stroke Council of the American Heart Association published a special report entitled, "Risk Factors in Stroke." A large number of variables were evaluated for their potential impact on stroke incidence (see box).[11] From this and other reports, hypertension, cardiac disease, and diabetes have been identified consistently as the primary medical risk factors for stroke; hypertension appears to be the most important. The risk of stroke seems to be related directly to the magnitude of blood pressure elevation.[12,13] Women do not appear to tolerate hypertension any better than men and there is no diminution of the ill effects of hypertension with advancing age.[14] Preliminary evidence suggests that isolated systolic hypertension in the elderly may engender less risk of stroke than sustained diastolic hypertension.[15]

Various forms of cardiac dysfunction (coronary artery disease, congestive failure, left ventricular hypertrophy, and dysrhythmias, especially atrial fibrillation) have a definite effect on stroke rate that appears independent of hypertension. Cardiac patients have two to five times the risk of stroke compared to age- and blood pressure–matched controls.[16,17] Diabetes mellitus is also an important risk factor for stroke. Stroke risk associated with diabetes does not diminish with age and actually appears to be greater for women than men. The risk of stroke in diabetic patients is associated strongly with hypertension.[11] These two risk factors are difficult to separate and probably are at least partially mediated through joint effects on the development of atherosclerosis of the cerebrovascular system.

The independent effects of elevated serum lipids and cigarette smoking on the single end-point of stroke are unclear. The effects of these variables appear significantly mediated through their influence on the development of atherosclerosis.[18] The amount and duration of cigarette smoking are the best correlates with extracranial cerebrovascular atherosclerosis. Interestingly, in the Framingham study smoking was identified as an independent risk factor for cerebral thromboembolic disease only in men below age 65.[19] Data from the Framing-

---

POTENTIAL STROKE RISK FACTORS*

Advanced age
Male sex
Race
Diabetes mellitus
Previous stroke
Carotid stenosis/ulceration
Transient ischemic attacks
Carotid bruit
Hypertension
Cardiac disease
Elevated hematocrit
Sickle cell anemia
Elevated blood cholesterol and lipids
Cigarette smoking
Oral contraceptives
Alcohol consumption
Family history of stroke

---

*Modified from Dyken ML, Wolf PA, Barnett HJ, et al. Risk factors in stroke. Stroke 15:1105-1111, 1984.

ham study, however, identified a combination of risk factors that purport to predict the 10% of the general population who will have at least one third of all strokes. The patients at especially high risk include those with all the following risk factors: elevated systolic blood pressure, elevated cholesterol, glucose intolerance, ECG-documented left ventricular hypertrophy, and cigarette smoking.[11,16]

Carotid Artery Disease
Asymptomatic Disease

The overall prevalence of significant extracranial carotid artery disease in unselected patients is very low. Less than 1% to 2% of persons under 60 years of age without significant atherosclerotic risk factors will have >50% internal carotid artery stenosis.[20] However, patients with advanced age, tobacco abuse, hypertension, diabetes, or demonstrable peripheral vascular disease have a much higher incidence of asymptomatic significant carotid artery stenosis[21] (see below).

Asymptomatic carotid ulceration has been implicated as a risk factor for stroke, especially in patients with large carotid atherosclerotic ulcerations. The evidence that carotid ulceration alone is a significant risk factor for stroke is not firmly established. Some studies have reported significant neurologic risks with such lesions[22]; others have not found them dangerous.[23] In addition, many strokes associated with asymptomatic ulcers have occurred many years after the diagnosis of carotid ulceration.[21] Whether the carotid ulceration was still present at the time of the eventual stroke is unknown in many cases.

The development and widespread application of noninvasive cerebrovascular testing have made possible serial quantitation of carotid stenosis in patients with cerebrovascular disease. There is now little doubt that as a group patients with asymptomatic carotid atherosclerosis have a low overall stroke incidence—in the range of 2% to 4%/year.[19,24] However, numerous studies have consistently shown an increased risk of stroke in patients with high-grade (>80%) asymptomatic internal carotid artery stenosis (Table 35-1). Presently no other anatomic risk factor has been implicat-

ed reliably as a short-term predictor of neurologic events in patients with asymptomatic carotid disease.

A number of older studies suggested that patients with asymptomatic carotid bruit were at an increased risk of stroke.[30,31] The major population-based studies from Framingham, Massachusetts,[19] and Evans County, Georgia,[24] have established clearly that asymptomatic cervical bruit, although a marker of neurologic risk, does not accurately predict the distribution or cause of subsequent neurologic events. Many of the patients who suffered strokes in these studies experienced the neurologic event in the vertebrobasilar distribution or the cerebral hemisphere opposite the carotid bruit, or they experienced a stroke secondary to cardiac embolism or subarachnoid or intracerebral hemorrhage. In addition to predicting neurologic events, the appearance of neck bruits appears to increase the risk of death from myocardial infarction at least two times.[23]

Transient Ischemic Attacks

Transient ischemic attacks (TIAs) are a prominent risk factor for stroke[11] but it is important to note that patients with TIAs have significantly more hypertension, cardiac disease, and diabetes than age-matched controls. Although TIAs may be associated with carotid artery disease, the importance of this association with respect to the occurrence of stroke must be viewed within the perspective that only about 10% of all strokes are preceded by a recognized TIA.[32] It is important to note that a significant percentage of TIAs occur in the complete absence of extracranial carotid artery

Table 35-1. Annual Stroke Risks in Patients With >80% Asymptomatic Internal Carotid Artery Stenoses

Author	Stroke risk (%)
Chambers and Norris[25] (1986)	5.5
Bogousslavsky et al.[26] (1986)	4.2
Hennerici et al.[27] (1987)	8.1
Moneta et al.[28] (1987)	12; 4*
Caracci et al.[29] (1989)	9

*Twelve percent, first year; 4%, second year.

disease. The best current information suggests that the risk of stroke associated with TIAs is highest in the first year after the TIA. Overall, about 10% of TIA patients will have a carotid distribution stroke within 1 year after an untreated TIA. The rate of stroke then decreases to give a cumulative risk of about 30% at 5 years.[33] Patients with multiple or crescendo TIAs appear to be at a considerably higher short-term risk.[34,35]

Previous Stroke

One of the few conclusions of stroke-related research in which there appears to be consensus is that patients with prior strokes are at much higher risk for a new cerebral infarction than patients without prior strokes.[11] The incidence of new strokes in patients with prior known cerebral infarction is about 10% per year.[36,37]

STROKE IN NONCEREBROVASCULAR SURGERY

The incidence and mechanism of stroke in patients undergoing noncerebrovascular surgery vary with the primary operative procedure.

Cardiac Surgery

If searched for assiduously, some type of neurologic complication can be found in up to 40% of cardiac surgery patients.[38] A large majority of these complications are short-term episodes of temporary and minor cognitive and psychiatric dysfunction. Less than 5% of the neurologic complications consist of a central, focal neurologic deficit (Table 35-2). The risk of stroke associated with cardiac surgery clearly increases with patient age and reaches the disturbing incidence of 8% to 10% in patients 70 years of age and older.[41,86,87] The overall risk of perioperative stroke with valve replacement is two to three times greater than the risk with coronary artery bypass (Table 35-2). An estimated 70% of strokes associated with cardiac surgery occur intraoperatively; the remaining 30% develop more than 24 hours postoperatively.[42,43,88] Intraoperative events are attributed most frequently to technical problems with aortic clamping or cannulation, inadequate venting of the heart of air and debris at the completion of the reconstruction, and occasionally hypoperfusion associated with cardiac bypass.

The role of extracranial cerebrovascular disease in the etiology of stroke associated with cardiac surgery is unclear. A careful review of the literature by Hart and Easton[89] concluded that there was no consistent evidence that cervical bruit alone was a marker for perioperative stroke in cardiac surgery patients. However, a more recent review by Reed et al.[43] from the Massachusetts General Hospital suggests that the presence of a cervical bruit increases the risk of stroke or TIA 3.9 times in coronary artery bypass patients although many of the strokes do not occur ipsilateral to the bruit.

Detectable carotid stenosis coexists with

Table 35-2. Incidence of Perioperative Strokes Following Noncerebrovascular Surgery

Procedure	References	No. of patients	Stroke (%)
Cardiac valve replacement	39,40	1,343	4.1
Coronary artery bypass only	39, 41-48	41,769	1.5
Infrarenal aortic aneurysm (nonrupture)	49-57	2,210	0.7
Infrarenal aortic aneurysm (ruptured)	50, 52, 55, 58-60	437	1.3
Aortofemoral graft (occlusive disease)	1, 49, 55, 57, 61	2,464	0.8
Infrainguinal graft	62-75	2,246	0.5
Thoracoabdominal aortic aneurysm (excludes aortic arch repairs)	76, 77	706	1.8
Other*	78-85	26,336	0.06

*Includes general surgical and subspecialty procedures (orthopedic, urology).

significant coronary artery disease in an estimated 15% of coronary disease patients. However, in the absence of neurologic symptoms, only about half of these patients have a >50% carotid stenosis.[90,91] Overall about 10% of cardiac surgery patients have a cervical bruit, but less than one third of the bruits are associated with a >50% stenosis of the internal carotid artery.[44,92]

Turnipseed, Berkoff, and Belzer[93] reported 16 neurologic complications following 170 cardiac surgical procedures. Eight percent of the 170 patients had a >50% carotid stenosis. Thirteen of the 16 neurologic complications occurred in patients with <50% carotid stenosis. Breslau et al.[94] reported two strokes in 102 cardiac procedures. Neither patient had a significant carotid lesion. Barnes et al.[44] prospectively performed noninvasive carotid studies in 449 patients undergoing cardiac or peripheral vascular surgery. As assessed by continuous-wave Doppler examination, 15% of the cardiac patients had a >75% internal carotid artery stenosis. There were six perioperative strokes in the 324 patients undergoing coronary surgery, only one of which occurred ipsilateral to a high-grade carotid stenosis. Other authors also have failed to demonstrate in cardiac surgery patients an increased risk of stroke ipsilateral to a >50% internal carotid artery lesion.[95]

On the other hand, Brener, Brief, and Alpert[39] found the incidence of TIA or stroke following cardiac surgery to be 1.9% in patients without carotid disease and 9.2% in those with a >50% internal carotid stenosis. It is not clear, however, whether all strokes occurred ipsilateral to the index carotid lesion. Interestingly, Kartchner and McRae[96] reported seven strokes in 41 cardiac surgery patients with positive findings on oculoplethysmographic (OPG) examinations, indicative of carotid stenosis. In 192 patients with negative findings on OPG examination or a carotid endarterectomy before cardiac surgery, stroke occurred in only two patients (1%). The study is difficult to interpret in that selection criteria for patients undergoing carotid endarterectomy are not stated, there is no documentation of the distribution of perioperative strokes with respect to the carotid lesions, and many patients in the study were symptomatic with a history of prior stroke or TIAs.

Thus there is no convincing evidence that asymptomatic extracranial carotid artery disease is a primary cause of perioperative stroke in the cardiac surgery patient. Clearly, many cardiac surgery patients have carotid atherosclerosis and it appears reasonable to evaluate these patients for significant carotid stenosis with noninvasive testing before their cardiac operation. Significant lesions should be surgically treated for the same indications as carotid lesions in other patients: >80% asymptomatic internal carotid stenoses or lesser disease if associated with TIAs. There is no evidence that prior carotid endarterectomy significantly reduces the overall perioperative stroke incidence in cardiac surgery patients.

Noncerebrovascular Vascular Surgery

Noncerebrovascular peripheral vascular surgery patients have a high incidence of extracranial cerebrovascular disease. About 20% of vascular surgery patients have a cervical bruit.[89] Using continuous-wave Doppler examinations, Hennerici et al.[21] found a 32.8% incidence of asymptomatic vertebral or carotid artery disease (>50% stenosis) in 325 patients undergoing peripheral vascular surgery. In 264 patients with severe coronary artery disease documented by angiography, these same investigators found similar carotid disease in only 6.8%. Barnes and Marszalek[90] detected >50% carotid stenosis in 17.2% of 116 patients undergoing peripheral vascular reconstruction and in 10.6% of 198 patients undergoing coronary bypass. Many vascular surgery patients are hypertensive, have suffered previous strokes, or have significant cardiac dysfunction—all of which are risk factors for stroke independent of carotid artery disease (see previous discussion).

Despite the extraordinary prevalence of extracranial vascular disease and associated risk factors for stroke in peripheral vascular surgery patients, the overall incidence of perioperative stroke in noncerebrovascular vascular surgery patients is surprisingly low and shows little variation among procedures. Perioperative neurologic deficits occur in less than 1% of peripheral vascular surgery patients as shown in Table 35-2. This information must be viewed from the perspective that cases summarized in Table 35-2 were not stratified for various medical risk factors for stroke and the frequency of prior carotid endarterectomy is unknown in these patients as is the severity of any associated carotid stenosis.

General Surgery

Perioperative stroke is also an infrequent complication of general and subspeciality surgical procedures. Landercasper et al.[78] recently reported an absence of strokes in 7517 consecutive patients without a prior history of stroke who underwent nonneurosurgical, noncardiac, and noncerebrovascular procedures while under general anesthesia. A very low perioperative stroke incidence also has been documented in general surgery patients in other reports (Table 35-2).

Although the overall risk of perioperative stroke in noncardiac, noncerebrovascular surgery populations appears to be between 0.3% and 0.7%, the subgroup of patients with a prior history of neurologic events appears to be at greatest risk. Of 8984 surgical patients reviewed by Knapp, Topkins, and Artusio,[79] 69 had a history of prior stroke and a new perioperative stroke developed in 1.5% of these patients. In a Danish study 6 of 279 operative patients (2.1%) with a prior cerebrovascular event suffered a postoperative stroke.[80] Finally, the study of Landercasper et al.[78] documented a 2.9% incidence of postoperative stroke in 173 consecutive general and noncerebrovascular surgery patients with a prior history of stroke. These authors estimated that the expected number of strokes in 173 similar patients observed for 15 days without surgery would be only 0.01 ± 0.5 (0.006%).

ETIOLOGY OF PERIOPERATIVE STROKE

The events leading to a perioperative stroke are not known with certainty. Acute hypotension in the setting of chronic hypertension has been implicated as a cause of stroke.[97] A patient who undergoes a difficult procedure associated with significant intraoperative blood loss and hypotension, followed by a postoperative neurologic deficit, will generally have the stroke ascribed to intraoperative hypotension. However, such patients are unusual. Severe alteration in blood pressure in direct proximity to stroke occurrence is an infrequent finding in perioperative cerebral infarction. Reviews of patients with perioperative cerebral infarction following aortoiliac procedures indicate neurologic events almost always occur after a variable lucid interval, not intraoperatively.[1,44,98] Hart and Hindman[99] reviewed the clinical features of 12 consecutive general surgery patients with perioperative stroke and found that although intraoperative hypotension was frequent, the onset of the neurologic deficit was intraoperative in only 17% of the cases; the deficit clearly occurred postoperatively in 83%. Larsen, Zaric, and Boyson[80] also found that all 6 of 2463 patients who suffered a perioperative stroke after noncardiac, noncerebrovascular surgery did so late in the postoperative period—between 5 and 26 days after surgery. The observation that intraoperative hypotension is not associated frequently with perioperative stroke is hardly surprising. Many hypotensive episodes occur in association with the use of anesthetic agents that may have cerebral protective effects. Furthermore, most cases of intraoperative hypotension are transient and may be hemodynamically insignificant.

The finding that most strokes following general and noncerebrovascular vascular surgery occur postoperatively contrasts with the primary intraoperative onset of perioperative stroke following cardiac surgery (see previous discussion). As noted, strokes following cardiac surgery appear related largely to intraoperative events; cerebral infarction following general and noncerebrovascular surgery must in most cases have other causes. Kelly and Kovacs[97] studied 26 patients in whom cerebral ischemia developed while the patients were hospitalized for an unrelated problem. Of the 14 patients who had invasive therapeutic or diagnostic procedures and a neurologic event not directly related to the procedure, one third were found to have a cerebral embolus from a cardiac source. Hart and Hindman[99] identified cardiogenic embolization as the underlying mechanism of stroke in 42% of their noncardiac, noncerebrovascular perioperative stroke patients. Eight of the 12 patients in their series of perioperative strokes had either atrial fibrillation, perioperative myocardial infarction, or known valvular vegetations.

The role, if any, of a perioperative hypercoagulable state in the occurrence of perioperative cerebral infarction is unknown. Recent evidence suggests that perioperative alterations in blood rheology and transient postoperative hypercoagulable states may contribute to the risk of postoperative stroke. Such speculation is consistent with the observation that perioperative strokes are nearly always thrombotic or embolic in origin. Blood rheology appears chronically altered in patients with previous strokes, TIAs, or significant risk factors for cerebrovascular disease.[100,101] Whole blood and plasma viscosities are elevated significantly in such patients as compared with normal controls. The effect appears to be independent of hematocrit level and primarily associated with elevated plasma fibrinogen and a decreased albumin/globulin ratio.

The postoperative state is associated with a number of alterations in the coagulation system. McDaniel et al.[102] found that in femorotibial bypass patients, increased platelet reactivity, increased factor VIII–related antigen levels, and decreased antithrombin III levels developed postoperatively. Other investigators have demonstrated increases in platelet count, factor VIII levels, and fibrinogen, together with decreased antithrombin III levels in patients following intra-abdominal aortic reconstruction.[103] In addition, plasma fibrinolysis appears relatively inhibited in the postoperative state.[104] Diabetic patients, who generally comprise between 30% and 50% of vascular surgery patients and a substantial portion of general surgery patients, frequently manifest baseline elevations of factor VIII, factor X, and fibrinogen, and increased platelet adhesiveness.[105] Specific acquired hypercoagulable conditions such as antiphospholipid antibodies clearly predispose surgical patients to postoperative thrombotic complications and are being recognized with increasing frequency.[106]

One can therefore postulate that there are perioperative increases in blood viscosity and coagulation factor abnormalities following vascular and general surgical procedures, which in certain patients may lead to a postoperative hypercoagulable state that results in a thrombotic or embolic stroke. Although a number of reports have addressed the association of hypercoagulability and early bypass graft failure, to our knowledge no study has specifically addressed the identification of perioperative alterations in blood viscosity or the coagulation system that may predispose surgical patients to stroke.

MINIMIZING PERIOPERATIVE STROKE

Despite the low incidence of perioperative stroke in noncerebrovascular surgery, consideration of the data presented herein suggests certain steps may decrease the risk of perioperative stroke.

Patient Selection

An important factor in reducing the incidence of perioperative stroke is careful patient selection. By the avoidance of all but essential surgery in stroke-prone patients (those patients with advanced age, especially greater than 75 years, history of recent myocardial infarction, previous stroke, atrial fibrillation, and known thrombotic tendencies), the incidence of perioperative stroke clearly can be reduced.

Intraoperative Management

Although many perioperative strokes do not occur intraoperatively, some obviously do. Certainly in cardiac surgery, extreme care must be used in manipulating the ascending and transverse aorta and the heart must be well flushed of air and debris before circulation is restored. Careful attention should be given to maintaining proper mean arterial pressure during cardiac bypass, and pump times should be kept as short as possible.

The noncardiac surgery patient should be maintained intraoperatively in as near normal a physiologic state as possible. Both mean arterial pressure and arterial carbon dioxide should be maintained within the patient's usual range.

Wide variations may alter cerebral autoregulation and increase susceptibility to stroke. Glucose levels should be maintained within normal ranges. Although prevention of hyperglycemia does not protect against stroke, it does appear to help minimize injury should ischemic cerebral infarction occur.[107]

Choice of anesthetic technique and agents may be of importance in high-risk patients. The major volatile anesthetic agents available—halothane, enflurane, and isoflurane—all produce cerebral vasodilatation and decrease cerebral oxygen consumption. Nitrous oxide also produces cerebral vasodilatation. Theoretically, the effects of these agents are cerebral protective but there is some concern that in patients with recent cerebral infarctions, such agents may result in a "steal" of blood from peri-infarction areas, resulting in extension of a previously stable cerebral infarction.[108]

Prophylactic Carotid Endarterectomy

Without question the available medical literature does not support the performance of carotid endarterectomy solely for decreasing the risk of stroke associated with an additional procedure. However, it must be noted that studies considering the association of asymptomatic carotid stenosis with perioperative stroke have not included large numbers of patients with a very high grade of carotid stenosis (>80%). Almost all studies to date have used >50% stenosis as the definition of an asymptomatic "high-grade" lesion. Current data suggest that the >80% asymptomatic lesions have the highest potential to result in a neurologic event during follow-up. Because carotid endarterectomy may be performed quite safely in patients with asymptomatic carotid disease (Table 35-3), it seems reasonable to perform carotid endarterectomy before another opera-

Table 35-3. Selected Series of Carotid Endarterectomies for Asymptomatic Internal Carotid Artery Stenoses

Author	No. of operations	Stroke (%)	Death (%)
Thompson et al.[109] (1978)	167	1.2	0
Burke et al.[110] (1982)	70	1.4	2.8
Hertzer et al.[111] (1986)	116	3.4	0.9
Moneta et al.[28] (1987)	56	1.8	0
Rosenthal et al.[112] (1987)	42	0	0
Caracci et al.[29] (1989)	100	1	1
Towne et al.[113] (1990)	211	2.4	1.9

Table 35-4. Mortality and Stroke in Patients Undergoing Combined Coronary Artery Bypass and Carotid Endarterectomy

Author	No. of patients	Stroke (%)	Death (%)
Bernhard et al.[114] (1972)	16	6.3	0
Okies et al.[115] (1977)	16	12.5	6.3
Craver et al.[116] (1982)	63	1.3	2
Hertzer et al.[117] (1983)	331	9	5.7
Jones et al.[118] (1984)	132	1.5	3
Lord et al.[119] (1985)	42	7.1	4.8
Perler et al.[120] (1985)	37	2.7	8.1
Babu et al.[121] (1985)	62	1.6	2.5
Minami et al.[122] (1988)	47	2.1	2.1
Cambria et al.[123] (1989)	51	2	2

tive procedure under the following circumstances. First, the patient should have either a recently symptomatic carotid lesion or a >80% asymptomatic lesion so that the performance of carotid endarterectomy can be justified on the basis of the carotid disease alone. Second, the patient should be a good operative risk and the operating surgeon should have a record of low stroke and death rates for carotid surgery. Third, the performance of carotid endarterectomy should not place the patient at severely increased risk resulting from the inherent delay in performing the other indicated operative procedure.

Combined Carotid/Coronary Surgery

The role of carotid endarterectomy in conjunction with coronary artery bypass is debated continually. A review of Tables 35-2 and 35-4 suggests that combining carotid endarterectomy with coronary artery bypass results in a moderate increase in perioperative stroke when compared with coronary artery bypass alone. This is hardly surprising since each operation carries an inherent risk of stroke. Clearly, combining the two procedures will neither diminish the risk of stroke associated with carotid endarterectomy nor result in prevention of "noncarotid" causes of stroke associated with coronary bypass surgery.

However, the position that combining the two procedures is never appropriate probably is incorrect. Patients with significant disease of both the coronary and carotid circulations probably have more severe atherosclerosis and therefore are at increased surgical risk regardless of whether the coronary and carotid problems are addressed simultaneously or in a staged fashion. Currently no randomized trial exists comparing staged to simultaneous coronary and carotid operations for all eligible patients within a single institution. Hertzer, Loop, and Beven[91] from the Cleveland Clinic randomized patients with unilateral >70% asymptomatic carotid stenosis requiring urgent coronary artery bypass. In this study, 129 patients were randomized to either combined coronary/carotid surgery or coronary artery

bypass followed by carotid endarterectomy during the same hospitalization or at a later date. The composite incidence of perioperative stroke in the group receiving delayed carotid surgery (14%) was worse than that for the group receiving a combined procedure (2.8%). However, the stroke rate associated with carotid endarterectomy for asymptomatic stenosis in the group with delayed carotid surgery was very high at 7.5%; therefore generalization of these results is difficult. In addition, the perioperative death rate for coronary artery bypass combined with carotid endarterectomy was 4.2% with a stroke rate of 2.8%; the death rate for the patients undergoing coronary artery bypass alone before carotid surgery was 3.4% with a stroke rate of 6.9%. These differences between the two groups were not statistically significant.

Available data therefore suggest that, for the majority of patients, combining coronary artery surgery with carotid endarterectomy will not result in a substantial improvement in the incidence of stroke following coronary artery bypass. No conclusions can be drawn for patients with severe bilateral carotid stenosis or those with symptomatic carotid disease who require urgent coronary revascularization. Combining coronary and carotid surgical procedures under those circumstances may be appropriate in centers with adequate expertise in both procedures.

CONCLUSION

Perioperative stroke following noncerebrovascular surgery is an infrequent problem. Its incidence is about 4% for cardiac valvular surgery, 1% to 2% for coronary artery bypass, and 0.5% to 1% for other surgical procedures. The risk of perioperative stroke is increased in older patients, patients with prior strokes and those with multiple risk factors for stroke. With the exception of cardiac procedures, most perioperative strokes do not occur intraoperatively but rather later in the postoperative period. There does not appear to be a consistent relationship between perioperative stroke and carotid bruit or asymptomatic carotid stenosis, although only a few patients with very high grade carotid stenosis have been studied. Prophylactic carotid endarterectomy in preparation for another procedure should be performed only when the extent of the carotid disease itself is adequate justification for carotid surgery and when the patient is not endangered by delaying the primary procedure.

REFERENCES

1. Carney WI, Stewart WB, DePinto DJ, et al. Carotid bruit as a risk factor in aortoiliac reconstruction. Surgery 81:567-570, 1977.
2. Mohr JP, Caplan LR, Melski JW, et al. The Harvard Cooperative Stroke Registry: A prospective registry. Neurology 28:754-762, 1978.
3. Hass WK, Fields WS, North RR, et al. Joint study of extracranial arterial occlusion. II. Arteriography, techniques, sites and complications. JAMA 203:159-166, 1968.
4. Heyman A, Wilkinson W, Heyden S, et al. Joint study of extracranial arterial occlusion. VI. Rapid differences in hospitalized patients with ischemic stroke. JAMA 222:285-289, 1972.
5. Bonita R, Stewart A, Beaglehole R. International trends in stroke mortality: 1970-1985. Stroke 21:989-992, 1990.
6. Brokerick JP, Phillips SJ, Whisnant JP. Incidence rates of stroke in the eighties: The end of the decline in stroke? Stroke 20:577-582, 1989.
7. Utilization of short stay hospitals: United States, 1981 annual summary. U.S. Department of Health and Human Services: Pub. No. (PHS)83-1733:13, 1983.
8. Gillum RF. Cerebrovascular disease morbidity in the United States, 1970-1983. Stroke 17:656-661, 1986.
9. Kuller LH. Incidence rates of stroke in the eighties: The end of the decline in stroke? Stroke 20:841-843, 1989.
10. Adelman SM. The national survey of stroke. Economic impact. Stroke 12(Suppl I):1-69, 1981.
11. Dyken ML, Wolf PA, Barnett HJ, et al. Risk factors in stroke: A statement for physicians by the Subcommittee on Risk Factors and Stroke of the Stroke Council. Stroke 15:1105-1111, 1984.
12. Kannel WB, Wolf PA, Verter J, et al. Epidemiologic assessment of the role of blood pressure in stroke: The Framingham study. JAMA 214:301-310, 1970.
13. Garraway WM, Whisnant JP. The changing pattern of hypertension and the declining incidence of stroke. JAMA 258:214-217, 1987.
14. Hypertension Detection and Follow-up Program Cooperative Group: Five year finding of the hypertension detection and follow-up program. III. Reduction in stroke incidence among persons with high blood pressure. JAMA 247:633-638, 1982.
15. Perry HM, Smith WM, McDonald RH, et al. Morbidity and mortality in the systolic hypertension in the elderly program (SHEP) pilot study. Stroke 20:4-13, 1989.
16. Wolf PA, Kannel WB, Verter J. Current status of risk factors for stroke. Neurol Clin 1:317-327, 1983.
17. Wolf PA, Dawber TR, Thomas HE Jr. Epidemiologic assessment of chronic atrial fibrillation and risk of stroke: The Framingham study. Neurology 28:973-977, 1978.
18. Whisnant JP, Homer D, Ingall TJ, et al. Duration of cigarette smoking is the strongest predictor of severe extracranial carotid artery atherosclerosis. Stroke 21:707-714, 1990.
19. Wolf PA, Kannel WB, Sorlie P, et al. Asymptomatic carotid bruit and the risk of stroke: The Framingham study. JAMA 245:1442-1445, 1981.
20. Colgan MP, Strode GR, Sommer JD, et al. Prevalence of asymptomatic cartoid disease: Results of duplex scanning in 348 unselected volunteers. J Vasc Surg 8:674-678, 1988.
21. Hennerici M, Aulich A, Sandmann W, et al. Incidence of asymptomatic extracranial arterial disease. Stroke 12:750-757, 1981.
22. Moore WS, Boren C, Malone JM, et al. Natural history of nonstenotic, asymptomatic ulcerative lesions of the carotid artery. Arch Surg 113:1352-1359, 1978.
23. Kroener JM, Dorn PL, Shoor PM, et al. Prognosis of asymptomatic ulcerating carotid lesions. Arch Surg 115:1387-1391, 1980.
24. Heyman A, Wilkinson WE, Heyden S, et al. Risk of stroke in asymptomatic persons with cervical bruits: A population study in Evans County, GA. N Engl J Med 302:838-841, 1980.
25. Chambers BR, Norris JW. Outcome in patients with asymptomatic neck bruits. N Engl J Med 315:860-865, 1986.
26. Bogousslavsky J, Despland P-A, Regli F. Asymptomatic tight stenosis of the internal carotid artery: Long term prognosis. Neurology 36:861-863, 1986.
27. Hennerici M, Hülshömer H-B, Hefter H, et al. Natural history of asymptomatic extracranial arterial disease: Results of a long term prospective study. Brain 110:777-791, 1987.
28. Moneta GL, Taylor DC, Nicholls SC, et al. Operative versus nonoperative management of asymptomatic high-grade internal carotid artery stenosis: Improved results with endarterectomy. Stroke 18:1005-1010, 1987.
29. Caracci BF, Zukowski AJ, Hurley JJ, et al. Asymptomatic severe carotid stenosis. J Vasc Surg 9:361-366, 1989.
30. Cooperman M, Martin EW, Evans WE. Significance of asymptomatic carotid bruits. Arch Surg 113:1339-1340, 1978.
31. Kanaly P, Peyton M, Cannon JP, et al. The asymptomatic bruit. Am J Surg 134:821-824, 1977.
32. Adams RD, Victor M. Principles of Neurology, 4th ed. New York: McGraw Hill, 1989, pp 617-692.
33. Dennis M, Bamford J, Sandercock P, et al. Prognosis of transient ischemia attacks in the Oxfordshire community stroke project. Stroke 21:848-853, 1990.

34. Estol CJ, Pessin MS. Anticoagulation: Is there still a role in atherothrombotic stroke. Stroke 21:820-824, 1990.

35. Mentzer RM, Finkelmeier BA, Crosby IK. Emergency carotid endarterectomy for fluctuating neurologic deficits. Surgery 89:60-66, 1981.

36. Terent A. Survival after stroke and transient ischemic attacks during the 1970's and 1980's. Stroke 20:1320-1326, 1989.

37. Sacco R, Wolf P, Kannel W, et al. Survival and recurrence following stroke. The Framingham study. Stroke 13:290-295, 1982.

38. Tufo HM, Ostfeld AM, Shekelle R. Central nervous system dysfunction following open-heart surgery. JAMA 212:1333-1340, 1970.

39. Brener BJ, Brief DK, Alpert J. A four year experience with perioperative noninvasive carotid evaluation of two thousand twenty-six patients undergoing cardiac surgery. J Vasc Surg 1:326-338, 1984.

40. Craver JM, Weintraub WS, Jones EL, et al. Predictors of mortality, complications, and length of stay in aortic valve replacement for aortic stenosis. Circulation 78(Suppl I):85-90, 1988.

41. Gardner TJ, Horneffer PF, Manolio TA, et al. Major stroke after coronary artery bypass surgery: Changing magnitude of the problem. J Vasc Surg 3:684-689, 1986.

42. Coffey CF, Massey EW, Roberts KB, et al. Natural history of cerebral complications of coronary artery bypass graft surgery. Neurology 33:1416-1421, 1983.

43. Reed GL, Singer DE, Picard EH, et al. Stroke following coronary-artery bypass surgery: A case control estimate of the risk from carotid bruits. N Engl J Med 319:1246-1250, 1988.

44. Barnes RW, Liebman PR, Marszalek PB, et al. The natural history of asymptomatic carotid disease in patients undergoing cardiovascular surgery. Surgery 90:1075-1081, 1981.

45. Bojar RM, Najafi H, DeLaria GA, et al. Neurological complications of coronary revascularization. Ann Thorac Surg 36:427-432, 1983.

46. Cosgrove DM, Loop FD, Lytle BW, et al. Primary myocardial revascularization: Trends in surgical mortality. J Thorac Cardiovasc Surg 88:673-684, 1984.

47. Montague NT III, Kouchoukos NT, Wilson TA, et al. Morbidity and mortality of coronary bypass grafting in patients 70 years of age and older. Ann Thorac Surg 39:552-557, 1985.

48. Shaw PF, Bates D, Cartlidge NEF, et al. Early neurological complications of coronary artery bypass surgery. Br Med J 291:1384-1387, 1985.

49. Treiman RL, Foran RF, Cohen JF, et al. Carotid bruit: A follow-up report on its significance in patients undergoing an abdominal aortic operation. Arch Surg 114:1138-1140, 1979.

50. Couch NP, Lane FC, Crane C. Management and mortality in resection of abdominal aortic aneurysms: A study of 114 cases. Am J Surg 119:408-415, 1970.

51. Fedde CW, Hobson RW II, Rich NM. Surgical management of 100 consecutive abdominal aortic aneurysms. Am J Surg 129:506-508, 1975.

52. Hicks GL, Eastland MW, DeWeese JA, et al. Survival improvement following aortic aneurysm resection. Ann Surg 181:863-869, 1975.

53. Crawford ES, Saleh SA, Babb JW III, et al. Infrarenal abdominal aortic aneurysm: Factors influencing survival after operation performed over a 25 year period. Ann Surg 193:699-709, 1981.

54. Pennell RC, Hollier LH, Lie JT, et al. Inflammatory abdominal aortic aneurysms: A thirty year review. J Vasc Surg 2:859-869, 1985.

55. Diehl JT, Cali RF, Hertzer NR, et al. Complications of abdominal aortic reconstruction: An analysis of perioperative risk factors in 557 patients. Ann Surg 197:49-56, 1983.

56. Cambria RP, Brewster DC, Abbott WM, et al. Transperitoneal versus retroperitoneal approach for aortic reconstruction: A randomized prospective study. J Vasc Surg 11:314-325, 1990.

57. Sedwitz MM, Hye RJ, Freischlag JA, et al. Zero operative mortality in 109 consecutive elective aortic operations performed by residents. Surg Gynecol Obstet 170:385-389, 1990.

58. Gaylis H, Kessler E. Ruptured aortic aneurysms. Surgery 87:300-304, 1980.

59. Lawrie GM, Morris GC Jr, Crawford ES, et al. Improved results of operation for ruptured abdominal aortic aneurysms. Surgery 85:483-488, 1979.

60. Hoffman M, Avelline JC, Plecha FR, et al. Operation for ruptured abdominal aortic aneurysms: A community wide experience. Surgery 91:597-602, 1982.

61. Szilagyi DE, Elliott JP Jr, Smith RF. A thirty year survey of the reconstructive surgical treatment of aortoiliac occlusive disease. J Vasc Surg 3:421-436, 1986.

62. Ray FS, Lape CP, Lutes CA, et al. Femoropopliteal saphenous vein bypass grafts: Analysis of 150 cases. Am J Surg 119:385-391, 1970.

63. Shore E, Foran RF, Golding A, et al. Femoral-popliteal occlusive disease: Saphenous vein bypass grafts below the knee: Analysis of 85 consecutive cases. Arch Surg 102:548-551, 1971.

64. Miller VM. Femoropopliteal bypass graft patency: An analysis of 156 cases. Ann Surg 180:35-38, 1974.

65. LoGerfo FW, Corson JD, Mannick JA. Improved results with femoropopliteal vein grafts for limb salvage. Arch Surg 112:567-570, 1977.

66. Ramsburgh SR, Lindenauer SM, Weber TR, et al. Femoropopliteal bypass for limb salvage. Surgery 81:453-458, 1977.

67. Naji A, Barker CF, Berkowitz HD, et al. Femoropopliteal vein grafts for claudication: Analysis of 100 consecutive cases. Ann Surg 188:79-82, 1978.

68. Naji A, Chu J, McCombs PR, et al. Results of 100 consecutive femoropopliteal vein grafts for limb salvage. Ann Surg 188:162-165, 1978.

69. Ferris EB, Cranley JJ. Use of umbilical vein graft as an arterial substitute. Arch Surg 114:694-697, 1979.

70. Hobson RW II, O'Donnell JA, Jamil Z, et al. Below-knee bypass for limb salvage: Comparison of autogenous saphenous vein, polytetrafluoroethylene, and composite Dacron-autogenous vein grafts. Arch Surg 115:833-837, 1980.

71. Prendiville EJ, Yeager A, O'Donnell TF, et al. Long term results with the above-knee popliteal expanded polytetrafluoroethylene graft. J Vasc Surg 11:517-524, 1990.

72. Klamer TW, Lambert GE Jr, Richardson JD, et al. Utility of inframalleolar arterial bypass grafting. J Vasc Surg 11:164-170, 1990.

73. Taylor LM Jr, Edwards JM, Porter JM. Present status of reversed vein bypass grafting: Five year results of a modern series. J Vasc Surg 11:193-206, 1990.

74. Bandyk DF, Kaebnick HW, Stewart GW, et al. Durability of the in situ saphenous vein arterial bypass: A comparison of primary and secondary patency. J Vasc Surg 5:256-268, 1987.

75. Hertzer NR, Beven EG, Young JF, et al. Incidental asymptomatic carotid bruits in patients scheduled for peripheral vascular reconstruction: Results of cerebral and coronary angiography. Surgery 96:535-543, 1984.

76. Crawford ES, Crawford JL, Safi HJ, et al. Thoracoabdominal aortic aneurysms: Preoperative and intraoperative factors determining immediate and long-term results of operations in 605 patients. J Vasc Surg 3:389-404, 1986.

77. Hollier LH, Symmonds JB, Pairolero PC, et al. Thoracoabdominal aortic aneurysm repair: Analysis of postoperative morbidity. Arch Surg 123:871-875, 1988.

78. Landercasper J, Merz BJ, Cogbill TH, et al. Perioperative stroke in 173 consecutive patients with a past history of stroke. Arch Surg 125:986-989, 1990.

79. Knapp RB, Topkins JF, Artusio JF. The cerebrovascular accident and coronary occlusion in anesthesia. JAMA 182:332-334, 1962.

80. Larsen SF, Zaric D, Boyson G. Postoperative cerebrovascular accidents in general surgery. Acta Anaesthesiol Scand 32:698-701, 1988.

81. Coventry MB, Beckenbaugh RD, Nolan DR, et al. 2,012 total hip arthroplasties: A study of postoperative course and early complications. J Bone Joint Surg 56A:273-284, 1974.

82. Eftekhar NS, Kiernan HA Jr, Stinchfield FE. Systemic and local complications following low-friction arthroplasty of the hip joint: A study of 800 consecutive operations. Arch Srug 111:150-155, 1976.

83. Mebust WK, Holtgrewe HL, Cockett ATK, et al. Transurethral prostatectomy: Immediate and postoperative complications. A cooperative study of 13 participating institutions evaluating 3,885 patients. J Urol 141:243-246, 1989.

84. Doerr FJ, Yildiz I, Fling LM. Pancreaticoduodenectomy: University experience and resident education. Arch Surg 125:463-465, 1990.

85. Blake R, Lynn J. Emergency abdominal surgery in the aged. Br J Surg 63:956-960, 1976.

86. Faro RS, Golden MD, Javid H, et al. Coronary revascularization in septuagenarians. J Thorac Cardiovasc Surg 86:616-620, 1983.

87. Horneffer PF, Gardner TJ, Manolio TA, et al. The effects of age on outcome after coronary bypass surgery. Circulation 76(Suppl V):V6-V12, 1987.

88. Gonzalez-Scarano F, Hurtig HI. Neurologic complications of coronary artery bypass grafting: Case control study. Neurology 31:1032-1035, 1981.

89. Hart RG, Easton JD. Management of cervical bruits and carotid stenosis in preoperative patients. Stroke 14:290-297, 1982.

90. Barnes RW, Marszalek PB. Asymptomatic carotid disease in the cariovascular surgical patient: Is prophylactic endarterectomy necessary? Stroke 12:497-500, 1981.

91. Hertzer NR, Loop FD, Beven EG. Surgical staging for simultaneous coronary and carotid disease: A study including prospective randomization. J Vasc Surg 9:455-463, 1989.

92. Ivey TD, Strandness DE, Williams DB, et al. Management of patients with carotid bruit undergoing cardiopulmonary bypass. J Thorac Cardiovasc Surg 87:183-189, 1984.

93. Turnipseed WD, Berkoff HA, Belzer FO. Postoperative stroke in cardiac and peripheral vascular disease. Ann Surg 192:365-367, 1980.

94. Breslau PJ, Fell G, Ivey TD, et al. Carotid arterial disease in patients undergoing cardiac surgery. J Thorac Cardiovasc Surg 82:765-767, 1981.

95. Furlan AJ, Craciun AR. Risk of stroke during coronary artery bypass graft surgery in patients with internal carotid artery disease documented by angiography. Stroke 16:797-799, 1985.

96. Kartchner MM, McRae LP. Carotid occlusive disease as a risk factor in major cardiovascular surgery. Arch Surg 117:1086-1088, 1982.

97. Kelly RE, Kovacs AG. Mechanism of in-hospital cerebral ischemia. Stroke 17:430-433, 1986.

98. Bernhard VM. Discussion of Turnipseed WD, Berkoff HA, Belzer FO. Postoperative stroke in cardiac and peripheral vascular disease. Ann Surg 192:367, 1980.

99. Hart R, Hindman B. Mechanisms of perioperative cerebral infarction. Stroke 13:766-773, 1982.

100. Coull BM, Beamer N, deGarmo P, et al. Chronic blood hyperviscosity in subjects with acute stroke, transient ischemic attacks and risk factors for stroke. Stroke 22:162-168, 1991.

101. Tanahashi N, Gotch F, Tomita M, et al. Enhanced erythrocyte aggregability in occlusive cerebrovascular disease. Stroke 20:1202-1207, 1989.

102. McDaniel MD, Pearce WH, Yao JST, et al. Sequential changes in coagulation and platelet function following femorotibial bypass. J Vasc Surg 1:261-268, 1984.

103. Collins GJ, Barber JA, Zajtchuk R, et al. The effects of operative stress on the coagulation profile. Am J Surg 133:612-616, 1977.

104. Griffiths NJ, Woodford M, Irving MH. Plasma fibrinolytic inhibitors after operation. Surg Gynecol Obstet 144:673-676, 1977.

105. Fuller JH, Keen H, Jarrett RJ, et al. Haemostatic variables associated with diabetes and its complications. Br Med J 2:964-966, 1979.

106. Ahn SS, Kalunian K, Rosove M, et al. Postoperative and thrombotic complications in patients with the lupus anticoagulant: Increased risk after vascular procedures. J Vasc Surg 7:749-756, 1988.

107. Pulsinelli WA, Levy DE, Duffy TE. Regional cerebral blood flow and glucose metabolism following transient forebrain ischemia. Ann Neurol 11:491-498, 1982.

108. Hindman BJ. Perioperative stroke: The noncardiac surgery patient. Int Anesthesiol Clin 24:101-134, 1986.

109. Thompson JE, Patman RD, Talkington CM. Asymptomatic carotid bruit: Long-term outcome of patients having endarterectomy compared with unoperated controls. Ann Surg 188:308-316, 1978.

110. Burke PA, Callow AD, O'Donnell TF, et al. Prophylactic carotid endarterectomy for asymptomatic bruit. Arch Surg 117:1222-1227, 1982.

111. Hertzer NR, Flanagan RA, O'Hara PJ, et al. Surgical versus nonoperative treatment of asymptomatic carotid stenosis. Ann Surg 204:163-171, 1986.

112. Rosenthal D, Rudderman R, Borrero E, et al. Carotid endarterectomy to correct asymptomatic carotid stenosis: Ten years later. J Vasc Surg 6:226-230, 1987.

113. Towne JB, Veiss DG, Hobson RW. First phase report of cooperative Veterans Affairs Asymptomatic Carotid Stenosis Study—Operative morbidity and morality. J Vasc Surg 11:252-259, 1990.

114. Bernhard VM, Johnson WD, Peterson JJ. Carotid artery stenosis: Association with surgery for coronary artery disease. Arch Surg 105:837-840, 1972.

115. Okies JE, MacManus W, Starr A. Myocardial revascularization and carotid endarterectomy: A combined approach. Ann Thorac Surg 23:560-563, 1977.

116. Craver JM, Murphy DA, Jones EL, et al. Concomitant carotid and coronary artery reconstruction. Ann Surg 195:712-719, 1982.

117. Hertzer NR, Loop FD, Taylor PC, et al. Combined myocardial revascularization and carotid endarterectomy: Operative and late results in 331 patients. J Thorac Cardiovasc Surg 85:577-589, 1983.

118. Jones EL, Craver JM, Michalik RA, et al. Combined carotid and coronary operations: When are they necessary? J Thorac Cardiovasc Surg 87:7-16, 1984.

119. Lord RSA, Graham AR, Shanahan MX, et al. Combined carotid coronary reconstructions—synchronous or sequential? Aust NZ J Surg 55:329-333, 1985.

120. Perler BA, Burdick JF, Williams GM. The safety of carotid endarterectomy at the time of coronary artery bypass surgery: Analysis of results in a high risk patient population. J Vasc Surg 2:558-562, 1985.

121. Babu SC, Shah PM, Singh BM, et al. Coexisting carotid stenosis in patients undergoing cardiac surgery: Indications and guidelines for simultaneous operations. Am J Surg 150:207-211, 1985.

122. Minami K, Sagoo KS, Breymann T, et al. Operative strategy in combined coronary and carotid artery disease. J Thorac Cardiovasc Surg 95:303-309, 1988.

123. Cambria RP, Ivarsson BL, Akins CW, et al. Simultaneous carotid and coronary disease: Safety of the combined approach. J Vasc Surg 9:56-64, 1989.

36

Complications With Repair of the Supra-aortic Trunks and Vertebral Arteries

Wesley S. Moore

Lesions of the supra-aortic trunks constitute approximately 6% of all operable lesions of the extracranial cerebrovascular system. Operations on these vessels probably are even fewer in number and represent an even smaller percentage of the overall operations performed for cerebrovascular insufficiency. For this reason the number of cases in any one series is few and the true complication rates associated with the operation are difficult to ascertain. The analysis is complicated further by the fact that there are two general categories for the surgical approach to the supra-aortic trunks: direct (transmediastinal or transthoracic) and indirect (extraanatomic). Older series in the literature were weighted more heavily toward the direct approach, which at the time carried a higher morbidity and mortality. Recent reports begin to develop a balance between direct and indirect repairs and also show a trend toward better results with direct repair than previously reported. To provide a contemporary perspective, the literature for this section has been limited to the last 12 years of reporting, with most of the reports in the last 5 to 7 years. The chapter is organized by analyzing complications associated with repair of specific arteries, including the innominate artery, right subclavian artery, left subclavian artery, common carotid arteries, and proximal vertebral artery. In those instances in which options exist between direct and extra-anatomic repairs, complication rates are subdivided. The general complications of mortality and stroke are discussed for

each approach, direct vs. indirect, and specific complication rates associated with the anatomic structures for each vessel are presented individually. Where sufficient data exist, either in individual reports or in a compilation of reports, complication rates are stated. Otherwise, individual potential complications are listed in order to draw the reader's attention to the risks and provide a basis for prevention. Finally, the chapter concludes with a discussion of the risk/benefit considerations for direct vs. extrathoracic repair of individually diseased vessels.

INNOMINATE ARTERY
Direct Repair

The surgical approach to direct repair of the innominate artery generally requires a median sternotomy. Alternatives of partial sternotomy with lateral extension (the trap door) or a cervical approach to distal lesions of the innominate artery are rarely used and compromise the safe exposure and hence control of the innominate artery. The options for repair include endarterectomy and aortoinnominate bypass grafting. There are no data in the literature that support an advantage of one procedure over the other. Theoretically, endarterectomy avoids the use of prosthetic graft material and hence the risk of late complications with infection. On the other hand, endarterectomy is a more technically demanding procedure, with the risk of atheromatous disruption at the level of the aortic arch producing either emboli or dissection. In addition, end-point problems, either

Table 36-1. Direct Innominate Repair

Series	No. of patients	No. of deaths	No. of strokes
Brewster et al.[1]	29	1 (3.4%)	2 (6.9%)
Carlson et al.[2]	34	2 (6%)	1 (3%)
Cherry et al.[3]	26	1	NR
Cormier et al.[4]	46	1	1
Crawford et al.[5]	18	0	0
Thompson et al.[6]	7	0	0
Vogt et al.[7]	34	5 (14.7%)	NR
Wylie and Effeney[8]	33	—	NR
TOTAL	227	10 (4.4%)	4* (3%)

NR, not recorded.
*Of 134.

proximally or distally, and perforation or rupture of the thinned residual adventitia of the large innominate artery increase the risk in the hands of surgeons who are not experienced with this procedure.

Eight series were reviewed, providing data from a composite of 227 innominate artery operations. The range of experience in these reports varied from 7 to 46 cases. The mortality rate for direct repair of the innominate artery averaged 4.4%, with a range of 0% to 15%. The perioperative stroke rate was 3%, with a range of 0% to 6.9% (Table 36-1).

Extrathoracic Repair

There are three principal options for the extra-thoracic bypass of an innominate artery occlusive lesion. These include the left subclavian–to–right subclavian bypass placed in a retromanubrial position, the left axillary–to–right axillary bypass placed subcutaneously over the sternum, or the left carotid–to–right carotid bypass.

A review of the literature for results specific to innominate artery occlusive disease using extra-anatomic bypass provides only limited data. Table 36-2 summarizes three series yielding only 49 cases with one death, for a mortality rate of 2%, and no strokes. Perhaps a better method of evaluating the risk of operation would be to look at a composite of all extrathoracic repairs, independent of the specific artery

being treated. Table 36-3 summarizes the results of nine series yielding 405 patients undergoing extrathoracic repair. There were three perioperative deaths (mortality, 0.7%) and nine postoperative strokes (stroke morbidity, 2.2%), which yields a combined operative mortality/stroke morbidity of 2.9%.

Table 36-2. Extrathoracic Innominate Repair

Series	No. of patients	No. of deaths	No. of strokes
Brewster et al.[1]	8	0	0
Schanzer et al.[9]	33	1	0
Vogt et al.[7]	8	0	0
TOTAL	49	1 (2%)	0

Table 36-3. Extrathoracic Repair—All Arteries

Series	No. of patients	No. of deaths	No. of strokes
Brewster et al.[1]	8	0	1
Crawford et al.[5]	99	1	2
Myers[10]	18	0	1
Rosenthal et al.[11]	32	0	0
Schanzer et al.[9]	33	1	0
Sterpetti et al.[12]	46	0	1
Thompson et al.[6]	67	0	0
Vogt et al.[7]	66	0	2
Ziomek et al.[13]	36	1	2
TOTAL	405	3 (0.7%)	9 (2.2%)

SUBCLAVIAN ARTERY
Direct Repair

Obstructive lesions of the origin of the left subclavian artery require a thoracotomy for direct repair. However, lesions of the right subclavian artery can be repaired through the cervical approach and therefore will be considered under the category of extrathoracic repair.

Direct repair of the left subclavian artery requires a third interspace thoracotomy for exposure of the origin of the left subclavian artery as it branches off from the aortic arch. The options for direct repair include open endarterectomy with tangential clamping of the aortic arch or bypass or replacement grafting with the prosthesis anastomosed end to side to the descending thoracic aorta.

Although the left subclavian artery is the most frequently diseased branch of the aortic arch, it is also the artery most likely to be treated with an extra-anatomic repair. Therefore the current reported operative experience with direct repair is limited. Table 36-4 summarizes the experience with two series in which specific details concerning results of thoracotomy for left subclavian repair could be identified. The cumulative experience was 49 cases with postoperative deaths yielding a mortality rate of 10%. Although three of the five deaths were caused by stroke, there were no nonfatal strokes reported.

Cervical Repair

The entire right subclavian artery can be exposed through a cervical approach. In addition, there are more distal lesions of the left subclavian artery that also are approachable directly through a supraclavicular incision. However, orifice lesions of the left subclavian artery require an extra-anatomic repair if the decision is made to avoid a thoracotomy. The options for repair include carotid-to-subclavian bypass, axilloaxillary bypass, and subclavian-to-carotid transposition.

Table 36-5 summarizes the cumulative experience in nine reported series, comprising 383 operations for cervical or extra-anatomic repair of the subclavian artery. There was one perioperative death for a mortality rate of 0.3%

Table 36-4. Left Subclavian Artery Direct Repair (Thoracotomy)

Series	No. of patients	No. of deaths	No. of nonfatal strokes
Thompson et al.[6]	6	3	0
Wylie and Effeney[8]	43	2	0
TOTAL	49	5 (10%)	0

Table 36-5. Cervical or Extra-anatomic Repair of Subclavian Artery

Series	No. of patients	No. of deaths	No. of strokes
Crawford et al.[5]	80	0	1
Myers et al.[14]	18	0	1
Rosenthal et al.[11]	32	0	0
Schanzer et al.[9]	33	1	0
Sterpetti et al.[12]	46	0	1
Thompson et al.[6]	67	0	0
Vogt et al.[7]	46	0	0
Wylie and Effeney[8]	40	0	0
Ziomek et al.[13]	21	0	0
TOTAL	383	1 (0.3%)	3 (0.8%)

and three postoperative strokes for a neurologic morbidity rate of 0.8%.

COMMON CAROTID ARTERY
Direct Repair

Direct repair of the right common carotid artery can be performed through a cervical approach and is discussed under cervical or extra-anatomic approaches. Direct repair of an orifice lesion of the left common carotid artery requires a transmediastinal approach, which is similar to the approach for an innominate artery stenosis. It also carries a similar operative mortality and neurologic morbidity.

Cervical or Extrathoracic Repair

The right common carotid artery can be approached through a cervical incision. If the artery is totally occluded, thromboendarterectomy with or without transposition to the right subclavian artery can be performed with restoration of blood flow through the common carotid artery. Often there will be associated carotid bifurcation atheromatous disease, which may be the mechanism for retrograde thrombosis. In that instance the carotid bifurcation requires repair as a part of disobliteration of the common carotid artery. This also is true for the left carotid artery. If the patient has a carotid bifurcation atheroma that produces retrograde thrombosis of the left common carotid artery, a retrograde thrombectomy combined with carotid bifurcation endarterectomy can produce restoration of blood flow to the left common carotid artery and carotid bifurcation. On the other hand, if the patient has a high-grade stenosis at the origin of the left common carotid artery, extrathoracic repair options include a subclavian-to-carotid bypass and a left carotid–to–subclavian transposition.

Operative mortality and neurologic morbidity are similar to the conventional carotid bifurcation endarterectomy and are a function of the indication for operation. Acceptable upper limits for mortality and neurologic morbidity rates as outlined by the Stroke Council for the American Heart Association are less than 3% for asymptomatic lesions, less than 5% for transient cerebral ischemia, and less than 7% for prior stroke with neurologic recovery.[15]

Repair of Proximal Vertebral Artery

The options for surgical repair of the proximal vertebral artery include transsubclavian endarterectomy of the vertebral artery orifice, vertebral-carotid transposition, and vertebral-subclavian angioplasty.

Four contemporary series were reviewed, providing a total of 580 operations in 538 patients (Table 36-6). There were 11 deaths for a mortality rate of 2% and six strokes for a neurologic morbidity rate of 1.1%. It is of interest that in the report by Branchereau and Magnan[17] providing an extensive experience with 191 operations, all of the postoperative strokes (two fatal and two nonfatal) occurred in combined vertebral/carotid artery surgery. Seven of the eight deaths occurred following the combination of vertebral/carotid artery surgery.

COMPLICATIONS RELATED TO TRANSSTERNAL/THORACOTOMY OPERATIONS

Unfortunately, the contemporary reports reviewed were incomplete with respect to the less major complications other than death or stroke. For this reason it is impossible to state an incidence rate. Complications that have been reported or potential complications are summarized below with a few words concerning prevention.

Wound Infection/Sternal Dehiscence

Fortunately, wound infection/sternal dehiscence is a rare complication. It is prevented by the usual careful handling of tissue and appropriate closure of either the thoracotomy or the sternotomy wound. Prophylactic antibiotics, both systemic and topical, are advisable.

Table 36-6. Vertebral Artery Repair

Series	No. of patients	No. of operations	No. of deaths	No. of nonfatal strokes
Berguer and Feldman[16]	35	35	0	0
Branchereau and Magnan[17]	179	191	8 (4.2%)	2[†] (1%)
Thevenet and Ruotolo[18]	290	320	2 (0.6%)	4 (1.2%)
Wylie and Effeney[8]	34	34	1 (2.9%)	0
TOTAL	538	580	11* (2%)	6[‡] (1.1%)

*Of 538.
†Of 191.
‡Of 580.

Innominate Vein Injury

At the time the sternotomy is performed, substernal tunnels from both the manubrium and xiphoid should have been completed by blunt digital manipulation. The air-powered sternotomy saw, with a shoe that protects underlying tissues, should prevent injury to the innominate vein. In the case of reoperation in the presence of prior sternotomy, this risk is increased.

Once the sternotomy has been completed, the innominate vein should be identified and carefully mobilized as the sternal retractor is opened. If the innominate vein is clearly in the way, such as in the instance of an innominate artery aneurysm, it may be divided temporarily between vascular clamps and then reapproximated at the conclusion of the procedure.

Aortic Clamp Injury

Although two aortic clamp injuries have been reported in one series involving the aorta/left subclavian artery junction,[6] this is a rare complication indeed. When the innominate artery or the left common carotid artery is being worked on, the aortic arch should be mobilized appropriately, both anteriorly and posteriorly, to provide the opportunity for careful manual palpation of the aorta in the region of the trunk orifices. Clamps should be selected carefully for partial aortic clamping. Various modifications of existing vascular clamps have been developed. For example, the so-called Wiley-J clamp has been modified to carry out minimal encroachment on the left common carotid artery while providing a maximal aortic cuff at the time of placement for innominate artery endarterectomy. I usually use a curved Glover clamp or a Satinsky clamp of appropriate size for the same purpose. In clamp placement it is important that blood flow to the left common carotid artery not be compromised when clamping the orifice of the innominate artery and vice versa. Similar precautions should be exercised with the left subclavian artery. It is worthwhile for the operating surgeon to remember that the subclavian artery has the least amount of collagenous connective tissue and therefore is a relatively fragile vessel. The aorta, on the other hand, should withstand partial clamping and the extension of endarterectomy into its orifice without difficulty, assuming that appropriate precautions, including proper mobilization and clamp selection, are observed.

Innominate Artery Perforation

One of the major concerns in the performance of innominate artery endarterectomy is the inadvertent perforation of the adventitia when circumferentially mobilizing the atheromatous plaque within the innominate artery. Should a posterior wall perforation occur that cannot be repaired directly either from within the artery or posteriorly, then it is best to simply ligate the innominate artery and proceed with the placement of an end-to-side graft to the ascending aorta with bypass to the distal innominate artery.

Embolization

Atheromatous stenoses of the origins of the innominate artery, left common carotid artery, and left subclavian artery are derived from plaque within the aorta itself that encroaches on the lumen. If the plaque is extensive within the arch of the aorta, attempts to place a partially occluding clamp may disrupt the plaque, producing either dissection of the aortic arch, fragmentation of the plaque with embolization, or potential aortic disruption. Careful attention should be paid to evaluating the extent of the plaque within the aorta before clamp application. If it is extensive in the arch, then it is best not to proceed with partial aortic clamping in that area but to use the ascending aorta as a site for placement of an end-to-side graft using the bypass principle.

Graft Thrombosis

Graft thrombosis of innominate artery, left common carotid artery, or left subclavian reconstructions should not occur. If it does, it is related directly to a technical error, including inadvertently sewing the graft shut at the time of the proximal anastomosis, or an intimal flap or dissection of the distal anastomosis. Careful attention should be paid to the placement of sutures of the proximal anastomosis. Once the suture line is complete, the anastomosis should be tested by flushing the graft to be sure that there are no incorrectly placed sutures. Distal intimal flap should be avoided by (1) direct inspection of the distal artery before anastomosis, (2) avoidance of an endarterectomized segment for distal anastomosis, and (3) careful placement of sutures to include both the intima and the adventitia.

Graft Infection

Graft infection in the mediastinum or the left chest is a disaster. Fortunately, it is a rare occurrence. The usual measures of prophylaxis against graft infection, including avoidance of skin contact, administration of systemic antibiotics, and application of topical antibiotics, should make this an unlikely occurrence. Should a graft infection occur, it is necessary to remove the graft in order to clear the septic focus. Graft excision preceded by extra-anatomic bypass should maintain flow to the critical vessel and allow the extraction of the septic focus.

Reperfusion/Hyperperfusion Syndrome

Patients who have multiple arch vessel occlusive lesions have temporarily lost cerebral autoregulation. The reestablishment of blood flow through multiple occlusive lesions or poor postoperative control of hypertension can lead to reperfusion cerebral injury. The severity of this injury can range from headache to seizures, cerebral hemorrhage, and death. The syndrome can be avoided by not reestablishing blood flow simultaneously to multiple occluded vessels. Rather, it is best to take them one at a time in a staged fashion. Careful pharmacologic control of blood pressure during the operation, particularly postoperatively, should prevent the complication.[19]

Hemomediastinum/ Hemothorax

Hemomediastinum/hemothorax is a preventable complication if the surgeon takes the time and effort to ensure excellent hemostasis before closure. Suction catheters should be used with a sternotomy incision and chest tubes should be used with left thoracotomy to remove any residual or continued bleeding.

Phrenic Nerve Injury

Phrenic nerve injury is a rare and preventable complication. Should it be necessary to open the pericardium to expose the ascending aorta, the phrenic nerve should be identified and carefully avoided.

Recurrent Nerve Injury

The recurrent laryngeal nerve can be injured in the mobilization of the subclavian artery or indirectly by injury to the vagus nerve. Careful identification of these structures will prevent the complication.

Pulmonary Complications

The complications of pneumonia or pneumothorax are associated with thoracotomy and appropriate prophylactic measures related to aggressive ventilatory physical therapy should be taken. Pneumothorax is prevented by the placement of a chest tube at the apex and the appropriate removal of the tube when the lung is expanded fully.

COMPLICATIONS RELATED TO EXPOSURE OF CERVICAL COMMON CAROTID ARTERY

Complications related to the cervical common carotid artery are similar to those associated with carotid bifurcation endarterectomy except that exposure of the cervical common carotid artery is lower in the neck and therefore less likely to produce injury to the spinal accessory or hypoglossal nerves. However, the vagus nerve is in the field of exposure and must be protected carefully. Anatomic structures that may incur injury include the jugular vein and lymphatic structures, particularly the thoracic duct. The cervical sympathetic chain, which is paravertebral in course, can be injured, producing Horner's syndrome. However, the dissection plane to expose the chain is considerably deeper than would be used ordinarily for mobilization of the common carotid artery.

Other complications include wound infection and arterial and graft thromboses.

COMPLICATIONS FROM REPAIR OF SUBCLAVIAN AND VERTEBRAL ARTERIES

Review of the literature documenting individual series of repairs provides a heterogeneous experience with respect to complications. Inevitably, all series report their experiences with respect to mortality and stroke morbidity. Individual series vary regarding completeness of reporting with respect to other nonfatal complications. Table 36-7 is a compilation of 11 series of repair of subclavian and vertebral arteries, providing an experience of 1108 patients undergoing 1158 operations. These series were selected because of their reasonable completeness with respect to other nonfatal complications. Individual complications, potential or actual, are discussed below. Where actual experience is indicated, the range and mean of the complication rate are presented.

Brachial Plexus Injury

The proximity of the brachial plexus to the subclavian artery represents an important relationship. Fortunately, the relationship is well recognized by most surgeons and the frequency of injury is low. Table 36-7 documents the experience with a range of injury rate from 0% to 1.6%. A total of four injuries in 1158 operations provides a mean complication rate of 0.3%. It should be pointed out that three of these four were temporary injuries and progressed to recovery. This is an easily preventable complication in the hands of the experienced surgeon.

Phrenic Nerve Palsy

Exposure of the subclavian and vertebral arteries involves exposure and division of the anterior scalene muscle. The phrenic nerve courses directly over the anterior scalene muscle and must be identified and protected. Even though direct injury to the nerve is rare, traction on the nerve may produce permanent malfunction with paralysis of the hemidiaphragm. Table 36-7 records an incidence rate ranging from 0% to 3%. A total of 14 instances

Table 36-7. Complications From Repair of Subclavian and Vertebral Arteries

Series	No. of patients	No. of operations	Brachial plexus injuries	Phrenic nerve palsies	Recurrent nerve palsies	Infections	Thromboses	Hemorrhages	Horner's syndrome cases	Lymph injuries
Berguer and Feldman[16] (1983)	34	35	—	1 (3%)	—	—	—	—	5 (14%)	4 (11%)
Brancherau and Magnan[17] (1990)	179	191	3 (1.6%)	1 (0.5%)	3 (2%)	1 (0.5%)	—	—	48 (25%)	—
Christensen[20] (1980)	32	32	—	1 (3%)	—	—	—	1 (3%)	7 (22%)	1 (3%)
Edwards and Mulherin[21] (1980)	157	159	—	—	2 (1%)	—	—	3 (2%)	—	1 (0.6%)
Luosto et al.[22] (1980)	98	100	1 (1%)	2 (2%)	3 (3%)	2 (2%)	7 (7%)	3 (3%)	1 (1%)	—
Roon et al.[23] (1979)	43	43	—	—	—	—	—	—	—	1 (2%)
Schroeder and Buchardt-Hansen[24] (1980)	60	63	—	1 (2%)	3 (5%)	2 (3%)	2 (3%)	2 (3%)	1 (2%)	3 (5%)
Sterpetti et al.[12] (1989)	46	46	—	1 (2%)	2 (4%)	—	—	—	2 (4%)	—
Thevenet and Ruotolo[18] (1984)	290	320	—	4 (1%)	7 (2%)	—	9 (3%)	2 (0.6%)	92 (28%)	22 (6%)
Thompson et al.[6] (1978)	67	67	—	—	—	1 (1%)	1 (1%)	—	—	1 (1%)
Wesolowski et al.[25] (1972)	102	102	—	3 (2%)	—	1 (1%)	1 (1%)	1 (1%)	—	—
TOTAL	1108	1158	4 (0.3%)	14 (1%)	20 (2%)	7 (0.6%)	20 (2%)	12 (1%)	156 (13%)	33 (3%)

in 1158 operations provides an overall incidence of 1%.

Recurrent Nerve Palsy

Vocal cord palsy can occur from injury to the recurrent laryngeal nerve or indirectly from trauma to the vagus nerve. Exposure of the subclavian and vertebral arteries carries a risk of injury to the recurrent laryngeal nerve as it courses around the subclavian artery. In addition, the medial exposure of the subclavian artery comes in close proximity to the carotid sheath and the vagus nerve.

Table 36-7 documents the experience with recurrent nerve palsy, which ranges from 0% to 5%. The total number of reported cases is 20 in 1158 operations, providing an overall incidence of 2%.

Infection

Superficial or deep wound infection is a relatively rare occurrence in well-vascularized cervical incisions. Table 36-7 documents the experience from the literature, which ranges from 0% to 3%. There have been seven reported cases of 1158 operations for an overall incidence of 0.6%.

Postoperative Thrombosis

Thrombosis of a reconstruction, whether graft or endarterectomy with angioplasty, is clearly technical in nature. Causes of thrombosis include intimal flap, kinking or extrinsic compression of the graft, inadequate graft diameter, or intraoperative outflow thrombosis. Causes for late occlusion include myointimal hyperplasia or extrinsic compression of a small-caliber graft.

Table 36-7 documents a total of 20 instances of operative thrombosis in 1158 operations, providing an average incidence of 2% with a range from 0% to 7%.

Postoperative Hemorrhage

Bleeding is also an infrequent complication associated with operations on the subclavian and vertebral arteries. Table 36-7 documents a range of occurrence from 0% to 3%. Twelve instances in 1158 operations provide an average occurrence rate of 1%.

Horner's Syndrome

The stellate ganglion lies immediately posterior to the vertebral subclavian junction. Aggressive mobilization of the subclavian vertebral junction can injure the ganglion, temporarily or permanently, leading to transient or permanent Horner's syndrome. Mobilization of the subclavian artery and the vertebral artery within the perivascular plane will avoid this complication.

Table 36-7 documents the range of occurrence of this complication in individual series (0% to 28%). There are 156 reported instances of Horner's syndrome, either temporary or permanent, in 1158 operations, providing an average incidence of 13%.

Lymphatic Injury

The tissues around the subclavian and vertebral arteries are rich in lymphatics. The scalene fat pad overlies the anterior scalene muscle and must be mobilized to gain exposure to the muscle before division. It is my practice to free the scalene fat pad along its inferior margin and to reflect it superiorly. Dividing these tissues between clamp and ligature helps to reduce the incidence of postoperative lymphatic leak. A major lymphatic structure that can provide a great deal of difficulty is the thoracic duct. Principally, this enters the internal jugular vein on the left side posteriorly. However, accessory thoracic ducts can enter the right jugular vein also. This structure should be sought carefully and either protected or divided between ligatures as needed.

Table 36-7 documents the occurrence of lymphatic injury in the 11 reported series (range, 0% to 11%). There have been 33 instances reported in 1158 cases, providing an average incidence of 3%.

COMPLICATIONS RELATED TO AXILLARY ARTERY EXPOSURE AND GRAFTING

There is an insufficient number of cases reported in the literature to provide an overall incidence of the various complications that can occur with axillary artery exposure and grafting. Therefore individual complications are described without an attempt to report incidence.

Important structures associated with the axillary artery and its exposure include the axillary vein, the brachial plexus, and the nerves to the pectoralis major muscle.

Skin Erosion With Graft Exposure

Skin erosion with graft exposure is unique to the axilloaxillary bypass graft, which takes a subcutaneous route across the sternum. Although this is an extremely rare complication, it has been reported and represents a major disadvantage of this surgical technique.

Venous Injury

Exposure of the axillary artery by an infraclavicular approach that splits the sternal and clavicular heads of the pectoralis muscle provides exposure of the artery, axillary vein, and adjacent nerves. Care must be taken to expose the vein, mobilize it properly, and protect it from injury.

Thrombosis and Emboli

Once mobilized, the axillary artery is quite mobile. Care must be taken not to exert undue traction on an attached graft in order to prevent distortion and kinking of the artery. If this is not done, the kinked artery can develop thrombosis or be the nidus of thromboembolism.

RISK/BENEFIT CONSIDERATIONS IN DIRECT VS. EXTRATHORACIC REPAIR

The ideal operation for repair of the supraaortic trunks and vertebral arteries is a direct repair without death or complication. Obviously the series always will fall short of the ideal. It is clear that direct repair using a mediastinal or thoracic approach carries somewhat higher morbidity and mortality rates. For this reason extra-anatomic repairs have become popular. For the most part extrathoracic repairs have been quite successful in achieving the desired clinical benefit with a reduced morbidity and mortality. However, there are some notable exceptions that deserve discussion. This section examines individual suprathoracic trunks and provides a recommendation for direct vs. extra-anatomic approach based on a risk/benefit analysis.

Innominate Artery

The average mortality rate for direct repair of the innominate artery is 5% with a 3% stroke rate. In contrast, extrathoracic repair of the innominate artery carries a 2% mortality and there have been no reported strokes (Table 36-2). Although on the surface this would appear to show an obvious advantage of the extrathoracic repair of the innominate artery, this must be balanced with the late results. In the instance of an innominate artery stenosis producing transient ischemic attacks, an end-to-side anastomosis for an extra-anatomic approach will continue to permit flow over the diseased innominate artery and allow for continued embolization. The only method to prevent this is a proximal ligation, which can be difficult through an extra-anatomic approach. In addition, late graft failure from a left subclavian–to–right carotid bypass or from carotid-to-carotid bypass is higher than in a direct innominate artery repair. For this reason it is my choice to carry out direct repair, either an endarterectomy or aortoinnominate bypass, rather than extra-anatomic repair. The benefits of long-term outcome in this instance outweigh the increased risk of direct sternotomy approach.

Left Common Carotid and Subclavian Arteries

The left common carotid, left subclavian, and right subclavian arteries lend themselves to extra-anatomic repair with a lower perioperative morbidity and mortality when compared with direct reconstruction and a perfectly satisfactory late patency rate. Operations such as carotid-subclavian bypass, subclavian-carotid transposition, carotid-subclavian transposition, and carotid-subclavian bypass have now been adequately tested with excellent long-term patency and function.

REFERENCES

1. Brewster DC, Moncure AC, Darling C, Ambrosino JJ, Abbott WM. Innominate artery lesions: Problems encountered and lessons learned. J Vasc Surg 2:99-112, 1985.
2. Carlson RE, Ehrenfeld WK, Stoney RJ, Wylie EJ. Innominate artery endarterectomy. Arch Surg 112: 1389-1398, 1977.

3. Cherry KJ, McCullough JL, Hallett JW Jr, Pairolero PC, Gloviczki P. Technical principles of direct innominate artery revascularization: A comparison of endarterectomy and bypass grafts. J Vasc Surg 9:718-724, 1989.

4. Cormier F, Ward A, Cormier J-M, Laurian C. Long-term results of aorto-innominate and aorto-carotid polytetrafluoroethylene bypass grafting for atherosclerotic lesions. J Vasc Surg 10:135-142, 1989.

5. Crawford ES, Stowe CL, Powers RW Jr. Occlusion of the innominate, common carotid, and subclavian arteries: Long-term results of surgical treatment. Surgery 94:781-791, 1983.

6. Thompson BW, Read RC, Campbell GS. Operative correction of obstructed subclavian or innominate arteries. South Med J 71:1366-1369, 1978.

7. Vogt DP, Hertzer NR, O'Hara PJ, Beven EG. Brachiocephalic arterial reconstruction. Ann Surg 196:541-552, 1982.

8. Wylie EJ, Effeney DJ. Surgery of the aortic arch branches and vertebral arteries. Surg Clin North Am 59(4):669-680, 1979.

9. Schanzer H, Chung-Loy H, Kotok M, Haimov M, Jacobson JH II. Evaluation of axillo-axillary bypass for the treatment of subclavian or innominate artery occlusive disease. J Cardiovasc Surg 28:258-261, 1987.

10. Myers KA. Reconstruction of vertebral artery stenosis. Aust NZ J Surg 47(1):41-48, 1977.

11. Rosenthal D, Ellison RG Jr, Clark MD, Lamis PA, Stanton PE Jr, Cudner MA, Daniel WW. Axillo-axillary bypass: Is it worthwhile? J Cardiovasc Surg 29:191-195, 1988.

12. Sterpetti AV, Schultz RD, Farina C, Feldhaus RJ. Subclavian artery revascularization: A comparison between carotid-subclavian artery bypass and subclavian-carotid transposition. Surgery 106:624-632, 1989.

13. Ziomek S, Quinones-Baldrich WJ, Busuttil RW, Baker JD, Machleder HI, Moore WS. The superiority of synthetic arterial grafts over autologous veins in carotid-subclavian bypass. J Vasc Surg 3:140-145, 1986.

14. Myers WO, Lawton BR, Jefferson FR, Kuehner ME, Sautter RD. Axillo-axillary bypass for subclavian steal syndrome. Arch Surg 114:394-399, 1979.

15. Beebe HG, Clagett GP, DeWeese JA, Moore WS, Robertson JT, Sandok B, Wolf PA. Assessing risk associated with carotid endarterectomy. Stroke 20:314-315, 1989.

16. Berguer R, Feldman AJ. Surgical reconstruction of the vertebral artery. Surgery 93:670-675, 1983.

17. Branchereau A, Magnan PE. Results of vertebral artery reconstruction. J Cardiovasc Surg 31:320-326, 1990.

18. Thevenet A, Ruotolo C. Surgical repair of vertebral artery stenoses. J Cardiovasc Surg 25:101-110, 1984.

19. MacGillivray DC, Valentine J, Rob CG. Reperfusion seizures after innominate endarterectomy. J Vasc Surg 6:521-523, 1987.

20. Christensen G. Reconstructive surgery on the vertebral artery. Neurosurg Rev 3:113-117, 1980.

21. Edwards WH, Mulherin JL. The surgical approach to significant stenosis of vertebral and subclavian arteries. Surgery 87:20-28, 1980.

22. Luosto R, Ketonen P, Harjola PT, et al. Extrathoracic approach for reconstruction of subclavian and vertebral arteries. Scand J Thorac Cardiovasc Surg 14:227-231, 1980.

23. Roon AJ, Ehrenfeld WK, Cook PB, et al. Vertebral artery reconstruction. Am J Surg 138:29-36, 1979.

24. Schroeder T, Buchardt-Hansen HJ. Arterial reconstruction of the brachiocephalic trunk and the subclavian arteries: 10 years' experience with a follow-up study. Acta Chir Scand 502:122-130, 1980.

25. Wesolowski A, Gillie E, McMahon JD, et al. New arteriographic and surgical techniques for vertebral arteriopathies. Cardiovasc Surg (Suppl II):III211-III219, 1972.

37

Prevention of Transient Ischemic Attacks and Acute Strokes After Carotid Endarterectomy: A Critique of Techniques for Cerebrovascular Protection During Carotid Endarterectomy

William H. Baker

Carotid endarterectomy is being scrutinized increasingly. Critics suggest that aspirin is equally effective in the prevention of stroke. They also suggest that surgery is unnecessarily risky. Although centers of excellence report stroke and mortality rates of 1% to 3% following carotid endarterectomy,[1,2] the Rand Corporation survey reported a combined stroke and mortality rate of almost 10% based on data from a variety of geographic areas of the United States.[3] Because of this current climate of doubt, it behooves all vascular surgeons to use the safest methods of cerebrovascular protection during operation. Although perioperative stroke rates also may be related to such factors as patient selection, anesthesia, and avoidance of cardiac complications, this chapter concentrates on those operative techniques that may correlate with intraoperative stroke.

TEMPORARY INDWELLING SHUNT

During the performance of a carotid endarterectomy, vascular clamps by necessity are applied to the common, external, and internal carotid arteries, resulting in cessation of flow in the ipsilateral internal carotid artery and a reduction of flow in the ipsilateral cerebral hemisphere. If collateral cerebral circulation is adequate, no neurologic sequelae result from this temporary reduction of flow. If cerebral collateral circulation is inadequate, the patient is at

risk for intraoperative stroke. In an effort to avoid stroke in patients in whom cerebral collateral flow is inadequate, surgeons have used a temporary indwelling shunt.[4] A variety of plastic tubes can be used to shunt blood from the common carotid artery to the distal internal carotid artery during the performance of endarterectomy. Whereas this technique does increase ipsilateral hemispheric flow during operation, the shunt itself may "snowplow" debris from the atheromatous intima into the ipsilateral cerebral circulation, causing hemispheric emboli. If air is inadvertently introduced during the insertion of a shunt, air emboli may result. Finally, the shunt itself is an encumbrance during the performance of endarterectomy. It can be easier to perform the operation without the presence of a plastic tube in the middle of the artery. Although the shunt does not preclude the performance of an adequate operation and in fact in some operations is easy to work around, it is simpler not to have it in the way. Furthermore, in some patients with a long tail of atheroma in whom the carotid bifurcation is situated quite high in the neck underneath the angle of the mandible, the operation is challenging even without the shunt in place. Using a temporary indwelling shunt in this situation is almost impossible. To protect the brain during the performance of carotid endarterectomy, some surgeons always use a temporary indwelling shunt,[4] most surgeons use a shunt selectively for all the reasons enumerated above,[5] and relatively few surgeons entirely avoid using a shunt.[6]

Surgeons who always use a shunt find it is the easiest way to perform the operation, arguing that the labyrinth of data concerning selective shunt usage is inconsistent. Thus, rather than sift through this maze of statistics to determine indications for shunt usage, they use the shunt in every case. These surgeons suggest that with constant shunt usage the surgeon becomes more proficient and accustomed to the shunt's presence in the operative field, and they do not find it an impediment to the performance of endarterectomy. They have developed techniques for its use even in the presence of a long atheroma impossibly located high in the neck. In these patients carotid endarterectomy is performed expeditiously in the internal carotid artery, the distal end-point is seen directly and tacked if necessary, and finally the distal end of the shunt is inserted under direct vision, taking care not to disturb the distal end-point. Insertion time may be somewhat prolonged in this group; the total time of decreased ipsilateral hemispheric blood flow is reduced markedly compared with that in patients in whom a shunt is not used. With a shunt in place, closure of the arteriotomy is said to be facilitated. If a long arteriotomy is required, a patch can be placed in a leisurely fashion since cross-clamping time is not important. Excellent results have been reported with this method.[4]

Criteria for Use

Most surgeons find that it is technically more pleasing to perform the operation without a shunt. Thus surgeons who recognize the occasional need for a shunt base their decisions for selective use on a variety of criteria.

One of the earliest criterion surgeons used was the observation of the back-bleeding from the internal carotid artery. Pulsatile blood flow that shot across the operative field clearly was adequate, whereas flow that seeped from the distal end of the internal carotid artery was inadequate. The exact distinction between adequate and inadequate is difficult to quantify using this method.

In an effort to quantify this back-bleeding, stump or distal internal carotid artery back pressures were measured. This method was used first by Moore and Hall[7] at the San Francisco V.A. Hospital and reported in 1969. Their initial and subsequent experiences with the measurement of stump pressure in patients undergoing operation using local anesthesia indicated that if the stump pressure was greater than 25 mm Hg, then the operation could be performed without risk of intraoperative neurologic deficit. Those patients with a reduced stump pressure were at an increased risk of intraoperative stroke. In the same city the University of California at San Francisco group suggested on the basis of their experience that the safe level of stump pressure was 50 mm Hg, not 25 mm Hg.[5] This latter pressure has become the accepted norm in this country. Most surgeons who practice this technique use mean pressure rather than systolic pressure.

This technique has its detractors also. Hobson et al.[8] reported that test occlusion will result in neurologic symptoms even with a back pressure greater than 50 mm Hg. Connelly, Kwaan, and Stemmer[9] have reported similar experiences. It would be interesting to know whether these authors tested the adequacy of carotid occlusion as reported by Archie.[10] During measurement of stump pressure, Archie occludes the internal carotid artery with the pickups. If indeed the pressure tracing does not become a straight line at zero, he repositions the clamp on the external carotid artery to ensure that all branches are occluded.

Electroencephalography also has been used successfully to determine which patient's require a temporary indwelling shunt. One champion of this technique is Callow[11] and his group at Tufts University Medical Center. The electroencephalogram is unquestionably accurate in detecting subtle abnormalities as they relate to cerebral circulation. Surgeons who use this technique to select patients for shunt usage find that up to one third require a shunt. This number is quite high considering the number of patients in whom a shunt is used while under local anesthesia and the observance of neurologic deficits.[12] Thus it must be concluded that the electroencephalogram is hypersensitive to subtle changes resulting from decreased perfusion. Surgeons using this technique undoubtedly will use the shunt more often, but they should feel secure that patients are carefully selected.

There are newer electroencephalograms in use that are easier for surgeons to interpret. They compress the tracings and interpret wave heights in numbers. Excellent results using this technique with carotid endarterectomy have been reported.[13]

Finally, the use of local anesthesia in helping to determine if a shunt is indicated is becoming increasingly popular. A field block is used to anesthetize the neck, a routine exposure is performed, and the carotid artery is clamped. If indeed the patient exhibits a neurologic deficit during the 3 to 5 minutes of test clamping, the clamps are removed and preparation is made for the use of a temporary indwelling shunt. Surgeons practicing this technique report that shunt usage is between 5% and 10%. Excellent results have been reported with the technique, but detractors point out that it is not suitable for all patients and that general anesthetic agents, although they are myocardial depressants, also depress the cerebral metabolic rate and may in themselves confer safety to the operation.

There are relatively few surgeons who never use a shunt. Initially our group opposed the use of shunts. We reasoned that the data were not precise in selecting who should and should not have a temporary indwelling shunt and we elected not to use shunts. During that time we measured stump pressures in all patients. Interestingly, we came to the conclusion that in patients with contralateral carotid occlusion and a stump pressure less than 50 mm Hg, the stroke rate was sufficiently high (11%) to demand the use of a temporary indwelling shunt.[14] In a subsequent publication our group reported an increased stroke risk in patients with a stump pressure less than 25 mm Hg, regardless of the status of the contralateral carotid artery.[15] These studies form the basis of our current pattern of selective shunt usage.

In the discussion of our initial results, we reasoned that if we had used a shunt in those patients with a low stump pressure and a contralateral carotid occlusion, the stroke rate in this subset would have been reduced from 11% to 2%. With the use of a shunt, seven patients who indeed had a stroke might have been spared this neurologic deficit. Overall this would have reduced the incidence of permanent neurologic deficit from 2% to 1.1%. This small reduction in stroke, although significant, especially for those seven patients, underscores that there is a preeminent role of other factors in the production of operation-related stroke.

AVOIDANCE OF INTRAOPERATIVE EMBOLIZATION

What are these other factors? Most surgeons agree that they are the avoidance of intraoperative embolization and the performance of a technically perfect operation. The incidence of intraoperative embolization is increased if the surgeon is rough in handling the carotid bifurcation before the application of appropriate vascular clamps. Evans[16] of Columbus, Ohio, suggests that those surgeons obtaining superior results with local anesthesia may do so because local anesthesia forces them to be gentle during the performance of the operation. We make a special effort not to dissect the carotid bulb until after the appropriate clamps have been placed to avoid the possibility of emboli. The incidence of embolization of air and atherosclerotic debris can be increased by the use of a temporary indwelling shunt unless the shunt is inserted perfectly.

THE TECHNICALLY PERFECT OPERATION

A technically superior operation can be performed with or without shunt usage. To assess our technical results in the operating room, we have used B-mode imaging increasingly. We find this technique to be superior to contrast radiology because of its ease of use and avoidance of the theatrics that sometimes accompanies intraoperative arteriography. Initially we found several defects that required correction. Because of the use of this technique, we routinely have carried the proximal extent of endarterectomy more caudad in the common carotid artery. This has resulted in a proximal shelf of atheroma that is less prominent. This monitoring technique, like operative arteriography and imaging of distal bypass grafts, forces the surgeon to be extremely meticulous, knowing that his operative result will be scrutinized immediately. This protects against the possibility of early postoperative occlusion.

Correction of Neurologic Deficits

What if the patient has a neurologic deficit in the immediate postoperative period? Is there a golden period in which the surgeon can boldly act before such a neurologic deficit becomes permanent? If the stroke is caused by intraoperative ischemia, clearly nothing can be done. If the stroke is the result of intraoperative embolization, any surgical actions taken postoperatively are akin to closing the barn door after the horse has escaped. Thus the surgeon can positively affect a postoperative stroke only if indeed there is a mechanical blockage in the internal carotid artery at the operative site.

Patients who awaken in the operating room with a neurologic deficit may or may not be reexplored. Clearly, a decade ago before the use of intraoperative scanning all patients with such a deficit were explored in our institution. It was assumed that they had an internal carotid artery occlusion, which, if corrected, may lead to total patient recovery. Kwaan, Connolly, and Sharefkin[17] have established that prompt restoration of flow results in total reversal of a neurologic deficit. In all likelihood the duration of this golden period is 1 to 2 hours. In some patients it is clearly much shorter. The patient who awakes with a stroke in the operating room can be quickly prepped and draped again, and the same instruments can be used to open the wound and inspect the artery. If no pulse is present distally, additional heparin is administered, clamps are applied, and the arteriotomy is opened. If indeed a pulse is present, an operative arteriogram or some other interrogation is carried out to prove that a technically adequate result has been achieved.

The patient who awakes in the operating room neurologically intact but in whom a deficit then develops in the recovery area is returned to the operating room. These patients are presumed to have had a carotid occlusion or an episode of embolization. The operation is carried out as already described. Even if a pulse is palpated, the carotid artery usually is opened since it must be completely assessed to rule out a source of emboli.

Those patients who awaken neurologically intact and later in their postoperative course have a transient ischemic attack are placed on a regimen of heparin. The carotid bifurcation is assessed usually with ultrasonography and contrast angiography. It is assumed that these patients have had a transient ischemic attack caused by embolization, and the source of an embolus must be ferreted out. If indeed a minor defect is seen arteriographically, the surgeon has the option of reexploration or treatment with anticoagulants over the next few weeks. Of course, major defects are corrected surgically.

It is difficult to assess whether the above plan is efficacious. Edwards et al.,[18] although advocating such a plan, cannot prove that it indeed helps their overall patient results. Other centers, including our own, have so few patients treated in such a manner that a retrospective review is meaningless.

CONCLUSION

The main methods used to avoid stroke during carotid endarterectomy are the use of an indwelling shunt during the performance of the operation to prevent intraoperative ischemia, avoidance of intraoperative embolization by gentle operative techniques, and performance of a technically perfect operation that prevents early postoperative occlusion. A variety of methods may safely predict who should and should not require a temporary indwelling shunt. Surgical technique that avoids trauma to the carotid bifurcation must be learned but cannot be monitored. Intraoperative arteriography, B-mode imaging, and other imaging techniques are of great assistance to detect defects that may lead to postoperative stroke and are recommended especially for those centers whose prior morbidity and mortality rates have been judged excessive. If indeed postoperative stroke occurs, especially after a period in which the patient is neurologically intact, immediate reexploration of a totally thrombosed carotid and reestablishment of cerebral blood flow may result in total or partial restoration of function.

REFERENCES

1. Callow AD, Mackey WC. Long term follow-up of surgically managed carotid bifurcation atherosclerosis: Justification for an aggressive approach. Ann Surg 210:308-316, 1989.
2. Sundt TM, Sharbrough FW, Marsh WR, et al. The risk-benefit ratio of intraoperative shunting during carotid endarterectomy: Relevancy to operative and postoperative results and complications. Ann Surg 203:196-204, 1986.
3. Winslow CM, Solomon DH, Chassin MR, et al. The appropriateness of carotid endarterectomy. N Engl J Med 318:721-727, 1988.
4. Thompson JE, Talkington CM. Carotid endarterectomy. Ann Surg 184:1-15, 1976.
5. Hays RJ, Levinson SA, Wylie EJ. Intraoperative measurement of carotid back pressure as a guide to operative management for carotid endarterectomy. Surgery 72:593, 1972.
6. Ott DA, Cooley DA, Chapa L, et al. Carotid endarterectomy without temporary intraluminal shunt: Study of 309 consecutive operations. Ann Surg 191:708-714, 1980.
7. Moore WS, Hall AD. Carotid artery back pressure: A test of cerebral tolerance to temporary carotid occlusion. Arch Surg 99:702-710, 1969.
8. Hobson RW, Wright CB, Jublett JW, et al. Carotid artery back pressure and endarterectomy under regional anesthesia. Arch Surg 109:682, 1974.
9. Connelly JE, Kwaan JH, Stemmer EA. Improved results with carotid endarterectomy. Ann Surg 186:334, 1977.
10. Archie JP. Technique and clinical results of carotid back stump pressure to determine selective shunting during cartoid endarterectomy. Presented at the 38th Scientific Meeting of the North American Chapter of the International Society for Cardiovascular Surgery. Los Angeles, Calif.: July 1990.
11. Callow AD. The Leriche Memorial Lecture. J Cardiovasc Surg 21:641-658, 1980.
12. Imparato AM, Ramirez A, Riles T, et al. Cerebral protection in carotid surgery. Arch Surg 117:1073-1078, 1982.
13. Tempelhoff R, Modica PA, Grubb RL, et al. Selective shunting during carotid endarterectomy based on two-channel computerized electroencephalographic compressed spectral array analysis. Neurosurgery 24:339-344, 1989.
14. Baker WH, Littooy FN, Hayes AC, et al. Carotid endarterectomy without a shunt: The control series. J Vasc Surg 1:50-56, 1984.
15. Littooy FN, Halstuk KS, Mamdani M, et al. Factors influencing morbidity of carotid endarterectomy without a shunt. Am Surg 50:350-353, 1984.
16. Evans WE. Personal communication, 1981.
17. Kwaan, JH, Connolly JE, Sharefkin JB. Successful management of early stroke after carotid endarterectomy. Ann Surg 190:676-678, 1979.
18. Edwards WH, Jenkins JM, Edwards WH Sr, et al. Prevention of stroke during carotid endarterectomy Am Surg 54:125-128, 1988.

38

Nonstroke Complications of Carotid Endarterectomy

David S. Sumner

Although stroke is the most widely emphasized complication of carotid endarterectomy, the outcome of this conceptually simple but technically demanding procedure can be marred by a number of other adverse events. Some of these complications are shared by other peripheral vascular operations but others are unique to the carotid bifurcation. A thorough knowledge of the potential hazards and a commitment to avoid the anatomic and physiologic pitfalls that lurk at every stage of the procedure will do much to ensure the patient a benign postoperative course and rapid recovery.

NERVE INJURY

The superior cervical triangle, bounded by the sternocleidomastoid, omohyoid, and digastric muscles, and areas immediately adjacent are richly endowed with a full complement of nerves, both cranial and cervical. Because the carotid bifurcation must be approached through this region, these nerves are susceptible to injury. Nerves lack the resilience of other tissues and are traumatized easily. They must be handled delicately, if at all, to avoid prolonged and sometimes permanent dysfunction.

Cervical Nerves

The transverse cervical nerve (or cervical cutaneous nerve) originates from the second and third cervical nerves and crosses the sternocleidomastoid muscle in a horizontal direction, deep to the platysma. At the anterior border of this muscle, it penetrates the deep fascia and

divides into ascending and descending branches to supply the skin of the anterolateral neck (Fig. 38-1). Thus branches of the transverse cervical nerve are encountered frequently when a longitudinal incision paralleling the anterior border of the sternocleidomastoid muscle is used. To gain access to the deeper tissues, often it is necessary to sacrifice one or more of these branches.[1-3] Numbness of the skin of the neck,

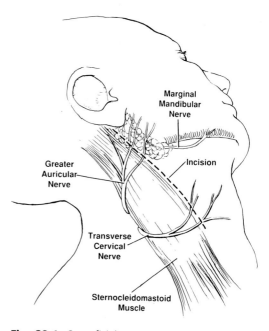

Fig. 38-1. Superficial nerves susceptible to injury during carotid endarterectomy.

471

which may be transient, is the only disability.[1,2] Male patients should be forewarned because numbness in this area may be disconcerting when they shave.[2] Some men complain of discomfort when they wear a collar and tie. In one series, only 4 of 30 patients (13%) with damage to the transverse cervical nerve complained of severe symptoms.[1]

When it is necessary to continue the dissection further up the neck to gain access to a high carotid bifurcation, the greater auricular nerve may be exposed (Fig. 38-1). This nerve also arises from the second and third cervical nerves, winds around the posterior border of the sternocleidomastoid muscle, and passes upward and anteriorly beneath the platysma. At the anterior border of the sternocleidomastoid muscle, it divides into anterior and posterior branches. The posterior component turns sharply cephalad to supply the skin over the mastoid process and the earlobe; the anterior components continue forward to the skin over the parotid gland. Injury to the posterior branch can be avoided by sweeping this portion of the nerve posteriorly with the sternocleidomastoid muscle as the tissues anterior to this muscle are divided.[1,2] Division of at least some of the anterior branches is inevitable when the dissection is carried up behind the parotid gland. Trauma to the posterior auricular nerve causes an annoying numbness of the earlobe, which can be permanent but may clear within 6 to 12 months.[2,4,5] As a result of the impaired sensation, pierced ears may be susceptible to infection.[6] Numbness over the angle of the jaw is of little consequence. Dehn and Taylor[1] report severe symptoms in only 3 of 26 patients (12%) with posterior auricular nerve injury.

Cranial Nerves

Whereas injuries to cervical nerves are seldom more than a nuisance, trauma to cranial nerves can cause significant disability. The cranial nerves subject to injury during carotid endarterectomy include the seventh (facial), ninth (glossopharyngeal), tenth (vagus), eleventh (spinal accessory), and twelfth (hypoglossal). Although these nerves rarely are severed, they may be traumatized during dissection, damaged by pressure exerted by retractors or

vascular clamps, crushed by inadvertent inclusion in a vascular clamp, or thermally injured by the electric cautery.[7] In many cases no explanation is apparent.

Facial Nerve

The marginal mandibular nerve descends below the angle of the mandible deep to the platysma, courses forward parallel and about 1 cm below the mandible, and then turns cephalad, crossing the facial artery, to supply motor fibers to the lower lip (Fig. 38-1). It is not visualized during carotid endarterectomy. Extending the neck and rotating the patient's head toward the opposite side tend to draw the nerve downward, closer to the operative field.[4] Incisions placed anterior to the earlobe and transverse cervical incisions increase the risk of damaging the marginal mandibular nerve.[4] Most injuries, however, are caused by pressure from self-retaining retractors. Directing the upper end of the incision toward the mastoid process, posterior to the earlobe, and careful use of retractors minimize the likelihood of trauma to this nerve.[7]

Damage to the marginal mandibular nerve causes drooping of the ipsilateral lip and facial asymmetry. Although symptoms are largely cosmetic, the ability to control saliva may be impaired. Several authors report restitution of nerve function in all patients within 6 weeks to 3 months of operation.[2,5,8] Eighty-six percent of the cases studied by Hertzer[3] recovered in a mean period of 3 months but 1 of 11 cases was permanent. In the series compiled by Massey et al.,[9] only 40% of patients with marginal mandibular paresis recovered within 1 year.

Hypoglossal Nerve

Emerging from the skull through a canal of the same name, the hypoglossal nerve descends between the internal jugular vein and the internal carotid artery along with the vagus nerve, to which it is closely bound. Near the angle of the mandible, it turns forward, crossing the internal and external carotid arteries, and disappears beneath the digastric and stylohyoid muscles to supply these structures and the intrinsic muscles of the tongue (Fig. 38-2). Positioned a few centimeters above the carotid bifurcation deep

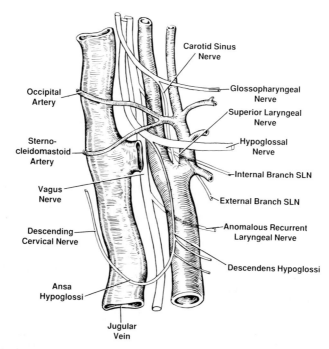

Fig. 38-2. Cervical nerves susceptible to injury during carotid endarterectomy. *SLN,* superior laryngeal nerve.

to the facial vein, a portion of the hypoglossal nerve is exposed during the course of most carotid endarterectomies. However, the nerve may not be seen when the bifurcation is quite low. As the hypoglossal nerve crosses the internal carotid artery, it gives off the slender descending hypoglossal nerve (descendens hypoglossi), which passes down the neck along the superficial surface of the common carotid artery. At about the midpoint of the neck, the descending branch of the hypoglossal nerve communicates with the more posteriorly located descending cervical nerve (a branch of C2 and C3) by means of a loop called the ansa cervicalis or ansa hypoglossi. Twigs from this loop supply the sternohyoid, sternothyroid, and inferior belly of the omohyoid muscles.

Injuries may occur during dissection or retraction, especially in cases with high-lying or extensive plaques in which a long length of the internal carotid artery must be exposed. The hypoglossal nerve is tethered posteriorly by a small, but constant, branch of the external ca-

rotid artery that supplies the sternocleidomastoid muscle. Further up the neck the occipital artery also crosses the hypoglossal nerve. Careful division and ligation of the sternocleidomastoid artery and small accompanying veins allow forward mobilization of the hypoglossal nerve without the need for undue traction.[4,7,10] (Cautery should not be used in the vicinity of the nerve and clamping always should be done under direct vision.) If necessary, the occipital artery also can be ligated.[7] Upward mobilization of the hypoglossal nerve is facilitated by dividing the descendens hypoglossi.[7] This nerve, together with the ansa hypoglossi, can be sacrificed with impunity. No deficits develop from division of these nerves. Often, however, sufficient mobility of the hypoglossal nerve can be obtained by keeping the plane of the common carotid dissection posterior to the descending branch, a maneuver that allows forward displacement of the entire hypoglossal complex.[2,8]

If one adheres to the techniques described

above, direct retraction of the hypoglossal nerve is unnecessary. Sufficient exposure can be obtained by applying the retractor to more superficial tissues. Even gentle retraction with a Silastic loop placed around the hypoglossal nerve is to be deplored. Retraction injuries to the hypoglossal nerve are more common when transverse incisions are used since this approach limits distal visualization.[4]

Deviation of the protruded tongue to the side of the dissection is the classic sign of hypoglossal nerve injury. Although most deficits are mild, patients may experience difficulty with swallowing, mastication, and articulation.[1,2,4,7] Several studies document return of function in all afflicted patients in 1 to 3 months.[1,2,8,11] Others report resolution of hypoglossal dysfunction in 60% to 88% of patients from 6 weeks to 12 months.[3,5,9,12]

Bilateral hypoglossal palsy is tolerated poorly. There is a risk of aspiration and upper airway obstruction that may on rare occasions require tracheostomy.[10,13-15]

Vagus Nerve

From the jugular foramen the vagus nerve passes vertically down the neck in the carotid sheath deep to and between the internal jugular vein and the internal and common carotid arteries (Fig. 38-2). A portion of the vagus is visualized during the course of most carotid dissections. If not seen, it can be palpated easily in the tissues posterior and lateral to the carotid artery. Rarely, the vagus may lie anterior to the internal and common carotid arteries and be mistaken for the much smaller descending hypoglossal nerve.[2,8] Within the chest the vagi give rise to the recurrent laryngeal nerves, which pass upward in the tracheoesophageal groove to supply the thyroarytenoid muscle of the larynx. On the right side the recurrent laryngeal nerve loops around the subclavian artery and, on the left, around the aortic arch. When the right subclavian artery arises from the aortic arch rather than from the innominate artery, the recurrent laryngeal nerve originates from the vagus in the neck and passes behind the common carotid artery to the larynx, where it is susceptible to clamp injury.[1,2,8,16]

Because the vagus is applied so closely to the internal carotid artery beyond the bulb, it is important to maintain a dissection plane immediately adjacent to the adventitia; otherwise, the vagus may be injured. (The vagus itself should never be manipulated directly.[7]) Below the bifurcation the vagus and common carotid artery are more widely separated. Yet even in this position, the nerve may be traumatized by inadvertent inclusion in the tips of clamps applied to the carotid artery or by prolonged pressure from vascular clamps resting on the nerve during the course of a carotid endarterectomy.[1,2] Fascicles destined for the recurrent laryngeal nerve are especially vulnerable since they tend to be located in the more medial portion of the nerve bundle, adjacent to the carotid artery.[1,17] Therefore to prevent injuries the entire jaw of the clamp should be visible during application. I have found a small "profunda clamp" to be ideal for the common carotid artery since it can be placed with the jaws almost parallel to the skin, allowing the tip to be seen at all times. The internal carotid artery may be controlled with a Silastic loop, a neurosurgical clamp (Heifitz clip), or a delicate renal pedicle clamp—all applied under direct vision. Self-retaining retractor blades should not be placed on the jugular vein, where they might damage the vein and rest on the vagus nerve.[7] Retraction of the jugular vein is achieved most safely by means of a 0 0 silk suture placed through the adventitia. It is also possible to damage the recurrent laryngeal nerve with the teeth of a retractor placed in the tracheoesophageal groove.[1,7] Finally, the surgeon always must keep in mind the possible aberrant locations of the vagus and recurrent laryngeal nerves.

Although the vagus innervates many organs in the thorax and abdomen, injuries in the neck are manifested exclusively by dysfunction of structures supplied by the recurrent laryngeal nerve. Paralysis of the ipsilateral vocal cord in the paramedian position produces hoarseness and impaired phonation in the lower frequency range. Coughing becomes inefficient. It is likely that many transient cases of vagal nerve injury are falsely attributed to damage caused by intubation during general anesthesia, which also may cause hoarseness.[1,2,7,18] Indirect or direct laryngoscopy is necessary to establish the diagnosis. Probably only 50% to 70% of patients with vocal cord paresis are symptomatic.[7,12]

In Hertzer's series[3] complete recovery of recurrent laryngeal function occurred in 83% of patients within an average period of 3 months. Sannella et al.[18] noted return of vocal cord function in 15 of 26 patients (58%) in 6 days to 8 months. Others report 100% recovery in 2 to 9 months.[2,8,9] In some cases speech may become normal despite persistent vocal cord paralysis.[18,19] If the paralysis does not resolve within 6 to 12 months, it may be necessary to inject the cord with Teflon to achieve permanent adduction. Bilateral injuries of the vagus nerve are of course very dangerous since they can result in upper airway obstruction.[7] Should this occur, tracheostomy may be required.

Superior Laryngeal Nerve

This nerve arises from the nodose ganglion of the vagus near the jugular foramen and passes down the neck medial and deep to the internal carotid artery (Fig. 38-2). Behind the external carotid artery, it splits into an internal branch that pierces the thyrohyoid membrane (where it receives sensory input from the laryngeal mucosa above the vocal fold) and into an external branch that innervates the cricothyroid muscle and inferior pharyngeal constrictor. Because of its small size and deep location, the superior laryngeal nerve is seldom identified. It is susceptible to injury during clamping of the internal and external carotid arteries or during dissection of the superior laryngeal artery, which lies quite close to the external branch.[1,4]

Injuries to this nerve may be overlooked easily because dysfunction is apparent only in patients who use their voices extensively. Only 20% of patients were symptomatic in one prospective study.[7] Lack of tension of the ipsilateral vocal cord impairs the production of high-pitched tones and leads to easy fatigability of the voice. Sensory loss may cause minor problems with swallowing.[4,8] The diagnosis of

injury may be inconclusive even with laryngoscopy but can be made by careful evaluation of speech patterns.[1,2] Most patients probably regain superior laryngeal function. Hertzer[3] noted complete recovery in two of four cases within 2 months; Aldoori and Baird[2] reported complete recovery in two of two patients at 8 months.

Glossopharyngeal Nerve

After exiting the skull through the jugular foramen, the glossopharyngeal nerve crosses the superficial surface of the internal carotid artery high in the neck, deep to the styloid process (Fig. 38-2). It parallels the stylopharyngeus muscles for a few centimeters, then dives beneath the hyoglossus muscle to innervate the tonsil and base of the tongue. The glossopharyngeal nerve elevates the larynx and pharynx during swallowing and receives sensory input from the mucous membranes of the pharynx, fauces, tonsils, and posterior tongue. Because of its remote location, it is seldom seen during routine carotid endarterectomy. Injuries may occur during mobilization of, or dissection above, the hypoglossal nerve, especially when division of the posterior belly of the digastric muscle or resection of the styloid process is required.[20] Retraction should be limited to the plane of the digastric muscle and extreme care should be taken to confine the dissection of the distal internal carotid artery to the periadventitial tissues. Symptoms range from mild dysphagia to severe incoordination of the swallowing mechanism and ablation of the gag reflex. Tracheostomy, intravenous hyperalimentation, enteric tube feedings, and even gastrostomy may be necessary when aspiration occurs.[3,20]

Spinal Accessory Nerve

Leaving the jugular foramen, the spinal accessory nerve turns posteriorly, passing in front of the jugular vein in two thirds of patients and behind in the remainder. It then enters or passes behind the upper sternocleidomastoid muscle, crosses the posterior triangle of the neck, and terminates in the trapezius muscle. Damage to this nerve during carotid endarterectomy is rare. Tucker et al.[21] reported four cases but found only three others in a literature review. In their experience symptoms first appeared 12 days to 2 months after operation. Pain in the shoulder is the initial complaint. Patients are unable to abduct their arms past 90 degrees, the shoulder droops, and there is atrophy of the superior portion of the trapezius muscle. Confirmation of the diagnosis may be obtained by electromyography. The mechanism of nerve damage is uncertain. Injuries do not appear to be related to high dissection; rather, they may be caused by excessive traction on the sternocleidomastoid muscle or by entrapment of the nerve in scar tissue formed during the postoperative period.[21] In most cases complete rehabilitation can be achieved with aggressive physical therapy.

Sympathetic Nerves

Injuries to the cervical sympathetic chain, which lies deep to the carotid sheath on the surface of the longus colli and longus capitis muscles, are exceedingly rare.[3,22,23] The resulting Horner's syndrome causes little disability.

Incidence of Nerve Damage

Although most surgeons reflecting on their personal series of carotid endarterectomies recall only a few cases of tongue deviation and a rare patient with vocal cord paralysis, the actual incidence of cranial nerve damage is appreciable, ranging from 4% to 18% in retrospective reviews and 13% to 39% in prospective studies (Table 38-1). The frequency with which injuries are detected depends on how carefully and how consistently patients are examined in the postoperative period. Thus information is apt to be more reliable when nerve function is assessed objectively by otolaryngologists.[5,7,12] Such testing is necessary to detect malfunction of the superior laryngeal nerve and to differentiate between vocal cord paresis and hoarseness caused by trauma related to tracheal intubation. Evaluation of integrated motor speech patterns by speech pathologists reveals the highest incidence of problems.[5,12] Although operative skill and the care exercised in avoiding the pitfalls described above will affect the incidence of cranial nerve injury, the outcomes listed in

Table 38-1. Incidence of Cranial Nerve Dysfunction Following Carotid Endarterectomy

Author	Cranial nerve dysfunction (%)				
	Marginal mandibular	Recurrent laryngeal	Superior laryngeal	Hypoglossal	Total‡
Retrospective					
Matsumoto et al.[8] (1977)	1.5	2.3	—	8.5	12.3
Massey et al.[9] (1984)	3.2	5.1	—	8.2	16.4
Theodotou and Mahaley[11] (1985)	1	1	—	2.6	4.7
Krupski et al.[23] (1985)	2.3	7.7	—	4.3	18
Kirshner et al.[24] (1989)	3.6	1.4	—	8.9	14.1
Hoyne[25] (1990)	0.7	1.5	—	0.7	4
Prospective					
Hertzer et al.[7] (1980)	2.5	5.8	2.1	5.4	15.8
Liapis et al.[5] (1981)	5.0	10.0	17.5	20.0	—
Evans et al.[12] (1982)*	—		14.6	5.6	16
speech pathologist†	—		35.0	11.0	39
Dehn and Taylor[1] (1983)	0	25.6	—	4.7	—
Aldoori and Baird[2] (1988)	5.8	5.8	3.8	13.5	25
Hertzer[3] (1989)	1.8	6.7	1.8	5.8	13.3

*Clinical assessment.
†Assessment by speech pathologist.
‡Total number of patients with nerve injuries.

Table 38-1 represent those of clinics with highly qualified and experienced surgeons. Krupski et al.[23] found no statistical difference in the frequency of nerve injuries associated with carotid endarterectomy performed in a university hospital, a private community hospital, and a V.A. hospital, in which the procedures were performed by supervised general surgery residents.

Prospective studies suggest that the tenth cranial nerve (recurrent laryngeal and superior laryngeal) is somewhat more likely to be damaged than the twelfth (hypoglossal). Both are injured more frequently than the seventh cranial nerve (marginal mandibular) and far more frequently than the ninth cranial nerve (glossopharyngeal). Paresis of the glossopharyngeal nerve was noted in 0.2%, 0.3%, 1.1%, and 1.5% of carotid endarterectomies in reports by Rosenbloom et al.,[20] Kirshner, O'Brien, and Ricotta,[24] Evans et al.,[12] and Hoyne,[25] respectively. However, most prospective studies do not include cases of glossopharyngeal dysfunction.[1,2,5,7] Multiple cranial nerve injuries are not uncommon and are recorded in most reports. Hertzer et al.,[7] for example, found involvement of two nerves in four (13.3%) and three nerves in one (3.3%) of 30 patients in whom cranial nerve injuries were detected.

Sensory loss in the distribution of the transverse cervical nerve has been reported in 70% to 89% of carotid endarterectomies and is almost inevitable when the incision parallels the anterior border of the sternocleidomastoid muscle.[1-3] Numbness of the earlobe caused by trauma to the posterior auricular nerve is only slightly less common, occurring in 40% to 60% of prospectively studied patients.[1,2]

Implications for Bilateral Carotid Endarterectomy

Injuries of both vagal and hypoglossal nerves may lead to catastrophic respiratory distress.[13-15] Although most cases of cranial nerve dysfunction eventually resolve, paresis may still be present at the time a contralateral carotid endarterectomy is being contemplated. In fact, in their preoperative evaluation of patients scheduled to undergo carotid endarterectomy,

Hertzer et al.[7] found a 5.7% prevalence of cranial nerve dysfunction. All of these patients previously had undergone a carotid endarterectomy or a coronary artery bypass. Because 30% to 40% of patients with persistent malfunction of the superior laryngeal or hypoglossal nerve may have no overt symptoms, the tongue should be examined carefully and laryngoscopy should be performed in the staging interval before the second carotid endarterectomy.[1,3,5,13] If either vocal cord paralysis or impaired function of the tongue is detected, the contralateral operation should be delayed until function returns or, if the operation is urgent, provisions should be taken to ensure an adequate airway.

WOUND HEMATOMAS

Several aspects of carotid endarterectomy are conducive to postoperative bleeding and hematoma formation: patients are subjected to routine anticoagulation with heparin during the procedure; many patients are pretreated with aspirin or other platelet-inhibiting agents; the neck is very vascular; and subcutaneous closure is limited to the platysma. The reported incidence of cervical hematoma varies from 0.7% to 13.7%,[23,25-27] but the median incidence probably hovers around 2% to 5%.[28-30] In one series, 9 of 41 cervical hematomas (22%) required reoperation.[23] Serious consequences of large hematoma formation include upper airway obstruction caused by deviation of the trachea, angulation of the internal carotid artery, and compression of cervical nerves.[18,26] Neglected hematomas are uncomfortable and cosmetically unsatisfactory, may liquify and drain spontaneously through the incision, and may serve as substrate for infection.[3] Although strokes have occurred in patients with hematomas, no firm evidence links the two events.[26]

As a rule all large hematomas should be evacuated promptly with the patient under local anesthesia. General anesthesia is not required and, because of difficulties encountered in intubating the deviated trachea, can be dangerous when hematomas are large.[28] In rare cases of critical airway compromise, it may be necessary to relieve the pressure by opening the wound at the bedside.[26] Cricothyroidotomy or tracheostomy is rarely necessary if there is no delay in removing the hematoma.[26] Once the neck is completely reopened, the hematoma can be removed under direct vision by manual extraction and irrigation with antibiotic solution. Care must be taken to avoid injury to the carotid arteries or cranial nerves. Bleeding points in the subcutaneous or muscular layers can be cauterized, larger vessels should be securely ligated, and suture line hemorrhage must be controlled with appropriately placed sutures. In our review of 20 hematomas that required reoperation, no bleeding points or only small, easily cauterized bleeders were encountered in 13 cases (65%); in the remainder (35%), ligation of a vessel or oversewing of a suture line defect was necessary.[29] Welling, Ramadas, and Gansmuller[26] found diffuse tissue bleeding in 57% of wounds requiring exploration for postoperative bleeding, suture line leaks in 35%, and specific arterial or venous bleeding points in 9%. Before wound closure it is advisable to irrigate the tissues thoroughly with dilute antibiotic solution to reduce the likelihood of infection.[3] A short course of antibiotic coverage also is recommended.

The best method of managing hematomas is to prevent their occurrence. Hemostasis should be maintained meticulously throughout the original dissection; at the end of the procedure, all parts of the wound should be inspected carefully for bleeding points. Closing a "wet" wound with the expectation that bleeding will cease is one way to invite wound hematomas. A little extra effort and a few minutes delay are time well spent.

Reversal of heparin by the administration of protamine is a controversial topic. Collagen in the media or adventitia exposed during endarterectomy is a very potent platelet activator. Because thrombi developing acutely (often within minutes) at the carotid bifurcation on this thrombogenic surface are responsible for about 19% of postoperative strokes,[31] surgeons understandably are reluctant to use any method that might encourage clot formation. The results of animal experiments clearly show that continuation of heparin anticoagulation after closure of the arteriotomy and restitution of flow ensures the development of a relatively nonthrombogenic platelet monolayer. Studies

by Ercius et al.[32] suggest that this monolayer is well established by 10 minutes, after which it is safe to administer protamine. Our study[29] and that of Treiman et al.[30] demonstrate that neutralizing heparin with protamine significantly decreases the incidence of wound hematoma without increasing the risk of stroke or postoperative transient ischemic attack. Protamine, however, is not an innocuous drug. If given too rapidly, it may cause hypotension. Although anaphylactic reactions are rare, they have resulted in death.[33] It is our policy to measure the activated clotting time (ACT) at the end of the procedure. If the ACT is significantly prolonged (more than 200 seconds) and if the wound continues to ooze, protamine is administered but only after flow has been restored for more than 10 minutes. We estimate the amount of circulating heparin by assuming a 90-minute heparin half-life and give no more than 1 mg of protamine/100 U of residual heparin, after which the ACT is measured again. Ordinarily only 20 to 30 mg is required. In the majority of cases, no protamine is needed.

Closed suction drainage of the wound with a silicone rubber catheter (Hemovac or Jackson-Pratt) may reduce the incidence of small hematomas but is not particularly effective when bleeding is substantial. Treiman et al.[30] observed hematomas in 8.6% of patients whose wounds were not drained and in 4% of those in whom a drain was used, but the difference was not statistically significant. Care must be taken in passing the drain through the subcutaneous tissues to avoid injuring the external jugular vein or one of its tributaries. Should an injury occur, the catheter must be withdrawn and repositioned.

Although there is a general impression that aspirin, dipyridamole, low-molecular-weight dextran, and other platelet-antiaggregating drugs increase bleeding during carotid endarterectomy, there is little evidence that they contribute significantly to the formation of hematomas. In our study, 40% of patients in whom hematomas developed were given aspirin preoperatively compared to 56% of a control group who did not experience postoperative bleeding.[29] Since aspirin appears to reduce platelet accumulation at the endarterectomy site and decreases mural thrombosis, some excess bleeding during carotid endarterectomy is a small price to pay for the added protection that aspirin might convey.[34,35]

Postoperative hypertension also has been implicated as a possible cause of hematoma. Kunkel et al.,[28] using 170 mm Hg as the criterion for hypertension, and Treiman et al.,[30] using a sustained blood pressure of 160 mm Hg or a single reading of 190 mm Hg, found that 47% and 44%, respectively, of patients in whom otherwise unexplained hematomas developed had experienced episodes of postoperative hypertension. Blood pressures greater than 200 mm Hg, sustained for more than 15 minutes, were recorded in the recovery room in 65% of patients in whom hematomas developed in the study of Welling, Ramadas, and Gansmuller.[26] Only 8% of the control subjects had hypertension. Hertzer[3] notes that the onset of some cervical hematomas may be attributed to transient elevation of blood pressure and venous distention that occur when patients "buck" at the time of endotracheal tube removal. The possibility of hypertension contributing to the formation of wound hematomas is therefore another argument for strict control of blood pressure during the early postoperative period.

WOUND INFECTION

Because the neck is so vascular and constitutes a clean surgical field, wound infections complicating carotid endarterectomy are extremely rare. In Thompson's series[27] only one patient developed a wound infection, an incidence of 0.09%. A large neck abscess extending to the carotid artery was reported by Mora, Hunter, and Malone[36] in a patient 3 weeks following carotid endarterectomy and 4 days after a dental extraction. The infection, which grew α-hemolytic streptococci, was attributed to bacteremia seeding a small perivascular hematoma. On the basis of this observation, the authors advocate delaying dental work or other manipulations that traumatize mucous membranes until primary wound healing is complete. If delay is not possible, prophylactic antibiotic coverage will reduce the likelihood of secondary infection.

Infected wounds should be opened widely, cleansed of devitalized tissues or residual hematoma, irrigated thoroughly with antibiotic solution, and closed with suction drainage. If a prosthetic patch has been used, it may be advisable to substitute one of autogenous vein. Systemic antibiotics, appropriate to the cultured organisms, should be administered.

RUPTURE OF VEIN PATCH ANGIOPLASTY

Vein patch angioplasty is being used with increasing frequency as a method for closing carotid arteries following endarterectomy. Some surgeons use this technique routinely; others reserve patches for recurrent stenoses, small arteries, and cases in which the endarterectomy must be carried far distally into the internal carotid artery. Although patches have been derived from external and internal jugular veins or from arm veins, most are harvested from greater saphenous veins at the ankle.

Rupture of a vein patch is a rare but catastrophic event. Ruptures usually occur on the second to the fifth postoperative day and characteristically present as a longitudinal tear in the center of the patch.[37-40] The patch at this point is usually described as having a necrotic appearance.[37,40] Anastomotic disruption and bleeding from a dislodged ligature on a side branch of the transplanted venous segment have also been described, but in most cases the suture line is intact.[39,41] Cultures of the angioplasty site are negative.[40] Because of the sudden massive bleeding, respiration may be compromised.[40] About half of the reported ruptures have been associated with temporary or permanent neurologic dysfunction.[37-39,42] Repair is accomplished by removing the damaged tissue and substituting a fresh autogenous vein patch.

All ruptures have occurred in saphenous vein patches taken from the ankle.[37-40] Based on their observation that 3 of 75 patches (4%) harvested from this site ruptured, whereas none of more than 600 patches derived from the saphenous vein at the groin suffered a similar complication, Riles et al.[40] have suggested that angioplasties should be fashioned from groin veins whenever possible. On the other hand, Hertzer et al.,[39] who preferentially used the ankle saphenous vein in 434 carotid endarterectomies, reported only three ruptures, for an incidence of 0.7% (and two of these were actually suture line problems). Archie, in discussing the article of Eikelboom et al.,[37] stated that only 1 of the 400 ankle saphenous veins (0.25%) used for carotid endarterectomy in his personal experience had ruptured. Moreover, reports of several large series comprising a total of 551 carotid endarterectomies performed with ankle saphenous vein do not mention this complication.[41,43-45] I have used ankle saphenous vein for patching 83 carotid endarterectomies since 1985 and have never seen a rupture or suture line problem.

There is no obvious reason why the saphenous vein at ankle level should be more prone to rupture than that at the groin. In the standing (or sitting) position, veins at the ankle are subjected to a greater hydrostatic pressure than those at the groin and therefore should be better equipped to sustain arterial pressure. Certainly, veins from the distal portions of the leg maintain their integrity when functioning as coronary artery bypass grafts or femorotibial bypasses. Even the much thinner walled internal jugular vein has been used by Seabrook et al.[41] at the Medical College of Wisconsin in a series of 76 patients without problems; Baker, commenting in the article of Seabrook et al.,[41] related an event-free experience with 32 external jugular vein patches. There are obvious advantages to using the ankle saphenous vein. It is readily accessible, anatomically constant, and easily harvested; its removal does not preclude using the more proximal segments for coronary or femorotibial bypasses. These considerations override the possible increased risk of rupture.

Why should a vein patch rupture in the absence of infection or obvious technical error? Kakkar[46] has shown that cephalic veins are capable of withstanding pressures of 430 mm Hg and that nonvaricosed saphenous veins do not burst until pressures exceed 600 mm Hg. Archie and Green[47] reported that the mean rupture pressure of ankle saphenous veins is 2900 ± 1375 mm Hg and that none burst below 700 mm Hg. Although smaller veins ruptured at lower pressures than larger veins, for veins of comparable diameter, rupture pressure was independent of location (ankle, knee, or thigh). Patches, however, are called upon to sustain greater stress than the intact vein when subjected to the same intraluminal pressure. Circumferential or hoop stress (τ)

equals the product of the intraluminal pressure (P) and the ratio of the internal radius of curvature (r_i) and the wall thickness (δ):

$$\tau = P \cdot \frac{r_i}{\delta}$$

Since the radius of the intact vein (1.5 to 3 mm) is considerably smaller than that of the reconstructed common carotid artery (5 to 7 mm), the stress may be doubled or tripled. Nonetheless, even with the most unfavorable combinations, only a small percentage of veins should be subjected to stress sufficient to cause them to burst.[47] To maintain a margin of safety, the venous patch should be trimmed to a width of 3 to 4 mm. Given the amount of space taken by the placement of sutures, patches of this width will increase the diameter of the reconstructed artery by about 1 mm or less.

Experimental studies have shown that the endothelial surface of a vein patch becomes fissured shortly after blood flow is reestablished.[48] This is followed by fragmentation of the internal elastic lamellae. It is possible that these early changes temporarily weaken the venous wall, providing a window of vulnerability to rupture. Other possible factors contributing to rupture may be hypertension; structural fatigue; venous desiccation, trauma, or ischemia (occurring during preparation); or the use of a poor-quality vein.[41,47] Obviously, varicose veins should not be used and segments with thin-walled valve sinuses should be avoided. By noting the location of side branches, the surgeon can split and trim the vein in such a way that they are not included in the patch. If a side branch is present, it should be sutured rather than ligated.

FALSE ANEURYSMS

Pseudoaneurysms developing at the site of a carotid endarterectomy are rare. At the Cleveland Clinic, only 4 of 2651 carotid reconstructions (0.15%) were complicated by a false aneurysm.[3] An incidence of 0.6% was reported by Thompson[27] and 0.25% by McCollum et al.[49] Branch and Davis,[50] after reviewing the literature, estimated the incidence at 0.3%. False aneurysms may occur as early as 9 days or as late as 15 years after carotid endarterectomy.[49,50] In the series reported by McCollum et al.,[49] the average time of presentation was 6.2 years, but more recent reviews suggest a median of about 4 to 6 months.[50,51]

Patients typically present with a pulsatile, often painful, cervical mass. Some have experienced transient ischemic attacks (TIAs) or strokes, attributable to emboli arising from the

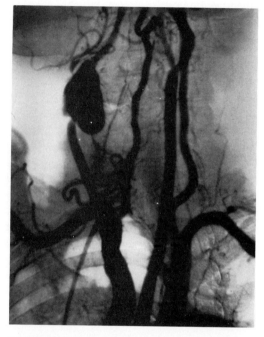

Fig. 38-3. Arteriogram showing recurrent false aneurysm following a carotid endarterectomy performed with a Dacron patch graft.

aneurysm.[52] Others may have signs of infection.[3,53,54] Hoarseness caused by a recurrent laryngeal nerve palsy has been reported.[55] The diagnosis can be made by duplex scanning and confirmed by arteriography, which of course is essential before operative intervention[56] (Fig. 38-3). When the aneurysm is filled with thrombus, arteriography may not reveal its true dimensions—a situation calling for the use of duplex scanning, computed tomography (CT) examination, or magnetic resonance imaging.

Dacron patches were used to close the original arteriotomy in 35 of 65 false aneurysms (54%) included in three reviews (Table 38-2).[50,51,54] Two others had been closed with Teflon and Ivalon patches, four with jugular vein patches, and three with saphenous vein patches. Isolated reports of false aneurysms following arterial homograft or synthetic graft replacement of the carotid bifurcation have appeared in the literature.[49,57,58] Because the majority of false aneurysms have been associated with patch angioplasties, the use of patches (especially those constructed of synthetic material) has been implicated as a risk factor for false aneurysms.[27,54,59] Branch and Davis,[50] however, concluded that the incidence of false aneurysm following Dacron patch angioplasty (0.33%) is not greatly different from that following primary closure (0.25%). They point out that most of the false aneurysms associated with Dacron patches occurred in the early days of carotid endarterectomy when silk was the only suture material available. Of 23 cases of false aneurysm

Table 38-2. Method of Original Arteriotomy Closure in 65 False Aneurysms Following Carotid Endarterectomy*

Method of closure			No. (%)
Patches (total)			44 (67.7)
Synthetic patches		37 (56.9)	
Dacron patch	35 (53.8)		
Teflon patch	1 (1.5)		
Ivalon patch	1 (1.5)		
Autogenous patches		7 (10.8)	
Internal jugular vein patch	3 (4.6)		
External jugular vein patch	1 (1.5)		
Saphenous vein patch	3 (4.6)		
Primary closure (no patch)			21 (32.3)
TOTAL			65

*Data from references 50, 51, and 54. Summary of 30 reports (1960-1986).

in which the suture material was specified, silk had been used in 19 (83%).[27,49,52,60] Whether the thin-walled jugular vein is more susceptible to aneurysm formation than other patch materials remains a topic of speculation.[54,60] There is at least one report of an aneurysm resulting from necrosis of a vein patch.[53]

As with false aneurysms in other areas, infection plays an important role.[3,50,51,53,54,56] About 10% of the false aneurysms associated with Dacron patches and 50% of those occurring with primary closure have been infected.[50] Many organisms have been identified, but staphylococcal species predominate.[50,51,54] Postoperative hypertension and technical errors complete the list of factors that may contribute to suture line breakdown. Damage incurred during shunt placement or the use of an improper endarterectomy plane are possible explanations for aneurysms that develop from rents in the arterial wall away from the suture line.[51]

Treatment

Because of the potential risk of embolization or rupture, operation is advised for all false aneurysms of the carotid bifurcation. Dissection is often difficult and hazardous because of the extensive scarring and the proximity of neural structures, which are often adherent to the aneurysm wall.[51,60] Especially vulnerable are the vagus and hypoglossal nerves. (It is always prudent to warn patients of the possibility of postoperative cranial nerve dysfunction.) To reduce the risk of embolization, manipulation of the aneurysm sac must be minimized during the initial dissection.[51,56] Before the sac is opened, the internal carotid, external carotid, and common carotid arteries are isolated and encircled with Silastic loops to ensure vascular control.[56] These vessels are best approached at sites remote from the aneurysm where scar tissue is less dense. Division of the posterior belly of the digastric muscle facilitates exposure of the distal internal carotid artery.[51] After vascular control has been obtained, the aneurysm is entered; the arteries are allowed to back-bleed; and, if a shunt is thought to be necessary, it is inserted between the common carotid and internal carotid arteries using care to avoid dislodging thrombus or injuring the

endothelium of the recipient vessels. Thrombus within the aneurysm sac is then evacuated; weakened or necrotic segments of the arterial wall are débrided; and, if indicated, prosthetic patch material is removed.[27,51,56] There is no need to remove all of the aneurysm wall; indeed, doing so may jeopardize neighboring structures.[56] The extent of débridement required in any given case is determined by the operative findings.

Unless the defect can be repaired expeditiously with a few sutures, shunting may be required to maintain cerebral perfusion during what can prove to be a prolonged period of potential cerebral ischemia.[56] The decision to use a shunt depends on the same factors that determine the necessity for shunting in routine carotid endarterectomy: carotid back-pressure less than 50 mm Hg, EEG changes developing during arterial clamping, CT findings, previous stroke, arteriographic evidence of inadequate collateralization, and the surgeon's personal preference.

In all cases there should be a high index of suspicion that infection may be a contributing factor.[51] Cultures of the thrombus, any prosthetic material, and degenerated arterial wall should be obtained.[50] Broad-spectrum antibiotics are administered until any organism that might be present is identified; at that time, administration of an antibiotic appropriate to the infection is begun.[50] When the tissues are grossly infected, some authors advocate postoperative irrigation with antiseptic or antibiotic solutions instilled through catheters left within the wound.[51,53]

A variety of methods have been used to treat pseudoaneurysms of the carotid bifurcation. When the aneurysm is small, the carotid wall is strong, and there is no evidence of infection, primary closure of a limited suture line defect or rent in the arterial wall may be possible.[50,54] Often, however, it is necessary to patch the defect or to replace an existing patch.[49,52,60] In the absence of infection, prosthetic material can be used; but if infection is present or even suspected, a patch of autogenous material (preferably saphenous vein) should be used and all preexisting prosthetic material removed.[50,51] Not infrequently, deterioration of the arterial wall precludes primary repair or patch grafting;

in this case, insertion of a bypass graft from the common carotid artery to the internal carotid artery is required.[27,54,56,59,60] If shunting is necessary, a segment of saphenous vein can be threaded on a plastic tube of the proper dimensions and the ends of this tube inserted into the orifices of the internal carotid and common carotid arteries, where it is secured by Silastic loops (Figs. 38-4 and 38-5). With the shunt in place, the distal suture line is completed first, followed by completion of the proximal suture line. Just before the last sutures of the proximal anastomosis are inserted, the graft is removed and the internal carotid and common carotid arteries are allowed to back-bleed.[56] Although implantation of the external carotid artery into the side of the graft is technically feasible, this artery can usually be ligated with impunity.[54,56]

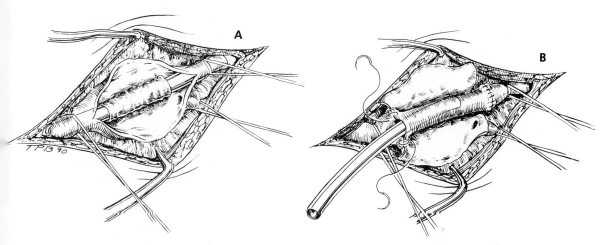

Fig. 38-4. Method of inserting a saphenous vein bypass graft during shunting of the carotid artery for reconstruction of a false aneurysm. **A,** The vein is threaded over the shunt. **B,** The shunt is removed after completion of the distal anastomosis and partial completion of the proximal anastomosis.

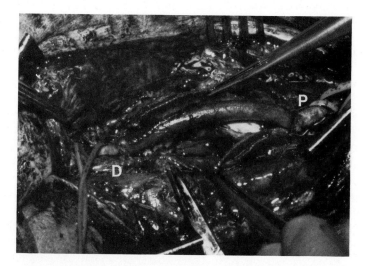

Fig. 38-5. Vein graft inserted between the common and internal carotid arteries for repair of a recurrent false aneurysm. Clamps are on the Dacron portion of the wall of the aneurysm. *P,* proximal anastomosis; *D,* distal anastomosis. (Same case as in Fig. 38-3.)

When scarring precludes distal control of the internal carotid artery, a balloon-tipped shunt of the Pruit-Inahara variety may be used. After the anastomoses are completed and flow is restored, the excess aneurysm wall is débrided and any infected prosthetic material removed. Regardless of the type of repair, a synthetic monofilament suture, such as polypropylene, should be used.[27]

Ligation of the contributing arteries followed by excision of the aneurysm is a rational approach when the internal carotid artery is occluded; otherwise this procedure should be undertaken only as a last resort.[51,56] Unfortunately, there may be no alternative in some patients with extensive infection in whom placement of an autogenous bypass is not feasible.[3] Of eight cases reviewed by Branch and Davis,[50] postoperative TIAs or stroke developed in two patients and two died of hemorrhagic infarcts.

Recurrent False Aneurysms

Hertzer[3] reported three patients and Branch and Davis[50] one patient in whom false aneurysms recurred after an initial repair of a false aneurysm with a saphenous vein patch. In each of these cases infection was the underlying cause. All four were treated with ligation and none developed a postoperative neurologic defect. Successful treatment of a recurrent false aneurysm with excision of an infected Dacron patch and replacement with a vein patch has also been described.[51] In my experience a secondary recurrence 4 years following Dacron patch repair of a primary recurrence required saphenous vein bypass grafting, and Ameli, Provan, and Keuchler[55] used Gore-Tex (W.L. Gore & Associates, Inc., Elkton, Md.) to bypass an aneurysm that developed 10 years after an initial pseudoaneurysm had been repaired with primary closure. These observations suggest that recurrent false aneurysms are more likely after patch angioplasty, especially when the initial false aneurysm is complicated by concomitant infection; but they may occur in the absence of infection even when primary closure is used.

Prevention

Although there is no certain way of preventing the occasional development of false aneu-

rysms, use of synthetic monofilament suture, precise placement of sutures, avoidance of an endarterectomy plane that weakens the residual arterial wall, and maintenance of rigorous aseptic technique will reduce the likelihood of this complication. When patching is required, it is probably best to use the saphenous vein rather than Dacron or the less sturdy jugular veins, but this remains a controversial point. Perioperative antibiotic coverage, especially when prosthetic patches are applied, diminishes the chance of infection developing and causing a false aneurysm.

POSTOPERATIVE HYPOTENSION AND HYPERTENSION

Although hypotension and hypertension can occur following any peripheral vascular operation, blood pressure instability appears to be especially common after carotid endarterectomy. This is even more remarkable when one considers that blood loss and fluid shifts, which are responsible for most postoperative circulatory problems in patients undergoing intraabdominal arterial procedures or extensive limb revascularizations, are relatively minimal during and after carotid endarterectomy. Although hypotension is generally rather benign, postoperative hypertension is often associated with neurologic deficits and mortality.

Etiology

The etiology of post–carotid endarterectomy blood pressure instability has been the subject of much speculation and considerable controversy. It is probable that there is no single cause and that the etiology in most cases is multifactorial.

Over the years the baroreceptor theory has received the most attention. Baroreceptors located in the adventitia of the internal carotid artery near its origin send afferent impulses along the carotid sinus nerve (Hering's nerve) to the glossopharyngeal nerve, which conveys these impulses to centers in the medulla oblongata (see Fig. 38-2). When the wall of the internal carotid bulb is stretched by an increasing intraluminal pressure, the cardioinhibitory center is stimulated and the vasomotor center is inhibited. The net effect is bradycardia, peripheral vasodilatation, and a fall in blood pressure.

Conversely, when stretch is reduced by a fall in intraluminal pressure, the frequency of baroreceptor firing is decreased and blood pressure falls. Thus a feedback mechanism is established to control transient fluctuations in blood pressure. Below pressures of 60 mm Hg, baroreceptors cease to discharge. Above 60 mm Hg, the rate of discharge increases commensurate with intraluminal pressure, reaching a peak at about 180 mm Hg, beyond which there is no further increase. Baroreceptors also respond to variations in pulse pressure. At a steady mean pressure, a fall in pulse pressure causes tachycardia and a rise in blood pressure. Within 1 or 2 days of a sustained change in blood pressure, baroreceptors become reset at the new level.

Post–carotid endarterectomy hypotension is explained as follows. Atheromatous plaques within the wall of the carotid artery reduce the stretch on the adventitia imposed by blood pressure and the pressure wave, causing the carotid sinus nerves to be reset at a lower level. Removal of the plaque allows the wall to stretch, stimulating the baroreceptors, which read the increased wall tension as an increased blood pressure (Fig. 38-6). The result is bradycardia and a fall in systemic blood pressure.[61-63] The observations of Angell-James and Lumley,[63] who recorded carotid sinus nerve impulses before and after carotid endarterectomy, lend support to this hypothesis. Blood pressure fell in three subjects with increased carotid sinus nerve activity, rose in two subjects with decreased nerve activity, and remained unchanged from preoperative levels in one subject with unchanged nerve activity. They also noted a direct relationship between baroreceptor activity and diameter of the carotid sinus. (A subsequent study by the same group revealed no long-term correlation between blood pressure and post–carotid endarterectomy baroreceptor function, as one would predict based on the rapidity with which the nerve sensitivity is reset.[64])

Several other facts implicate the carotid sinus as having a role in the genesis of postoperative hypotension, namely (1) hypotension seldom occurs when the carotid sinus is denervated during the operative procedure[61] and develops frequently only when efforts are made to avoid injury to the nerve[61,65]; (2) infiltration

of the carotid sinus with local anesthetic reverses postoperative hypotension[63,65]; and (3) bradycardia, another manifestation of increased baroreceptor activity, commonly accompanies the hypotension.[61,62] Even when nerve-sparing operations are performed, hypotension does not always occur, possibly because of differences in the physical properties of the plaque or because the stimulation of the ipsilateral carotid sinus nerve is overridden by baroreceptors on the opposite side or within the aortic arch.[61]

It is more difficult to explain post–carotid endarterectomy hypertension on the basis of altered carotid sinus nerve function. A commonly cited theory is that of reduced barore-

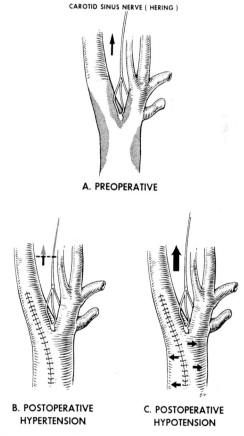

CAROTID SINUS NERVE (HERING)

A. PREOPERATIVE

B. POSTOPERATIVE
HYPERTENSION

C. POSTOPERATIVE
HYPOTENSION

Fig. 38-6. Baroreceptor mechanism for post–carotid endarterectomy hypertension and hypotension. (From Hertzer NR. Nonstroke complications of carotid endarterectomy. In Bernhard VM, Towne JB, eds. Complications in Vascular Surgery, 2nd ed. Philadelphia: WB Saunders, 1985, pp 739-752.)

ceptor activity caused by deliberate resection of the carotid sinus nerve or inadvertent damage to the nerve during dissection of the carotid bifurcation[63,65] (Fig. 38-6). That hypertension occurs more commonly following bilateral carotid endarterectomy is perhaps indirect evidence for this theory.[66]

A number of investigators, however, report no relationship between operative manipulation of the carotid sinus and the development of postoperative blood pressure instability.[62,67,68] Wade et al.,[69] using the Valsalva maneuver to evaluate baroreceptor function,[70] found that only four of eight patients undergoing bilateral carotid endarterectomy showed any appreciable diminution of function; postoperative hypotension developed in none of these patients. These studies were done 1 to 4 weeks after operation, at which time the baroreceptors should have been reset; therefore the findings may not be pertinent to the issue of postoperative hypertension. Moreover, Wade et al.[69] and Appenzeller and Descarries[71] found that baroreceptor function decreased with advancing age (>40 years) and that about one third of patients with chronic cerebrovascular disease had no baroreceptor responses whatsoever. It is possible, of course, that these observations reflect stiffening of the carotid bulb caused by aging or atherosclerosis rather than any change in the potential sensitivity of the carotid baroreceptors. In this context, it must be remembered that carotid sinus hypersensitivity, sufficient to cause transient cardiac arrest, may be seen in elderly patients with carotid plaques.[72,73]

Because alterations in baroreceptor activity do not adequately explain all cases of post–carotid endarterectomy blood pressure instability, other mechanisms have been investigated. Skydell et al.[74] suggested that loss or interference with normal cerebrovascular autoregulation (resulting from cerebral hypoxia, temporary carotid occlusion, or anesthetic agents) may cause cerebral edema, increased intracranial pressure, and—as a result—hypertension. Smith[75] proposed a central nervous system Goldblatt phenomenon based on his observation that the ratio of renin in the internal jugular vein to that in systemic arteries was significantly increased in four of six patients in whom postoperative hypertension developed. However, within 24 hours, the ratios reverted to normal levels in all patients despite the persistence of hypertension. Ahn, Marcus, and Moore[76] confirmed the increase in the cerebral/systemic renin ratios in samples drawn immediately after clamp release but found no correlation with postoperative hypertension. In their study, patients with post–carotid endarterectomy hypertension had an increase in cranial and peripheral norepinephrine levels, which was most pronounced immediately after clamp release and 2 to 6 hours postoperatively. No increase in norepinephrine levels occurred in normotensive patients. On the basis of these findings, they suggested a central nervous system sympathomimetic mechanism as the cause of postoperative hypertension, theorizing that the mechanism is activated by cerebral hypoperfusion, subclinical cerebral edema, and elevation of intracranial pressure.

Incidence

The reported incidence of hypertension following carotid endarterectomy ranges from almost nil to 62%.[61,77] This variation in part can be attributed to widely differing criteria for what constitutes hypertension. Other factors include differences in the population being studied and possibly the surgical technique employed. Towne and Bernhard,[67] who classified as hypertensive only those patients in whom there was a sustained elevation of the systolic blood pressure over 200 mm Hg during the postoperative period that required pharmacologic control, reported an incidence of 19%. On the other hand, Lehv, Salzman, and Silen[68] found that 56% of patients experienced postoperative hypertension when the criterion was an elevation greater than or equal to 15 mm Hg above the mean preoperative systolic pressure sustained over a 12-hour period. A similarly high incidence of 58% was reported by Skydell et al.[74] who defined postoperative hypertension as an increase in systolic blood pressure greater than 35 mm Hg over baseline or any blood pressure elevation requiring administration of nitroprusside. Therefore all studies dealing with post–carotid endarterectomy hypertension must be interpreted in light of the criterion employed.

Post–carotid endarterectomy hypotension

is usually defined as a greater than 40 mm Hg fall in systolic blood pressure or a systolic pressure less than 100 mm Hg requiring volume expansion or vasopressors.[61,62,65] In several studies, hypotension was rarely seen, occurring in 0% to 4% of patients.[67,74,76] Others reported an incidence ranging from 28% to 52%.[61,62,65] Those who observed a high incidence of postoperative hypotension found a low incidence of postoperative hypertension and vice versa.

Onset and Duration

Hypertension in the study of Bove et al.[62] first appeared 0 to 15 hours after operation (mean, 1.4 hours), reached a peak at an average of 2.3 hours, and lasted from 1 to 24 hours (mean, 5.6 hours). Towne and Bernhard[67] reported that hypertension resolved in less than 4 hours in 31% of patients and lasted more than 24 hours in 20%.

Hypotension was most severe at an average of 5.3 hours after carotid endarterectomy in those patients studied by Bove et al.[62] Time of onset ranged from 30 minutes to 11 hours (mean, 1.4 hours), and the duration ranged from 1 to 24 hours (mean, 14.8 hours). An occasional patient will continue to be hypotensive for several days.[61]

Risk Factors for Hypertension

Preoperative hypertension, prior contralateral carotid endarterectomy, and neurologic deficits present at the time of operation have been identified as factors predisposing to post–carotid endarterectomy hypertension.

Reflecting the general composition of the population with cerebrovascular disease, preoperative hypertension was present in 62% of the patients studied by Towne and Bernhard.[67] Of these, 35% were normotensive on medication, whereas the remainder were uncontrolled, either because they were not being treated (20%) or were inadequately treated (45%). Eighty percent of the patients who developed post–carotid endarterectomy hypertension (a sustained elevation of systolic blood pressure over 200 mm Hg) were hypertensive preoperatively, whereas only 57% of those who did not become hypertensive in the postoperative period were hypertensive preoperatively. Looked at in another way, only 10% of normotensive

patients became hypertensive after carotid endarterectomy, but 25% of those who were hypertensive and 30% of those with uncontrolled hypertension developed the complication. These results were statistically significant. Although other investigators have noted a similar relationship,[62,65,78] some have failed to find a correlation between preoperative and postoperative hypertension.[68,74]

Schroeder, Sillesen, and Engell[78] studied 56 patients who underwent staged bilateral carotid endarterectomies. After the second operation, 39% of the patients became hypertensive compared with only 23% after the first operation (p <.05). When the second procedure was done within 3 weeks of the first, 48% of the patients developed hypertension; but when the operations were staged at a longer interval, only 8% became hypertensive. Satiani, Vasko, and Evans[66] also noted a trend toward higher blood pressure after the second operation, but, unlike the observations of Schroeder, Sillesen, and Engell, the increase was significant only in those patients whose procedures were separated by more than 60 days.

Lehv, Salzman, and Silen[68] reported the appearance of post–carotid endarterectomy hypertension in 68% of patients in whom there was a preoperative neurologic deficit or an altered level of consciousness. In contrast, only 28% of neurologically intact patients developed hypertension. This report was based on operations performed between 1966 and 1968; currently, few of the patients included in this study with overt neurologic problems would be considered candidates for carotid endarterectomy. Other authors have found no association between preexisting neurologic deficits and post–carotid endarterectomy hypertension.[65,74]

Three of 10 patients with postoperative hypertension in the series of Cafferata, Merchant, and DePalma,[65] had undergone surgical denervation of the carotid sinus during the course of carotid endarterectomy, which prompted these investigators to suggest a causative relationship. The opposite conclusion was reached by Towne and Bernhard,[67] who observed an almost identical incidence of postoperative hypertension in patients in whom the carotid sinus nerves were completely divided (23.8%)

and in those in whom every effort was made to preserve the nerves (24.1%).

Diabetes mellitus, use of isoflurane anesthesia, peripheral pulse deficits, preoperative TIAs, and ipsilateral carotid stenosis were identified as statistically significant risk factors for post–carotid endarterectomy hypertension by Skydell et al.[74] Most studies fail to demonstrate a correlation between postoperative hypertension and blood loss or replacement, fluid administration, anesthetic used, antihypertensive medications, diabetes, associated peripheral vascular or coronary artery disease, degree of ipsilateral or contralateral internal carotid stenosis, or indications for operation.[62,65,67,68] Towne and Bernhard,[67] however, noted that 94% of postoperatively hypertensive patients had either preoperative hypertension or >75% stenosis of the internal carotid artery, or both. Similar findings were present in only 78% of those in whom hypertension did not develop.

Risk Factors for Hypotension

The observations of Tarlov et al.[61] suggest that preoperative hypovolemia, manifested by a low central venous pressure, contributes to the development of post–carotid endarterectomy hypotension. According to Cafferata, Merchant, and DePalma,[65] hypotension developed in about 50% of patients who underwent operations designed to spare the carotid sinus nerve, irrespective of their preoperative blood pressure status. Similar results (a 40% incidence of hypotension) were reported by Tarlov et al.[61] when this nerve was spared. Although Bove et al.[62] observed a higher preoperative blood pressure and pulse pressure in patients in whom postoperative hypotension developed than in those who remained normotensive, others have not noted this association.[65]

Morbidity and Mortality

In the series reported by Towne and Bernhard,[67] 10.2% of patients who developed post–carotid endarterectomy hypertension suffered neurologic deficits (three permanent, two temporary) on the day of surgery, whereas only 3.4% of those who remained normotensive did so. These events, however, were all thromboembolic and could not be attributed directly to

hypertension. Nonetheless, the development of postoperative hypertension was the first indication of an impending neurologic problem in several patients. The only deaths in the series occurred in the postoperatively hypertensive patients.

An even more striking association between postoperative hypertension and deteriorating neurologic status was reported by Lehv, Salzman, and Silen,[68] who noted that 47% of these patients demonstrated worsening of preexisting neurologic deficits, appearance of new deficits, or altered level of consciousness. In contrast, none of the normotensive patients experienced neurologic problems. On the other hand, Satiani, Vasko, and Evans[66] found no association between postoperative strokes and postoperative hypertension, although strokes were statistically more frequent (20%) in patients who were being treated with antihypertensive medications before operation than in those not receiving antihypertensive medication (5%). Hypertension is also thought to increase the risk of postoperative intracerebral hemorrhage (see below).[79,80]

In the series reported by Bove et al.,[62] no strokes occurred in patients who were normotensive postoperatively, but 10% of the hypertensive patients and 7% of the hypotensive patients suffered neurologic deficits. Of 195 patients undergoing carotid endarterectomy in the series reported by Owens and Wilson,[81] postoperative hypotension developed in 18 (9%), and five (28%) of these patients suffered neurologic deficits (three strokes and two TIAs). Half of the strokes in the entire series were attributed to hypotension. Severe intraoperative hypotension, which can be devastating, accounted for 19% of the perioperative strokes reported by Imparato et al.[82] In general, however, hypotension does not seem to be a major risk factor for postoperative stroke, but it may have adverse consequences in those patients with significant coronary artery occlusive disease.[61,65]

Treatment and Prevention

Control of hypertension preoperatively is the single most important method for preventing this complication in the postoperative period. When carotid endarterectomy is elective, a few days or even weeks spent adjusting to antihypertensive medication is time well spent. Although there is no conclusive evidence supporting the efficacy of operations that preserve the nerve supply to the carotid bifurcation, surgeons who use this technique seem to have a lower incidence of postoperative hypertension.[61,65] The technique involves studiously avoiding dissection of the tissues in the area between the internal carotid and external carotid arteries. Control of the external carotid artery is obtained distal to the origin of the superior thyroid artery, and control of the internal carotid artery is secured several centimeters beyond the bifurcation distal to the carotid bulb. The arteriotomy is made toward the lateral side of the internal carotid artery. This technique has the added advantage of minimizing troublesome bleeding from the highly vascular tissues between the two arteries.

Dangerously high levels of blood pressure occurring in the postoperative period can be managed by an intravenous drip of sodium nitroprusside or nitroglycerine. Use of an intra-arterial pressure monitor is critical to the safe titration of these drugs to prevent sudden severe depression of blood pressure and potentially hazardous pressure swings. Once the patient is able to tolerate oral intake, oral administration of antihypertensive agents should be commenced, especially if the patient was taking these drugs preoperatively. Towne and Bernhard[62] recommend institution of aggressive treatment if the systolic blood pressure rises above 200 mm Hg. They strive to maintain the systolic blood pressure between 160 to 200 mm Hg. Others begin therapy when the systolic blood pressure exceeds 180 mm Hg or when the diastolic pressure rises above 100 mm Hg.[65,76] Even tighter pharmacologic control has been advocated by Baker,[83] who attempts to keep postoperative blood pressures lower than 110% of the highest recorded preoperative systolic pressure and higher than 90% of the lowest recorded preoperative pressure. The dangers of moderate elevations of blood pressure probably do not justify such stringent control.[66]

Maintaining an adequate blood volume by the judicious infusion of fluids before and during operation is the best method for avoiding post–carotid endarterectomy hypotension.[61] Management based on the central venous pressure or preferably the pulmonary wedge pressure will permit this to be done without risking fluid overload. Although complete denervation of the carotid sinus has been shown to reduce the incidence of hypotension, this technique is not recommended since it may predispose to postoperative hypertension.[61] Bradycardia and hypotension occurring during operative manipulation of the carotid bifurcation are effectively controlled by the injection of 1 ml or less of 1% lidocaine (without epinephrine) into the tissues between the internal carotid and external carotid arteries. Such injections do not affect the incidence of postoperative hypertension or hypotension.[62]

Since post–carotid endarterectomy hypotension is ordinarily benign, most patients who are alert, conversant, and who display no neurologic deficit probably do not require treatment.[65] Patients in whom the pulmonary wedge or central venous pressures are low can often be managed by the administration of fluid therapy alone.[61,62,65] More recalcitrant cases, in which hypotension is largely caused by peripheral vasodilatation, require a carefully monitored intravenous drip of phenylephrine hydrochloride (Neo-Synephrine) or epinephrine. In the series reported by Bove et al.,[62] 47% of the hypotensive patients were treated with vasopressors, 28% received fluid therapy alone, and 25% received no specific treatment. Treatment is usually reserved for patients with systolic blood pressures less than 100 mm Hg. Cafferata, Merchant, and DePalma[65] and Angell–James and Lumley[63] have demonstrated that post–carotid endarterectomy hypotension can be reversed by the injection of lidocaine into the region of the carotid sinus through a cannula left in place at the time of surgery. Blood pressure begins to rise within 5 minutes of instillation and the effect is maintained for 45 to 90 minutes. Because of the relative infrequency of serious postoperative hypotension, this technique has not gained wide acceptance.

HYPERPERFUSION SYNDROME

Autoregulation of the cerebral vasculature tends to maintain cerebral blood flow at a relatively constant level (about 50 ml/100 gm of tissue/min) over a wide range of perfusion pressures, extending from 60 mm Hg to 160 mm Hg.[84,85] Below 60 mm Hg, resistance vessels become maximally dilated, autoregulatory function is lost, and flow becomes directly responsive to changes in perfusion pressure. Distal to a tight stenosis of the internal carotid artery, blood pressures are reduced, the extent of the reduction depending not only on the hemodynamic effects of the stenosis, but also on the adequacy of the collateral circulation. When perfusion pressures are low, compensatory dilatation of the cerebrovascular bed usually maintains blood flow at near normal levels (or at slightly reduced levels compared with those of the opposite hemisphere). Autoregulation, however, is impaired to a variable extent.[86] When blood flow is restored after a tight stenosis has been removed, flow to the ipsilateral hemisphere is increased compared with the preoperative flow level. Removal of the obstruction subjects the low resistance (passive) vascular bed to systemic pressure without the protective effect of autoregulation. Flow may increase by 100% to 400% within hours after release of the occluding clamps and may remain elevated for several days.[87-90] (Hyperperfusion either does not occur or is much less pronounced when stenoses are less severe and when they are not associated with a significant pressure gradient.[89,90]) Autoregulation begins to return within days and by 3 months postoperatively is completely restored.[86] During the period of post–carotid endarterectomy hyperemia, however, the cerebral microvasculature is subjected to abnormally high pressures, leading directly or indirectly to a constellation of adverse events (headache, seizures, cerebral hemorrhage), which have been ascribed to the hyperperfusion syndrome.

Headache

Although headache has been reported in 42% of patients following carotid endarterectomy, severe headaches are rare.[91,92] Of interest are those severe headaches of a pulsatile, throbbing nature that present suddenly 36 to 72 hours after an uneventful carotid endarterectomy.[93] These headaches are ipsilateral to the side of endarterectomy; involve the temple, forehead, and retrobulbar region; are often accompanied by nausea; and are clinically indistinguishable from classic migraine. The patient may experience paresthesias or minor neurologic deficits in the face or arm on the side opposite the endarterectomy.[92] Attacks occur regularly for days to weeks (lasting for 4 to 8 hours) and then spontaneously subside, disappearing entirely after 1 to 6 months.[92] Typically, the headaches respond poorly to analgesics and ergotamine. Although some patients have a history of migraine, others do not.[92,94] There is no consistent relationship to postoperative hypertension, but severe hypertension has been reported in conjunction with postoperative headache.[95] The degree of preoperative carotid stenosis, however, does appear to have a significant effect on the incidence of post–carotid endarterectomy headache. In the study of Akers et al.,[96] 30% of patients operated on for high-grade carotid obstruction (>70% diameter reduction) developed severe headaches but only 7% of the patients with lesser degrees of stenosis did so.

The cause remains unclear, but it has been postulated that headache results from postoperative distention of cerebral vessels previously protected by a stenotic plaque from normal pressure levels.[93] The delayed onset several days after endarterectomy is not easily explained by this mechanism. A disturbance of autoregulation may be responsible and fits with the self-limited nature of the headache. Some authors attribute headache to manipulation of the carotid sinus or damage to the sympathetic chain, which may alter regional cerebral blood flow.[91,92]

Seizures

Focal motor seizures complicate from 0.4% to 1.3% of carotid endarterectomies.[97,98] Seizures typically occur in patients with longstanding severe chronic ischemia who undergo correction of high-grade carotid stenosis.[97,98] Of ten patients reported by Reigel et al.,[98] five had unilateral stenoses exceeding 98%, three had bilateral high-grade stenosis, and two had high-grade stenosis and contralateral occlusion. Although about 40% of patents who develop seizures have had a prior stroke, stroke does not appear to be a risk factor. Also, preoperative and postoperative hypertension have not been implicated as risk factors (although in at least one report seizures were preceded by severe hypertension).[95,97] CT scans obtained after seizures are negative or show no change from preoperative studies.[98] Likewise, postoperative carotid arteriograms have demonstrated patency of the reconstruction and provide no explanation for the seizures.

Seizures are almost invariably preceded by severe headaches that occur ipsilateral to the side of endarterectomy on the first to the seventh postoperative day. Seizure activity begins on the third to the eleventh postoperative day and involves the side opposite that of the carotid endarterectomy. Periodic lateralizing epileptiform discharges (PLEDs) are consistently recorded on the EEG.[98] Generalized convulsions may follow focal seizures, and postictal paralysis is common.[97,98] The seizures are frequently difficult to control, requiring diazepam and phenobarbital in addition to phenytoin. Although the majority of patients recover without neurologic sequelae and remain seizure free on an appropriate medication regimen, 3 of 18 patients (17%) reviewed by Youkey et al.[97] developed intracerebral hemorrhage, two of whom died. Reigel et al.[98] reported a 44% incidence of cerebral infarction following seizure but did not indicate how many patients died.

Using the xenon-133 technique, Reigel et al.[98] measured cerebral blood flow before and after carotid endarterectomy in six patients who subsequently developed seizures.[98] Flow increased in all six from an average pre-endarterectomy level of 34 ml/100 gm of brain tissue/min to 88 ml/100 gm/min after clamp release. In four of the six patients, the post–endarterectomy flow rate was three to four times baseline. Similar observations had previously been made by Sundt et al.[99] who noted an increase of more than 100% in regional cerebral blood flow in all of their patients with postoperative seizures. Thus, like postoperative headache, seizure ac-

Table 38-3. Incidence of Perioperative Myocardial Infarction and Mortality in Patients Undergoing Carotid Endarterectomy*

Author	No.	Total no. of MI (%)	No. of fatal MI (%)	Total no. of deaths (%)	No. of fatal MI/ total no. of MI (%)	No. of fatal MI/ total no. of deaths (%)
Thompson et al.[109] (1970)	748	—	5 (0.7)	20 (2.7)	—	5/20 (25.0)
Riles et al.[113] (1979)	683	16 (2.3)	5 (0.7)	—	5/16 (31.3)	—
Ennix et al.[108] (1979)	1391	21 (1.5)	13 (0.9)	29 (2.1)	13/21 (61.9)	13/29 (44.8)
Hertzer and Lees[111] (1981)	390	—	6 (1.5)	10 (2.6)	—	6/10 (60.0)
O'Donnell et al.[110] (1983)	509	13 (2.6)	3 (0.6)	5 (1.0)	3/13 (23.1)	3/5 (60.0)
Till et al.[107] (1987)	389	5 (1.3)	3 (0.8)	9 (2.3)	3/5 (60.0)	3/9 (33.3)
Rubin et al.[106] (1988)	8535	—	60 (0.7)	135 (1.6)	—	60/135 (44.4)
Kirshner et al.[24] (1989)	1035	23 (2.2)	2 (0.2)	14 (1.4)	2/23 (8.7)	2/14 (14.3)
Yeager et al.[112] (1989)	249	10 (4.0)	1 (0.4)	3 (1.2)	1/10 (10.0)	1/3 (33.3)
TOTAL WITH COMPLETE DATA†	3573	72 (2.0)	22 (0.6)	60 (1.7)	22/72 (30.6)	22/60 (36.7)

MI, myocardial infarction.
*Excludes concomitant or staged carotid endarterectomy and CABG.
†Total of references 24, 107, 108, 110, 112.

tivity seems to be a manifestation of hyperperfusion. Lack of cerebral autoregulation even in the normotensive patient would subject fragile terminal vessels to increased pressure, causing local edema or pericapillary microhemorrhage. Although Wilkinson, Adams, and Wright[100] have suggested that post–carotid endarterectomy seizures are caused by emboli arising from the operative site, arteriographic and CT scan evidence does not support this theory.

Patients who have undergone carotid endarterectomy for poorly collateralized high-grade stenosis and who develop severe postoperative headaches should be observed closely for seizure activity.[98] If EEG evidence of epileptiform discharges are noted or if seizures occur, a regimen of anticonvulsant medication (phenytoin, diazepam, phenobarbital) should be instituted. Some advocate instituting phenytoin administration with the onset of headache.[97] Treatment is continued for a minimum of 3 to 6 months or longer if the EEG remains abnormal. Because of the risk of intracerebral hemorrhage, patients with seizures should undergo CT scanning. For the same reason, anticoagulants should be avoided if at all possible.

Cerebral Hemorrhage

Revascularization of totally occluded or severely stenotic internal carotid arteries in patients with acute strokes has long been known to result in a high incidence of fatal postoperative cerebral hemorrhage.[101,102] In these cases restoration of blood flow at systemic pressure to the acutely ischemic tissues adjacent to a previously infarcted area of brain is the generally accepted treatment mechanism.[103] Although operations on totally occluded arteries and on patients with acute stroke have largely been abandoned, cerebral hemorrhage continues to account for approximately 20% of perioperative strokes.[80,82]

In two recent reports, the incidence of post–carotid endarterectomy cerebral hemorrhage was 0.6% and 0.7%, respectively.[80,90] Salient facts emerging from these reports were (1) hemorrhage occurred on the side ipsilateral to the endarterectomy between the first and thirteenth postoperative day, (2) all patients in whom hemorrhage developed had undergone

operation for high-grade carotid stenosis and most had lesions that compromised the lumen by >90%, and (3) there was no apparent relationship between the occurrence of hemorrhage and age, preoperative hypertension, preoperative CT scan findings, or history of cerebral infarction. Postoperative hypertension with systolic blood pressures of 200 to 240 mm Hg was present in 6 of the 11 patients (55%) in the series of Pomposelli et al.[80] and was also present in two patients reported by Caplan et al.[79] Although hypertension undoubtedly increases the risk of hemorrhage, it is clearly not a prerequisite.

In 9 of 14 patients (64%) with cerebral hemorrhage reported by Piepgras et al.,[90] cerebral blood flow increased more than 100% following endarterectomy. This contrasts to a 12% incidence of hyperperfusion in the general population of patients undergoing carotid endarterectomy. These findings, coupled with the observation that hemorrhage develops only in those patients in whom a severe stenosis has been corrected, strongly suggests that lack of autoregulation and restoration of blood flow to a region of the brain previously shielded from normal (or hypertensive) pressures is in some way responsible for the breakdown in the blood-brain barrier. It is not clear, however, why the patient usually has several symptom-free days before the catastrophe occurs. Although headache and seizures may precede the event, hemiparesis is the most common presentation.[80]

There is no certain way of preventing cerebral hemorrhage, but careful attention to blood pressure control lessens the stress placed on the cerebrovascular bed. In patients who have suffered a stroke, it is probably advisable to delay operation for 4 to 6 weeks, especially when the CT scan shows marked contrast enhancement, indicating breakdown of the blood-brain barrier or excessive regional perfusion.[104] Once cerebral hemorrhage develops, the mortality rate is high (36% in the report of Pomposelli et al.[80]) but complete recovery is possible. Blood pressure control is the mainstay of treatment. Craniotomy is reserved for patients with a progressing deficit and a hematoma that can be evacuated.

Other Complications of Hyperperfusion

Akers et al.[96] noted that 92% of patients who underwent carotid endarterectomy for high-grade lesions experienced increased fatigue, lethargy, and somnolence for 6 to 8 weeks following operation. In contrast only 5% of patients with less severe lesions had similar symptoms. Moreover, 22% of those with high-grade lesions developed postoperative psychiatric disturbances, including paranoid ideation and depression—symptoms also noted by Reigel et al.[98] They attributed these findings to metabolic derangement associated with cerebral hyperperfusion.

Inappropriate antidiuretic hormone secretion, characterized by marked hyponatremia, low serum osmolality, and inappropriately high urine osmolality, has been reported following carotid endarterectomy.[105] Reperfusion injury to a small area of persistent ischemia was postulated to be the cause.

POSTOPERATIVE MYOCARDIAL INFARCTION

Myocardial infarction remains a major cause of death in the first 30 days following carotid endarterectomy (Table 38-3).[24,106-113] In some series cardiac events have been responsible for as many as 60% of the deaths.[110,111] Roughly 2% of patients undergoing carotid endarterectomy experience a myocardial infarction in the postoperative period, of which approximately one third are fatal. Over a 14-year period, our group performed 535 carotid endarterectomies. Seven deaths occurred during the first 30 postoperative days (1.3% mortality), three (43%) of which were caused by myocardial infarction. Following bilateral carotid endarterectomy, T wave inversions in leads I, II, aV$_1$, and V$_2$ through V$_6$ have been observed in the absence of isoenzyme changes or clinical evidence of myocardial infarction.[114] It has been postulated that these changes are caused by increased cardiovascular sympathetic activity resulting from bilateral denervation of the carotid sinuses. Thus not all post–carotid endarterectomy ECG changes signify a myocardial infarction.

Patients with symptomatic coronary artery disease (CAD) (angina pectoris, congestive heart failure, and arrhythmias) are 3 to 16 times more likely to suffer a myocardial infarction than those without symptoms and are far more likely to die of the event (Table 38-4). In the absence of symptoms, an abnormal ECG showing evidence of an old myocardial infarction or nonspecific ST-T wave changes is less consistently predictive.[110-112] Hypertension also has little effect, but diabetes appears to increase the risk of perioperative myocardial infarction.[24,112,113,115] Asymptomatic patients who have had a myocardial infarction in the past may not have an appreciably elevated risk.[108]

Because of the widespread distribution of atherosclerotic plaques, it comes as no surprise that many patients with carotid artery disease

Table 38-4. Incidence of Post–carotid Endarterectomy Myocardial Infarction and Fatal Myocardial Infarction in Patients With and Without Symptoms of CAD*

Author	Symptomatic CAD			No symptoms of CAD		
	No.	Total no. of MI (%)	No. of fatal MI (%)	No.	Total no. of MI (%)	No. of fatal MI (%)
Riles et al.[113] (1979)	284	14 (4.9)	5 (1.8)	399	2 (0.5)	0 (0.0)
Ennix et al.[108] (1979)	85	11 (12.9)	11 (12.9)	1306	10 (0.8)	2 (0.2)
Hertzer and Lees et al.[111] (1981)	160	—	5 (3.1)	175	—	1 (0.6)
O'Donnell et al.[110] (1983)	274	11 (4.0)	3 (1.1)	235	2 (0.9)	0 (0.0)
Yeager et al.[112] (1989)	114	7 (6.1)	1 (0.9)	135	3 (2.2)	0 (0.0)
TOTAL WITH COMPLETE DATA†	757	43 (5.7)	20 (2.6)	2075	17 (0.8)	2 (0.1)

MI, myocardial infarction.
*Excludes concomitant or staged carotid endarterectomy and CABG.
†Total of references 108, 110, 112, 113.

also have lesions in their coronary arteries. The almost ubiquitous nature of coronary involvement in this group is, however, somewhat unexpected. To gain insight into the problem, Hertzer et al.[115] performed coronary arteriograms on 506 consecutive patients who were being evaluated for carotid endarterectomy, regardless of the presence or absence of cardiac symptoms. As shown in Table 38-5, 93% of the patients had angiographic evidence of CAD; and in 34%, the lesions were classified as severe. As anticipated, the prevalence of severe disease was higher in symptomatic that in asymptomatic subjects, but it was disquieting to discover that almost 18% of patients who had no clinical symptoms or signs of cardiac disease also had severe coronary lesions. Similar findings were reported by Rokey et al.,[116] who performed exercise thallium-201 scintigraphy and exercise radionuclide ventriculography on 50 consecutive patients with cerebrovascular symptoms. Positive scans were found in 15 of 16 patients (94%) with symptoms suggestive of cardiac disease and in 14 of 34 patients (41%) without cardiac symptoms. Thus it seems prudent to maintain a high index of suspicion for the presence of CAD in all patients being considered for carotid endarterectomy, even in the absence of overt cardiac symptoms.

Prevention

Based on their observation that almost 13% of patients with symptoms of CAD died of myocardial infarction following carotid endar-terectomy, whereas only 0.2% of patients without cardiac symptoms undergoing the same procedure did so, Ennix et al.[108] recommended an aggressive approach to the diagnoses of CAD in symptomatic patients (Table 38-4). Noting that only 2.6% of a parallel series of patients who had either undergone coronary artery bypass grafting (CABG) before or at the time of carotid endarterectomy suffered a postoperative myocardial infarction and that only 0.6% died of a cardiac event, they believed that consideration should be given to concomitant CABG in all patients in whom significant correctable CAD was disclosed during the preoperative workup.

Adopting a similar stance, Hertzer and colleagues[115,117,118] at the Cleveland Clinic recommend obtaining coronary arteriograms before undertaking carotid endarterectomy in patients with an abnormal ECG or angina pectoris. Patients who are asymptomatic or have mild stable angina first undergo cardiac screening with stress ECG and thallium-201 scintigraphy; those with positive findings are then referred for coronary arteriography. Staged or simultaneous CABG is advocated when severe correctable coronary lesions are found. In patients with neurologic symptoms and stable cardiac disease, carotid endarterectomy is performed several days before elective CABG. Combined procedures are reserved for those with active neurologic symptoms and diffuse or unstable CAD. Hertzer and his associates argue not so much that this approach reduces the

Table 38-5. Angiographic Classification of CAD in 506 Patients With Cerebrovascular Disease*

Angiographic classification	Clinical indications of CAD		
	None no. (%)	Suspected no. (%)	Total no. (%)
Normal coronary arteries	27 (13.5)	9 (2.9)	36 (7.1)
Mild to moderate CAD	93 (46.5)	49 (16.0)	142 (28.1)
Advanced but compensated CAD	45 (22.5)	109 (35.6)	154 (30.4)
Severe correctable CAD	32 (16.0)	109 (35.6)	141 (27.9)
Severe inoperable CAD	3 (1.5)	30 (9.8)	33 (6.5)
TOTAL	200 (100)	306 (100)	506 (100)

*Modified from Hertzer NR, Young JR, Beven EG, et al. Coronary angiography in 506 patients with extracranial cerebrovascular disease. Arch Intern Med 145:849-852, 1985. Copyright 1985, American Medical Association.

short-term mortality of carotid endarterectomy, but that it significantly reduces long-term mortality, almost equating it in their experience to that of post–carotid endarterectomy patients without significant CAD. (Approximately 25% to 60% of all long-term deaths following carotid endarterectomy are attributable to cardiac causes.[109,111,112,119]) After preliminary coronary arteriography in a series of 295 patients presenting to the Cleveland Clinic with cerebrovascular disease, 71 patients underwent CABG either as a staged procedure or in conjunction with 293 carotid endarterectomies, with an overall perioperative mortality for the two procedures of 1.8%.[118] In a follow-up study of patients presenting for treatment of cerebrovascular disease, actuarial survival at 5 years (including perioperative risk) was 91% for those with normal coronary arteries or with mild to moderate CAD and 76% for those who also underwent CABG (Fig. 38-7). These results were superior to the 5-year survival of 60% for patients with advanced but compensated CAD and 41% with severe uncorrected or

inoperable coronary disease.[3] A similar beneficial effect of CABG on late mortality in patients following carotid endarterectomy has been noted by Bernstein et al.[120]

Most surgeons, however, are less inclined to recommend coronary arteriography in patients presenting for carotid endarterectomy and are more restrictive in their indications for CABG (see Ch. 3). First, roughly 50% of all patients with carotid lesions have symptoms of CAD, a history of myocardial infarction, or ECG changes; even in this group, the risk of a fatal myocardial infarction is relatively low, ranging from 0.9% to 3.1% in most series (Table 38-4). In patients without cardiac symptoms or signs, the risk of a fatal cardiac event is far less than 1%. Therefore it is doubtful that general application of aggressive diagnostic measures designed to detect severe CAD can be justified on a cost-benefit basis, even if restricted to all patients with symptomatic CAD.[110,112] Second, CABG is not without risk in patients with cerebrovascular disease. A collective review of 26 series of 1345 conjointly performed carotid endarterectomies and CABG disclosed a cumulative operative mortality of 5.7%, a 3.8% incidence of perioperative myocardial infarction, and a 3% incidence of perioperative stroke.[121] Admittedly, these procedures were performed on seriously ill patients, so the relatively high incidence of complications is perhaps acceptable. Also, it must be recognized that there are individual series with very low complication rates.[121] Nonetheless, the combined procedure is not to be undertaken without serious consideration of alternatives.

Riles and Pasternack[122] reported three post–carotid endarterectomy myocardial infarctions (7% incidence, none fatal) in 26 patients with angiographically demonstrated CAD. Fifty-one percent had a history of a previous myocardial infarction; 60% had angina at rest; and 81% experienced angina with exertion. As a result of this favorable experience, combined carotid endarterectomy and CABG grafting is rarely performed at their center. When the combined procedure is done, the indication is always one of protecting the bypass patient from stroke rather than protecting the patient with carotid artery disease from myocardial

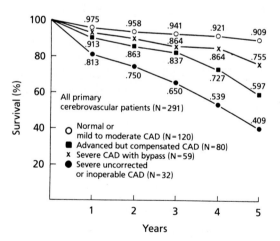

Fig. 38-7. Cumulative 5-year post–carotid endarterectomy survival of patients presenting to the Cleveland Clinic for therapy of extracranial carotid lesions, all of whom underwent coronary arteriography and were treated accordingly. (From Hertzer NR. Postoperative management and complications following carotid endarterectomy. In Rutherford RB, ed. Vascular Surgery, 3rd ed. Philadelphia: WB Saunders, 1989, pp 1451-1471.)

infarction. They attribute their low complication rate to the use of local rather than general anesthesia, close monitoring during surgery, and administration of coronary protective drugs when indicated. Similarly, surgeons at the University of Oregon believe that extensive screening designed to identify potential CABG candidates is rarely indicated, the exception being patients with unstable angina.[112] Unlike the Cleveland Clinic group, they found no appreciable difference in the long-term survival of patients following carotid endarterectomy regardless of their preoperative cardiac symptoms or whether they had undergone preceding or subsequent CABG.

O'Donnell et al.[110] reserve combined carotid endarterectomy and CABG for patients with crescendo angina or decubitus angina who have symptomatic carotid artery disease or asymptomatic bilateral stenoses, ipsilateral stenosis and contralateral occlusion, or unilateral high-grade stenosis. They advocate the use of the Goldman risk factor index[123] to help select patients for coronary arteriography. In class II and class III patients with or without stable angina, surgery is delayed while attempts are made to reduce risk factors, such as congestive heart failure or cardiac arrhythmias, by medical treatment. If these measures do not permit reclassification to class I, radionuclide studies and exercise or cold pressor tests are performed. If these tests indicate significant myocardial ischemia, the patients are referred for coronary arteriography. Class IV patients are not subjected to carotid endarterectomy. Included among the tests that may be used to identify the patient at risk for a postoperative cardiac event are exercise ECG (ST depression), exercise thallium-201 scanning (perfusion defect), dipyridamole thallium-201 scanning (perfusion defect or redistribution), radionuclide arteriography (ejection fraction and wall motion), and B–mode scanning (wall motion and ejection fraction).[124] Of these, dipyridamole thallium-201 scanning appears to be the most sensitive.

In addition to the proper selection of patients for carotid endarterectomy, careful management of anesthesia and close scrutiny of hemodynamic parameters by means of radial artery pressure monitors and Swan-Ganz catheters is essential. Although blood pressure must be maintained at a level high enough to ensure coronary and cerebral perfusion, hypertension, which increases the afterload, left ventricular work, and metabolic requirements of the myocardium, must be avoided.[110] In fact, there is evidence that the use of vasopressors during operation increases the risk of postoperative myocardial infarction.[113] On the other hand, the judicious use of β-blockers, inotropic agents, and coronary vasodilators will reduce the likelihood of postoperative myocardial infarction.[112]

In summary, concomitant carotid endarterectomy and CAD bypass is seldom indicated in patients presenting with cerebrovascular disease, but close attention to the identification of CAD and its preoperative and postoperative management is necessary if the incidence of postoperative myocardial infarction is to be minimized. The decision as to whether to perform carotid endarterectomy as a staged procedure before or at the time of CABG in patients with symptomatic or asymptomatic carotid disease presenting primarily for myocardial revascularization is another issue, which is beyond the scope of this chapter.

REFERENCES

1. Dehn TCB, Taylor GW. Cranial and cervical nerve damage associated with carotid endarterectomy. Br J Surg 70:365-368, 1983.
2. Aldoori MI, Baird RN. Local neurological complications during carotid endarterectomy. J Cardiovasc Surg 29:432-436, 1988.
3. Hertzer NR. Postoperative management and complications following carotid endarterectomy. In Rutherford RB, ed. Vascular Surgery, 3rd ed. Philadelphia: WB Saunders, 1989, pp, 1451-1471.
4. Verta MJ, Applebaum EL, McClusky DA, Yao JST, Bergan JJ. Cranial nerve injury during carotid endarterectomy. Ann Surg 185:192-195, 1977.
5. Liapis CD, Santiani B, Florance CL, Evans WE. Motor speech malfunction following carotid endarterectomy. Surgery 89:56-59, 1981.
6. Sundt TM Jr. Exposure of the high carotid bifurcation. Postgraduate course #17: Peripheral Vascular Surgery. Presented at the Meeting of the American College of Surgeons. San Francisco: Oct. 9, 1990.
7. Hertzer NR, Feldman BJ, Beven EG, Tucker HM. A prospective study of the incidence of injury to the cranial nerves during carotid endarterectomy. Surg Gynecol Obstet 151:781-784, 1980.

8. Matsumoto GH, Cossman D, Callow AD. Hazards and safeguards during carotid endarterectomy: Technical considerations. Am J Surg 133:458-462, 1977.

9. Massey EW, Heyman A, Utley C, Haynes C, Fuchs J. Cranial nerve paralysis following carotid endarterectomy. Stroke 15:157-159, 1984.

10. Imparato AM, Bracco A, Kim GE, Bergmann L. The hypoglossal nerve in carotid arterial reconstruction. Stroke 3:576-578, 1972.

11. Theodotou B, Mahaley MS Jr. Injury of the peripheral cranial nerves during carotid endarterectomy. Stroke 16:894-895, 1985.

12. Evans WE, Mendelowitz DS, Liapis C, Wolfe V, Florence CL. Motor speech deficit following carotid endarterectomy. Ann Surg 196:461-464, 1982.

13. Gutrecht JA, Jones HR Jr. Bilateral hypoglossal nerve injury after bilateral carotid endarterectomy. Stroke 19:261-262, 1988.

14. Satiani B, Liapis C, Pflug B, Vasko JS, Evans WS. Role of staging in bilateral carotid endarterectomy. Surgery 84:784-792, 1978.

15. Bageant TE, Tondini D, Lysons D. Bilateral hypoglossal-nerve palsy following a second carotid endarterectomy. Anesthesiology 43:595-596, 1975.

16. Stewart GR, Mountain JC, Colcock BP. Non-recurrent laryngeal nerve. Br J Surg 59:379-381, 1972.

17. Miehlke A. Rehabilitation of vocal cord paralysis. Studies using the vagus recurrent hypass anastomosis, type ramus posterior shunt. Arch Otolaryngol 100:431-441, 1974.

18. Sannella NA, Tober RL, Cipro RP, Pedicino JF, Donovan E, Gabriel N. Vocal cord paralysis following carotid endarterectomy: The paradox of return of function. Ann Vasc Surg 4:42-45, 1990.

19. Welch EL, Geary JE. Vocal cord paralysis following carotid endarterectomy. J Cardiovasc Surg 20:393-394, 1979.

20. Rosenbloom M, Friedman SG, Lamparello PJ, Riles TS, Imparato AM. Glossopharyngeal nerve injury complicating carotid endarterectomy. J Vasc Surg 5:469-471, 1987.

21. Tucker JA, Gee W, Nicholas GG, McDonald KM, Goodreau JJ. Accessory nerve injury during carotid endarterectomy. J Vasc Surg 5:440-444, 1987.

22. Bryant MF. Complications associated with carotid endarterectomy. Am Surg 42:665-669, 1976.

23. Krupski WC, Effeney DJ, Goldstone J, Deuel M, Webb RL, Etheredge SN, Ehrenfeld WK, Stoney RJ. Carotid endarterectomy in a metropolitan community: Comparison of results from three institutions. Surgery 98:492-499, 1985.

24. Kirshner DL, O'Brien MS, Ricotta JJ. Risk factors in a community experience with carotid endarterectomy. J Vasc Surg 10:178-186, 1989.

25. Hoyne RF. Review of 272 consecutive carotid endarterectomies in a smaller community. Surg Gynecol Obstet 170:522-526, 1990.

26. Welling RE, Ramadas HS, Gansmuller KJ. Cervical wound hematoma after carotid endarterectomy. Ann Vasc Surg 3:229-231, 1989.

27. Thompson JE. Complications of carotid endarterectomy and their prevention. World J Surg 3:155, 1979.

28. Kunkel JM, Gomez ER, Spebar MJ, Delgado RJ, Jarstfer BS, Collins GJ Jr. Wound hematomas after carotid endarterectomy. Am J Surg 148:844-847, 1984.

29. Gooley NA, Sumner DS. Wound hematomas following carotid endarterectomy. The effect of protamine and aspirin [abstr]. J Cardiovasc Surg 28:80, 1987.

30. Treiman RL, Cossman DV, Foran RF, Levin PM, Cohen JL, Wagner WH. The influence of neutralizing heparin after carotid endarterectomy on postoperative stroke and wound hematoma. J Vasc Surg 12:440-446, 1990.

31. Imparato AM, Riles TS, Lamparello PJ, Ramirez AA. The management of TIA and acute strokes after carotid endarterectomy. In Bernhard VM, Towne JB, eds. Complications in Vascular Surgery, 2nd ed. Orlando, Fla.: Grune & Stratton, 1985, pp 725-738.

32. Ercius MS, Chandler WF, Ford JW, Burkel WE. Early versus delayed heparin reversal after carotid endarterectomy in the dog: A scanning electron microscopy study. J Neurosurg 58:708-713, 1983.

33. Gupta SK, Veith FJ, Ascer E, Wengerter KR, Franco C, Amar D, El-Gaweet E-S, Gupta A. Anaphylactoid reactions to protamine: An often lethal complication in insulin-dependent diabetic patients undergoing vascular surgery. J Vasc Surg 9:342-350, 1988.

34. Findlay JM, Lougheed WM, Gentill F, Walker PM, Glynn MFX, Houle S. Effect of perioperative platelet inhibition on postcarotid endarterectomy mural thrombus formation: Results of a prospective randomized controlled trial using aspirin and dipyridamole in humans. J Neurosurg 63:693-698, 1985.

35. Ercius MS, Chandler WF, Ford JW, Swanson DP, Burke JC. Effect of different aspirin doses on arterial thrombosis after canine carotid endarterectomy: A scanning electron microscope and indium–111 labeled platelet study. Neurosurgery 14:198-203, 1984.

36. Mora W, Hunter G, Malone J. Wound infection following carotid endarterectomy. J Cardiovasc Surg 22:47-49, 1981.

37. Eikelboom BC, Ackerstaff RGA, Hoeneveld H, Ludwig JW, Teeuwen C, Vermeulen FEE, Welten RJT. Benefits of carotid patching: A randomized study. J Vasc Surg 7:240-247, 1988.

38. Katz MM, Jones GT, Degenhardt J, Gunn B, Wilson J, Katz S. The use of patch angioplasty to alter the incidence of carotid restenosis following thromboendarterectomy. J Cardiovasc Surg 28:2-8, 1987.

39. Hertzer NR, Beven EG, O'Hara PJ, Krajewski LP. A prospective study of vein patch angioplasty during carotid endarterectomy: Three-year results for 801 patients and 917 operations. Ann Surg 206:628-635, 1987.

40. Riles TS, Lamparello PJ, Giangola G, Imparato AM. Rupture of the vein patch: A rare complication of carotid endarterectomy. Surgery 107:10-12, 1990.

41. Seabrook GR, Towne JB, Bandyk DF, Schmitt DD, Cohen EB. Use of the internal jugular vein for carotid patch angioplasty. Surgery 106:633-638, 1989.

42. Rosenthal D, Archie JP Jr, Garcia-Rinaldi R, Seagraves MA, Baird DR, McKinsey JF, Lamis PA, Clark MD, Erdoes LS, Whitehead T, Pallos LL. Carotid patch angioplasty: Immediate and long-term results. J Vasc Surg 12:326-333, 1990.

43. Archie JP Jr. Prevention of early restenosis and thrombosis-occlusion after carotid endarterectomy by saphenous vein patch angioplasty. Stroke 17:901-905, 1986.

44. Sundt TM Jr, Whisnant JP, Houser OW, Fode NC. Prospective study of the effectiveness and durability of carotid endarterectomy. Mayo Clin Proc 65:625-635, 1990.

45. Clagett GP, Patterson CB, Fisher DF Jr, Fry RE, Eidt JF, Humble TH, Fry WF. Vein patch versus primary closure for carotid endarterectomy: A randomized prospective study in a selected group of patients. J Vasc Surg 9:213-223, 1989.

46. Kakkar VV. The cephalic vein as a peripheral vascular graft. Surg Gynecol Obstet 128:551-556, 1969.

47. Archie JP Jr, Green JJ Jr. Saphenous vein rupture pressure, rupture stress, and carotid endarterectomy vein patch reconstruction. Surgery 107:389-396, 1990.

48. Awad IA, Little JR. Patch angioplasty in carotid endarterectomy: Advantages, concerns, controversies. Stroke 20:417-422, 1989.

49. McCollum CH, Wheeler WG, Noon GP, DeBakey ME. Aneurysms of the extracranial carotid artery. Twenty-one years' experience. Am J Surg 137:196-200, 1979.

50. Branch CL Jr, Davis CH Jr. False aneurysm complicating carotid endarterectomy. Neurosurgery 19:421-425, 1986.

51. Graver LM, Mulcare RJ. Pseudoaneurysm after carotid endarterectomy. J Cardiovasc Surg 27:294-297, 1986.

52. Buscaglia LC, Moore WS, Hall AD. False aneurysm after carotid endarterectomy. JAMA 209:1529, 1969.

53. Motte S, Wautrecht JC, Bellens B, Vincent G, Dereume JP, Delcour C. Infected false aneurysm following carotid endarterectomy with vein patch angioplasty. J Cardiovasc Surg 28:734-736, 1987.

54. Ehrenfeld WK, Hays RJ. False aneurysm after carotid endarterectomy. Arch Surg 104:288-291, 1972.

55. Ameli FM, Provan JL, Keuchler PM. Unusual aneurysms of the extracranial carotid artery. J Cardiovasc Surg 24:69-73, 1983.

56. Rhodes EL, Stanley JC, Hoffman GL, Cronenwett JL, Fry WJ. Aneurysms of extracranial carotid arteries. Arch Surg 111:339-343, 1976.

57. Lougheed WM, Elgie RG, Barnett HJM. The results of surgical management of extracranial internal carotid artery occlusion and stenosis. Can Med Assoc J 95:1279-1293, 1966.

58. Ribet M, Florin MF, Debus JP. Faux anéurysme carotidien après mise en place d'une prosthese: Resection et greffe veineuse. Presse Med 76:725-726, 1968.

59. Welling RE, Taha A, Goel T, Cranley J, Krause R, Hafner C, Tew J. Extracranial carotid artery aneurysms. Surgery 93:319-323, 1983.

60. Smith RB III, Perdue GD, Collier RH, Stone HH. Post-operative false aneurysms of the carotid artery. Am Surg 36:335-341, 1970.

61. Tarlov E, Schmidek H, Scott RM, Wepsic JG, Ojemann RG. Reflex hypotension following carotid endarterectomy: Mechanism and management. J Neurosurg 39:323-327, 1973.

62. Bove EL, Fry WJ, Gross WS, Stanley JC. Hypotension and hypertension as consequences of baroreceptor dysfunction following carotid endarterectomy. Surgery 85:633-637, 1979.

63. Angell-James JE, Lumley JSP. The effects of carotid endarterectomy on the mechanical properties of the carotid sinus and carotid sinus nerve activity in atherosclerotic patients. Br J Surg 61:805-810, 1974.

64. Dehn TCB, Angell-James JE. Long-term effect of carotid endarterectomy on carotid sinus baroreceptor function and blood pressure control. Br J Surg 74:997-1000, 1987.

65. Cafferata HT, Merchant RF Jr, DePalma RG. Avoidance of postcarotid endarterectomy hypertension. Ann Surg 196:465-472, 1982.

66. Satiani B, Vasko JS, Evans WE. Hypertension following carotid endarterectomy. Surg Neurol 11:357-359, 1979.

67. Towne JB, Bernhard VM. The relationship of post-operative hypertension to complications following carotid endarterectomy. Surgery 88:575-580, 1980.

68. Lehv MS, Salzman EW, Silen W. Hypertension complicating carotid endarterectomy. Stroke 1:307-313, 1970.

69. Wade JG, Larson CP Jr, Hickey RF, Ehrenfeld WK, Severinghaus JW. Effect of carotid endarterectomy on carotid chemoreceptor and baroreceptor function in man. N Engl J Med 282:823-829, 1970.

70. Sharpey-Schafer EP. Effects of Valsalva's manoeuvre on the normal and failing circulation. Br Med J 1:693-695, 1955.

71. Appenzeller O, Descarries L. Circulatory reflexes in patients with cerebrovascular disease. N Engl J Med 271:820-823, 1964.

72. Solti F, Mogan ST, Renyl-Vamos F, Moravcik A. The association of carotid artery stenosis with carotid sinus hypersensitivity: Transitory cerebral ischaemic attack provoked by carotid sinus reflex. J Cardiovasc Surg 31:693-696, 1990.

73. Schellack J, Fulenwider JT, Olson RA, Smith RB III, Mansour K. The carotid sinus syndrome: A frequently overlooked cause of syncope in the elderly. J Vasc Surg 4:376-383, 1986.

74. Skydell JL, Machleder HI, Baker JD, Busuttil RW, Moore WS. Incidence and mechanism of post-carotid endarterectomy hypertension. Arch Surg 122:1153-1155, 1987.

75. Smith B. Hypertension following carotid endarterectomy: The role of cerebral renin production. J Vasc Surg 1:623-627, 1984.

76. Ahn SS, Marcus DR, Moore WS. Post-carotid endarterectomy hypertension. Associated with elevated cranial norepinephrine. J Vasc Surg 9:351-360, 1989.

77. Towne JB. Blood pressure instability following carotid endarterectomy. In Ernst CB, Stanley JC, eds. Current Therapy in Vascular Surgery. Philadelphia: BC Decker, 1991, pp 101-104.

78. Schroeder T, Sillesen H, Engell HC. Staged bilateral carotid endarterectomy. J Vasc Surg 3:355-359, 1986.

79. Caplan LR, Skillman J, Ojemann R, Fields WS. Intracerebral hemorrhage following carotid endarterectomy: A hypertensive complication? Stroke 9:457-460, 1978.

80. Pomposelli FB, Lamparello PJ, Riles TS, Craighead CC, Giangola G, Imparato AM. Intracranial hemorrhage after carotid endarterectomy. J Vasc Surg 7:248 255, 1988.

81. Owens ML, Wilson SE. Prevention of neurologic complications of carotid endarterectomy. Arch Surg 117:551-555, 1982.

82. Imparato AM, Riles TS, Lamparello PJ, Ramirez AA. The management of TIA and acute strokes after carotid endarterectomy. In Bernhard VM, Towne JB, eds. Complications in Vascular Surgery, 2nd ed. Orlando Fla.: Grune & Stratton, 1985, pp 725-738.

83. Baker WH. In discussion of Towne JB, Bernhard VM. The relationship of postoperative hypertension to complications following carotid endarterectomy. Surgery 88:580, 1980.

84. Lassen NA. Cerebral blood flow and oxygen consumption in man. Physiol Rev 39:183-238, 1959.

85. Strandgaard S, Paulson OB. Cerebral autoregulation. Stroke 15:413-416, 1984.

86. Russell D, Dybevold S, Kjartansson O, Nyberg-Hansen R, Rootwelt K, Wiberg J. Cerebral vasoreactivity and blood flow before and 3 months after carotid endarterectomy. Stroke 21:1029-1032, 1990.

87. Schroeder T, Holstein PE, Engell HC. Hyperperfusion following endarterectomy. Stroke 15:758, 1984.

88. Powers AD, Smith RR. Hyperperfusion syndrome after carotid endarterectomy: A transcranial Doppler evaluation. Neurosurgery 26:56-60, 1990.

89. Schroeder T, Sillesen H, Sorensen O, Engell HC. Cerebral hyperperfusion following carotid endarterectomy. J Neurosurg 66:824-829, 1987.

90. Piepgras DG, Morgan MK, Sundt TM, Yanagihara T, Mussman LM. Intracerebral hemorrhage after carotid endarterectomy. J Neurosurg 68:532-536, 1988.

91. Messert B, Black JA. Cluster headache, hemicrania, and other head pains: Morbidity of carotid endarterectomy. Stroke 9:559-562, 1978.

92. Pearce J. Headache after carotid endarterectomy. Br Med J 2:85-86, 1976.

93. Appenzeller O. Cerebrovascular aspects of headache. Med Clin North Am 62:467-480, 1978.

94. Leviton A, Caplan L, Salzman E. Severe headache after carotid endarterectomy. Headache 15:207-210, 1975.

95. Dolan JG, Mushlin AI. Hypertension, vascular headaches, and seizures after carotid endarterectomy. Arch Intern Med 144:1489-1491, 1984.

96. Akers DL, Brinker MR, Engelhardt TC, Kerstein MD. Postoperative somnolence in patients after carotid endarterectomy. Surgery 107:684-687, 1990.

97. Youkey JR, Clagett GP, Jaffin JH, Parisi JE, Rich NM. Focal motor seizures complicating carotid endarterectomy. Arch Surg 119:1080-1084, 1984.

98. Reigel MM, Hollier LH, Sundt TM Jr, Piepgras DG, Sharbrough FW, Cherry KJ. Cerebral hyperperfusion syndrome: A cause of neurologic dysfunction after carotid endarterectomy. J Vasc Surg 5:628-634, 1987.

99. Sundt TM, Sharbrough FW, Piepgras DG, Kearns TP, Messick JM Jr, O'Fallon WM. Correlation of cerebral blood flow and electroencephalographic changes during carotid endarterectomy with results of surgery and hemodynamics of cerebral ischemia. Mayo Clin Proc 56:533-543, 1981.

100. Wilkinson JT, Adams HP Jr, Wright CB. Convulsions after carotid endarterectomy. JAMA 244:1827-1828, 1980.

101. Wylie EJ, Hein MF, Adams JE. Intracranial hemorrhage following surgical revascularization for treatment of strokes. J Neurosurg 2:212-215, 1964.

102. Bruetman ME, Fields WS, Crawford ES, DeBakey ME. Cerebral hemorrhage in carotid artery surgery. Arch Neurol 9:458-467, 1963.

103. Meyer JS. Importance of ischemic damage to small vessels in experimental cerebral infarction. J Neuropathol Exp Neurol 17:571-585, 1958.

104. Ropper AH, Kehne SM. Contrast enhancement CT scan and post-endarterectomy hemorrhage. Stroke 17:898-900, 1986.

105. Magovern JA, Sieber PR, Thiele BL. The syndrome of inappropriate secretion of antidiuretic hormone following carotid endarterectomy. J Cardiovasc Surg 30:544-546, 1989.

106. Rubin JR, Pitluk HC, King TA, Hutton M, Kieger EF, Plecha FR, Hertzer NR. Carotid endarterectomy in a metropolitan community: The early results after 8535 operations. J Vasc Surg 7:256-260, 1988.

107. Till JS, Toole JF, Howard VJ, Ford CS, Williams D. Declining morbidity and mortality of carotid endarterectomy. The Wake Forest University Medical Center experience. Stroke 18:823-829, 1987.

108. Ennix CL Jr, Lawrie GM, Morris GC Jr, Crawford ES, Howell JF, Reardon MJ, Weatherford SC. Improved results of carotid endarterectomy in patients with symptomatic coronary disease: An analysis of 1,546 consecutive carotid operations. Stroke 10:122-125, 1979.

109. Thompson JE, Austin DJ, Patman RD. Carotid endarterectomy for cerebrovascular insufficiency: Long-term results in 592 patients followed up to thirteen years. Ann Surg 172:663-679, 1970.

110. O'Donnell TF Jr, Callow AD, Willet C, Payne D, Cleveland RJ. The impact of coronary artery disease on carotid endarterectomy. Ann Surg 198:705-712, 1983.

111. Hertzer NR, Lees CD. Fatal myocardial infarction following carotid endarterectomy. Three hundred thirty-five patients followed 6-11 years after operation. Ann Surg 194:212-218, 1981.

112. Yeager RA, Moneta GL, McConnell DB, Neuwelt EA, Taylor LM Jr, Porter JM. Analysis of risk factors for myocardial infarction following carotid endarterectomy. Arch Surg 124:1142-1145, 1989.

113. Riles TS, Kopelman I, Imparato AM. Myocardial infarction following carotid endarterectomy: A review of 683 operations. Surgery 85:249-252, 1979.

114. Baur HR, Pierach CA. Electrocardiographic changes after bilateral carotid endarterectomy. N Engl J Med 291:1121-1122, 1974.

115. Hertzer NR, Young JR, Beven EG, Graor RA, O'Hara PJ, Ruschhaupt WF III, de Wolfe VG, Maljovec LC. Coronary angiography in 506 patients with extracranial cerebrovascular disease. Arch Intern Med 145:849-852, 1985.

116. Rokey R, Rolak LA, Harati Y, Kutka N, Verani MS. Coronary artery disease in patients with cerebrovascular disease: A prospective study. Ann Neurol 16:50-53, 1984.

117. Graor RA, Hertzer NR. Management of coexistent carotid artery and coronary disease. Stroke 19:1441-1444, 1988.

118. Hertzer NR, Beven EG, Young JR, O'Hara PJ, Ruschhaupt WF III, Graor RA, de Wolfe VG, Maljovec LC. Coronary artery disease in peripheral vascular patients. A classification of 1000 coronary angiograms and results of surgical management. Ann Surg 199:223-233, 1984.

119. DeWeese JA, Rob CG, Satran R, Marsh DO, Joynt RJ, Summers D, Nichols C. Results of carotid endarterectomies for transient ischemic attacks—five years later. Ann Surg 178:258-264, 1973.

120. Bernstein EF, Humber PB, Collins GM, Dilley RB, Devin JB, Stuart SH. Life expectancy and late stroke following carotid endarterectomy. Ann Surg 198:80-86, 1983.

121. Cambria RP, Ivarsson BL, Akins CW, Moncure AC, Brewster DC, Abbott WM. Simultaneous carotid and coronary disease: Safety of the combined approach. J Vasc Surg 9:56-64, 1989.

122. Riles TS, Pasternack PF. Management of concomitant carotid and coronary arterial occlusive disease. In Ernst CB, Stanley JC, eds. Current Therapy in Vascular Surgery, 2nd ed. Philadelphia: BC Decker, 1991, pp 142-145.

123. Goldman L, Caldera DL, Nussbaum SR, Southwick FS, Krogstad D, Murray B, Burke DS, O'Malley TA, Goroll AH, Caplan CH, Nolan J, Carabello B, Slater EE. Multifactorial index of cardiac risk in noncardiac surgical procedures. N Engl J Med 297:845-850, 1977.

124. Yeager RA. Basic data related to cardiac testing and cardiac risk associated with vascular surgery. Ann Vasc Surg 4:193-197, 1990.

39

Recurrent Carotid Stenosis

D. Eugene Strandness, Jr.

Carotid endarterectomy is a procedure designed to eliminate the source of emboli, remove a site where thrombosis can occur, and provide long-term patency of the involved segment. The operation itself removes the atherosclerotic plaque in a cleavage plane and leaves behind a portion of the media of the artery and its investing adventitia. This procedure starts in motion a series of events that are often uncertain and impossible to appreciate. Although the most desired result is complete resurfacing of the endarterectomized area with endothelium, it is not at all clear as to what extent this occurs. What is known is that a unique lesion, generally referred to as myointimal hyperplasia, subsequently develops in a subset of patients. The lesion can develop quickly (within weeks) and is usually complete in terms of its maturation by 2 years after carotid endarterectomy. The recurrent lesion resembles the type of change that occurs when arteries have been injured by some direct means. In fact, in the experimental animal the balloon injury model is usually employed to study this phenomenon of recurrent stenosis.

Although the purpose of this chapter is to discuss this lesion in the carotid artery, it must be recognized that the same or a similar type of recurrent lesion develops wherever the arterial wall is injured. The injury can be caused by balloon angioplasty, laser-assisted balloon angioplasty, or direct arterial surgery, be it by construction of a bypass graft or carotid endarterectomy.

MATERIALS AND METHODS

We at the University of Washington School of Medicine became interested in this problem because of the increased availability of duplex ultrasonic scanning, which made it possible to study patients in a sequential manner after completion of carotid endarterectomy. The application of duplex ultrasonic scanning involves the combined use of imaging and pulsed Doppler to investigate flow velocity changes that occur across bifurcation. Our previous validation studies have shown that as the artery becomes progressively narrowed, the velocity within that segment of artery increases in a predictable manner, permitting the classification of the degree of stenosis into broad but useful categories.[1]

The categories used for screening and follow-up purposes are as follows:

1. *Normal*. The normal carotid bulb is characterized by the presence of boundary layer separation in the posterolateral portion of the bulb. In this region flow reversal will be seen. Peak velocities in the artery should not exceed 125 cm/sec, with the end-diastolic flow always above 0 when the recording is made near the flow divider or in the internal carotid artery itself. If one chooses to measure frequency instead of velocity, the peak systolic frequency should not exceed 4 KHz when the transmitting frequency is 5 MHz and the angle of the incident sound beam is kept at or very close to 60 degrees with the long axis of the artery.

2. *1% to 15% narrowing*. Vessels in this

category exhibit minimal disease, which is characterized by the filling of the posterolateral aspect of the carotid bulb without impingement of the plaque on the flow stream itself. This classification is recognized by the absence of boundary layer separation in the carotid bulb and a normal peak systolic velocity and frequency. Some spectral broadening may be evident.

3. *16% to 49% stenosis.* With this degree of narrowing the plaque is beginning to impinge on the flow stream of the internal carotid artery. There is some increase in the peak systolic velocity, but it is still below 125 cm/sec. A major feature of the spectral display is spectral broadening throughout the entire pulse cycle.

4. *50% to 79% stenosis.* For this degree of narrowing the peak systolic velocity exceeds 125 cm/sec (peak systolic frequency exceeds 4 KHz) and marked spectral broadening is noted.

5. *80% to 99% stenosis.* With this very tight lesion the peak systolic velocity is well above 125 cm/sec. A new variable is taken into account at this point: end-diastolic velocity. When the end-diastolic velocity exceeds 145 cm/sec (or end-diastolic frequency is >4.5 KHz), the lesion is placed in this category.

6. *Total occlusion.* For these lesions the flow in the common carotid artery will often fall to 0 at end-diastole. In 34 cases of total occlusion of the internal carotid artery, this occurred in 32 (D.E.S., unpublished data, 1991). No flow can be detected within the internal carotid artery beyond the carotid bulb.

The accuracy of this method for both screening patients suspected of having carotid artery disease and for evaluating patients following carotid endarterectomy has been evaluated in several different studies in our laboratory.[1-4] For preoperative screening purposes duplex scanning has a sensitivity of over 90% and a specificity of 90%. Since carotid endarterectomy itself produces changes in the carotid bulb, it is necessary to establish if duplex scanning has a similar accuracy during follow-up. In order to be certain of our results, we have divided our studies into those performed in the early postoperative phase (within the first 30 days) as compared with those done at later postoperative intervals. In the immediate postoper-

ative period duplex scanning should be used only to determine if the vessel is patent. Changes occur in the carotid bulb during this period that make interpretation more difficult. In addition, if a carotid patch is used routinely, a new geometry is created that may make the vessel difficult to examine. In our center we do not patch carotid arteries unless a technical problem demands it.

We evaluated 36 patients (30 men, 6 women) who had been studied postoperatively with duplex scanning within 3 months of arteriography.[2] Forty-four operated segments were available for comparison. The follow-up period ranged from 1 week to 10 years (mean, 28 months). The distribution of the disease in the carotid bulb at the time of the arteriography is shown in Table 39-1.

When the results of duplex scanning were compared with those of arteriography, the following findings were noted: (1) one normal side was placed in the 16% to 49% stenosis category; (2) two of the five with a 1% to 15% stenosis finding were placed in the 16% to 49% stenosis category; (3) in the 16% to 49% stenosis group, one was labeled as having 1% to 15% stenosis, 16 were correctly classified, and four were placed in the 50% to 99% stenosis group; (4) in the 50% to 99% stenosis category 14 were correctly classified, with one placed in the 16% to 49% stenosis group; and (5) the two occlusions were correctly categorized. The overall accuracy of duplex scanning by stenosis category was 80%. If only the >50% stenoses and occlusions are considered, duplex scanning was accurate in 94% of the cases.

The correlation between duplex scanning and arteriography shows how useful duplex

Table 39-1. Disease Distribution as Determined by Arteriography

Percent diameter reduction	No. of sides	%
Normal	1	2.3
1% to 15%	5	11.4
16% to 49%	21	47.7
50% to 99%	15	34.1
Total occlusion	2	4.5

scanning is in this population. It is important to realize that if only the >50% stenoses and occlusions are considered as significant, then only four sides that were shown by arteriography to have lesser degrees of narrowing would have been placed in this stenosis category.

STUDY POPULATION

Interest in restenosis began with our initial report, which appeared in 1982.[3] We had the opportunity of performing studies on 76 patients (89 operations) at the Seattle Veterans Administration Hospital. This patient population was unique in that an operative arteriogram had been performed in all patients to verify the initial technical result after carotid endarterectomy. A total of nine patients had a patch placed; in six cases this was because the surgeon believed that the internal carotid artery was too small to be closed primarily. In the remaining three cases the arteriogram revealed a defect that required reopening the artery and patching.

A total of 32 sides (36%) at one or more examinations showed >50% stenosis in the carotid bulb. Serial follow-up studies were possible on 22 of the 32 sides with a >50% stenotic lesion. Twelve of these arteries showed persistent stenosis of >50%, whereas nine appeared to improve to the 16% to 49% stenosis category. One artery had progressed to total occlusion. It was estimated on the basis of this study that a persistent restenosis rate of 19% was likely. Recurrent neurologic symptoms developed in eight patients appropriate to the operated segment. In these eight patients, the degree of stenosis was >50% in four and <50% in three. The remaining patient had exacerbation of the neurologic deficit related to an internal carotid artery occlusion.

The next study, which we reported in 1985, was the result of a prospective follow-up study of 107 men and 27 women (145 sides) that extended up to 4 years.[4] During follow-up nine late deaths occurred, of which two were stroke related (1.4%). Focal symptoms developed in 12 patients on the operated side, six of which were strokes (one lacunar). Transient ischemic attacks (TIAs) referable to the operated side developed in seven patients, but in only two

instances were these associated with >50% stenosis. During the follow-up period recurrent stenosis developed in 32 patients (22%). The lesions appeared to regress in seven, resulting in a persistent restenosis rate of 17%. It appeared that women had a significantly higher risk of restenosis ($p < .01$). By life-table analysis restenosis developed early and appeared to be complete and stable by 24 months following carotid endarterectomy.

In a subsequent follow-up (mean, 4 years) the restenosis rate in 301 patients was 31% at 7 years. Regression was observed in 10%, resulting in a persistent restenosis rate of 21%.[5] TIAs occurred in 12% of the restenosis patients and stroke in 3%. The cumulative incidence of ischemic events was not significantly different between those patients with and those patients without restenosis. It was concluded that a conservative approach is warranted when restenosis occurs since ischemic events were rarely associated with a stenotic lesion in the operated segment.

If the restenotic lesion is largely benign, is it likely in its course of development to progress to a total occlusion? In a study of 200 patients with serial duplex scans and a mean follow-up of 31 months, five occlusions developed.[6] One occlusion developed in the perioperative period; the other four were detected at times ranging from day 61 to day 702. The late occlusion rate was found to be 2.5%. In three of these four patients occlusion was accompanied by the development of a stroke.

DISCUSSION

Since carotid endarterectomy removes in toto the lesion for which the operation is indicated, the end result should be preservation of patency and endothelial integrity to prevent recurrent neurologic events. It is now clear that problems following carotid endarterectomy that are of concern to the surgeon can and do occur. In the studies reported here the restenosis rate is approximately 20% for the development of >50% stenosis. The restenotic lesion is proliferative and usually smooth and does not appear to degenerate to become analogous to the complicated plaque for which the operation was originally indicated.

It appears that the histologic appearance of the lesion explains its benign nature. Although it may narrow the artery by an amount that is worrisome, the lesion does not appear to ulcerate and thus provide a site for thrombi to develop. Although not yet determined, even high-grade lesions do not seem to have the same propensity for progressing to a total occlusion. This fact is important because although total occlusions can occur without producing ischemic events, the incidence of ischemic events is much higher with total occlusions than with stenotic lesions alone. As noted, of the four occlusions that occurred in the late postoperative period, three were associated with the development of a stroke.

Are our results supported by other studies in the literature? Sanders et al.[7] reported serial studies up to 24 months after operation using both duplex scanning and intravenous digital subtraction arteriography. At 3, 6, 12, and 24 months, the rate of significant restenosis was 6%, 12%, 6%, and 8%, respectively. The rate of persistent restenosis was 14.8% in women and 4.1% in men. It is of interest that in 40% of the patients with significant restenosis at 3 months, the stenosis increased to a higher degree of narrowing during the first year postoperatively. Very little change was observed in the second year of follow-up.

In a recent report by Green et al.,[8] 686 patients were studied within 4 weeks of operation and every 6 months thereafter. In this group three patterns of residual disease were described: (1) plaque proximal to the carotid bulb without flow abnormalities, (2) plaques proximal to the carotid bulb with a <50% diameter reduction, and (3) elevated flows consistent with >50% stenosis distal to the operated site but without visible plaque. It is important to recognize that the disease discovered during follow-up was defined in this study as residual disease and not as a recurrent myointimal hyperplastic lesion. The incidence of ischemic events in the long term was strikingly higher for those patients with proximal plaque that narrowed the artery by >50%. In this group the stroke rate was 9% as compared with 1.5% for those patients with no residual disease and 1.6% in those with a proximal

plaque not associated with any flow disturbances. It is not clear from this study how the recurrent lesion differs in behavior from what the authors define as a residual lesion.

In order to place our studies and those of others into proper perspective, it is necessary to review the study procedures performed, their accuracy, what they can define, and finally the natural history of newly discovered lesions after operation.

The ultrasound studies consist of two major components—imaging studies and velocity studies. Although both are performed with the same instrument, the interpretation of each is different. Ideally, the imaging component provides the anatomic location of the recurrent or residual lesion and depicts its morphology and surface character. During the evolution of the studies performed by us and by others the technology was improving, particularly in terms of achieving better resolution with most imaging instruments. Yet, even with improved resolution, one has to consider those changes likely to be seen and those that are difficult to visualize. Calcification, which is a common finding in complicated plaque, is only a marker and tells the observer nothing about such factors as surface continuity and ulceration. Although there is little doubt that irregularity can be observed, it is not possible to go one step further and definitively note the presence or absence of ulceration. If the lesion appears to be homogeneous, it is probably a fibrous plaque, particularly if no calcification is evident. Fibrous lesions also tend to be smooth, which is the typical appearance of the recurrent myointimal lesion.

Velocity information is essential in defining the degree of stenosis. For patients who present with carotid artery disease, the degree of narrowing is the most powerful predictor of subsequent events. Does the same reasoning apply to recurrent stenosis? Only a guarded opinion can be given with regard to this probability. Statistically, it appears in our studies that the recurrent high-grade lesion (here defined as a >50% stenosis) does not carry the same prognosis. However, in the study by Green et al.[8] the residual lesion that narrows the artery by >50% in the region proximal to the carotid bulb carries a poorer prognosis. This leads to an important question: How should a recurrent stenosis be defined as compared with a residual lesion?

In our first study[3] the fact that the operation was not completed until the operative arteriogram was determined to be normal would suggest that all stenoses that develop after operation qualify as recurrent lesions. If the same criteria used during the preoperative screening process were used for recognition of a residual lesion, then it is likely that the discovery of a similar lesion at the first postoperative study would indicate that the lesion is truly a residual plaque that was not removed in its entirety at operation. This distinction is obviously important not only in classifying the types of lesions encountered, but also in permitting an estimation of the risk the lesion poses to the patient.

A potentially important alternative to standard carotid endarterectomy with primary closure is patching the artery. Would the addition of a venous or synthetic patch reduce the incidence of early restenosis? Eikelboom et al,,[9] in a randomized series of 129 patients, showed that patching significantly reduced the restenosis rate as determined by duplex scanning. The benefits of patching were most evident in women. A later study from the same institution by Ten Holter et al.[10] followed up the long-term outcome of 172 patients in whom the artery was closed primarily as compared with 167 in whom venous patches were used to close the artery. The rate of significant (>50% diameter reduction) early restenosis for the arteries closed primarily was 14.5% for men and 24.4% for women in the first year postoperatively. In those patients in whom arteries were patched the restenosis rates were 3.4% for men and 4.3% for women. This difference in restenosis rates was not evident after the first year postoperatively, which suggests that later recurrences, which may be secondary to atherosclerosis, are not affected by patching.

These results suggest that patching reduces the incidence of restenosis that results from myointimal hyperplasia. Should a practice of patching be adopted on the basis of these studies? This issue is complex and not easily resolved. The major potential problem with venous patches is the low but definite incidence of patch blowout, which is a disastrous complication. Another concern is whether the use of a patch will make the long-term clinical results of carotid endarterectomy better in terms of patient outcome. This issue will be difficult to resolve because there is little evidence to support the idea that early restenosis subjects the patient to a higher risk for late ischemic events.

If for the moment the exact nature of the lesion discovered postoperatively is disregarded, what should be the strategy in the management of the patient? We believe that these patients should be managed conservatively until the patient becomes symptomatic. Given the fact that a recurrent lesion will develop in 10% to 20% of patients, it seems prudent to simply observe the patient.

Finally, can follow-up studies of the operated segment be justified given the benign prognosis of the recurrent lesion? Cook, Thompson, and Barnes[11] considered this issue in 120 consecutive patients who had undergone carotid endarterectomy between the years 1983 and 1988. The incidence of recurrent symptoms was 6%. Postoperative duplex studies were performed in 63 patients (78 operated sides). Two arteries had evidence of residual disease and were excluded from further analysis, leaving 76 arteries for analysis. Significant recurrent stenosis (>50%) developed in 14 arteries (18.2%). In 12 of the 14 stenotic arteries, stenosis did not lead to ischemic events and did not require reoperation. Ipsilateral symptoms developed in the remaining two arteries. In the group of 62 arteries without recurrent high-grade lesions, ipsilateral symptoms developed in four but none underwent reoperation. When the results in the two groups were compared by life-table analysis, there did not appear to be an increased risk of ischemic events in patients with restenosis. The authors concluded that although duplex scanning may be of use in follow-up examinations of the contralateral carotid artery, its routine use to identify patients with recurrent stenosis may not be justified.

Although aspirin is routinely given to patients with carotid artery disease both before and after operation, there is little evidence to support its use as a method of preventing recurrent stenosis. It is this author's view that at the present time there are no proven pharmacologic methods available for the prevention of recurrent stenosis. With the interest in low-molecular-weight heparin and angiotensin converting enzyme (ACE) inhibitors as modifiers of this response, research with these substances in coming years with regard to the prevention of myointimal hyperplasia will be of interest.

REFERENCES

1. Langlois Y, Roederer GO, Chan ATW, et al. Evaluating carotid artery disease: The concordance between pulsed Doppler/spectral analysis and angiography. Ultrasound Med Biol 9:51-63, 1983.
2. Roederer GO, Langlois Y, Chan ATW, et al. Post-endarterectomy carotid ultrasonic duplex scanning concordance with contrast angiography. Ultrasound Med Biol 9:73-78, 1983.
3. Zierler RE, Bandyk DF, Thiele BL, et al. Carotid artery stenosis following endarterectomy. Arch Surg 117:1408-1415, 1982.
4. Nicholls SC, Phillips DJ, Bergelin RO, et al. Carotid endarterectomy: Relationship of outcome to early restenosis. J Vasc Surg 2:375-381, 1985.
5. Healy DA, Zierler RE, Nicholls SC, et al. Long-term follow-up and clinical outcome of carotid restenosis. J Vasc Surg 10:662-669, 1989.
6. Healy DA, Clowes AW, Zierler RE, et al. Immediate and long-term results of carotid endarterectomy. Stroke 20:1138-1142, 1989.
7. Sanders EACM, Hoeneveld H, Eikelboom BC, et al. Residual lesions and early recurrent stenosis after carotid endarterectomy. J Vasc Surg 5:731-737, 1987.
8. Green RM, McNamara J, Ouriel K, et al. The clinical course of residual carotid artery disease [abstr]. Presented at the Annual Meeting of the Society for Vascular Surgery. Los Angeles, Calif.: June 4-5, 1990.
9. Eikelboom BC, Ackerstaff RGA, Hoeneveld H, et al. Benefits of carotid patching: A randomized study. J Vasc Surg 7:240-247, 1988.
10. Ten Holter JBM, Ackerstaff RGA, Thoe Schwartzenberg GWS, et al. The impact of vein patch angioplasty on the long-term surgical outcome after carotid endarterectomy. A prospective follow-up study with serial duplex scanning. J Cardiovasc Surg 31:58-65, 1990.
11. Cook JM, Thompson BW, Barnes RW. Is routine duplex exam after carotid endarterectomy justified [abstr]. Presented at the Annual Meeting of the Southern Association for Vascular Surgery. Acapulco, Mexico: January 24-27, 1990.

Index

A

Abdominal aortic aneurysm; *see* Aortic aneurysm

Abdominal aortic branch reconstruction, 172-179

Abdominal disease
aortic surgery with, 147-150
chylous ascites and, 385

ABI; *see* Ankle/brachial index

Above-knee amputation
healing of, 314, 318
selection criteria for, 317

Above-knee femoropopliteal bypass, 288-289

Abscess, infrainguinal, 253

Access, vascular, 389-402; *see also* Vascular access for dialysis

Accreditation
for testing laboratories, 12
for vascular laboratory, 10

Activated clotting time, 478

Activated partial thromboplastin time, 120

Acute tubular necrosis
as erroneous description of renal function, 42
ischemia and, 47

Adenosine monophosphate, cyclic, 61

Adenosine triphosphate, 332

Adhesion of bacteria to graft, 229-230

Adrenergic receptors, erection and, 162

Aggregation, platelet; *see* Platelet aggregation

Agkistrodon rhodostoma venom as anticoagulant, 128-129

Air embolus, 405

Albumin
fluid shifts and, 44
postbypass edema and, 375

Algorithm for renovascular hypertension, 187

Aliasing, 17

Allergic reaction
dextran and, 128
heparin-induced, 121
to sclerotherapy, 354
to thrombolytic agents, 438

Alopecia, heparin-induced, 121

Alternate route bypass graft, 217-222
axillofemoral, 217-221
thoracofemoral, 221

ε-Aminocaproic acid, 437

Aminoglycoside
renal toxicity from, 47

Aminoglycoside—cont'd
septic foot and, 308

Ampicillin for septic foot, 308

Amplatz filter, 363

Amputation
aortoenteric fistula and, 248
lower extremity, 313-329
diabetes mellitus and, 301-329
failure to heal of, 318-319
flexion contractures in, 321
late complications from, 322-324
level of, 314-317
medical profile of patient with, 313-314
pain and, 320-321
preoperative preparation for, 314
pulmonary complications of, 321
rehabilitation and, 324
stump infection in, 319-320
thromboembolic complications of, 321-322

Anaphylaxis
dextran and, 128
sclerotherapy and, 354

Anastomosis; *see also* Anastomotic *entries*
aortic, rupture of, 251-253
autogenous graft failure and, 264
axillofemoral bypass and, 217-218
direct venous reconstruction and, 340
femoral, 228
femorofemoral graft and, 220
hemorrhagic complications of, 7
infrainguinal graft failure and, 286
lympholymphatic, 371
lymphovenous, 368-370

Anastomotic aneurysm, 87-99
clinical manifestations of, 94
Dacron graft and, 70-72
incidence of, 87-88
location of, 88-89
pathogenesis of, 89-94
polytetrafluoroethylene graft and, 78
suture line failure and, 79-80
treatment of, 95-97
umbilical vein graft and, 80-81

Anastomotic neointimal hyperplasia, 55-64
intimal thickening and, 59-61
polytetrafluoroethylene graft and, 76, 78
prevention of, 61-62
synthetic graft healing and, 57-59
vein graft healing and, 55-57

Anastomotic pannus ingrowth, 66-67

Anastomotic stenosis
aortic reimplantation and, 193
Dacron graft and, 73-74
intraoperative, 265-266
renal arterial, 189
umbilical vein graft and, 81

Ancrod
clinical application of, 128-129
heparin-induced arterial thrombosis and, 104
pharmacology of, 128

Anemia, 297

Anesthesia
carotid endarterectomy and, 468
perioperative stroke and, 450
pulmonary disease and, 37
sclerotherapy and, 349

Aneurysm
anastomotic, 87-99; *see also* Anastomotic aneurysm
aortic; *see* Aortic aneurysm
cholecystitis and, 148
false; *see* Pseudoaneurysm

Aneurysmal aortorenal vein graft, 199
rupture of, 200

Aneurysmectomy, aortic, 143

Angina, intestinal, 140

Angiography
aortic graft infection and, 238
coronary, 23-24
for preoperative risk assessment, 25
heparin-induced arterial thrombosis and, 102
impotence testing and, 166-167
for peripheral arterial testing, 19
problems with, 18

Angioneogenesis, sclerotherapy and, 350

Angioplasty
aortic bifurcation graft limb occlusion and, 208-210
laser, 427-428, 430
patch, 481
percutaneous transluminal
autologous graft failure and, 267-268
failure of, 411-414
infrainguinal graft failure and, 282-283, 286
local complications with, 410-412
prevention of complications with, 414-417
risk management and, 33